D1295645

Diagnostics of Endocrine Function in Children and Adolescents
4th, revised and extended edition

Diagnostics of Endocrine Function in Children and Adolescents

4th, revised and extended edition

Editors

Michael B. Ranke Tübingen
Primus-E. Mullis Bern

109 figures and 80 tables, 2011

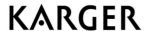

Basel · Freiburg · Paris · London · New York · Bangalore ·
Bangkok · Shanghai · Singapore · Tokyo · Sydney

Michael B. Ranke, MD
Pediatric Endocrinology Section
University Children's Hospital
University of Tübingen
Tübingen, Germany

Primus-E. Mullis, MD
Pediatric Endocrinology, Diabetology &
Metabolism
University Children's Hospital
Inselspital
Bern, Switzerland

Library of Congress Cataloging-in-Publication Data

Diagnostics of endocrine function in children and adolescents / editors,
Michael B. Ranke, Primus-E. Mullis. -- 4th, rev. and extended ed.
   p. ; cm.
  Includes bibliographical references and indexes.
  ISBN 978-3-8055-9414-1 (hard cover : alk. paper) -- ISBN 978-3-8055-9415-8
(E-ISBN)
  1. Pediatric endocrinology. I. Ranke, Michael B. II. Mullis, P.-E.
  [DNLM: 1. Endocrine System Diseases--diagnosis. 2. Adolescent. 3.
Child. 4. Hormones -- analysis . WS 330]
  RJ418.D535 2011
  618.92'4--dc22

                            2010052495

1st edition published in 1992 as *Functional Endocrinologic Diagnostics in Children and Adolescents* by
J & J Verlag, Mannheim

2nd edition published in 1996 as *Diagnostics of Endocrine Function in Children and Adolescents* by
Barth Verlag (Edtion J & J), Heidelberg

3rd edition published in 2003 as *Diagnostics of Endocrine Function in Children and Adolescents*
3rd revised and extended edition by S. Karger Publishers, Basel

Bibliographic Indices. This publication is listed in bibliographic services, including Current Contents® and Index Medicus.

© Copyright 2011 by S. Karger AG, P.O. Box, CH–4009 Basel (Switzerland)
www.karger.com
Printed in Switzerland on acid-free and non-aging paper (ISO 9706) by Reinhardt Druck, Basel
ISBN 978–3–8055–9414–1
e-ISBN 978–3–8055–9415–8

Contents

Preface

Since the first appearance of the first edition of this book in 1992, there have been a multitude of new developments which have influenced the diagnostic approach in children and adolescents with endocrine disorders. The encouraging response to the first three editions of this book encouraged us to adhere to the original format of the chapters, which are a combination of in-depth discussion of the diagnostic process, practical conclusions, and expert advice based on extensive experience. The new developments, as considered by the authors of this volume, refer to practically all the traditional areas of pediatric endocrinology not only the rapidly advancing field of molecular genetics and steroid metabolism. Several chapters have been revised completely and all have been updated by authors who had contributed to the previous editions as well as a large number of new authors. In addition, new chapters dealing with the muscle-bone unit and bone metabolism have also been incorporated, since the editors felt that this emerging field will broaden our understanding of the links between growth, hormones and metabolism. It was also considered that this major new area of pediatric endocrinology is related to physiological changes and disorders occurring during the neonatal phase of term and preterm babies.

We hope that this 4th revised edition on the diagnostics of endocrine function will continue to support clinicians in their attempts to reach evidence-based, rapid diagnostic solutions as the basis of advice and therapy for their patients. We thank the contributing authors for their devotion to this project. The editors are particularly grateful to Thomas Nold (Karger Publishers) who has encouraged us throughout the complex process of the production of this 4th edition.

Michael B. Ranke, Tübingen
Primus-E. Mullis, Bern

Preface to the Third Edition

When the first edition of this volume appeared in 1992, it soon became clear that a second edition would follow in order to incorporate the new developments in pediatric endocrinology. The second edition was published in 1996, and further, significant expansions in knowledge have made this new edition necessary. These include the discoveries in molecular genetics which dominated the biosciences in the past decade. It cannot be denied, however, that the prime professional challenges for the physician are to identify clinical symptoms, arrive at a definite diagnosis, and select the most appropriate treatment for each individual patient.

The encouraging response to the first two editions of this book and the readers' appreciation of its value at various stages of the diagnostic process have led to our decision to adhere to the original format of the chapters, which are a combination of in-depth discussion of the diagnostic process, succinct, practical conclusions, and expert advice deriving from extensive experience. One unique feature of this third edition is that, in light of the wealth of new information and recent discoveries in some fields, most of the contributors offer the readers completely revised chapters. Thus, this edition incorporates several aspects which could not be dealt with previously, such as new information on congenital hyperinsulinaemic states, steroid analysis by GCMS, specific elements in the prematurely born and the neonate, bone development, and the influence of weight changes on the diagnostic process.

This edition also offers improved flow charts which illustrate the differential diagnoses of frequently-encountered disorders that, understandably, continue to be the subject of debate.

It is my sincere hope that the new information, coupled with all of the improvements and revisions, will enhance the value of this book as a guide and reference work in the field of endocrine diagnostics in children and adolescents. I would like to thank all the contributing authors for their co-operation, thoroughness and patience. I am also grateful to Priscilla Herrmann (University Children's Hospital, Tubingen, Germany) and Thomas Nold (Karger Publishers, Basel, Switzerland) for their support of this project, without which the production of this third edition would not have been possible.

Michael B. Ranke, Tübingen, June 2003

Preface to the Second Edition

The first edition of this volume received a favorable response from readers, who also provided many constructive suggestions for improvements. These and the many new developments in pediatric and adolescent endocrinology have led to a completely revised and expanded second edition. New chapters relating to molecular genetics, imaging methods using radionuclides, sequential hormone measurements, and the measurement and diagnostic relevance of urinary growth hormone have also been added to expand the coverage of areas that were not exhaustively treated in the first edition. An appendix of flow charts illustrating the differential diagnosis of frequently encountered hormonal and metabolic disorders has also been included at the end of the volume to provide physicians with quick guidance on how to deal with complex diagnostic situations.

It is my hope that these revisions will further enhance the value of the book as a practical guide and reference to the diagnosis of endocrine and metabolic disorders in pediatric and adolescent patients. My thanks go to the contributing authors for their collaboration in this project, as well as to Dr. Susan Kentner of Edition .J & J for her tireless editorial support, without which the production of this second edition would not have been possible.

Michael B. Ranke, Tübingen, July 1996

Preface to the First Edition

In terms of sheer numbers, hormonal disorders in children and adolescents occupy a significant place in pediatrics. Research in pediatric endocrinology has progressed to the point where it is now possible to arrive at a precise diagnosis of the most important endocrine disorders, classify them exactly according to pathophysiology, and provide treatment based on rational criteria. New molecular genetic techniques have increased our understanding of a variety of pathologic conditions, and the ability to produce hormones biosynthetically has rapidly broadened the spectrum of therapeutic methods at our disposal.

In light of these developments, it seems particularly important for the physician to be able to proceed from the observation of clinical symptoms to the correct diagnosis and the appropriate therapy by following a series of rational diagnostic steps. In most textbooks of pediatrics, methods of diagnosing endocrine disorders in children and adolescents are given little space with no mention of specific details. The objective of this volume is therefore to describe in depth methods for the functional diagnosis of the most important hormonal disorders occurring in pediatric age groups. Special emphasis is placed on evaluating the methods discussed in terms of their clinical relevance. Normal values for hormonal parameters and test results are presented, together with a discussion of methodologic problems and more recent techniques that have not yet become firmly established diagnostic procedures. The intention is to provide a judicious mixture comprising not only knowledge based on long-established diagnostic procedures and confirmed test results, but also reflecting the personal experience of the contributing authors with a variety of newly developed and less well-established test procedures. This combination provides a picture of the problems associated with functional endocrinologic diagnostics that is at once extremely varied, but always relevant to actual clinical practice.

I thank all the authors for contributing their knowledge and expertise to realize this volume. Special thanks also go to Dr. Susan Kentner, who has guided the publication of the volume with experience and patience.

Michael B. Ranke, Tübingen, January 1992

Before Using This Book

The pediatrician is frequently confronted with disorders of endocrine function and deviations from normal growth patterns. Diagnosing such conditions often demands detailed knowledge of childhood developmental processes, profound clinical experience, and an understanding of the intricate interaction of metabolic and endocrine factors. At the same time, we are fortunate in having a diverse and well-validated arsenal of diagnostic methods at our disposal.

This volume presents the diagnostic approaches, test procedures, and normative data required to establish diagnoses for a broad spectrum of endocrine disorders. It is hoped that the reader will use this book to obtain reference values for various diagnostic parameters. In this regard, however, it is appropriate to provide a few preliminary words of caution on how to evaluate the information presented in this volume:

(1) The diagnostic approaches outlined here are based on the profound experience of the authors and reflect the state of the art. Nevertheless, other diagnostic paths not discussed in this volume, that are based on different traditions and experience, may also be useful.

(2) Test results may depend on a variety of circumstances related to the individual tested and the test modalities. With regard to the latter, for example, the time of day at which a test is administered may be of particular importance. Specific normative data need to be established for procedures performed at special times during the day owing to circumstances within a particular clinical setting. In special situations, certain requirements (e.g., fasting state) must be fulfilled.

(3) Standard hormone measurements are performed today in many laboratories, and often a multitude of assays are available for the same hormone. Assay performance and the quality of the results obtained can therefore vary considerably depending on the laboratory and the assay used. Reference data are therefore only valid for the method used and for the laboratory that has established them. The data published in this volume can thus only be taken as guidelines for normative data when different methods are employed.

(4) In general, it is important that those interpreting the results of hormone measurements be familiar with the methods used, the conditions under which they are employed, and the quality of the results obtained with them. If the clinician has no

control over the characteristics of a particular assay (e.g., because an outside laboratory is performing it), he or she should obtain the relevant information from the laboratory. In particular, it should be kept in mind that an assay that works well for adults may not be appropriate for children, e.g., because of differences in the relevant range of concentrations or because of other interfering factors specific to the child's developmental stage.

(5) Each investigator should make an effort to establish normative data with the methodology at his or her disposal. As a minimal requirement, investigators should acquire sufficient experience to develop a 'feeling' for the results of a given method in order to be able to judiciously evaluate the figures supplied by the laboratory performing the assay. The latest fashions in methodology may not necessarily serve the needs of either the investigator or the patients – neither do shortcuts imposed by economic considerations. The reader is therefore urged to study not only the tables included in this book, but also the methodological analyses presented by each author in order to gain the critical confidence required to counsel and treat patients

Ranke MB, Mullis P-E (eds): Diagnostics of Endocrine Function in Children and Adolescents, ed 4.
Basel, Karger, 2011, pp 1–31

Laboratory Measurements of Hormones and Related Biomarkers: Technologies, Quality Management and Validation

Martin W. Elmlinger

Nycomed GmbH, Konstanz, Germany

Laboratory measurements have become an essential part of medical diagnostics. In pediatric endocrinology, measurements of hormones and related biomarkers like growth factors are practically indispensable. They initially allow the evaluation of the pathological stage and differential diagnosis of a patient. In the following, they are used to monitor and predict a therapeutic success and outcome. Thus, measurements of hormones and growth factors must be valid and reproducible in both technical and medical terms. The laboratory must warrant the technical validity and reproducibility of the hormone measurements through standardized laboratory procedures and adequate quality standards and quality management. It is, however, the responsibility of the treating physician, first to choose the right laboratory parameters to be examined, and second to ensure adequate test circumstances including the time of sampling, influence of nutrition and cyclic factors, co-medication and shipment of the sample. The physician/pediatrician is responsible for interpretation of the laboratory results and the use of this medical information in patient care.

During the last two decades, laboratory diagnostics in endocrinology and in general have undergone a technological revolution in several ways. The major trends are the following.

Multiplex Techniques and Miniaturization

Multiplex techniques represent a current megatrend in laboratory diagnostics with the aim of saving time and resources upon the release of the diagnostic result, and of doing multiparametric analysis at one go. Multiplex panels can include up to ten-thousands of parameters. This goes along with miniaturization to reduce the sample volume needed for testing and thereby reduces invasiveness.

These techniques are based on either protein or antibody microarrays or chips, coated beads, glass fibers, or microcapillary discs. The immunological methods amongst them make use of the classical interaction of an antigen (analyte) with an immobilized antibody, or vice versa. Other than that, immobilized RNA, DNA, cDNA, aptamers, etc. are used. These methods do not play a significant role in endocrine routine diagnostics and are not discussed here.

Nevertheless, singleplex immunoassays like ELISA or RIA still play a central role in the endocrinology laboratory, due to their robustness and high sensitivity. One reason why they have not been replaced by multiplex techniques yet is the possible interference of different antibodies in multiplex, especially bead-based techniques. These interferences can lower the sensitivity and specificity of the methods. Thus, today multiplex and chip technologies are used in screening approaches in biomedical sciences and drug discovery, rather than in quantitative routine diagnostics.

Plasmon resonance as a principle of antigen detection is not used in clinical routine, but it can be helpful in the screening of binding properties of antibodies, such as binding strength and kinetics during the development of immunoassays.

Significant progress, however, has been achieved by making use of intelligent modifications in the detection systems and washing technology.

Automation, Integrated Care Systems and Theranostics

The pressure of reducing costs and laboratory staff and the necessity to speed up laboratory measurements, has fueled the development of fully automated diagnostic platforms. These are often assembled of modules, which can be used in different combinations, in order to increase the degree of automation and the capacity of measurements. They are used in large laboratories with a high daily throughput of samples. Midsized or small-sized automated platforms are also available for smaller laboratories. These systems are available for clinical chemistry, as well as immuno-diagnostic testing. The development of such high-technology platforms is, however, only possible in larger companies with an appropriate financial background. Sample and patient registration, sample injection from original vessels, dilution and the whole analytical procedure, including quality management, data handling and data transfer, as well as a customized standardized data output are managed automatically by the system. Automated data management can even include preliminary evaluation of data on the basis of relevant reference ranges.

The next step of innovation includes the implementation of integrated care systems, as driven by the big players in diagnostic industry (e.g. Siemens, Abbott, Philips, Roche), who combine imaging and laboratory diagnostics and link them with an integrated concept of medical care. A typical feature of those integrated systems is a seamless data flow from bedside to the laboratory and back to the treating physician. The whole analytic procedure, but also the data management and transfer can be perfomed in a fully regulated environment (see 'Quality management', below).

Another kind of development is reflected by theranostics, which means the co-development of a drug with a specific diagnostic to pre-test the individual patient for responsiveness and thereby to optimize the therapy.

Biomarkers in Personalized Medicine

Personalized medicine makes use of biomarkers in several ways with the aim to find and optimize drug therapies for the individual patient. Generally spoken, the goal is to treat the right patient population with the right drug at the right dose regimen, in order to achieve a maximum response. Before a patient is treated, stratification biomarkers can be measured, if appropriate, to choose the right therapy or to adjust a dosage. Genetic predisposition like mutations of the 21-hydroxylase gene, which goes along with a high 17OH-progesterone level, is evaluated in the molecular diagnostics of adrenogenital syndrome (AGS). Other typical stratification biomarkers are individual expression levels or polymorphisms of drug transporters or metabolizers (e.g. cytochrome P450). Disease biomarkers are markers which reflect a relevant pathway of the respective pathomechanism. If this marker or set of markers responds adequately to a drug therapy, it can be also used as a pharmacodynamic biomarker. The serum level of insulin-like growth factor-1 (IGF-1) and of its major circulating binding protein IGFBP-3 are types of these of biomarkers. They are used to diagnose and assess the degree of the human growth hormone (hGH)-deficient state, and to measure responsiveness and predict the outcome of hGH therapy of a patient. They are also used in the differential diagnosis of growth disorders in order to elucidate the etiology of the disease. In addition, IGF-1 and IGFBP-3, i.e. their ratio, can serve as safety biomarkers of hGH therapy.

Point of Care Diagnostics

Cost pressure in the health care sector, the development of diagnostic techniques which can also be operated by nursing staff, and the demand for immediate measuring of results (e.g. in intensive care) are all factors contributing to the increasing use of point of care testing (POCT) equipment. While comparable with conventional laboratory methods in terms of accuracy and specificity, these instruments save time and reduce laboratory staff costs. POCT instruments are expected to find still wider use in the future, as they are available even in pocket-sized formate to be used anywhere.

Measuring blood glucose, HbA1c, and insulin in outpatient facilities are examples. Another approach to be used in outpatient facilities is standardized analysis strips to measure, for example, IL-6 in neonatal sepsis, critical biomarkers in stroke/cardiac disease management, e.g. brain natriuretic protein, luteinizing hormone and parameters of infection serology. Some strips like hCG strips for pregnancy testing are means of self-observation, which can be used even at home. Most of these technologies are based on antibody techniques.

Thereby, the markers can be measured from different fluids (blood, urine, etc.) mostly without any sample preparation and consuming a minimum of sample. During the last years POCT methods have become more reliable from a technical point of view and are comparable to classical laboratory techniques, including the integration in quality management systems [book recommendation: Luppa PB, Schlebusch H: Patientennahe Labordiagnostik, Heidelberg, Springer, 2008].

New Assays and Compartments

Tremendous progress has been achieved in the number and quality of parameters that can be measured from body fluids. Commercial providers constantly try to implement new assays on automated platforms, thereby massively increasing their analytical menus. However, the quality of singleplex assays is also continuously being improved, e.g. by switching from RIA to ELISA, and by increasing the sensitivity through technical improvement, e.g. high-sensitivity cortisol. It is also an important goal of today's diagnostics development to identify body fluids that can be gained less invasively, e.g. saliva to measure cortisol.

Quality Management

As the major part of the diagnostic and therapeutic decisions in pediatric endocrinology relies on hormone measurements, the latter must be valid and reproducible in both technical and medical terms. This request can be fulfilled by implementation of standardized quality management systems (QMS). A QMS is defined as the whole of all measures suitable for achieving the quality of a product or a service (analysis) that has been agreed upon or required for a certain purpose. An efficient and adequate QMS can be proven if the laboratory accepts an accreditation procedure, i.e. a proof of competence by an independent third party. The practice of licensing of diagnostic laboratories by national governments is handled differently in different countries. The use and management of internal and external quality controls (e.g. Ringversuche) represents a minimum of QMS in the clinical laboratory in Germany. With the goal of international harmonization, international standards like CLIA, (http://www.cms.hhs.gov/clia/), ISO9000, EN45000 and/or GLP (Good Laboratory

Practice) have been set up to ensure the quality of laboratory diagnostics across borders. Coordinating institutions like the WELAC (Western Europe Laboratory Accreditation Cooperation) are the drivers of implementation of the quality standards in diagnostic laboratories.

Immunoassay Methods to Measure Hormones and Growth Factors

Bioassays

Bioassays were the first available methods of determining hormone concentrations. A historical example is the measurement of human growth hormone (hGH) concentration using the growth of the proximal epiphyseal cartilage of the femur of hypophysectomized rats [1].

Today, in vivo and in vitro bioassays are only used in two areas:

Firstly, in the standardization of hormone preparations; examples are establishing the international reference preparation (IRP) for recombinant human growth hormone [2] and for human leptin [3] by reference laboratories of the World Health Organization. Here, bioassays complement physical and biochemical methods such as gravimetry, high-performance liquid chromatography (HLPC), protein microsequencing, mass spectrometry and immunoassays. The best approximation of the real IRP is attained by averaging the concentrations gained by the various methods.

Secondly, bioassays are sometimes used to relate the biological activity of a hormone in the serum of patients, e.g. of TSH [4] or of hGH to its measured concentration. Through the introduction of an automatic cell counter the measurement of the biological activity of hGH using the proliferation assay on rat Nb2 lymphoma cells [5] has reached a precision comparable to that of immunoassays. Since the introduction of the stabile GH receptor transgenic cell line BA/F3-GHR [6], the GH bioactivity can even be measured directly with GH receptor-mediated cell proliferation, instead of indirectly by prolactin receptor-mediated cell proliferation as with Nb2 cells. However, bioassays are not used in routine clinical diagnostics.

Radioreceptor Assays

Radioreceptor assays (RRA) make use of the specific binding of the respective hormone to a membrane (peptide hormone) receptor or cytoplasmatic (steroid or thyroid hormone) receptor. A major difference to bioassays is that here only the binding and not the biological activity of the hormone is examined. The quantitative evaluation is thus comparable to that of immunoassays. Lymphocytes are mostly used as target cells as they are usually easy to handle [7]. As receptor binding is generally weaker than binding to specific antibodies, RRA is very prone to disturbances. For example, the presence of soluble GH-binding proteins is a serious hindrance for the GH RRA [8]. RRA also plays a role in testing the receptor binding potential of synthetic steroid variants or analogs [9].

Immunofunctional Assays

Immunofunctional assays are variants that involve binding of the ligand to be measured to the binding site of its natural receptor, and subsequent recognition of the ligand bound by a specific monoclonal antibody that serves for quantitative detection. This kind of assay has been developed, for example, for leptin, GH and IGFBP-3 [10–12].

In situ Methods

The use of labeled antibodies and antibody sandwiches for detecting immobilized antigens in microtome sections of tissues (immunohistochemistry), in cells (cytochemistry) and after transfer (blotting) onto carrier membranes in an electric field (dotblot, Western immunoblot), generally belongs to basic research areas but is also used in infection serology. The antibodies can be labeled with an enzyme, a dye or a fluorophor.

Immunoassays

Antibody Production

An important part of the humoral immune answer to foreign immunogens (cells, antigens, haptens) is the production and secretion of specific antibodies by B lymphocytes. Antibodies can thus be produced by repeated immunization (boostering) of animals with pure antigen or hapten solutions using Freund's adjuvans. The antiserum can be directly used or is purified and enriched by affinity-chromatography using a protein-A or protein-G column. The IgG fraction obtained contains polyclonal antibodies directed against various epitopes (fig. 1).

The antigen-binding $F(ab)_2$ and the F_c region are the functionally important areas of the IgG molecule (150 kDa). The former consists of a light (V_L) and a heavy chain (V_H), which together form the antigen-binding slot like a keyhole. Due to the enormous number of possible antigens (10^8), the composition of the 110 amino acids in the V area is highly variable, especially in the three hypervariable regions (V_H). In contrast, the amino acid composition in the C-regions is largely constant as these are responsible for complement and macrophage activation.

The method of producing monoclonal antibodies devised by Köhler and Milstein (Nobel Prize, 1984) is based on the following principle: after immunizing mice with a particular antigen, antibody-producing B cells are gained from their spleen and immortalized into hybridoma through fusion with a mouse myeloma cell line. The hybridoma cell line thus unites the potential immortality of the myeloma cells and the ability of the B cells to produce a single kind of specific antibodies. Through separating the individual hybridoma, re-cloning and testing

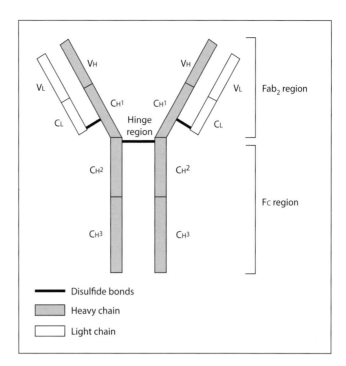

Fig. 1. Antibody structure (IgG).

for specificity, particular cell clones can be gained which produce IgG for specific epitopes. These can then be used to produce large quantities of specific antibodies in bioreactors or in mouse ascites (in Germany, the latter is forbidden by the Law for Protection of Animals).

Today, genetic engineering enables the cDNAs which encode the bond-specific Fab parts of IgGs to be cloned and recombinantly expressed. By cloning, targeted modifications can be brought into the protein expressed. Nowadays one often only uses the specific F(ab)2 or Fab fragments instead of the whole IgG molecule. As long as stocks of the genetically programmed organisms (*Escherichia coli*, eucaryotic cells) are preserved, monoclonal antibodies are producible in nearly unlimited quantities and constant high quality, in contrast to polyclonal antibodies.

Antigen Production
Pure antigens can either be produced by sequential chromatographic steps from biomaterials (body fluids, cell lysates) or, nowadays much more commonly, from lysates after recombinant expression of cloned cDNA sequences in *E. coli* or in eucaryotic (insect, mouse, monkey) cells. Recombinant proteins can be produced in unlimited amounts and constant quality. The choice of the expression system depends on the respective protein. *E. coli* can easily express large amounts of relatively small peptide hormones, but is often unable to produce complicated high-molecular-weight proteins with disulfide bonds in correct folding. In this case,

eucaryotic expression in mammalian or insect cell systems with specific vectors have to be used.

Principles

Immunoassays are an in vitro implementation of the specific, high-affinity bonding between antibodies (IgG) and their antigens. According to the law of mass action, a steady state develops between the concentrations of the bound and free antigens [Ag] and antibodies [Ab]. An important step in the immunoassay is therefore the subsequent removal of the unbound component in order to evaluate the amount of bound antigens or antibodies:

$$[Ag] + [Ab] \underset{K1}{\overset{K2}{\rightleftarrows}} [Ag\text{-}Ab] \qquad K_{eq} = \frac{K1}{K2}$$

Berson and Yalow's [13] discovery of the radioimmunoassay (RIA) for measuring insulin in 1959 opened a new chapter in the history of hormone measurements and replaced the hitherto used bioassay and the precipitation tests (radial double diffusion, immunoelectrophoresis, rocket immunoelectrophoresis) which were based on making the precipitates directly visible at the point of equivalence. The rapid success of immunoassays was promoted by improved techniques for producing antibodies and for their chromatographic purification. Later, recombinant expression of antigens led to further improvements. Further, various labeling and detection techniques (radionuclides, enzymes, coupling through biotine/streptavidine, dyes, fluorophores, chromophores, etc.) have been developed and intelligent methods of phase separation (adsorption techniques; fixed phases: microplates, coated tubes, beads) have been implemented. Depending on whether reagents are used in limited or in excess amounts, one speaks of competitive or noncompetitive immunoassays. The usability of the RIA is limited by the half-life of the radionuclide used (e.g. ^{125}I, t½ = 60 days) and by the problem of radioactive waste disposal. Nevertheless, the RIA is a robust and inexpensive technique.

Competitive versus Noncompetitive Assays

The competitive radioimmunoassay (RIA) is based on the competitive reaction between a determined amount of radioactive ^{125}I-antigen [Ag*] and an unknown amount of 'cold' antigen [Ag] with a limited amount of antibodies [Ab] in the sample.

The separation of the unbound components is mostly done by precipitation and subsequent centrifugation of the antigen-antibody complex with the help of a secondary antibody and addition of a precipitation catalyst (such as polyethylene glycol). In the competitive assay (fig. 2, 3) the initial amount of antigen in the sample is inversely proportional to the bound radioactivity. As in practice neither K_{eq} nor [Ab] are known, a standard dilution series is used for calibration: bound and free [Ag*] (% bound) are plotted against the concentration of the used antigen in a standard graph.

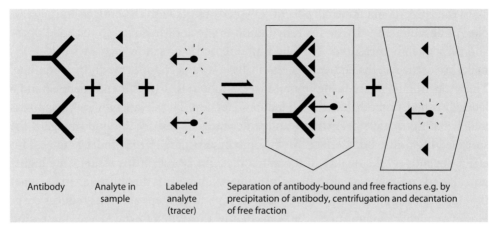

| Antibody | Analyte in sample | Labeled analyte (tracer) | Separation of antibody-bound and free fractions e.g. by precipitation of antibody, centrifugation and decantation of free fraction |

Fig. 2. Principle of the competitive RIA.

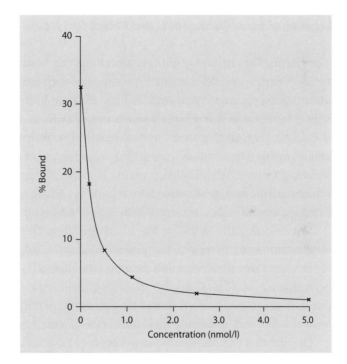

Fig. 3. Calibration (dose-response) graph of the competitive RIA.

Since only the availability of one of the components is limited, noncompetitive assays are less labile than competitive ones with respect to the precision of the used amounts and the purity of labeled antigen and antibody. They are, however, more prone to disturbances through cross-reactions and nonspecific binding.

In 1968, Miles and Hales [14] achieved a further step by developing noncompetitive (single-site) immunoradiometric assays (IRMA) using labeled antibodies.

In the IRMA a marginal surplus of ^{125}I-[Ab*] reacts with the antigen in the sample. All unsaturated ^{125}I-[Ab*] is fully bound to the antigens fixed to the solid phase and subsequently measured. Two-site immunometric or sandwich assays (fig. 4, 15) make use of the fact that antigens generally have several epitopes for antigen bonding. The antigen initially binds the immobilized antibody [Ab1], is then separated and a labeled second antibody [Ab2] is added for detection. The advantages are an approximately ten times higher sensitivity and wider range than RIA. A disadvantage is the so-called high-dose hook effect which sometimes occurs in the binding curve. This effect depends on the quality of the antibodies. A variant of this assay is the highly sensitive coated-tube assay in which the primary antibody is directly fixed to the reaction tube. This simplifies and abbreviates the separation steps and thus reduces costs. However, higher amount of tracer is needed in this type of assay. Here, the bound radioactivity is proportional to the amount of antigens in the sample.

Labeling of Assay Components and Detection Systems

The chemical reaction conditions attending the labeling of antigens or antibodies with ^{125}I (e.g. by the chloramine-T method) or with enzymes or biotin or streptavidin must first be optimized and standardized for each individual antigen. Today, labeling with ^{3}H, ^{131}I or ^{57}Co has largely fallen out of fashion. Label addition or subtraction should be controlled with a view to avoiding conformational changes of the molecules. Furthermore, radiolysis resulting from the use of radioactive markers can cause serious damage of the labeled protein. The specific activity (mCi/μg protein) of the tracer must be known. Bound radioactivity is measured in counts per minute (cpm) using a gamma (or beta) counter with inbuilt correction for counting efficiency.

The following drawbacks spoke in favor of developing nonradioactive markers for assay components along with the requisite alternative detection systems: (1) health risks, (2) stringent regulations for radiation protection and removal of radioactive waste and hence higher costs for isotope laboratories, (3) limited automation and speed limitations due to long incubation periods and long counting periods (counting error = $\sqrt{}$ accumulated counts), and (4) limited shelf-life of labeled components due to radioactive decay.

The fact that radioimmunoassays are still in use today can be attributed to the following advantages: (1) assays are robust, (2) their analytical sensitivity can be manually increased by increasing the amounts of specimen or antibodies, e.g. for hormones with very low serum concentration such as sex steroids, (3) sparing in the consumption of limited polyclonal antibodies, and (4) commercial assays are relatively inexpensive, a particularly significant aspect in less-affluent countries.

Nonradioactive methods (table 1) involve labeling of either the antigen or the antibody, depending on the format of the assay. This involves either direct conjugation of the respective component with an enzyme, fluorophore or chromophore, or indirect conjugation through labeling with biotin or streptavidin/avidin. Due to the catalytic

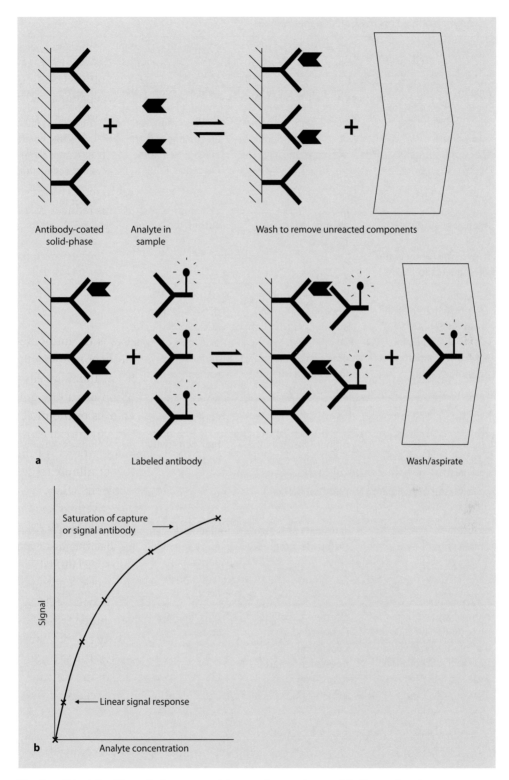

Antibody-coated   Analyte in   Wash to remove unreacted components
solid-phase   sample

a   Labeled antibody   Wash/aspirate

Saturation of capture
or signal antibody →

Signal

← Linear signal response

b   Analyte concentration

Fig. 4. **a** Principle of two-site immunometric assay (reagent excess). **b** Respective dose-response curve.

Table 1. The most common nonradioactive detection techniques

	Colorimetry	Direct fluorometry	Chemiluminescence	Time-resolved fluorescence
Principal	enzyme-bound antigen competes for the Ab-binding site end-point spectrophotometry of color strength.	comparable to RIA. fluorophores (e.g. fluorescein, rhodamine) act directly as labels or are enzymatically produced. Fluoresence is measured	light emission in the course of a chemical reaction catalyzed by an enzyme. Variant: electrochemilumi-nescence (ECL)	delayed measurement of the emitted light from the excited fluorophore use of lanthanides with extremely large Stokes' shift, decay times and quantum yields (e.g. Europium)
Assay format and type	manual or automated ELISA 96-well microtiter plates alternative: tab-ELISA	automated assays, EIA, ELISA	automated assays	DELFIA system as automated assay or manual microtiter plate assay
Substrates	2,2´-azino-bis(ethylbenzothiazoline-6-sulfonate) (ABTS), o-phenylenediamine OPD), 3,3´,5,5´-tetramethyl-benzidine (TMB)	4-methylumbelliferyl phosphate (4-MUP) stimulation with light of 365 nm wavelength, emission at 448 nm (measurement of the Stokes' shift)	adamantyl 1,2-dioxetane or in ECL: simultaneous oxidation of tripopyl-amine and ruthenium-II, chelate label of the antigen at the anode, excited Ru-II emits light	None
Sensitivity/range	range of spectrophotometer: – 2.0 OD peroxidase-based assays more sensitive	higher sensitivity than colorimetry through repeated excitation and photomultiplying	high sensitivity wide range	high sensitivity wide range
Advantages	robust simple	sensitivity as high as isotope techniques	minimal background quick signal generation, high specific activity	delayed measurement minimizes interference from fluorescent molecules in the sample
Drawbacks	narrow range, but can be extended by choosing a photometry wavelength next to the absorption peak	interference of the fluorescence with background fluorescence and quenching	only for automated systems	not known

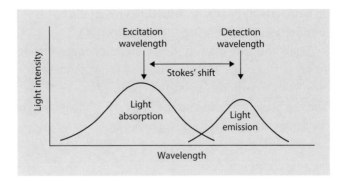

Fig. 5. Principle of fluorescent measurement (Stoke's shift).

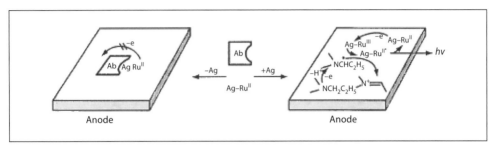

Fig. 6. Homogeneous immunoassay electrochemilumunescence (ECL) principle. (From Wild: Immunoassay Handbook, fig. 12.17.)

effect in the enzyme immunoassay (EIA), it is possible for small amounts of bound enzyme to metabolize large quantities of substrate, depending on reaction time which results in an amplification of the signal generated. EIAs are therefore highly sensitive, but also prone to interference.

Most Commonly Used Enzyme Immunoassays

Alkaline phosphatase, hydrolyses phosphate esters of primary alcohols, phenols and amines. Horseradish peroxidase, which initially oxidizes by reacting with the substrate H_2O_2, is then in turn able to oxidize other substrates, causing a change in their absorption spectra (fig. 5) and thus forming a colored, fluorescent or luminescent derivative.

Another widely used immunoassay principle is electrochemiluminescence (ECL) (fig. 6). The measurement of ECL, which allows homogeneous immunoassays with great sensitivity, is nowadays widely used in automated immunoassay platforms. It is based on the simultaneous oxidation of a tripopylamine and a ruthenium-II, Rhu(II), chelate label of the antigen at the anode. As an intermediate product, an excited state of Ru(II) is generated, which subsequently emits light that is detected and quantified. The immunoassay is carried out by causing the ruthenium label to bind to antibodies on suspendable beads, or sometimes magnetic beads. The ECL system is used in large immunoassay systems (e.g. Roche's Elecsys®).

Small antigens often undergo steric changes through conjugation with enzymes. To avoid this, such antigens can be conjugated with a spacer like biotin, a vitamin of only 244 Da, which couples the enzyme by way of the linkers avidin or streptavidin. The egg protein avidin and the bacterial (*Staphylococcus aureus*) streptavidin have an enormous affinity (10^{15} l/mol) to biotin.

Separation Techniques of Solid from Fluid Phase in Heterogeneous Assays

The separation of the antibody-bound antigen from the free antigen fraction is a decisive step in heterogeneous immunoassay techniques, having a major influence on the accuracy and reproducibility of the assay. A distinction is made between fluid-phase and solid-phase separation techniques. Which method is used depends on the analyte, amongst other factors. Assays in which one component is coupled to a solid phase are easier and quicker to perform and are therefore by far the most frequently used.

In fluid-phase assays, especially in RIA, the bound and unbound hormone fractions are separated by precipitation techniques using polyethylene glycol or secondary antibody or a combination of the two. The high-molecular-weight complexes formed hereby can easily be pelleted by centrifugation and the fluid phase can subsequently be decanted. The technically demanding and time-consuming gel filtration and electrophoresis techniques are hardly used in clinical practice. The same applies to absorption on dextran-coated charcoal for steroid measurements.

In solid-phase assays, either antigen or antibody is bound to glass, plastic or magnetic beads (microparticle-capture enzyme immunoassay, MEIA) or large spheres. Another widespread technique is immobilization on polystyrene tubes (coated tube assay) or 96-well microtitration plates (ELISA) (fig. 7, 8). A variant in terms of performance is available in the tab ELISA which uses an anti-IgG-coated tab to bind the Ag-Ab complex. Automated processes sometimes make use of sophisticated phase separation techniques, e.g. evasion of the fluid phase through rotation of the test tube (fig. 9), for instance in the Siemens Immulite® system [16].

Solid-phase assays are generally more sensitive and less dependent on the affinity of the antibody than fluid-phase assays since a stationary layer forms above the solid phase in which the probability of a reassociation between antigen and antibody is greater than in the fluid phase, even in cases of antibodies with low affinity.

Calibration Curve Fitting

A calibration curve is used to determine the analyte concentration in samples from the strength of the signal produced in an immunoassay. It represents a plot of calibrator

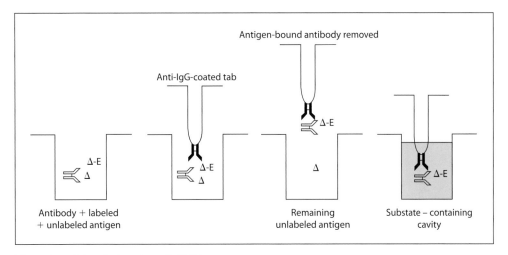

Fig. 7. Principle of microtiter tab-ELISA.

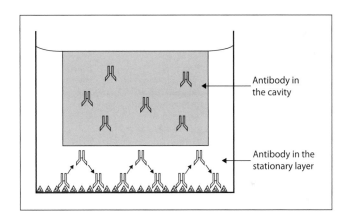

Fig. 8. Increased probability of a reassociation in an assay between bound antigen and antibody in the stationary layer above the solid phase.

concentration against signal level. Nowadays, the calculation process is commonly computerized. The computer calculates a mathematical algorithm, which has to match the calibration curve as closely as possible across the concentration range (fig. 10).

Instead of the two variables (analyte concentration and signal level) dose-response metameters are often used, which are functions of these variables. For example, the logarithm of the analyte concentration is plotted against the percent bound. If it is possible functions linearize the plot in order to enable the use of a simple linear regression analysis. This function, however, alters the error structure. Thus, ideally weighted regression should be used. In principal, the various curve fitting techniques are categorized in two ways [17]: Empirical or interpolatory methods, and regression methods.

Frequently used curve fitting methods are the linear interpolation, spline fitting, polynomial regression, and the logit-log transformation method.

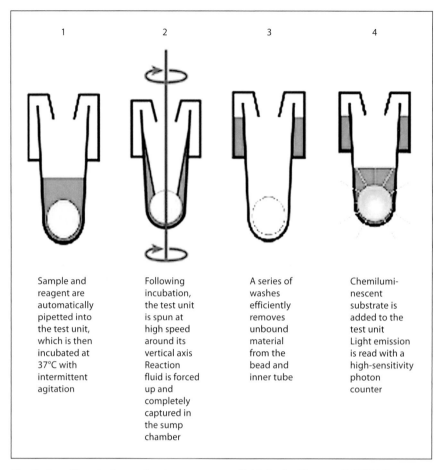

1	2	3	4
Sample and reagent are automatically pipetted into the test unit, which is then incubated at 37°C with intermittent agitation	Following incubation, the test unit is spun at high speed around its vertical axis Reaction fluid is forced up and completely captured in the sump chamber	A series of washes efficiently removes unbound material from the bead and inner tube	Chemilumi-nescent substrate is added to the test unit Light emission is read with a high-sensitivity photon counter

Fig. 9. Specific spinning technology to remove fluids in the Siemens IMMULITE system.

Homogeneous Immunological Techniques

Agglutination assays, which nowadays are rarely used, require no separation step and are therefore suited for automation. They are based on the immobilization of the antibody on cells (e.g. sheep erythrocytes) or latex particles. Upon contact with a ligand agglutination takes place. Nephelometry is likewise based on the formation of high-molecular complexes, with light scattering serving as a quantitative measure.

Technical Trends in Immunoassays
As mentioned above miniaturization, automation, new detection systems, multiplexing on beads (e.g. Luminex® technology), chips or arrays are the major trends of making immunoassays more efficient, more rapid and cheaper. They are mainly based on the classical antigen-antibody interaction.

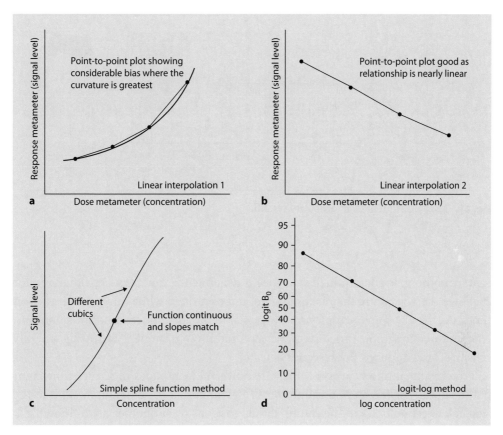

Fig. 10. Types of calibration curve fittings. **a** Linear interpolation 1. **b** Linear interpolation 2. **c** Simple spline function. **d** logit-log method.

An elegant variant of multiplexing, miniaturized (nanoliter scale!) immunoassay systems is the Gyros® system, which is based on a disc designed in the format of a compact disc (CD). The CD contains microcapillary segments with integrated microcolumns filled with streptavidin-coated beads to couple biotinylated proteins.

The Gyros system (fig. 11) is an open, parallel nanoliter microfluidic analysis system [18] which allows the development of new assays if suitable biotinylated antigens are available. The streptavidin-coated beads are activated with biotinylated capture reagents as the first step in the immunoassay. Capillary action is used to draw liquids into a distribution channel, filling a volume definition chamber. A hydrophobic barrier prevents the liquid from moving further into the microstructure. Spinning the CD generates centrifugal force causing the distribution channel to empty, leaving behind a precisely defined liquid volume. A second spin, at higher speed, creates a *g* force sufficient to drive the liquid over the hydrophobic barrier and through the

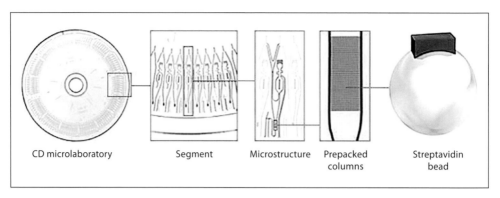

Fig. 11. Gyros disc formate microcapillary system.

capture column. Predetermined spin speeds generate the exact flow rate required for each step, i.e. to capture the maximum amount of protein while minimizing reaction times. As the CD spins, samples are processed in parallel under uniform conditions. After automatic sample processing, the captured protein is quantified using a highly sensitive, laser-induced fluorescence detector.

Protein and antibody arrays, which are powerful techniques in terms of throughput, flexibility, speed and consumption of low amounts of sample may replace the singleplex technologies in the future. Either antigens or antibodies are immobilized. In open systems, specifically customized sets of analytes can be assembled to measure whole biomarker panels of parameters of a certain medical indication. However, today they are mainly used in research and screening approaches, e.g. in the screening of IgE-binding proteins in allergy [19].

The use of biosensorics like the principle of plasmone resonance [20], which generate a physical signal from any kind of highly specific interaction between biomolecules (antibody-antigen, DNA-DNA, DNA-RNA, DNA-protein or receptor and ligand) are still restricted to research use.

For small biomolecules, e.g. steroids or peptides, advanced physical methods of mass spectrometry that are highly specific and sensitive are often used in combination with liquid chromatography (LC/MS; MALDI). These methods are discussed in detail later in this book.

Performance and Validation of Immunoassays: Preanalytical Phase
The preanalysis phase begins with a decision to carry out a laboratory test on a patient and ends with the delivery of the required specimen to the laboratory.

Technical Validation of Immunoassays
To be able to assess the measuring results the pathologist or clinical chemist requires knowledge of certain technical characteristics of the assay employed, as will be

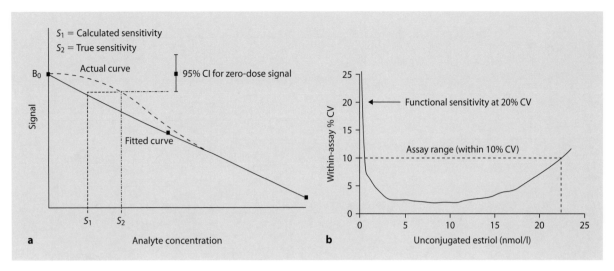

Fig. 12. Analytical (**a**), and functional (**b**) sensitivity of immunoassays.

described in the following. In making a diagnosis, the clinician needs to have maximum confidence in the technical reliability of the results.

The analytical sensitivity (fig. 12a) of an assay is generally determined by repeated tests on a blank sample. It is defined as three times the standard deviation from the mean analyte concentration found in the blank test series. In practice there is often a discrepancy between the fitted calibration curve and the dose-response curve in the measuring range below the calibrator, and calculated sensitivity (S1) and true sensitivity (S2) therefore often differ quite significantly.

A more practicable approach is therefore to determine the functional sensitivity (fig. 12b), which is defined as the smallest concentration for which the coefficient of variation (CV) is below a set figure, usually 20%. For this purpose, a precision profile must be prepared showing precision (y-axis) as a function of concentration.

Precision (fig. 13) is a dimensionless quantity which gives the degree of agreement between at least two successive measurements; it is limited by random errors. Its opposite is imprecision, which is expressed as the standard deviation or coefficient of variation (CV) of the results of a series of at least 10 successive measurements. A distinction is made between the percentual intra-assay CV of successive measurements within a test series and the percentual interassay CV of the results of at least 10 different test series, laboratories or measuring days: $\%CV = (SD/mean) \times 100 = $ relative SD.

While double measurements as they are commonly used in laboratories lead to no statistically significant improvement of precision, they make it easier to recognize outliers, especially in the case of manual methods. Therefore, automated methods often perform single measurements only. The assay drift describes systematic errors which only become apparent over time such as trends in the results of measurements

Accuracy	Precision		Error type
Optimum	Optimum	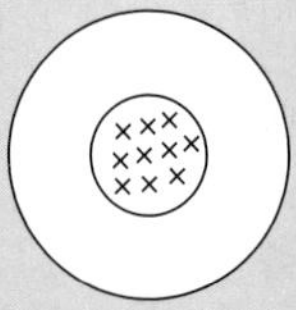	–
Good	Bad	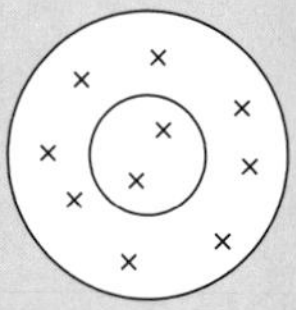	Coincidental error
Bad	Good	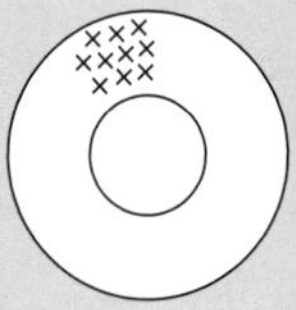	Systematic error
–	–	Wrong target used	Gross error

Fig. 13. Illustration of accuracy and precision (target model).

performed on standards or calibrators over months or years (see chapter: quality assurance).

Accuracy (fig. 13) is defined as the degree of agreement between the best estimate of a quantity and its true value (result of an immunoassay as compared with the value obtained with a reference preparation. Accuracy is limited by systematic errors. The following table illustrates the nature of accuracy and precision.

The detection limit is the smallest concentration of an analyte which produces a measuring signal that can be distinguished from that of a blank sample with a defined statistical reliability. Most assays perform reliably in a measuring range beginning 10 blank-value SDs above the detection threshold (fig. 12).

The specificity of an immunoassay is its ability to selectively determine the concentration of a single component (e.g. thyroxin) within a mixture of chemically related substances (e.g. serum). Most assays are multistage, the specificity of which is at best as good as their most selective step. Specificity is limited by antibody cross-reactivity (fig. 14) which can be determined by spiking tests on chemically related substances. Interfering companion substances may also detract from the specificity of an assay.

Elmlinger

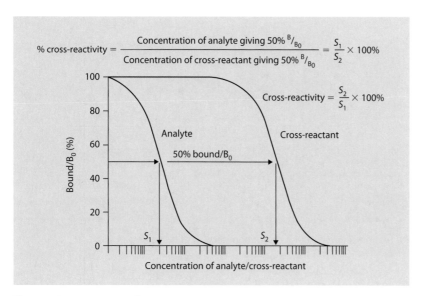

$$\% \text{ cross-reactivity} = \frac{\text{Concentration of analyte giving 50\% } {}^B/_{B_0}}{\text{Concentration of cross-reactant giving 50\% } {}^B/_{B_0}} = \frac{S_1}{S_2} \times 100\%$$

$$\text{Cross-reactivity} = \frac{S_2}{S_1} \times 100\%$$

Fig. 14. Crossreactivity of an immunoassay.

Recovery (expressed as a percentage) expresses the proportion of added analyte which can still be detected by the measurement. It is defined as the ratio of the incremental increase in measured analyte concentration to the predicted increase after addition of a known amount of analyte to the sample. It is usually determined by spiking blank samples or samples containing three different low-range concentrations of analyte. The recovery gives an indication of the quality of calibration of an assay and also reveals matrix effects. Studies on the parallelism of dilution are based on precisely defined standards (e.g. an IRP). They provide information on the affinity of the antibody employed and also on matrix effects, since the matrix is being diluted as well. It is recommended to use fractional (100, 90, ..., 10) rather than doubling dilutions (100, 50, ...3,125...) to avoid pipetting errors.

In order to compare two assays designed to measure the same hormone or growth factor one has to apply both to as many standards as possible, covering the entire working range in the process. Then the results of the two methods are plotted against each other and analyzed graphically and mathematically (fig. 15). The Pearson product correlation coefficient, which can be inferred from the scatter plot, is prone to interference and does not give a true picture of the data distribution. The scatter produced by most assays is dependent on concentration. Thus, the difference plot presented by Bland and Altmann [22] yields proportional information on the reliability of an assay also in the low concentration range. Which regression method is most suitable for calculating the intercept and slope must be decided case by case. Linnet [23] has written a good review article on this issue.

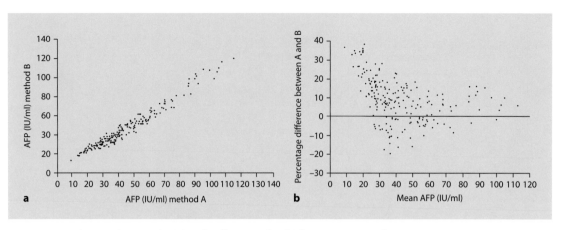

Fig. 15. Scatter plot (**a**) and Difference plot (**b**) for comparison of two assays.

Immunoassay Quality Management and Quality Assurance

The aim is for clinical laboratories to only supply results which permit meaningful estimates of the true value and show minimum scatter. In addition to the permanent internal quality control inherent to every assay, there are also regular external quality inspections which provide information on the precision and accuracy of measurements as compared with those of other laboratories. All measures taken must be accurately documented in suitable computer programs and must also be understandable to outsider observers such as calibration or licensing authorities.

Internal quality control includes the regular maintenance and operational testing of pipettes and instruments, consistency in the use of standard operation procedures and in reagent quality, and of course the use of specially trained staff. The best way to ensure the certifiability of operations in a medical laboratory is to have the laboratory accredited according to an international standard for quality management (DIN ISO 9001, ISO 15189, ISO 17025, CLIA, or GLP).

However, the laboratory staff has virtually no influence on the preanalysis phase (table 2). In the event of deviations the troubleshooting will initially be limited to variable parameters (e.g. quality of commercial assays or of the control preparation). Internal quality control procedures are usually based on measurements of commercial control preparations followed by longitudinal evaluation. Many laboratories additionally have in-house quality controls such as a standardized serum pool. If this is used over a long period of time, the analyte must be guaranteed to be sufficiently stable, which is checked by repeated testing. In contrast to commercial preparations which come in successive charges, a serum pool will often be available over years or even decades. Commercial control preparations usually have a matrix which differs from those of samples submitted to the laboratory so that matrix-related systematic errors therefore may often go undetected.

Table 2. Preanalytical steps and responsibilities

Steps	Remarks	Supervised by
Appointment and patient preparation	time of specimen collection nutritional status of patient co- medication requirements for laboratory parameters	physician
Choice of the primary specimen, e.g. blood, 24-hour urine, spontaneous urine, saliva, feces, liquor	suitable specimen storage (e.g. with anticoagulants, such as EDTA, citrate, LiCl)	physician
Unequivocal labeling and documentation of specimen	type of sample, date of collection, name (code), age, sex, tentative diagnosis	physician
Preparation of secondary specimen (e.g. serum)	e.g. centrifugation, portioning	physician /laboratory
Intermediate storage and shipment to laboratory	laboratory must be competent to deal with the parameter in question; cooling/freezing, knowledge of possible mechanism of decay of the analyte	physician /laboratory
Specimen processing	documentation of specimen and patient data on a computer in a regulated invironment (e.g. GLP), immediate portioning, preservation if necessary and submission for laboratory testing storage of residual specimen as backup	laboratory

As a general rule, each assay should be controlled at three different concentration levels (fig. 16). Assays often also come with technical calibrators, but these should be used in addition and should not replace control preparations. Results from control preparations should be evaluated immediately after completion of the assay, since the outcome decides on whether the patient's data can be released. The results are documented in control charts, which today are available in special quality control computer programs or included in the software of laboratory information managing systems.

Here, time, expressed in terms of days, is plotted against a concentration interval measured. The central line represents the target value for the sample, while the upper and lower warning limits represent two, and the upper and lower control limits three standard deviations from the target value. These analyte specific limits are often specified by the manufacturer, but they must nevertheless be verified by evaluation over a preliminary testing period of at least 20 assay days and corrected as necessary. Subsequently measured values should then oscillate within these limits. As a rule, the sum of three standard deviations should not exceed 15% of the mean value. In the event of values

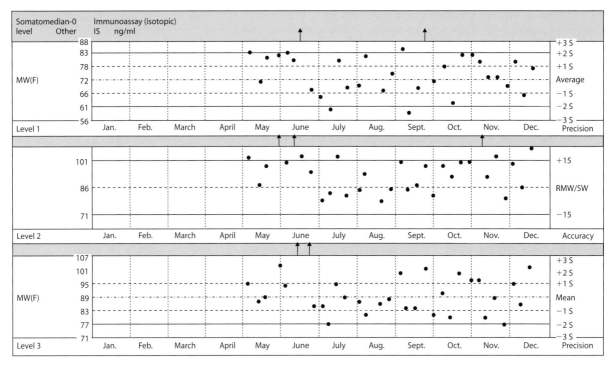

Fig. 16. Example for a control chart of IGF-1.

exceeding the 3S (SDs) limit, seven successive values showing a continuous upward or downward trend, or of seven successive values coming to lie on one side of the central line there is probably a systematic error. Computer programs in such cases will give an optical or acoustic alert signal and advise to reject the sample and eliminate the error.

External quality control requires spot-check measurements of one sample pair per analyte several times a year. It also involves an assessment of the measuring techniques employed by the laboratory and a comparison with other measuring techniques commonly used for the parameters in question as well as with the results of numerous other laboratories participating in the quality control program (inter-laboratory testing). Participation in such programs is not mandatory in all countries. The control preparation is made available to the participating laboratories by state-certified centers (in Germany, e.g. by DGKL, Instand e.V.), and the results are sent back to the center for evaluation. The outcome is usually communicated to the participants in the form of a Youden plot (fig. 17) (see also http://www.medcalc.be/manual/youdenplot. php). If the results found by the laboratory are within a predefined tolerance range around the target value, the participant is presented with a certificate confirming the accuracy of his measurements.

Value pairs are read as coordinates and entered into the plot as dots each representing a laboratory. All results which fall within a predefined square are considered to

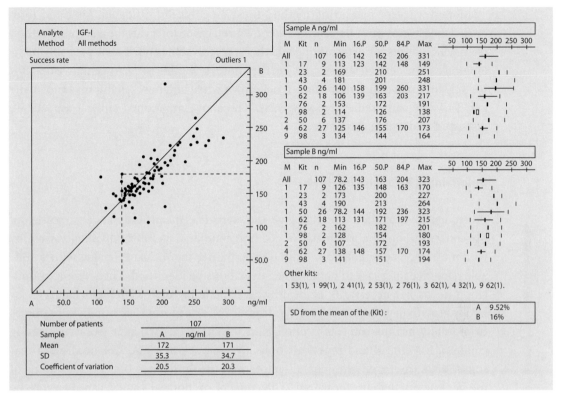

Fig. 17. Youden plot for external quality control.

have met the requirements. Values located outside the square but close to the diagonal are indicative of systematic errors. Values far from the diagonal are grossly imprecise. With some programs, the participants are informed on the number and types of methods employed by all participants. Technical and method-specific calibrators are also used for the validation of hormone assays.

Clinical Validation of Hormone Measurements and Diagnosis
Immunoassays are used for diagnosis, quantification (example: TSH in screening of the newborn) and monitoring (example: IGF-1 measurement before and after growth hormone therapy) of endocrine diseases. Before the physician can make a clinical interpretation of the results they must have been fully validated by the pathologist, clinical chemist and laboratory staff. Diagnoses can only be made on the basis of accurate and precise measurement data. Laboratory data can only be interpreted properly if due consideration is given to other clinical parameters of the patient as well as to factors that might have influenced the assay (e.g. medication, nutrition, weight, cachexia, infections, circadian rhythms etc.). Some laboratory parameters such as a basal growth hormone value (pulsatile secretion) are of little informative value when considered alone.

Moreover, every measuring method must be clinically validated. First and foremost, laboratories must determine their own reference intervals for a certain method from which limits for determining whether a given value is normal or probably pathological can be derived statistically. Furthermore, to be able to verify tentative diagnoses (e.g. thyroxin deficiency), it must be known when and how reliably an abnormally low T4 value can predict hypothyreosis. The above-mentioned clinical aspects are discussed in detail in this book.

Determining Reference Intervals

Prerequisites: reference intervals give the statistical mean and range of scatter of the concentration of a parameter (e.g. a hormone), i.e. its interindividual variability within a reference population. Only by comparing the measured value with a suitable reference interval can pathological deviations be identified. The reference population needs not necessarily be healthy, as is demonstrated by reference curves for bodily growth in girls with Turner syndrome [24]. An appropriate number of samples from totally healthy subjects is often hard to obtain in particular from very young children, for ethical and practical (only low amount of blood can be drawn) reasons. Furthermore, environmental factors may also influence the concentrations of the parameters that are measured. The concept of 'normal values' can therefore be regarded as obsolete. However, it is necessary for reference populations to be composed of precisely defined reference individuals with due consideration to age, sex, body weight, pregnancy, state of health and all other factors that might have an influence on the parameter in question. In the time from birth to adulthood, the hormone balance undergoes drastic changes as the body grows and the gonads develop. Reference intervals for hormones in children must therefore be defined for small age intervals and according to different stages of sexual development. Reference intervals also depend on ethnic and cultural factors (e.g. dietary habits and physical activity). For example, it is not permissible to apply reference intervals defined for Japanese children directly to Central European children.

Reference values are also assay-specific (fig. 18). Ideally, every laboratory should determine its own reference intervals. The minimum requirement is that results should always be assessed on the basis of reference values obtained with the same type of assay and for a representative reference population.

Statistical Methods

The most common approach is to perform a parametric calculation of the reference intervals of a normal distribution of either the values of reference individuals directly or of the output of a logarithmic normalizing transformation performed on

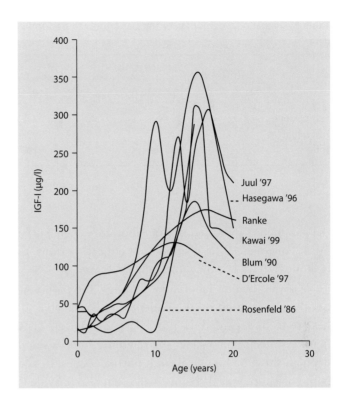

Fig. 18. Comparison of 50th percentiles for IGF-1 evaluated by different commercial and in-house assays.

those values. The exact procedure is set forth as a proposal in the Guidelines of the International Federation of Clinical Chemistry (IFCC) [25].

If there is a sufficient number of individuals per group, the central 95% CI is used (2.5th to 97.5th percentile), corresponding to the mean value of ± 1.96 SD. This method is relatively safe when it comes to assessing individual values, and it excludes extreme outliers. Another robust method makes use of the median to estimate the arithmetic mean and defines the SD as the difference between the 90th and 10th percentile divided by 2.563. The age curves for the arithmetic mean and standard deviation are commonly smoothed by means of a spline-fitting algorithm. Depending on which cut-off is postulated for the assessment of patient data, one can then calculate different percentiles and depict them graphically.

Interpretation of Laboratory Test Results

As already mentioned, an assessment of laboratory data by the physician presupposes that the conditions at the time of sampling (time of day, preanalysis), the patient's status (dietary habits, medication, if any) as well as possible interfering factors are known and verifiable. Furthermore, it is the physician's responsibility to ensure that

Table 3. Scenario to demonstrate the basic tools to perform clinical interpretation of laboratory data

	Disease status		Total
	diseased (n)	healthy (n)	
Test positive	95 (a)	2 (b)	97 (a+b)
Test negative	5 (c)	98 (d)	103 (c+d)
Total	100 (a+c)	100 (b+d)	–

the parameters indicated on the laboratory sheet suffice to verify the tentative diagnosis. For financial (and sometimes ethical) reasons, the range of parameters should be limited to what is diagnostically necessary.

When evaluating laboratory findings, the pathologist and clinical chemist must use the information on the patient that is available to them to decide whether values are to be regarded as 'normal', 'pathological', 'critical' or 'ambiguous'. In deciding they must also consider the reference intervals and corresponding cut-off limits distinguishing pathological from normal values. In addition to this information, the pathologist or clinical chemist will often also provide the physician with recommendations for further tests, and in some cases even for an appropriate therapy.

Diagnostic procedures involving single measurements of hormones or simulation tests must be examined by the clinician in terms of their clinical sensitivity, specificity, relevance and predictive value.

This will be illustrated in the following scenario (table 3) by comparing a cohort of 100 patients with confirmed endocrine disease with a cohort of 100 healthy patients. All patients are immunoassayed for a defined hormone parameter:

The clinical sensitivity measures how well the test detects those patients with the endocrine disease. It is expressed as the proportion of true positives that are correctly identified out of the 100 persons with the disease:

Sensitivity = a/(a + c); 95% in the example.

The clinical specificity measures how well the test correctly identifies those patients who do not have the disease. It is expressed as the proportion of true negatives that are correctly identified out of the 100 healthy patients:

Specificity = d/(b + d); 98% in the example.

The false-positive rate is the proportion of demonstrably unaffected individuals falsely identified as having the disease:

False-positive rate = 1 – specificity.

The decisive criterion in clinical practice, however, is how reliably a positive result can predict that the endocrine disease really is present. This quantity gives the likelihood in the test population of a positive test result being true. The positive predictive value (PPV) is the likelihood that a patient with a positive test result actually has the endocrine disease, i.e. the proportion of patients with positive test results who are correctly diagnosed:

PPV = a/(a + b); 97.5% in the example.

The negative predictive value (NPV) is the likelihood that a patient with a negative test result does not have the endocrine disease:

NPV = d/(c + d); 95.1% in the example.

In contrast to the incidence, which gives the proportion of new cases of a disease (e.g. diabetes mellitus) within a population, the prevalence gives the proportion of persons in that population who already have the disease at a given point in time. In the above example the prevalence of the disease would be:

P = diseased persons/diseased persons + healthy persons = 50%.

This value does probably not represent the true prevalence of the disease in the population, which is normally far lower. The clinical utility of a diagnostic test, and hence of PPV and NPV, can be severely restricted by the prevalence of the disease in question.

On the Critical Use of Laboratory Data in Clinical Diagnostics

The number of laboratory parameters that can be measured and for which reimbursement is provided has increased considerably over the past years, but is now limited by the financial limitations of the public health care systems. This makes it increasingly difficult for physicians to select the right parameters for diagnosis.

In matters of quality control, the physician must be able to trust in the reliability of the laboratory. Quality management systems are used in every diagnostic laboratory today. Nevertheless, he should not trust laboratory results blindly, since errors can also go undetected in the laboratory. In cases of doubt, improbable measuring results must be checked, or it may even be necessary to generate a new sample. This presupposes a continuous dialogue between the physician and the laboratory. At the same time, for cost reasons, laboratory diagnostics should be reduced to the minimum of what is necessary. To avoid false-positive, or worse still, false-negative results, physicians must command a wide experience and continuously train their knowledge.

Last but not least, it should be pointed out that a clinical diagnosis can be accomplished and refined, rather than be replaced by measuring meaningful laboratory parameters.

References

1　Evans HM, Simpson ME, Marx W, Kibrick E: Bioassay of pituitary growth hormone: width of the proximal epiphyseal cartilage of the tibia in hypophysectomized rats. Endocrinology 1943;32:13–16.

2　Bristow AF, Jespersen AM: The Second International Standard for somatropin (recombinant DNA-derived human growth hormone): preparation and calibration in an international collaborative study. Biologicals 2001;29:97–106.

3　Robinson CJ, Gaines Das R, Woollacott D: The first international standard for human leptin and the first international standard for mouse leptin: comparison of candidate preparations by in vitro bioassays and immunoassays. J Mol Endocrinol 2001;27:69–76.

4　Persani L, Ferretti E, Borgato S, Faglia G, Beck-Peccoz P: Circulating thyrotropin bioactivity in sporadic central hypothyroidism. J Clin Endocrinol Metab 2000;85:3631–3635.

5　Binder G, Benz MR, Elmlinger M, Pflaum CD, Strasburger CJ, Ranke MB: Reduced human growth hormone (hGH) bioactivity without a defect of the GH-1 gene in three patients with rhGH responsive growth failure. Clin Endocrinol (Oxf) 1999;51:89–95.

6　Ishikawa M, Nimura A, Horikawa R, Katsumata N, Arisaka O, Wada M, Honjo M, Tanaka T: A novel specific bioassay for serum human growth hormone. J Clin Endocrinol Metab 2000;85:4274–4279.

7　Kiess W, Butenandt O: Regulation of GH binding to specific cellular receptors in vitro-a new model of growth regulation in vivo. Horm Metab Res 1987;19:171–176.

8　Baumann G: Growth hormone binding proteins and various forms of growth hormone: implications for measurements. Acta Paediatr Scand 1990(suppl);370:2–80.

9　Asai D, Shimohigashi Y: The assessment of xenoestrogens by competitive receptor binding assays. Nippon Rinsho 2000;58:2486–2490.

10　Strasburger CJ, Wu Z, Pflaum CD, Dressendorfer RA: Immunofunctional assay of human growth hormone (hGH) in serum: a possible consensus for quantitative hGH measurement. J Clin Endocrinol Metab 1996;81:2613–2620.

11　Lammert A, Kiess W, Bottner A, Glasow A, Kratzsch J: Soluble leptin receptor represents the main leptin binding activity in human blood. Biochem Biophys Res Commun 2001;283:982–988.

12　Lassarre C, Duron F, Binoux M: Use of the ligand immunofunctional assay for human insulin-like growth factor (IGF) binding protein-3 (IGFBP-3) to analyze IGFBP-3 proteolysis and IGF-I bioavailability in healthy adults, GH-deficient and acromegalic patients, and diabetics. J Clin Endocrinol Metab 2001;86:1942–1952.

13　Berson SA, Yalow RS: Assay of plasma insulin in human subjects by immunological methods. Nature 1959;184:1984.

14　Miles LEM, Hales CN: Labelled antibodies and immunological assay systems. Nature 1968;219:186–189.

15　Addison GM, Hales CN: The immunoradiometric assay; in Kirkham KE, Hunter WM (eds): Radioimmunoassay Methods. Edinburgh, Churchill-Livingstone, 1970, pp 447–461.

16　Babson AL, Olson DR, Palmieri T, Ross AF, Becker DM, Mulqueen PJ: The IMMULITE assay tube: a new approach to heterogeneous ligand assay. Clin Chem 1991;37:1521–1522.

17　Box FEP, Hunter WG: A useful method for model-building. Technometrics 1962;4:301–318.

18　Andersson P, Jesson G, Kylberg G, Ekstrand G, Thorsén G: Parallel nanoliter microfluidic analysis system. Anal Chem 2007;79:4022–4030.

19　Templin MF, Stoll D, Schwenk JM, Pötz O, Kramer S, Joos TO: Protein microarrays: promising tools for proteomic research. Proteomics 2003;3:2155–2166.

20　Schultz JS: Biosensors. Scientific American, August 1991;48–55.

21　Gordon Malan P: Immunological Biosensors; in Wild D (ed): The Immunoassay Handbook. London, Macmillan Press, 1994, p 131 (UK).

22　Bland JM, Altmann DG: Statistical methods for assessing agreement between two methods of clinical measurement. Lancet 1986;i:307–310.

23　Linnet K: Evaluation of regression procedures for method comparison studies. Clin Chem 1993;39:424–432.

24 Rongen-Westerlaken C, Corel L, van den Broeck J, Massa G, Karlberg J, Albertsson-Wikland K, Naeraa RW, Wit JM: Reference values for height, height velocity and weight in Turner's syndrome. Swedish Study Group for GH treatment. Acta Paediatr 1997; 86:937–942.

25 International Federation of Clinical Chemistry Scientific Committee, Clinical Section: Expert Panel on Theory of Reference Values and International Committee for Standardization in Haematology. 5. Statistical treatment on the theory of reference values: determinations of reference limits. J Clin Chem Clin Biochem 1987;25:645–656.

Prof. Martin W. Elmlinger
Nycomed International Management GmbH
Thurgauerstrasse 130
CH-8152 Glattpark-Opfikon, Zurich (Switzerland)
Tel. +41 505 44 555 1228, Fax +41 505 44 555 1455, E-Mail martin.elmlinger@nycomed.com

Ranke MB, Mullis P-E (eds): Diagnostics of Endocrine Function in Children and Adolescents, ed 4.
Basel, Karger, 2011, pp 32–52

Molecular Genetics and Bioinformatics Methods for Diagnosis of Endocrine Disorders

Amit V. Pandey · Primus-E. Mullis

Pediatric Endocrinology, Diabetology and Metabolism, Department of Clinical Research, University of Bern, and University Children's Hospital Bern, Bern, Switzerland

Diagnostic and preventive clinical medicine has undergone major changes due to advancements in molecular genetics, especially the molecular biological tools that allow detection of complex abnormalities in the genetic makeup of an individual. No field of medicine has benefitted more and contributed to the molecular genetics advancements than endocrinology. Modern endocrinology has changed from simple measurement of hormones to analysis of every aspect of hormone synthesis and action, ranging from biosynthesis of hormones, genes and proteins involved in hormone synthesis, interaction of hormones with their receptors as well as regulation of genes involved in hormone biosynthesis and action pathways in a cellular and tissue-specific manor. A modern endocrinology laboratory routinely applies the latest molecular biological methods to identify and characterize inherited metabolic disorders.

Endocrinology has also contributed to the advancement and practice of molecular genetics and endocrinologists have been among the early adaptors of modern techniques of molecular biology as these became available. Initial attempts by endocrinologists to identify, characterize and purify hormones and their receptors had led to attempts for identification and cloning of genetic sequences for hormones. Human growth hormone and insulin have been among the first molecules to be studied at genetic level and cloned in bacteria for production as recombinant molecules [1–3]. Moreover, insulin and human growth hormone were the first two recombinant proteins to be produced for clinical use and their success led to establishment of biotechnology industry starting with Genentech in San Francisco, Calif., USA. A further boost to adaptation of modern analysis methods came in the form of polymerase chain reaction (PCR) which allowed endocrinologists and molecular geneticists to diagnose rare endocrine disorders and explain the causative anomalies at molecular level. Genes for steroid metabolizing enzymes were among the first to be cloned and analyzed at genetic level in patients. A major advantage of molecular biological methods is that these allow detection of rare genetic disorders where biochemical laboratory measurements are not clear as well as in pediatric and neonatal diagnosis where sample size is often limited. The latest advancement in the field has been the availability of human genome sequence. An almost complete catalogue of human genes has allowed endocrinologists to identify new targets for candidate genes for many genetic disorders and subsequent sequencing of genetic material from patients had led to identification of the exact molecular basis of many hormonal and metabolic defects.

Sample Preparation and Basic Analytical Methods

Linkage studies are used to indicate the probability with which an endocrine disorder is associated with a particular gene. In presence of known polymorphisms linkage association studies can be performed rapidly. However, such studies do not provide the exact location of the disorders/mutations and, therefore, no functional conclusion could be obtained solely from linkage analysis. Therefore, identification of the exact location of the mutations is of importance to clinical laboratories as a wide variation in severity of disease could be seen in endocrine disorders, often due to the wide nature of point mutations in the target gene with each mutation resulting in a specific effect. The ultimate test of functional genomics characterization of a disease comes from identification of the exact location of mutations followed by biochemical characterization of genetic defects performed with recombinant genes/proteins that replicate the patient DNA sequences in experimental setup. Many different techniques are available for the identification of genetic disorders related to endocrine disruption. A pure DNA/RNA sample is required to perform laboratory diagnosis using molecular biological methods and procuring a sufficient quantity of genetic material is a first step in proceeding with genetic analysis. Nowadays, amplification of genetic material is carried out in laboratories by using polymerase chain reaction. This allows relatively smaller sample amounts to be used in analysis and, therefore, several different analysis approaches could be used on relatively small amounts of DNA obtained from blood or tissue samples. Traditional cloning and target identification methods are no longer employed since availability of a complete human genome sequence has provided necessary sequence information about almost all genes. Therefore, in the current version of this book, traditional cloning strategies based on protein sequences or partial sequence information have been omitted.

When DNA analysis is to be performed by an external laboratory, it is usually sufficient to send a small blood sample (5 ml of EDTA treated blood) in unfrozen form so that the diagnostic laboratory can isolate DNA according to method of its choice. Modern diagnostic techniques employ DNA amplification based methods and require only a small amount of DNA for most diagnostic methods. It is important to obtain blood samples from not only the patients but from as many family members as possible. Parents and siblings provide additional information about the nature and inheritance pattern of the disease and genotype-phenotype correlations within family members may provide important information about the effect of sequence anomalies and mutations. Family studies can provide molecular and physiological relevance of new disorders before advanced cloning and expression techniques are used to test a hypothesis about functional testing of the gene products. However, not all disorders can be effectively categorized by genetic analysis alone and often changes found in genetic analysis are widespread (commonly referred to as polymorphisms). When DNA analysis is to be performed in the laboratory of the investigator then in-house DNA isolation and purification techniques are employed to prepare genomic DNA/RNA from blood/tissue samples.

DNA Preparation

Proper handling of patient samples is of great importance in molecular laboratory diagnostics. Pediatric endocrinology has especially benefited from modern diagnostic methods that require only a small amount of sample as opposed to older methods that performed restriction digestion and Southern blot analysis directly on patient DNA and required 15–20 ml of whole blood to provide enough genetic material for testing. With the PCR based detection methods it has become possible to reduce the sample amount and often 1–2 ml of blood will be enough to provide sufficient DNA for sequencing of candidate genes. For even smaller sample volumes, especially in neonatology and pediatrics, DNA can be extracted from a spot of blood on a Guthrie card [4]. Dried blood specimens can be collected by applying a few drops of blood on a filter paper which is air dried and put in a plastic bag with some desiccating material to reduce humidity. A good laboratory practice is to prepare the DNA as soon as sample is available. Often whole blood is used for this purpose and fresh blood samples are preferable to isolate the DNA. However, frozen blood samples can also be used for DNA isolation but yields will often be less than when fresh samples are used. An EDTA-based blood collection method is preferable over heparin-based anticoagulation as it is compatible with most DNA isolation methods.

Several protocols for preparation of DNA from blood samples are available [5]. The classical methods involve isolation of nucleated cells from whole blood by differential gradient centrifugation and selective lysis of erythrocytes. In these procedures care must be taken to remove the proteins from DNA as excess proteins in DNA samples often lead to degradation of DNA over time, even when stored frozen. A phenol-chloroform based separation has been used successfully to remove proteins from DNA. Upon mixing with phenol-chloroform reagent and subsequent centrifugation, proteins are found in the organic phase or at the interphase while DNA remains in aqueous phase. Soluble DNA from aqueous phase is precipitated using ethanol and propanol and dissolved in small amounts of water or buffer and stored at –70°C. There are several commercial DNA extraction kits based on selective binding of DNA as the basis for isolation. Generally, a silica-based matrix is used for selective binding of DNA after the cell lysis and several washing steps employing different buffers are used to remove proteins and other containments. Purified DNA is then eluted in small amounts of water or buffer and stored at −70°C.

RNA Preparation

In many cases isolation of RNA is also required as it may cut down the analysis time by providing full-length coding sequencing for mutational analysis, especially in cases when the genomic transcript contains many introns or is very long. Afterwards mRNA could be used in a reverse transcriptase reaction to produce cDNA which is suitable for amplification by PCR and sequencing. This approach has the disadvantage that some genes may not be transcribed in blood samples and tissues are often not available. Moreover, RNA is difficult to handle as it degrades rapidly, so immediate processing is required. Some commercially available storage solutions (e.g. RNA Later) can minimize RNA degradation and allow shipment of blood/tissue samples in normal cold storage (4°C) or even at room temperature. When purifying RNA sample for genetic analysis, one has to consider the source of the sample and the pros/cons of individual purification methods [5].

The single-step RNA isolation methods based on guanidine isothiocyanate (GITC)/phenol/chloroform extraction are very popular because they require much less time than older methods (e.g. $CsCl_2$ ultracentrifugation). Many commercial reagents based on phenol/chloroform extraction method are available (e.g. Trizol). The entire procedure takes less than 2 h to produce high-quality total RNA. Silica gel-based purification methods like RNeasy are available as a kit from several suppliers. These kits use a silica membrane embedded in a spin-column to selectively bind RNA. These methods are also quick and do not involve the use of phenol. The yield from spin columns is usually lower compared to phenol/chloroform extraction methods. To prepare mRNA from the total RNA, oligo-dT-based affinity purification is used. The use of oligo-dT-based affinity binding to selectively bind poly (A)+ RNA results in enrichment of mRNA and greatly reduces rRNA and other RNA contaminations. The mRNA enrichment is essential for preparing of cDNA by reverse transcription.

Primer Design for Sequencing and PCR

A primer is a short synthetic oligonucleotide which is used in many DNA-based molecular techniques like PCR, DNA sequencing and nucleic acid hybridization. Primers are designed to have a sequence which is the reverse complement of a region of the target DNA so that it can anneal to the target sequence. It is advisable to use primer design software tools available at bioinformatic resources rather than relying on manual design. These tools may reduce the cost and time involved in experimentation by lowering the chances of failed reaction due to wrong primers. Primer3Plus provides a web interface to the popular Primer3 program with a task-oriented approach. Several different options for primer design are available including sequencing and cloning

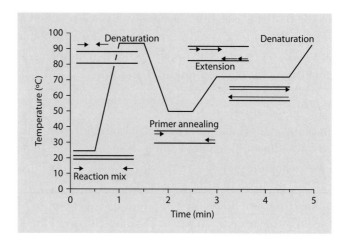

Fig. 1. An overview of polymerase chain reaction. See text for details.

as well as design of probes for Northern analysis, etc. The Primer3Plus web interface is available at http://www.bioinformatics.nl/cgi-bin/primer3plus/primer3plus.cgi. An important step in successful diagnostic or amplification experiments is to check the specificity of primers. A primer homology search or BLAST (explained in following sections) against all known human sequences to check for alternative priming sites is required. Primers that display 'significant' homology to alternative targets should be discarded. Two main criterions in selecting primers are to discard sequences where alternative sites have more than 90% homology to the primary site and more than 7 consecutive nucleotides homologous to other targets are present at the 3′ end of the primer. The primer blast tool available at NCBI can screen for mismatches and alternative binding sites (http://www.ncbi.nlm.nih.gov/tools/primer-blast/).

PCR

The polymerase chain reaction (PCR) is a technique widely used in molecular biology where a piece of DNA is amplified by in vitro enzymatic replication [6]. The original DNA molecules are replicated by the DNA polymerase enzyme and resulting in doubling the number of DNA molecules (fig. 1). Then each of these molecules is replicated in a second 'cycle' of replication, resulting in four times the number of the original molecules. Each of these molecules is then replicated in a third cycle. This process is known as a 'chain reaction' in which the original DNA template is exponentially amplified. With PCR it is possible to amplify a single piece of DNA, or a very small number of pieces of DNA, over many cycles, generating millions of copies of the original DNA molecule. The PCR usually consists of a series of 25–35 repeated temperature change cycles in 3 temperature steps [5]. The cycling is often preceded by a single temperature step (hold) at a high temperature (>90°C), and followed by one hold at the end for the final product extension or storage. A basic PCR reaction could be described as follows:

Pandey · Mullis

(1) Initialization step: This step consists of heating the reaction to a temperature of 92–94°C, which is held for 1–2 min.

(2) Denaturation step: This is the first cycle in the reaction and consists of heating the reaction to 92–96°C for 20–30 s to denature the DNA template by disrupting the hydrogen bonds between complementary bases and produces single-stranded DNA.

(3) Annealing step: Temperature is lowered to 50–65°C for 30–45 s to allow annealing of primers to the single-stranded DNA templates.

(4) Extension/elongation step: Usually performed at 72°C but may depend on type of DNA polymerase used in reaction. At this step the DNA polymerase synthesizes a new DNA strand that is complementary to the template sequence by adding nucleotides that are complementary to the template in the 5′ to 3′ direction, The time of extension depends on the DNA polymerase and the length of the DNA fragment and generally approximated 1,000 bp/min.

(5) Final elongation: This single step is occasionally performed at a temperature of 68–72°C for 5–15 min after the last PCR cycle to ensure that any remaining single-stranded DNA is fully extended.

(6) Final hold: This step at 4–15°C for an indefinite time may be employed for short-term storage of the reaction. The PCR products may be analyzed by agarose gel electrophoresis by comparing against standard molecular weight markers.

DNA Sequencing

DNA sequencing is still the most reliable method to confirm a genetic defect and provide the exact location and nature of the disorder. Sequencing of DNA is no longer performed in individual laboratories and has been relegated to central facilities of outsourced to private companies providing sequencing services. Most facilities employ the chain termination based approach initially developed by Sanger. Modern fluorescence dye based methods involve labeling of the chain terminator nucleotides with fluorescent tags, this allows sequencing in a single reaction where each of the four chain terminators are labeled with fluorescent dyes with different wavelengths of fluorescence emission (fig. 2). The dye-terminator sequencing method are carried out by automated high-throughput DNA sequence analyzers that can take multiple samples in microwell plates and perform unattended analysis. Typically, 600–800 bp can be analyzed in single runs. The automated and efficient sequencing technology has allowed comparison of normal and patient DNA sequences without manually reading the chromatograms. One efficient tool for automated mutation analysis from DNA sequence traces is Mutation Surveyor software from Softgenetics (http://www.softgenetics.com/mutationSurveyor.html). Mutation Surveyor, is available for academic labs with simultaneous reading of 48 samples from Sanger Sequencing traces provided by automated dye terminator sequencers. Mutation Surveyor can locate genetic variants, SNPs and Indel mutations between reference traces and sample/patient traces and has a several reporting possibilities for both research and laboratory diagnostics.

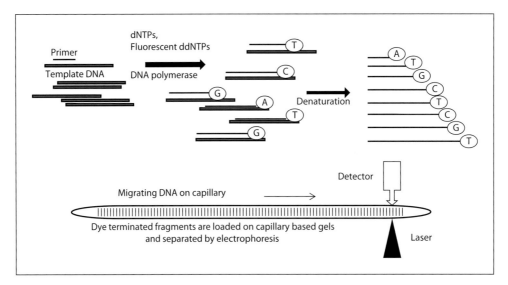

Fig. 2. Principle of dye termination DNA sequencing. Modern fluorescent dye terminator-based sequencers can read at four different wavelengths for each type of nucleotide allowing a single gel/capillary to be used for detecting all four nucleotide types in the DNA. Different fragment lengths of DNA get terminated once a ddNTP is incorporated during the PCR stage and the fluorescent scanner reads each fragment and identifies the end nucleotide. A DNA sequence is generated by listing the end-terminal nucleotide for each fragment.

Reverse Genetics in the Diagnosis of Endocrine Disorders

Direct analysis based on biochemical parameters is often difficult and in most cases could not be performed due to unavailability of tissue samples. Molecular genetic methods have led to development of several different tools that can be used in the detection of endocrine disorders. A powerful technique to narrow down causes of diseases with unknown genetic basis is linkage analysis. It involves identification of genes based on information about its location on chromosomes. Chromosomes are long stretches of DNA sequences where different genes are located next to each other in a long row. Genetic linkage occurs when particular genetic alleles for genes are inherited jointly. Genetic loci on the same chromosome are physically close to one another and tend to stay together during meiosis, and are thus genetically linked. This is called autosomal linkage. Alleles for genes on different chromosomes are usually not linked, due to independent assortment of chromosomes during meiosis.

Because there is some crossing over of DNA when the chromosomes segregate, alleles on the same chromosome can get separated and passed on to different daughter cells. The alleles that are farther apart on the chromosome have higher chance of this crossing over, as it is more likely that a cross-over will occur between those genes. The relative distance between two genes is calculated from the offspring of an organism

Pandey · Mullis

Table 1. A list of common endocrine disorders for molecular genetic testing with OMIM links

Organ	Disorder	Gene defect	OMIM
Adrenal	congenital adrenal hyperplasia	21-hydroxylase	+201910
		11β-hydroxylase	#202010
		17-hydroxylase	#202110
		3β-HSD	+201810
		P450 reductase	#201750, #207410
	hypoaldosteronism	C-18 hydroxylase	
		aldosterone synthetase	
Bone	phosphophatemic rickets		#193100, #241520
Kidney	vitamin D resistance		#277440
Thyroid	congenital goiter	thyroid peroxidase	
		thyroglobulin	
	congenital hypothyroidism	TSH receptor	#275200
	thyroid hormone resistance	T3 receptor	
Testes	male limited precautious puberty	LH receptor	#176410
	hypogonadotrophic hypogonadism		#146110
	Kallmann syndrome	KAL gene	+308700
Genitalia	intersex	androgen receptor	#300068
	pseudohermaphroditism	5α-reductase	#264600
		SRY	#400044
		TDF	#400044
Pituitary	isolated GHD	GH-1	#262400
		GHRH receptor	*139191
	combined pituitary hormone deficiency	PIT-1	#613038

Table 1. Continued

Organ	Disorder	Gene defect	OMIM
	GH, TSH, Prl	PIT-1 (POU1F1)	
	GH, TSH, Prl and LH/FSH	PROP-1	#262600
	GH, TSH, Prl and LH/FSH ACTH	HESX-1	
	with/without midline defects		
	GH, TSH, Prl and LH/FSH ACTH	LHX-3	#221750
	with cervical spine shortening		
	GH, TSH, Prl and LH/FSH ACTH	LHX-4	#262700
	with flattening of sella		
	diabetes insipidus central	vasoprasin	
	diabetes insipidus renal	vasoprasin receptor	#304800
		aquaporin-2	#125800
Dwarfism	GH resistance, high GH low IGF-1	GH receptor	#262500

showing two linked genetic traits, and then finding the percentage of the offspring in cases when the two traits are not found together. The percentage of descendants that does not show both traits is directly proportional to the distance between the two genes. Thus, the more distant the genetic loci are, the more often recombination takes place. A recombination of 1% is roughly equal to a distance of 1 million bases. The maximal theoretical recombination frequency is 50%, which is the same as when two genes are located on two different chromosomes. This recombination frequency corresponds linearly up to a distance of 2 million bp but becomes nonlinear when distances are greater that 4–5 million bp and at that point double recombinations are more likely to happen.

Linkage mapping is an important technique for the identification of disease-causing genes. In a normal population, genetic markers may be found in many different combinations and the frequencies of these combinations are derived from the frequencies

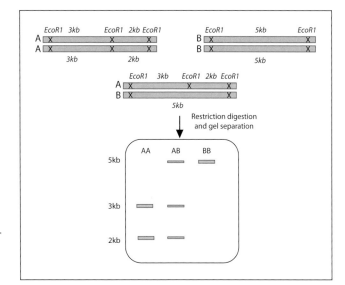

Fig. 3. An overview of the RFPL principle. A point mutation causing abolition of one *EcoR1* site results in different fragment lengths that could be resolved by gel electrophoresis. An example of WT, heterozygous and homozygous mutation is shown here.

of the individual genes in the population. Linkage analysis is performed to check if any particular combinations of polymorphic alleles are inherited in the disease that is being studied. Therefore, only those genetic loci that show some sequence variation in the populations are used for linkage analysis. When some combination of alleles appears more frequently in patients, the chances of those polymorphic sites being close to the gene that may be causing the disease are considered higher. Therefore, for mapping the candidate genes for endocrine disorders it is important to study as many members of the family and relatives over several generations, as possible. The chances that data will show linkage between two loci should be computed statistically from the observed parameters and the number of individuals in the study. The odds are then calculated for chances of linkage over the chances against the linkage. The $\log_{10}$ of these odds called the LOD score is typically 3 times or higher if the data are truly showing a linkage pattern.

Restriction Fragment Length Polymorphism
Restriction fragment length polymorphism (RFLP) was the simplest and earliest method to detect SNPs. SNP-RFLP is based on availability of several different restriction enzymes and their specificity towards unique restriction sites. By digesting genomic DNA and determining the fragment lengths generated after digestion by electrophoresis, it is possible to determine whether or not the restriction enzymes cut the DNA at the expected restriction sites (fig. 3). Several online restriction digestion tools can provide in silico digestion pattern and expected fragment lengths that can be compared with actual results. Two such tools are *BioTools* available at http://biotools.umassmed.edu/tacg/WWWtacg.php and *NEBcutter* found at http://tools.

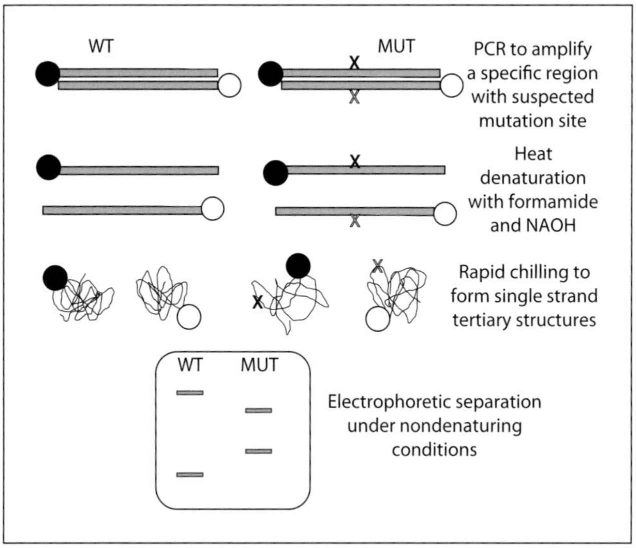

Fig. 4. An example of SSCP analysis. Single nucleotide changes will cause altered folding of single-stranded DNA. In SSCP analysis, DNA is first denatured and then cooled rapidly to promote folding of single-stranded DNA. Gel electrophoresis is then used to compare differences in movement against the WT allele.

neb.com/NEBcutter2/index.php. A failure to cut the genomic sample results in an identifiably larger than expected fragment implying that there is a mutation at the point of the restriction site which is protecting that restriction site from nuclease activity. Unfortunately, several factors like the complexity of human genome, the requirement for specific endonucleases and the fact that the exact mutation cannot often be resolved in a single experiment, as well as limitations associated with nature of gel electrophoresis based assays make RFLP a poor choice for high throughput analysis and it is being replaced by chip based SNP genotyping assays.

Single-Strand Conformation Polymorphism (SSCP) Analysis
Single-stranded DNA (ssDNA) folds to form a secondary structure that is dependent on DNA sequence and, therefore, most single basepair mutations will alter the shape of the folded structure. When DNA is subjected to gel electrophoresis, the secondary structure of ssDNA will determine its mobility (fig. 4). Therefore, gel electrophoresis of ssDNA can be used to differentiate between SNP alleles based on different pattern of mobility due to differences in structure changes [7]. The ssDNA conformation polymorphism analysis involves the PCR amplification of the target DNA sequence containing suspected polymorphisms. The double-stranded DNA obtained after PCR amplification is then denatured by application of heat and formaldehyde to produce ssDNA. A denaturing loading buffer and rapid cooling on ice is used to keep the two strands of DNA separate before entering the electrophoretic gel. The ssDNA is then subjected to nondenaturing gel electrophoresis and allowed to fold into a secondary structure. Both the gel and running conditions are optimized to allow formation of complex structures from each strand. Differences in DNA sequences

will alter the tertiary conformation that can be detected as a difference in the mobility of ssDNA. After electrophoresis, a mutation is detected by a shift in the band with mutation when compared to the two bands from the control DNA. Two bands with a migration shift are indicative of homozygous mutation and four bands with altered migration are indicative of heterozygous mutations. This method had been widely used because it is simple to perform, inexpensive and can be performed in most laboratories using commonly available equipment. Earlier, a radiolabeling approach during PCR was used to detect the bands but silver staining procedures are now used for detection with similar sensitivity. However, compared to other SNP genotyping methods now available, the sensitivity of ssDNA conformation analysis is lower. It has been reported in many studies that the ssDNA conformation is highly dependent on temperature and it is not generally clear what temperature is to be used as ideal for this analysis. Quite often the assay will be performed under different temperature settings in different laboratories. Moreover, the length of fragments that could be examined is somewhat restricted, as the sensitivity of this assay decreases when sequences longer than 200 bp are analyzed [8]. Therefore, sequences longer than 400 bp should be divided into two or more sequences as necessary for SSCP analysis either by generating overlapping sequences by PCR or by digestion with restriction enzymes to generate smaller fragments. For SSCP analysis PCR conditions should be optimized to reduce artifacts and PCR products should be checked separately before SSCP analysis is performed.

Denaturing Gradient Gel Electrophoresis

The denaturing gradient gel analysis is used to separate PCR products for mutation analysis. In this system, a linear gradient of increasing concentration of a denaturing agent is used for gel formation. When DNA starts moving it gets denatured as it migrates through the gel with increasing denaturant concentration. When a partial denaturation of DNA is achieved, the movement of DNA is slowed down [9]. This denaturing point is dependent on the sequence of the PCR fragments being analyzed and under optimal conditions mutation will result in altered migration pattern compared to standard sequence. Formation of gradient gels requires density gradient mixers and casting systems linked with a peristaltic pump or gravity based setups to cast the gels with a linear gradient of denaturant. Usually, one of the PCR primers in this analysis is designed with a stretch of guanine and cytosine bases at the 5′-end to form a tight hydrogen bond based coupling at one end that holds the PCR fragments together and avoids complete denaturation even at higher end of denaturant concentration in the gel.

Temperature Gradient Gel Electrophoresis

The temperature gradient gel electrophoresis (TGGE) or temperature gradient capillary electrophoresis (TGCE) method is based on the same principle as denaturing gradient gel electrophoresis in that the partially denatured DNA is more restricted and moves slower during gel electrophoresis and a temperature gradient is used to apply selection. This allows the separation of DNA by its melting temperature which is dependent on its sequence. To adapt this property for SNP detection, two DNA fragments are used: the target DNA which may contain the SNP site being tested, and an allele-specific normal DNA fragment [10]. The normal DNA fragment is identical to the target DNA being tested except for the potential SNP site, which is unknown in the target DNA. The fragments are first denatured and then re-annealed. If the target DNA has the same sequence as the normal allele then homo-duplexes will be formed and both will have the same melting temperature. When this type of sample is separated on the gel with a temperature gradient, only one band will appear. If the target DNA has a polymorphic allele, four products will form after the renaturation step: homo-duplexes consisting of target DNA, homo-duplexes consisting of normal DNA, and hetero-duplexes of each strand of target DNA hybridized with the normal DNA. These four products will have a difference in melting temperatures and will appear as four bands after the denaturing gel electrophoresis. Detection of heterozygous alleles is an advantage of TGGE over DGGE.

Ligase Chain Reaction (LCR)
The LCR technique is an adaptation of PCR that uses thermostable ligase to amplify a standard sequence based on repetitive ligation of two oligonucleotides [11]. It can be adopted for detecting point mutations to diagnose known disease causing alleles [12]. A thermostable DNA ligase is used to ligate adjacent oligos covering the left and right side of a known mutation (fig. 5). Two sets of oligos can be designed that anneal to one DNA strand with one oligo ending with or starting at the potential mutant site and a second set of two oligos are designed similarly for the second strand. Only the wild-type sequence will permit joining of two oligos by ligation and a mismatch due to point mutation will prevent annealing of oligos to the template DNA and will not allow DNA ligase to join adjacent oligos. Once the wild-type DNA allows ligation of oligos, that sequence becomes the target for next round of annealing and ligation, resulting in exponential increase in ligated oligos for the wild-type sequence. In case a high-risk point mutation is suspected, LCR can be used to detect that mutation in a relatively shorter time period compared to PCR and sequencing.

Single Nucleotide Polymorphism Genotyping

Genotyping provides a measurement of the genetic variation between members of a species. Single nucleotide polymorphisms (SNP) are the most common type of genetic variation found among members of a species. A SNP is a single basepair mutation at a specific locus; usually consisting of two alleles (the rare allele frequency is ≥1% to be called polymorphic). SNPs are often linked to of many human

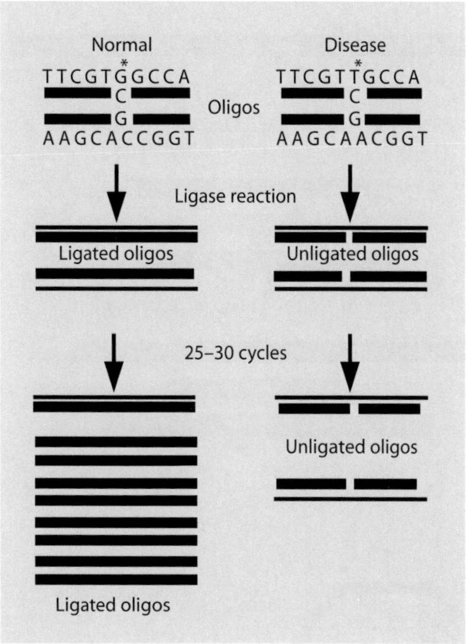

Fig. 5. Principle of LCR. LCR is a fast and powerful method of detecting known mutations. Two oligos are designed for each strand of the DNA sequences that cover the suspected mutation site and one oligo for each strand either end or begins with a potential mutation site. In the mutated allele, oligos will not align to template and ligase will be unable to join two oligos. Several cycles of this reaction are performed with a thermostable ligase resulting in selective amplification of ligated oligos for the WT sequence, while the mutated sequence is not amplified.

diseases and since SNPs are evolutionarily conserved, they have become popular as markers to be used in disease linkage association studies in place of microsatellites [13].

SNP Microarrays

The high-density oligonucleotide SNP arrays are formed by spotting several hundred thousand probes on small chips, allowing for large numbers of SNPs to be probed simultaneously [14]. Since SNP alleles are only different to normal alleles by one nucleotide the target DNA could potentially to hybridize to mismatched probes and result in false-positives (fig. 6). To minimize the false-positives, several redundant probes for each SNP are employed during spotting. Different probes for the same SNPs are designed to have the SNP site in different physical locations and also contain mismatches to the SNP allele to provide negative controls. Specific homozygous and heterozygous alleles are identified based on differential hybridization patters for many redundant probes. Oligonucleotide microarray methods have often lower specificity and sensitivity compared to more refined techniques but the amount of SNPs that can be checked in a single analysis is of great advantage. The Affymetrix Human SNP 6.0 GeneChip performs a genomewide assay that can test over 1.8 million markers for genetic variations including 906,600 human SNPs, including those obtained from HapMap project and 946,000 probes for copy number variations covering known copy number changes in the Toronto Database of Genomic Variants

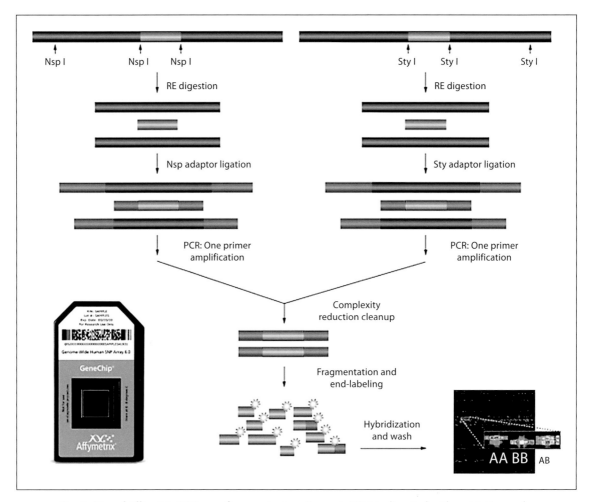

Fig. 6. Use of Affimatrix SNP array for genotyping. Genomic DNA is digested with restriction endo-nucleases, PCR amplified and labeled with fluorescent tags and hybridized on oligonucleotide array. After washing to remove unbound DNA, chips are read using fluorescence scanners and SNPs are identified based on binding to known sequences.

(DGV) (Affymetrix 2009). This allows performing whole genome association studies and copy number variation polymorphisms.

For the assay, 500 ng of genomic DNA is digested with Nsp 1 and Sty 1 restriction enzymes and then ligated to adaptors recognizing the 4-bp overhangs. A generic primer specific to adaptor sequence is used to amplify the adaptor ligated DNA fragments giving products of 200–1,100 bp. The PCR products for each restriction digestion are combined, fragmented, end labeled and hybridized to SNP microarray. Chips are processed according to manufacturer guidelines and read on a fluorescence scanner. Binding pattern of WT and mutant alleles allows detection of different SNPs.

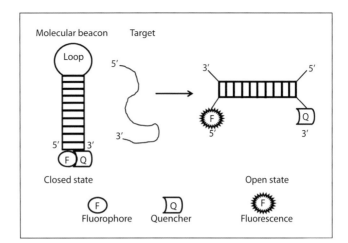

Fig. 7. Molecular beacons for mutation detection. See text for details.

Molecular Beacons for SNP Detection

SNP detection through molecular beacons is based on target specific single-stranded oligonucleotide probes with fluorescent tags. The oligonucleotides are designed to form a hairpin and stem of due to self-complementary regions at both end and the probe sequence is located in between to form a loop. This design strategy makes a hairpin-like structure in the natural, unbound state. At one end of the probe a fluorophore is attached and at the other end a quencher is attached. Due to the hairpin-shaped closed loop structure of the probe, the fluorophore comes close to the quencher and. therefore, in the native form the probe is not fluorescent (fig. 7). The beacon is designed in a way such that the loop sequence in the probe is complementary to the target sequence in the genomic DNA [15]. When the probes are hybridized with the target DNA the beacons with complementary sequences on the target anneal to form duplexes. The length of the probe sequence in the beacon favors the denaturation of the hairpin structure to form a more stable complex with the target sequence on the target DNA. This conformational change results in the fluorophore getting away from the quencher and the probe-target hybrid becomes fluorescent. However, if the probe sequence gets in contact with a variation in the target sequence, even by a single nucleotide, the beacon stays in the hairpin form with the fluorophore and quencher in close proximity and no fluorescence is emitted. This property of the molecular beacons permits the design of specific probes against WT and variant alleles for detection of SNPs. The molecular beacon can be designed against both WT and mutant allele and labeled with different fluorophores to allow detection of both alleles in the same assay to identify the genotype of an individual. If only the WT probe's fluorescence is detected during the assay then the individual is homozygous to the wild type. If only the mutant probe's wavelength is detected then the individual is homozygous to the mutant allele. When both fluorescences are detected, then both the WT and mutant alleles are detected permitting the diagnosis of heterozygous alleles.

Target Gene Hypothesis

The completion of the human genome project along with techniques to amplify DNA/RNA has allowed direct target-driven approaches to identify the suspected genes responsible for genetic disorders in patients. A small amount of blood sample is needed to isolate the DNA/RNA that is subjected to PCR to amplify the candidate genes which are then studied for abnormalities by sequence analysis. Once a defect has been identified, the target gene from patients can be cloned directly, or often the mutation/disordered can be replicated by changing the normal gene that is already available in laboratories in the form of standard DNA libraries. It is then possible to deduce the amino acid sequence of proteins and predict its structural and biophysical properties. Recombinant genes with artificially introduced mutations/defects are introduced in bacteria/yeast/mammalian cells to generate proteins, which are then studied to identify enzymatic or biochemical disruptions to gain information about possible causes of disease [16]. In cases where structural information of proteins is available, an in silico modeling approach could be used to predict the effects of mutations [17, 18].

Bioinformatics Methods for Sequence Analysis and Disease Information

Several approaches to analyze DNA sequence information are used in modern diagnostic laboratories. Initially, the gene sequences from patients are compared with standard sequences from databases and then specific properties are analyzed using special tools and databases to evaluate any changes that are observed in sequences from patients.

Basic Alignment Search Tool (BLAST)
The BLAST is the most powerful technique to analyze DNA or protein sequences by comparing a query sequence against whole databases (http://www.ncbi.nlm.nih.gov/blast). The BLAST can perform several different searches including nucleotide to nucleotide search (Blast N), protein to protein searches (Blast P) or searching a nucleotide entry against protein sequence databases (Blast X). After a sequence from patient DNA has been obtained, BLAST is the first tool that a researcher uses to compare that sequence against standard sequences. A specialized version of BLAST called 'align two sequences (bl2seq)' can be used to align patient DNA against standard sequences from databases (refseq) for both nucleotide or translated protein sequences to identify the differences.

Genetics and Disease Databases
Genetic, functional, clinical and structural information can be accessed freely from public databases in Europe (European Bioinformatics Institute (EBI), http://www.ebi.ac.uk), United States (National Center for Biotechnology Information (NCBI), http://www.ncbi.nlm.nih.gov) or National Institute of Genetics (NIG) in Japan (http://www.

Table 2. A list of bioinformatics tools and web resources for diagnosis and research on human genetic disorders

Resource name	Function	Address
NCBI	US central database	http://www.ncbi.nlm.nih.gov
EBI	European central database	http://www.ebi.ac.uk
UCSC Genome Browser	reference sequence of human	http://genome.ucsc.edu
OMIM	database of human genes and phenotypes	http://www.ncbi.nlm.nih.gov/omim/
BLAST	search/alignment of genes/proteins	http://www.ncbi.nlm.nih.gov/blast
LALIGN	precise two sequence alignment	http://ch.embnet.org/software/LALIGN_form.html
BioTools	restriction digestion of DNA	http://biotools.umassmed.edu/tacg4/
NEB Cutter	New England Biolabs DNA cutter	http://tools.neb.com/NEBcutter2/index.php
Sequence editor	sequence conversion	http://www.fr33.net/seqedit.php
Sequence massager	DNA sequence cleanup	http://www.attotron.com/cybertory/analysis/seqMassagerhtm
Primer3Plus	primer design tool	http://www.bioinformatics.nl/primer3plus
CLUSTALW	multiple sequence alignment	http://ebi.ac.uk/clustalw
UniProt	main portal for proteins	http://www.uniprot.org/
KEGG	pathway centric database	http://www.genome.jp/kegg/
SNP analysis	Affymetrix human SNP array	http://www.affymetrix.com

nig.ac.jp). These three databases are the main portals for all genetic sequence information and are synchronized every day to reflect the same information across all three repositories. Primary DNA sequences are submitted by individual researchers or sequencing projects and are assigned an accession number. These primary sequences are often redundant and contain several copies of same sequence submitted by different laboratories. Therefore, a separate Refseq project had been established to provide a reference sequence for each molecule in a nonredundant dataset that is verified, checked for accuracy and catalogued as reference sequences, where each gene or protein has only one entry. The refseq entries are distinguished from other entries by a distinct accession number scheme. The refseq entries follow a 2 + 6 numbering system, a two letter code indicating the type of reference sequence followed by an underscore and a six-digit number. Experimentally determined sequences have entries have NM_123456 for mRNA, NP_123456 for protein and NT_123456 for genomic DNA. Refsequence entries catalogued from genome sequencing efforts have the pattern XM_123456 for model mRNA and XP_123456 for model protein sequences. The refsequence entries contain additional information about the gene/protein like major publications, corresponding biological process, gene structure etc.

University of California Santa Cruz Genome Browser
The UCSC genome browser (http://genome.ucsc.edu) is probably the most useful site for complete genome assemblies and human genetic makeup informatics. The genome browsers can zoom and scroll over single chromosomes to locate and show individual genes with links to expression pattern, homology to other species and related genes. The BLAT tool (not to be confused with BLAST) provides precise information about gene structure and intron-exon boundaries by mapping a DNA sequence over genome.

OMIM
The Online Mendelian Inheritance in Man is a database of diseases and genes. It was initiated by Dr. Victor A. McKusick, and published in printed form for 12 editions and has later been adopted to online version. Every disease and gene is assigned a six-digit number with first digit being related to method of inheritance: 1 for autosomal dominant, 2 for autosomal recessive, 3 for X-linked phenotype, 4 for Y-linked phenotype, 5 for mitochondrial and 6 for autosomal phenotype catalogued after 1994 for both autosomal-dominant and autosomal-recessive phenotypes. An asterix represents an entry with known sequence, a number symbol (#) indicates a descriptive phenotype entry, a plus sign indicates a gene of known sequence and phenotype, a percentage (%) sign indicates that entry has a confirmed Mendelian phenotype where molecular basis of disease and gene are not known. The OMIM database can be searched using simple text based queries or from links to reseq entries for genes or proteins.

GeneReviews and Genetest
GeneReviews are expert-authored, peer-reviewed, current disease descriptions that apply genetic testing to the diagnosis, management, and genetic counseling of patients and families with specific inherited conditions. The reviews are authored and reviewed by known experts in diagnosis of specific diseases. The articles are peer reviewed and updated by the authors every 2–3 years. Significant changes to clinically relevant information are updated on a more frequent basis. GeneReviews can be searched by disease name, gene symbol, title or author names, etc. Reviews are linked

to related literature in PubMed. Genetests is a publicly funded resource created for cataloguing of medical genetics laboratories.

GeneCards and GeneLoc

GeneCards (http://www.genecards.org) is a searchable, integrated database of human genes that provides genetic and functional information on all known human genes. Information catalogued under a GeneCard includes gene name aliases, orthologies, disease relationships, mutations and SNPs, RNA expression data, gene function, pathways, protein, protein-protein interactions, related drugs and compounds and direct links to suppliers of research reagents and tools such as primers, antibodies, proteins, clones, expression assays and RNAi reagents. GeneLoc records DNA sequence, physical map positions and associated sequences.

Pathway Focused Databases

Genes involved in particular biochemical pathways can be viewed and researched at pathway focused databases. The major portal for such information is Kyoto Encyclopedia of Genes and Genomes (KEGG) (http://www.genome.ad.jp/kegg). A complete overview of biochemical processes and genes involved in individual steps could be obtained at KEGG database. Links from the subheadings in KEGG databases provide information gathered from other databases.

Indications for Performing Molecular Genetic Diagnosis in Pediatric Endocrinology

Our knowledge of genetic disorders responsible for hormonal/endocrine disorders is rapidly increasing. A comprehensive list of all possible indicators for analysis in pediatric endocrinology is hard to achieve and will be very long to include in any single publication. At present, many inherited genetic disorders seen in endocrinology have well-established molecular genetic analysis indications and molecular genetic analysis can provide risk analysis for the chances of inheriting the disorder and possibly its outcome in affected family members. Some of the commonly diagnosed disorders include various forms of pituitary hormone deficiency and congenital adrenal hyperplasia caused by defects in steroid metabolizing enzymes like CYP17A1 and CYP21A2. It is imperative that genetic analysis should be preceded by a proper clinical and biochemical laboratory diagnosis including hormonal values for all standard tests. Molecular genetic analysis can help and compliment the laboratory and clinical analysis and remove ambiguity when clinical and hormonal diagnosis could not resolve the cause of disorder. Especially in neonatal cases, conventional testing is often difficult to perform due to limitations on sample size and viability of other clinical procedures, but underling endocrine deficiencies would nevertheless be life threatening. In such cases, genetic analysis takes the form of emergency testing and a well-established laboratory following standard operating procedures is imperative to provide results in time.

Modern automated sequencers in combination with rapid DNA isolation and PCR based protocols can still take 2–3 days for providing the results of genetic analysis.

References

1   Goeddel DV, Heyneker HL, Hozumi T, Arentzen R, Itakura K, Yansura DG, Ross MJ, Miozzari G, Crea R, Seeburg PH: Direct expression in *Escherichia coli* of a DNA sequence coding for human growth hormone. Nature 1979;281:544.
2   Goeddel DV, Kleid DG, Bolivar F, Heyneker HL, Yansura DG, Crea R, Hirose T, Kraszewski A, Itakura K, Riggs AD: Expression in *Escherichia coli* of chemically synthesized genes for human insulin. Proc Natl Acad Sci USA 1979;76:106.
3   Itakura K, Hirose T, Crea R, Riggs AD, Heyneker HL, Bolivar F, Boyer HW: Expression in *Escherichia coli* of a chemically synthesized gene for the hormone somatostatin. Science 1977;198:1056.
4   Makowski GS, Davis EL, Aslanzadeh J, Hopfer SM: Enhanced direct amplification of Guthrie card DNA following selective elution of PCR inhibitors. Nucleic Acids Res 1995;23:3788.
5   Sambrook J, Russell DW: The Condensed Protocols from Molecular Cloning : A Laboratory Manual. Cold Spring Harbor, Cold Spring Harbor Laboratory Press, 2006.
6   Mullis KB, Faloona FA: Specific synthesis of DNA in vitro via a polymerase-catalyzed chain reaction. Methods Enzymol 1987;155:335.
7   Orita M, Iwahana H, Kanazawa H, Hayashi K, Sekiya T: Detection of polymorphisms of human DNA by gel electrophoresis as single-strand conformation polymorphisms. Proc Natl Acad Sci USA 1989;86:2766.
8   Balogh K, Patocs A, Majnik J, Racz K, Hunyady L: Genetic screening methods for the detection of mutations responsible for multiple endocrine neoplasia type 1. Mol Genet Metab 2004;83:74.
9   Fischer SG, Lerman LS: Length-independent separation of DNA restriction fragments in two-dimensional gel electrophoresis. Cell 1979;16:191.
10 Nollau P, Wagener C: Methods for detection of point mutations: performance and quality assessment. IFCC Scientific Division, Committee on Molecular Biology Techniques. Clin Chem 1997;43:1114.
11 Landegren U, Kaiser R, Sanders J, Hood L: A ligase-mediated gene detection technique. Science 1988; 241:1077.
12 Kalin I, Shephard S, Candrian U: Evaluation of the ligase chain reaction (LCR) for the detection of point mutations. Mutat Res 1992;283:119.
13 Konrad M, Schaller A, Seelow D, Pandey AV, Waldegger S, Lesslauer A, Vitzthum H, Suzuki Y, Luk JM, Becker C, Schlingmann KP, Schmid M, Rodriguez-Soriano J, Ariceta G, Cano F, Enriquez R, Juppner H, Bakkaloglu SA, Hediger MA, Gallati S, Neuhauss SC, Nurnberg P, Weber S: Mutations in the tight-junction gene claudin 19 (CLDN19) are associated with renal magnesium wasting, renal failure, and severe ocular involvement. Am J Hum Genet 2006;79:949.
14 Hoheisel JD: Microarray technology: beyond transcript profiling and genotype analysis. Nat Rev Genet 2006;7:200.
15 Abravaya K, Huff J, Marshall R, Merchant B, Mullen C, Schneider G, Robinson J: Molecular beacons as diagnostic tools: technology and applications. Clin Chem Lab Med 2003;41:468.
16 Flück CE, Tajima T, Pandey AV, Arlt W, Okuhara K, Verge CF, Jabs EW, Mendonca BB, Fujieda K, Miller WL: Mutant P450 oxidoreductase causes disordered steroidogenesis with and without Antley-Bixler syndrome. Nat Genet 2004;36:228.
17 Janner M, Pandey AV, Mullis PE, Flück CE: Clinical and biochemical description of a novel CYP21A2 gene mutation 962_963insA using a new 3D model for the P450c21 protein. Eur J Endocrinol 2006;155: 143.
18 Petkovic V, Godi M, Pandey AV, Lochmatter D, Buchanan CR, Dattani MT, Eble A, Flück CE, Mullis PE: Growth hormone (GH) deficiency type II: a novel GH-1 gene mutation (GH-R178H) affecting secretion and action. J Clin Endocrinol Metab 2010; 95:731–739.

Dr. Amit V. Pandey
Pediatric Endocrinology, Diabetology and Metabolism
Department of Clinical Research, University of Bern
Tiefenaustrasse 120c, CH–3004 Bern (Switzerland)
Tel. +41 31 308 8044, Fax +41 31 308 8028, E-Mail amit@pandeylab.org

Ranke MB, Mullis P-E (eds): Diagnostics of Endocrine Function in Children and Adolescents, ed 4.
Basel, Karger, 2011, pp 53–67

Sonographic Measurement of Endocrine Tissue

Hans P. Haber · Andreas Neu

Universitätsklinik für Kinder- und Jugendmedizin, Tübingen, Deutschland

Sonographic examination has become a standard technique in endocrinological diagnostics. The judgment of the structure and size of endocrine glands is part of daily clinical routine. With modern technical equipment, e.g. high-resolution scanners, computerized processing of the signal images of different organs has reached a very high standard. Standardized sections and an adequate pool of normal data make it possible to classify gland size as normal or pathological in relation to age or different body measurements.

Nevertheless, the use of sonography in endocrinological diagnostics is subject to some critical restrictions. Depending on their personal experience, examiners tend to use the most careful critical judgment in determining size in general and in interpreting measured data in particular. The choice of the right section, the precise differentiation of glands from surrounding tissue, and the correct position of the calipers are essential for successful examination. At the same time, these factors also represent a source of error. As this chapter shows, the choice of valid reference data can also be a cause of problems because of the variety of values available.

Examiners employing sonographic investigation agree that the measurement of different organs is helpful, first of all in establishing pathological deviations from the average range and, secondly, in providing further controls in monitoring the progress of a disease.

To achieve reliability in the determination of size, two conditions should be met:

1 The measurement should include sufficient documentation, i.e. the images must show how the measurements were obtained. In this way, examination results can be reproduced even if the sonographer changes.
2 Interpretation of the measurements should not be restricted to an uncritical consultation of tables of normal values. Rather, the relation of the gland under investigation to the surrounding organs and the overall impression should always be part of the evaluation and the basis for the examiner's assessment.

Thyroid Gland

General Considerations

Measuring the size of the thyroid gland is technically simple and needs no special preparation. The thyroid gland is easily found owing to its superficial location and is well marked with respect to surrounding structures. The examination requires little time. Measurements for purposes of documentation and the observation of clinical changes do not cause any problems and can be accomplished with normal technical equipment.

Technical Requirements

Usually, the examination is performed with a linear scanner and frequencies of 5–10 MHz. Scanners with high-resolution power are especially necessary in cases requiring an evaluation of internal structure. In such cases, changes of up to 0.5 mm can be seen. For examining newborns, special short scanners are employed, since otherwise it is not possible to bring the scanner into a longitudinal position because of the newborn infant's short neck.

Sonographic examination of the thyroid gland is performed with the patient in a supine position. It may be helpful to tip the head backward by means of a head or neck pillow. This causes the sternocleidomastoid muscle to move dorsally, thus allowing complete access to the lateral parts of the thyroid.

The presentation is carried out in both horizontal and longitudinal sections parallel to the axes of the organ (fig. 1). Documentation should also include the large neck vessels, which aid in pinpointing the anatomical location and facilitate reproduction.

For volumetry, both lobes are measured: the length, width, and the depth of each lobe are multiplied by a factor of 0.5 (fig. 2). The total volume represents the sum of both lobes [1] and is expressed in milliliters.

Evaluation: Normal Findings

Normally, the contour of the thyroid gland is smooth; both lobes form ellipsoids. The inner structure is finely granulated and homogeneous and shows medium echodensity. The thyroid gland of the newborn is of lower echodensity than that of older children. Frequently, one can observe an asymmetry of the two lobes, the right lobe being slightly larger [2].

The volume of the thyroid gland increases continuously from the neonatal age to adolescence; growth is insignificant in children older than 16 years [2, 3].

In childhood, there is no relevant difference between male and female probands with regard to the volume of the thyroid gland [1, 4]. However, for girls, a smaller increase in size during puberty has been described [2, 3].

The volume of the thyroid gland also correlates with age, body weight, height, body surface area, and pubertal stage [1–4]. It is noteworthy that different authors prefer different parameters: correlations with body surface area [2, 5] or height [1] are considered to be more precise than the other parameters. However, in normal clinical

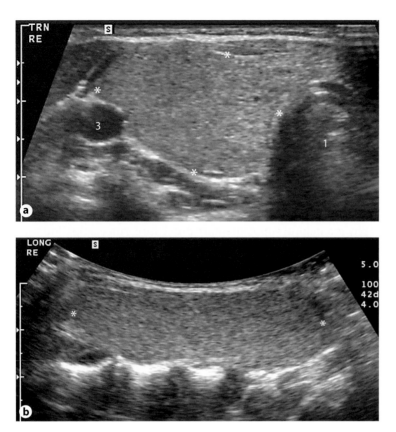

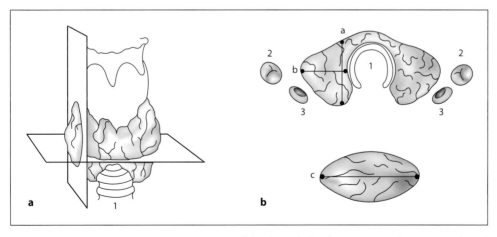

Fig. 1. Sonographic sections through thyroid gland (right lobe). **a** Transverse section. **b** Longitudinal section.

Fig. 2. a Anatomical planes used in volumetry of the thyroid gland (Maier 1984). **b** Sections *a*, *b*, and *c* of both lobes are multiplied according to the formula $a \times b \times c \times 0.5$ and the product is expressed in milliliters. 1 = Trachea; 2 = jugular vein; 3 = carotid artery.

practice, the correlation to age or weight [6] seems to provide adequate precision (fig. 3, 4). Some approximate data can provide a general guideline: the volume of the normal thyroid gland in neonates is 1 ml, in 4-year-old children 2 ml, and in children of school age 8 ml [7].

Diagnostic Values

There is no doubt that sonographic volumetry is to be preferred to volume determination by palpation [8, 9]. More often than not, thyroid volume is overestimated rather than underestimated when the palpation method is used [10]. Reproduction of sonographic volumetry is simple and leads to false results in only 12% of cases at most [8]. Especially in distinguishing between normal size and a slight enlargement of the thyroid gland, sonography is a helpful supplementary procedure, since palpation very often fails in this borderline range.

While volumetry of the thyroid gland appears to be simple, its interpretation proves to be deceptively difficult. The range of normal values is enormously wide and varies from author to author, with differences of more that 100%. One main reason for these divergences can be traced to the varying degrees of iodization in the different geographic areas covered by the available studies. Even in geographically comparable regions, however, the interpretation of what constitutes normality varies. A sensible approach would seem to be for examiners to establish standards for their own population and to let themselves be guided by these data.

Figure 4 shows the normal range of values for the volume of the thyroid gland in different age groups. The examination is based on the results for more than 200 children and adolescents.

Special Aspects

Normal data for children older than 5 years are available in a large number of studies [2–4, 9], but there is a lack of data for younger children, especially for infants and newborns [11]. The examination of this age group requires some technical skill and should therefore be carried out by an experienced sonographer.

External influences on thyroid volume, such as menstrual cycle and seasonal variations have been described, but are irrelevant for normal clinical practice.

Uterus

General Considerations

Sonographic examination of the female genital organs has become a standard technique and is a useful tool in endocrinological diagnostics when carried out with sufficient experience and preparation. Though preparations are simple, they should not be neglected, since the diagnostic value of the examination depends largely on these measures.

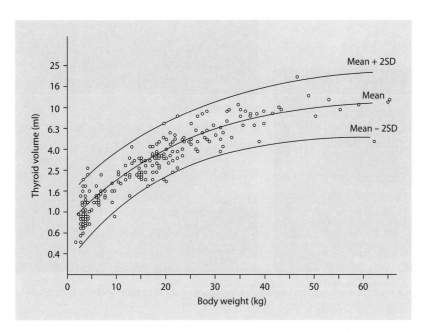

Fig. 3. Normal ranges for thyroid volume (sum of the right and the left thyroid lobe volumes) in relation to body weight (author's data; n = 204). Ranges are expressed as mean ± 2 SD (calculated after logarithmic transformation).

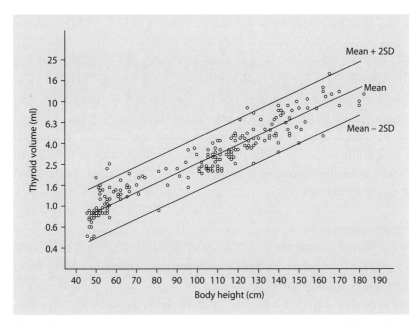

Fig. 4. Normal ranges for thyroid volume (sum of the right and the left thyroid lobe volumes) in relation to body height (author's data; n = 204). Ranges are expressed as mean ± 2 SD (calculated after logarithmic transformation).

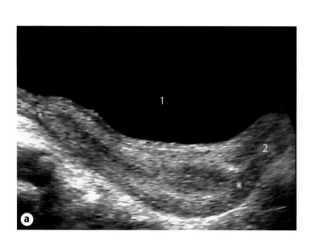
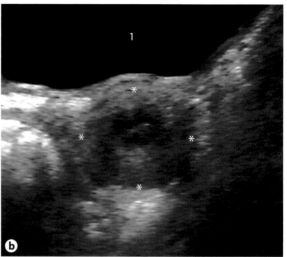

Fig. 5. Sonographic sections through the uterus (marked by*). **a** Longitudinal section. **b** Transverse section.

Technical Requirements

Examination of the uterus can be done with either a sector scanner or a linear scanner. In general, the best presentation is gained by using a 3.5- to 5-MHz sector scanner.

The most important preliminary to the examination is making sure that the patient's bladder is full. In general, the fuller the bladder, the better the image. Therefore, it is advisable to invest enough time in waiting until the bladder is full, rather than performing the examination when the bladder is not full enough.

The examination is performed in a supine position. Two sections, the transversal section and the longitudinal section through the corresponding axes of the uterus, are necessary to determine the volume of the organ (fig. 5). The volume is calculated according to the ellipsoid formula (fig. 6).

Evaluation: Normal Findings

The shape of the uterus varies depending on the age of the child. During the neonatal period and infancy, it is drop shaped. By the age of 8 years, it acquires a tubular form and reaches the typical pear shape during puberty [12].

The relation of cervix to corpus is 2:1 in the prepubertal stage and 1:2 postpubertally [see 12, 25]. The typical angle between the uterine corpus and the cervix can be seen only after puberty.

The transversal section always shows an oval form, which sometimes presses against the bottom of the bladder. Very often, the longitudinal axis is tilted slightly to the left of the medial axis of the body.

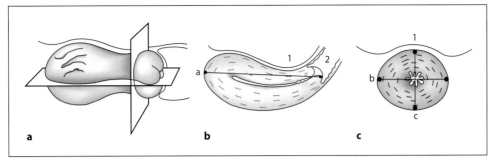

Fig. 6. Sections used to determine volume V (in ml) of the uterus according to the formula V = a × b × c × 0.5. **a** Anatomical planes. **b** Longitudinal section. **c** Transverse section. 1 = Urinary bladder; 2 = vagina.

Table 1. Uterine and ovarian volume (mean (SD)) in relation to Tanner score (breast stage) (author's data; n = 178)

Tanner score	Uterine volume, ml	Ovarian volume, ml
B1	1.0 (0.3)	0.7 (0.4)
B2	2.3 (0.6)	1.6 (0.9)
B3	10.3 (6.1)	3.5 (1.8)
B4–5	24.6 (14.4)	7.4 (4.8)

The contour of the organ is smooth and the structure fine, with low echodensity. After puberty, a zone of higher echodensity in the centre that represents the mucosa is apparent and is clearly seen, especially premenstrually.

Uterine length and uterine volume are significantly correlated to both age and pubertal stage [13–16] (table 1).

To determine the size of the uterus, length and volume are also taken into account. During infancy [12] and early childhood, a small decrease in size can be seen, whereas in later childhood a continuous, slow increase in length and volume is found up to puberty [15, 17]. Around the age of 10 years, both length and volume start to increase steeply, until they reach adult dimensions at about the age of 16 years [18].

With increasing age, the range for standard values broadens. The variations in normal values have been confirmed by several authors [12, 18]. One main reason for these variations is the fact that there is no clearly defined level at which the horizontal section should be positioned. Therefore, volume and length can generally be used as well. In practice, length is considered to be the more reliable parameter, especially in older girls. Usually, uterine length and volume are related to age or to Tanner classification [14, 18]. It is helpful to use diagrams that show mean values as well as standard deviations (fig. 7, 8).

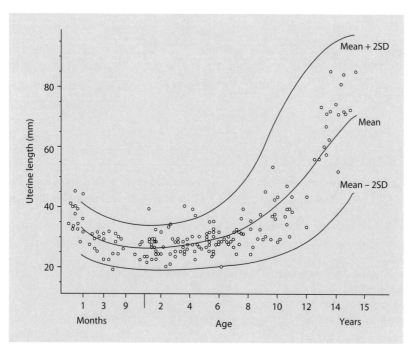

Fig. 7. Normal values for uterine length (in mm) in relation to age (author's data; n = 178). Ranges are expressed as mean ± 2 SD (calculated after logarithmic transformation).

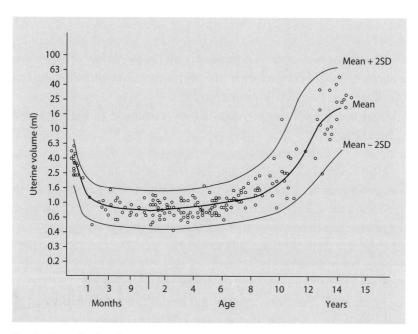

Fig. 8. Normal values for uterine volume (in ml) in relation to age (author's data; n = 178). Ranges are expressed as mean ± 2 SD (calculated after logarithmic transformation).

Haber · Neu

Doppler evaluation of the uterine artery is a useful complementary parameter to follow puberty, although it requires experienced hands. In prepubertal girls, the Doppler spectral pattern shows absent blood flow during diastole. At the end of puberty, there is a broad systolic flow waves with continuous flow signal during diastole [19].

Diagnostic Value
Ultrasound imaging of uterus and ovaries is a convenient, noninvasive diagnostic tool for various forms of endocrine abnormalities, such as premature thelarche and pubarche, precocious puberty, pubertal delay, isolated vaginal bleeding, or hirsutism [20, 21]. Ultrasonographic measurement of uterine size offers a reliable means of distinguishing between isolated premature thelarche and early stages of central precocious puberty [20, 22, 23]. The mean uterine volume is significantly greater in children with precocious puberty than in controls. In contrast, no significant differences are found between children with premature thelarche and the control group [22].

Special Aspects
Transvaginal sonography is assuming increasing importance in gynecological practice. The advantage of this method of examination is that the examiner does not have to wait for the bladder to be full. In general, however, this technique is not necessary in order to determine genital size in girls and should be used for special investigations only.

Ovaries

General Considerations
Much more than ultrasound examination of the uterus, sonographic imaging of the ovaries can cause problems for the sonographer. The position of the ovaries varies, and it is not easy to distinguish the ovaries from surrounding structures. Therefore high-resolution equipment is necessary to identify the ovaries in a child. After menarche, the identification of the organ is much easier because of the growing number of follicular cysts.

Despite these difficulties, sonography of both the ovaries and the uterus has become a standard technique in endocrinological diagnostics for children and adolescents.

Technical Requirements
The scanners used for the ovaries are the same as for examination of the uterus.

To locate the ovaries, a full urinary bladder is of even more importance than in the examination of the uterus. Otherwise, air-containing intestines located between the ovaries and the scanner make access to the organ impossible. If difficulties in finding the ovaries are encountered, it may be helpful to use the uterine body as the guiding

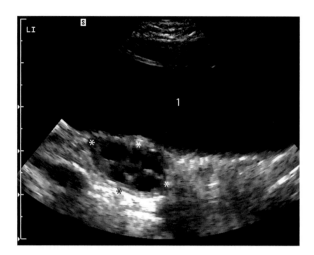

Fig. 9. Longitudinal section through the ovary (marked by *).

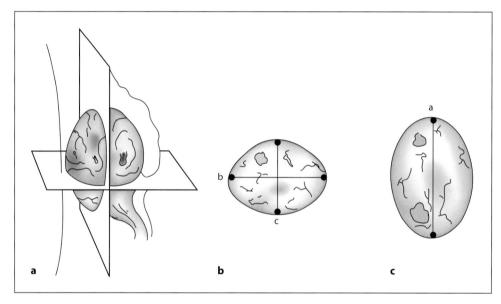

Fig. 10. Sections used to determine volume V (in ml) of the ovaries according to the formula $V = a \times b \times c \times 0.5$. **a** Anatomical planes. **b** Transverse sections b and c. **c** Longitudinal section a.

structure. From the longitudinal axis of the uterus, the scanner is tilted laterally until the ovary appears on the screen. Sometimes, it is also advisable to locate the ovary from the contralateral side by pointing the scanner diagonally through the bladder. The standard sections are transversal and longitudinal parallel to the axes of the organ (fig. 9). Whatever access is chosen, the patient must be supine.

Ovarian volume is calculated from the measurements of the ovary's three dimensions (fig. 10).

Haber · Neu

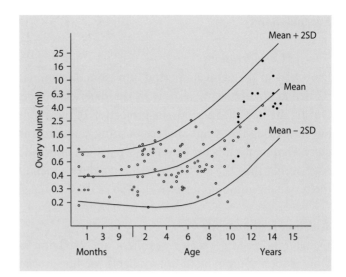

Fig. 11. Normal values for ovary volume (mean value of the right and the left ovarian volumes) in relation to age (author's data; n = 94). Ranges are expressed as mean ± 2 SD (calculated after logarithmic transformation).

Evaluation: Normal Findings

The shape of the ovary is oval with a smooth contour and an inhomogeneous structure. The echodensity is low and frequently small cysts can be seen. Ovarian follicles can be detected from the age of early infancy onward. They increase progressively in size and number after the age of 8.5 years [23]. Three to four small cysts (average diameter, 5 mm) can be considered normal at any age.

Ovarian volume is relatively stable in early childhood [24] and shows only little increase before puberty [13, 16, 25]. Because of this relative stability, it is correct to define all ovaries smaller than 1 ml in volume as prepubertal.

During puberty, a steep increase in volume occurs [15], and ovarian growth continues even after menarche [26]. The average volume of the ovaries in a young adult is approximately 6.5 ml [18].

Ovarian maturation is influenced by age only [15, 17]. The two ovaries show no difference in their internal structure, nor is there any relation to weight or menstrual cycle phase [27]. There is a positive correlation between Tanner score and ovarian volume [18] (table 1). Normal values related to age are shown in figure 11.

Diagnostic Value

Together with uterine size, ovarian volume is a reliable indicator of the degree of development in girls [21, 25], despite the technical difficulties mentioned above. The experience of the examiner seems to be more important for this examination than for other ultrasound examinations.

Special Aspects

The remarks on transvaginal ultrasound made with respect to examination of the uterus also apply to sonographic examination of the ovaries.

Adrenal Gland

General Considerations

Especially in the neonatal period, ultrasound examination of the adrenal gland is of particular interest with respect to the diagnosis of congenital adrenal hyperplasia. During the neonatal period, the projection of the adrenal gland is technically simple, but measuring the gland and establishing standard values for size cause some difficulty. Frequently, it is the examiner's personal impression, i.e. his or her prior experience, rather than the actually measured values which forms the basis for interpreting the results in sonographic examination of the adrenal gland.

Technical Requirements

Usually, 5–7.5 MHz sector scanners are used for examining the adrenal gland. Only if such equipment is not available are linear scanners of the same frequencies employed.

Longitudinal and transversal sections are carried out with the scanner in the axillary line. During the procedure, the patient is in a supine position or is turned slightly to the right or the left side. Sometimes, positioning the sector scanner medially in the epigastric region can result in better projection. However, even an experienced sonographer with good equipment does not always succeed in attaining adequate demonstration. Owing to anatomical conditions, an approach from the left side poses problems in adolescents and adults more often than one from the right side [28].

To determine size, different parameters were tested [29], including transverse and anteroposterior diameters, circumference and area in the transversal plane, and longitudinal length. All these parameters seems to reflect in some way the size of the adrenal gland. For practical purposes, the distance between the cranial pole of the gland and the upper renal pole, which is referred to as 'longitudinal length' or 'thickness,' can be regarded as the easiest to determine as well as the most reproducible [30] (fig. 12).

Documentation of the method used to determine size is more necessary for the adrenal gland than for other organs. The projection should include the upper renal pole and the liver or spleen.

Evaluation: Normal Findings

Generally, the adrenal gland rests on the upper renal pole like an inverted cup. The shape of the organ shows great variety and in most cases is either crescent shaped or resembles a reclining 'Y' (fig. 12).

The younger the child, the more clearly the medulla can be distinguished from the cortex. The projection of the medulla is like a small bench. The medulla has a high echodensity, while the cortex has a fine structure with very low echodensity.

Owing to the involution of the fetal zone, an early decrease in adrenal size is observed [31]. During the first 36 h of life, the average length is about 12.5 mm in

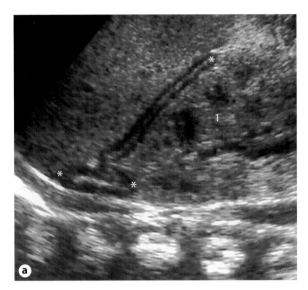 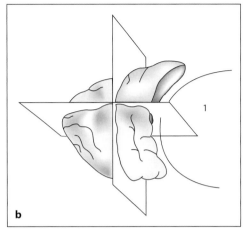

Fig. 12. a Longitudinal section through the adrenal gland (marked by *). **b** Anatomical planes of the adrenal gland. 1 = Kidney.

newborns, which is not much smaller than in adults [30]. As a result of physiological shrinking, the gland diminishes to a length of 4–6 mm within the first 3–5 days [32]. Further shrinking occurs during the first weeks. The size of the organ decreases by 40% within 6 weeks [29]. For this reason and also because of the increase in subcutaneous fat, projection is difficult even in infancy.

Diagnostic Value

Ultrasonographic determination of the size of the adrenal gland should be considered critically. Clinically, it can be useful in particular during the neonatal period. A positive relation between adrenal steroid levels and size of the gland has been proven for this period of life [33].

Usually, pathologically enlarged glands can be discovered by the experienced examiner. Enlarged, lobulated adrenals with abnormal echogenicity are found in children with congenital adrenal hyperplasia (CAH) due to 21-hydroxylase deficiency [34]. Mean length measurements of 20 mm or greater and mean width measurements of 4 mm or greater suggest the diagnosis of neonatal CAH [35]. However, one should not rely solely on ultrasound diagnostics: normal size does not exclude a diagnosis of CAH [35].

References

1 Ueda D: Sonographic measurement of the volume of the thyroid gland in healthy children. Acta Paediatr Jpn Overseas Ed 1989;31:352.

2 Mueller-Leisse C, Troeger J, Khabirpour F, Poeckler C: Schilddrüsenvolumen-Normwerte: Sonographische Messungen an 7- bis 20jährigen Schülern. Dtsch Med Wochenschr 1988;113:1872.

3 Kaloumenou I, Alevizaki M, Ladapoulos C, Antoniou A, Duntas LH, Mastorakos G, Chiotis D, Mengreli C, Livadis S, Xekouki P, Dacou-Voutetakis C: Thyroid volume and echostructure in schoolchildren living in a iodine-replete area: relation to age, pubertal stage, and body mass index. Thyroid 2007; 17:875.

4 Ivarsson SA, Persson PH, Ericsson UB: Thyroid gland volume as measured by ultrasonography in healthy children and adolescents in a non-iodine deficient area. Acta Paediatr Scand 1989;78:633.

5 Svensson J, Nilsson PE, Olsson C, Nilsson JA, Lindberg B, Ivarsson SA: Interpretation of normative thyroid volumes in children and adolescents: is there a need for a multivariate model? Thyroid 2004; 14:536.

6 Tajtakova M, Hancinova D, Tajtak J, Malinovsky E, Varga J, Langer P: Goiter prevalence and thyroid volume by ultrasonographic volumetry in two groups of school children and adolescents from east Slovakia. Endocrinol Exp 1989;23:85.

7 Klingmüller V, Fiedler C, Otten A: Besonderheiten der Schilddrüsensonographie im Säuglings- und Kindesalter. Radiologe 1992;32:320.

8 Igl W, Lukas P, Leisner B, Fink U, Seiderer M, Pickardt CR, Lissner J: Sonographische Volumenbestimmung der Schilddrüse: Vergleich mit anderen Methoden. Nuklearmedizin 1981;20:64.

9 Gutekunst R, Smolarek H, Hasenpusch U, Stubbe P, Friedrich HJ, Wood WG, Scriba PC: Goitre epidemiology; thyroid volume, iodine excretion, thyroglobulin and thyrotropin in Germany and Sweden. Acta Endocrinol (Copenh) 1986;112:494.

10 Skvor J: Palpacni a sonograficke hodnoceni velikosti stitne zlazy. Cesk Pediatr 1993;48:415.

11 Perry RJ, Hollman AS, Wood AM, Donaldson MD: Ultrasound of the thyroid gland in the newborn: normative data. Arch Dis Child Fetal Neonatal Ed. 2002;87:F209–F211.

12 Bundscherer F, Deeg KH: Die sonographische Beurteilung der Uterusentwicklung im Kindesalter. Monatsschr Kinderheilkd 1988;136:246.

13 Haber HP, Mayer EI: Ultrasound evaluation of uterine and ovarian size from birth to puberty. Pediatr Radiol 1994;24:11.

14 Orbak Z, Sagsöz N, Alp H, Tan H, Yildirim H, Kaya D: Pelvic ultrasound measurements in normal children: relation to puberty and sex hormone concentration. J Pediatr Endocrinol Metab 1998;11:525.

15 Herter LD, Golendziner E, Flores JA, Becker E Jr, Spritzer PM: Ovarian and uterine sonography in healthy girls between 1 and 13 years old: correlation of findings with age and pubertal status. Am J Roentgenol 2002;178:1531.

16 Badouraki M, Christoforidis A, Economou I, Dimitriadis AS, Katzos G: Sonographic assessment of uterine and ovarian development in normal girls aged 1 to 12 years. J Clin Ultrasound 2008;36:539.

17 Salardi S, Orsini LF, Cacciari E, Bovicelli L, Tassoni P, Reggiani A: Pelvic ultrasonography in premenarcheal girls: relation to puberty and sex hormone concentrations. Arch Dis Child 1985;60:120.

18 Ivarsson SA, Nilsson KO, Persson PH: Ultrasonography of the pelvic organs in prepubertal and postpubertal girls. Arch Dis Child 1983;58:352.

19 Ziereisen F, Heinrichs C, Dufour D, Saerens M, Avni EF: The role of Doppler evaluation of the uterine artery in girls around puberty. Pediatr Radiol 2001;31:712.

20 Griffin IJ, Cole TJ, Duncan KA, Hollmann AS, Donaldson MDC: Pelvic ultrasound measurements in normal children. Acta Paediatr 1995;84:536.

21 Garel L, Dubois J, Grignon A, Filiatrault D, Van Vliet G: US of the pediatric female pelvis: a clinical perspective. Radiographics 2001;21:1393.

22 Haber HP, Wollmann HA, Ranke MB: Pelvic ultrasonography: early differentiation between isolated premature thelarche and central precocious puberty. Eur J Pediatr 1995;154:182.

23 Herter LD, Golendziner E, Flores JA, Moretto M, Di Domencino K, Becker E Jr, Spritzer PM: Ovarian and uterine findings in pelvic sonography: comparison between prepubertal girls, girls with isolated thelarche, and girls with central precocious puberty. J Ultrasound Med 2002;21:1237.

24 Stanhope R, Adams J, Jacobs HS, Brook CG: Ovarian ultrasound assessment in normal children, idiopathic precocious puberty, and during low dose pulsatile gonadotrophin-releasing hormone treatment and hypogonadotrophic hypogonadism. Arch Dis Child 1985;60:116.

25 Orsini LF, Salardi S, Pilu G, Bovicelli L, Cacciari E: Pelvic organs in premenarcheal girls; real-time ultrasonography. Radiology 1984;153:113.

26 Deutlinger J, Bernaschek G: Normgrössen des inneren Genitales bei Mädchen vor und nach der Menarche. Wien Klin Wochenschr 1986;98:465.

27 Cohen HL, Tice HM, Mandel FS: Ovarian volumes measured by US: bigger than we think. Radiology 1990;177:189.

28 Yamakita N, Yasadu K, Miura K: Delineation of adrenal in controls and non-tumorous adrenal disorders by real-time ultrasonic scanner. Ultrasound Med Biol 1986;12:107.

29 Scott EM, Thomas A, McGarrigle HH, Lachelin GC: Serial adrenal ultrasonography in normal neonates. J Ultrasound Med 1990;9:279.

30 Leidig E: Sonographie der Nebennieren-Erkrankungen des Neugeborenen. Ultraschall 1988;9:155.

31 Hauffa BP, Menzel D, Stolecke H: Age-related changes in adrenal size during the first year of life in normal newborns, infants and patients with congenital adrenal hyperplasia due to 21-hydroxylase deficiency: comparison of ultrasound and hormonal parameters. Eur J Pediatr 1988;148:43.

32 Grunert D, Leidig E (eds): Pädiatrische Ultraschalldiagnostik. Workbook, Elementary and Intermediate Levels. Tübingen, 1989.

33 Matsumura I, Hashino M, Maruyama S, Yanaihara T, Nakayama T: Relation between size of fetal and neonatal adrenal glands and steroid levels in maternal and neonatal serum. Nippon Sanka Fujinka Gakkai Zasshi 1987;39:2125.

34 Al-Alwan I, Navarro O, Daneman D, Daneman A: Clinical utility of adrenal ultrasonography in the diagnosis of congenital adrenal hyperplasia. J Pediatr 1999;135:71.

35 Sivit CJ, Hung W, Taylor GA, Catena LM, Brown-Jones C, Kushner DC: Sonography in neonatal congenital adrenal hyperplasia. Am J Roentgenol 1991;156:141.

Prof. Dr. Hans P. Haber
Universitätsklinik für Kinder- und Jugendmedizin
Hoppe-Seyler-Strasse 1
DE–72076 Tübingen (Germany)
Tel. +49 7071 298 3781, Fax +49 7071 295 328, E-Mail peter.haber@med.uni-tuebingen.de

Ranke MB, Mullis P-E (eds): Diagnostics of Endocrine Function in Children and Adolescents, ed 4.
Basel, Karger, 2011, pp 68–84

In vivo Diagnostic Methods of Imaging and Testing of Endocrine Function with Radionuclides

Christoph Reiners · Jamshid Farahati · Michael Lassmann

Department of Nuclear Medicine, University of Würzburg, Würzburg, Germany

Radionuclides may be applied to image different organs and to test their functions. Historically, radioactive isotopes of iodine were initially used for the diagnosis of thyroid diseases. Today, different radionuclides are available for scintigraphy and testing of thyroid function as well as of other endocrine glands such as the parathyroids or adrenals. Clinically most relevant in children and adolescents are scintigraphy of the thyroid, of the parathyroids and of pheochromocytoma.

Thyroid

Pathophysiologic Background

The thyroid develops during organogenesis from the entoderma of the pharyngeal pouch. Its descent along the thyroglossal duct is normally completed during the 7th week of gestation, and its final position is anterior to the second or third tracheal cartilage [Pintar et al., 1991]. Frequently, a remnant of the thyroglossal duct in the form of a pyramidal lobe pointing cranially from the isthmus of the left lobe may be found. Descent disorders may result in dystopia of the thyroid; possible locations of thyroidal tissue are shown in figure 1.

Histologically, the thyroid gland consists of follicles approximately 25–50 µm in diameter containing colloid, which is produced by the epithelial cells of the follicles. Blood vessels, lymphatic ducts, and parafollicular C cells are located between the follicles.

Normal functioning of the thyroid depends on an adequate nutritional supply of iodide. The synthesis of thyroid hormones begins after the 12th week of gestation

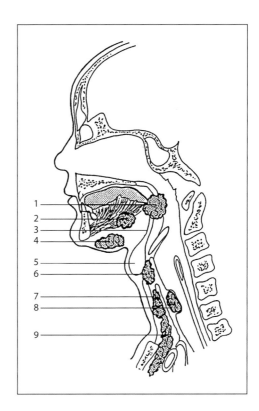

Fig. 1. Normal and dystopic locations of thyroid tissue. 1 = Base of the tongue; 2 = intralingual; 3 = thyroglossal duct; 4 = sublingual; 5 = thyroglossal cyst; 6 = prelaryngeal; 7 = normal; 8 = intratracheal; 9 = substernal [Reiners, 1994].

[Pintar et al., 1991]. In childhood, the thyroid requires from 50 µg iodide daily in newborns to 100 µg in children 1–3 years of age and 150 µg in children 7–9 years of age. In puberty, as in adulthood, 200 µg iodide daily are needed [Arbeitskreis Jodmangel, 2008].

Iodide, which is ingested with nutrition, is nearly completely resorbed in the intestines. The metabolism of iodine in the thyroid includes several steps [Taurog, 1991]. First, the sodium-iodide symporter (NIS) of the epithelial cell [Dadachova et al., 2004] actively takes up iodide from the blood stream against a concentration gradient in a process known as 'trapping.' Monovalent anions of similar volume (approximately 4 $\times 10^{-23}$ cm^3) such as perchlorate or pertechnetate may compete with the iodide anion during trapping. Inside the follicular epithelial cells, iodide is quickly oxidized to elementary iodine (iodination). Iodine is then incorporated into tyrosyl remnants of thyroglobulin (iodization). Iodine-containing thyroglobulin is secreted into the follicular lumen, where synthesis of the thyroid hormones tetraiodothyronine (T_4) and triiodothyronine (T_3) from their precursors monoiodotyrosine and diiodotyrosine takes place. These reactions are catalyzed by peroxidase.

Under the influence of thyroid-stimulating hormone (TSH) secreted by the pituitary, the thyroid hormones T_4 and T_3 are taken up again from the follicular colloid into the follicular epithelial cells and secreted into the bloodstream. The metabolism of iodine in the thyroid is additionally influenced by TSH-independent autoregulation [Nagataki, 1991], which guarantees the normal production of thyroid hormones in spite of variations in iodine intake ranging from micrograms to milligrams. High doses of iodine (more than ten milligrams) may lead to a blockade of iodine uptake and hormone synthesis and secretion. Small children are quite vulnerable to this effect, so that iodine overload may lead to hypothyroidism.

Scintigraphy in the Diagnosis of Thyroid Disorders

Radiopharmaceuticals
Today, technetium-99m (^{99m}Tc, physical half-life 6.0 h) is generally used for scintigraphy because of its optimal radiation quality and its general availability. [99m]Tc in the form of pertechnetate is trapped by the thyroid gland in the same manner as iodide. However, unlike radioiodine, ^{99m}Tc pertechnetate is not subsequently organified. After trapping, pertechnetate is released from the thyroid and may be displaced by perchlorate.

Normally, scintigraphy is performed between 20 and 30 min after intravenous injection of a tracer activity of ^{99m}Tc pertechnetate. Because of the relatively high blood background of ^{99m}Tc pertechnetate, its uptake into the salivary glands and its excretion with saliva, the interpretation of ^{99m}Tc scans may sometimes pose difficulties, especially in the case of gland dystopia. However, a gustatory stimulus using lemon juice and rinsing of the mouth with water may wash out salivary activity, so that uptake in ectopic tissue may be proven even with ^{99m}Tc pertechnetate (fig. 2).

Despite its sometimes restricted availability and higher cost, iodine-123 (^{123}I, physical half-life 13.2 h) may be preferred for thyroid imaging in children, especially if ectopic tissue has to be localized. Scanning after a tracer activity of ^{123}I sodium iodide is usually performed between 4 and 6 h after injection. At that time, the ratio of organ to background activity is ten times higher with ^{123}I than with ^{99m}Tc pertechnetate, owing to the organification of iodine.

The appropriate activity to be administered in children based on body weight according to the recent recommendations of the European Association for Nuclear Medicine are calculated according to the tables given by Lassmann et al. [2007]. Selected weight-dependent activities and the corresponding thyroid-absorbed doses are listed in table 1. The effective dose for an administration of 80 MBq ^{99m}Tc pertechnetate is 1 mSv and for 20 MBq of [123]I 4.4 mSv. [131]I was at one time used for thyroid scanning. However, today it should no longer be employed for routine imaging because of its very high radiation dose to the thyroid gland. The only indication for scintigraphy with ^{131}I in children is whole-body scanning after radioiodine therapy and follow-up of thyroid cancer. Usually, whole-body scans are performed 2–3 days after the administration of the diagnostic or therapeutic activity.

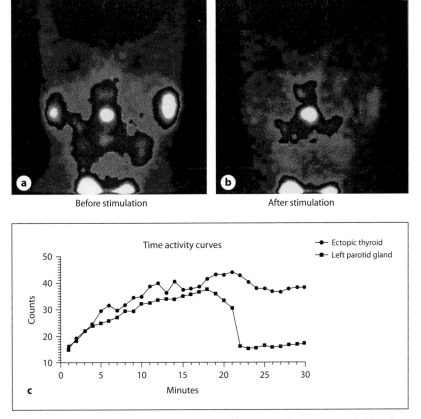

Before stimulation   After stimulation

Fig. 2. a–c Gamma camera scintigrams with ^{99m}Tc pertechnetate in a child with ectopic thyroid tissue at the base of the tongue. **a** Visualization of ectopic thyroid tissue and activity in the salivary glands. **b** Flushing of salivary gland activity after oral administration of lemon juice permits clearer visualization of ectopic thyroid. **c** Time activity curves of thyroid (upper curve) and the salivary glands (lower curve); there is remarkable displacement of activity from the salivary gland by lemon juice after 20 min.

Indications

The indications for thyroid scintigraphy in childhood include [Clerc et al., 2008]:

1 Differential diagnosis of neck masses.
2 Localization of ectopic thyroid tissue.
3 Differential diagnosis of hypothyroidism.
4 Differentiation of organification defects.

Figure 3 summarizes the methods and procedures to be used in the differential diagnosis of thyroid conditions (see also the diagnostic algorithms in 'Appendix B, charts 1, 2').

Generally, thyroid scintigraphy is not indicated in children with diffuse goiter. Only if there are lesions detected by sonography scintigraphy is indicated as an additional

Table 1. Activities to be administered and thyroid absorbed doses in thyroid scintigraphy for typical activities of ^{99m}Tc and ^{123}I, according to weight; the absorbed dose is calculated for an iodine uptake of 35% [International Commission on Radiological Protection 1988, 1998; Lassmann et al., 2007]

	Weight	^{99m}Tc ($T_{1/2}$ 6 h)	^{123}I ($T_{1/2}$ 13.2 h)
Recommended activity	3 kg	10 MBq	3 MBq
	10 kg	15 MBq	3 MBq
	20 kg	27 MBq	5 MBq
	55 kg	65 MBq	15 MBq
	adults	80 MBq	20 MBq
Thyroid absorbed dose	3 kg	2.2 mGy	129 mGy
	10 kg	1.8 mGy	69 mGy
	20 kg	1.5 mGy	55 mGy
	55 kg	1.8 mGy	105 mGy
	adults	1.7 mGy	90 mGy

diagnostic examination. Malignant lesions, which may occur even in childhood with an incidence of 0.5 in 100,000 children, typically present with low echogenicity in ultrasound examinations. If the correlation of such a lesion in scintigraphy is a cold node, fine-needle biopsy is indicated, which has been proven to be a safe, sensitive and specific technique for detection of thyroid malignancies in children [Corrias et al., 2001].

A study by Paltiel et al. [1992] investigated the most frequent diagnoses in a group of 246 children scanned with ^{123}I sodium iodide; these are summarized in table 2. In this series, 88% of the patients evaluated for neck masses clinically believed to be extrathyroidal had a normal thyroid as confirmed by scintigraphy. In these cases, the neck mass could be removed with no negative impact on the thyroid hormone status. In 9% of the cases, the mass proved to be an ectopic thyroid. In 23% of the 31 children presenting with a solitary thyroid nodule, thyroid cancer was found after surgery. The relative frequency of solitary thyroid nodules due to malignant disease in children depends on the nutritional iodine supply; in iodine-deficient regions such as Germany with a high frequency of benign nodules, the prevalence of malignant lesions will be lower. Nevertheless, a solitary thyroid nodule has to be taken seriously in a child. If there is no indication for removing it immediately by surgery, it must be followed up closely by ultrasonography.

About 80% of children with thyroid carcinoma present with lymph node metastases and 10–15% with pulmonary metastases at postoperative staging [Paltiel et al.,

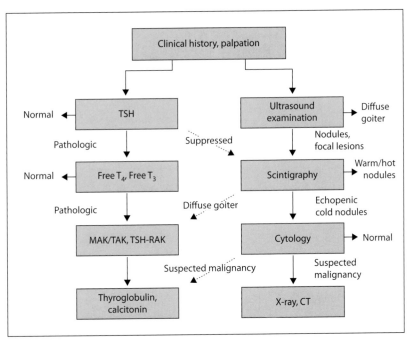

Fig. 3. Methods and procedures employed in the differential diagnosis of thyroid conditions. TSH = Thyroid-stimulating hormone; TRH = thyroid-releasing hormone; T_4 = tetraiodothyronine; T_3 = triiodothyronine; MAK = thyroid microsomal antigen autoantibodies; TAK = thyroglobulin autoantibodies; TSH-RAK = thyroid-stimulating hormone receptor autoantibodies; CT = computerized tomography. Modified from Reiners [1990].

1994]. Postoperative ^{131}I whole-body scanning is mandatory in cases of differentiated thyroid cancer.

Hypothyroidism in children may be caused by anatomical defects, functional disorders, or iodine deficiency [Clerc et al., 2008]. Anatomical defects include athyrosis and ectopic thyroid tissue. In some cases, a normal gland may be present together with thyroid gland dystopia, or there may be dystopia alone without a thyroid in the normal location. It is therefore important to know before surgery whether a mass at the base of the tongue represents all of the thyroid tissue detected in the patient or whether there is in addition a normal thyroid in the neck.

Functional abnormalities of the thyroid in children include inborn errors of thyroid hormonogenesis and peripheral hormone resistance, as well as a lack of TSH. Functional abnormalities in the newborn which have been acquired during fetal life may be due to iodine deficiency or iodine overload and goitrogenic substances, as well as diaplacental transfer of antibodies in Graves' disease of the mother.

Clerc et al. [2008] reviewed the literature with respect to the etiology of congenital hypothyroidism. In totally 1,489 cases, 43.2% presented with ectopic and 25.5% with eutopic glands; the remaining 31.2% suffered from athyrosis.

Table 2. Most frequent diagnoses of thyroid disorders in a group of 246 children scanned with ^{123}I sodium iodide

Diagnosis	%
Extrathyroidal masses	18
Thyroglossal duct cysts	16
Ectopic thyroid tissue	12
Hashimoto thyroiditis	8
Benign thyroid nodules	7
Normal thyroid	6
Benign diffuse goiter	5
Thyroid malignancy	4
Transient hypothyroidism	4
Hypothyroidism of unknown etiology	4
Athyrosis	3
Postradiation hypothyroidism	3
Graves' disease	3
Miscellaneous	7

Data from Paltiel et al. [1992].

Table 3. Withdrawal of thyroid-specific medication prior to thyroid scintigraphy

Medication	Withdrawal time prior to scintigraphy
Iodide	4–6 weeks
Levothyroxine	4–6 weeks
Liothyronine	10–14 days
Perchlorate	1–2 days
Lithium	1–2 days
Thiamazol	2–4 days
Carbimazol	2–4 days

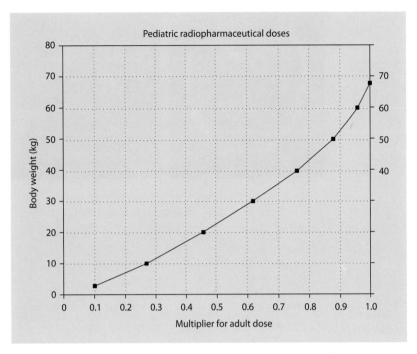

Fig. 4. Reduction scheme for perchlorate according to Piepsz et al. [1990].

Preparation of the Patient

Usually, the patient does not need to be prepared for thyroid scintigraphy with ^{99m}Tc pertechnetate or ^{123}I iodide. However, depending on the substance, thyroid-specific medication should be withdrawn for the intervals shown in table 3.

Particularly in the case of the follow-up of thyroid cancer with ^{131}I whole-body scanning [Franzius et al., 2007], suppressive treatment with thyroid hormones must be stopped for a period long enough to induce endogenous TSH stimulation (usually 4 weeks off T_4 and at least 2 weeks off T_3).

Alternatively, rhTSH may be used to stimulate ^{131}I uptake exogenously without withdrawal of thyroid hormone medication [Luster et al., 2009].

Investigation Procedure

In children, scintigraphy is justified only after sonography of the thyroid has been performed. Today, a gamma camera with computer and high-resolution collimator is used for scintigraphy of the thyroid with ^{99m}Tc and ^{123}I [Mahlstedt et al., 1989; Dietlein et al., 2007]. Depending on the age of the patient, scintigraphy is performed in the sitting position or supine with the neck in hyperextension. Imaging is performed 20–30 min after intravenous injection of ^{99m}Tc pertechnetate or 4–6 h after intravenous or oral administration of ^{123}I iodide. Imaging time varies between 5 and 15 min. Anatomical reference points such as the clavicles and the cricoid cartilage, as

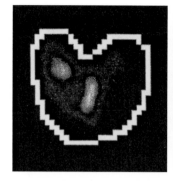
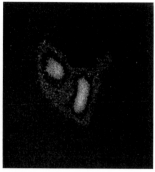

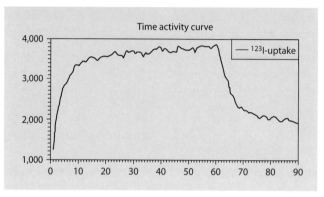

Time activity curve

Fig. 5. Depletion test in a child with Pendred's syndrome and nodular goiter due to dyshormogenesis. Time activity curve shows more than 50% depletion of the thyroid activity shortly after oral administration of potassium perchlorate applied after 60 min.

well as any palpable masses, should be marked on the scan. Calibration of the camera for quantitative measurements of uptake with the activity in the syringe before injection is recommended.

The activity to administer for scintigraphic studies of children should be calculated according to the recommendations of the European Association of Nuclear Medicine [Lassmann et al., 2007, also available at https://www.eanm.org/scientific_info/dosagecard/dosage_card.php?navId = 548]. The reference activities for adults are 80 MBq ^{99m}Tc pertechnetate and 20 MBq ^{123}I iodide. The EANM recommends using not less than 10 MBq ^{99m}Tc pertechnetate and 3 MBq ^{123}I iodide [Lassmann et al., 2007].

For the differential diagnosis of inborn errors of hormonogenesis, a depletion test may be of importance [Dige-Petersen, 1997; El-Desouki, 1995; Hildtich et al., 1982; Meller et al., 1997]. The inborn enzymatic defect may be responsible for organification defects of iodide. This may be detected if an organification blocker such as perchlorate is given immediately after the administration of radioactive iodide (fig. 5). In the case of an organification defect, a considerable amount of iodine taken up by the thyroid will be flushed out after perchlorate. Depletion tests using injectable forms of perchlorate were recommended at one time. Since perchlorate for injection is no longer available in some countries such as Germany, a test using oral administration may be performed: At an interval of 60 min after intravenous injection of a tracer activity of ^{123}I iodide, which has been calculated according to the EANM dosage card, we administer a fraction of the adult dose of 1 g perchlorate orally, using the reduction scheme shown in figure 4. For oral administration, a small infusion tube is used. If the child is not cooperative, a gastric catheter may be used.

Interpretation

Up to present, no age-related reference data for thyroid uptake measured with ^{99m}Tc pertechnetate or ^{123}I iodide have been established. As a general guideline, reference values for adults of roughly 5% for maximal basal ^{99m}Tc uptake and 1.5–2% for maximal ^{99m}Tc uptake under suppression ofTSH may be used. However, in the case of dyshormonogenesis, the depletion test may be interpreted in children as follows (fig. 5): 60 min after intravenous injection of ^{123}I iodide, a body weight-related dose of perchlorate should deplete not more than approximately 10% of the activity from the thyroid [El-Desouki, 1995; Meller et al., 1997; Meller et al., 1998]. In the case of a child with deafness due to Pendred's syndrome as demonstrated in figure 5, typical depletion of more than 50% is caused by a complete organification defect.

Influence of Drugs and Interference Factors

Sufficient knowledge of the patient's medication is mandatory for the correct interpretation of in vivo studies with radionuclides. In addition to different diseases, thyroid hormones, iodine-containing drugs, X-ray contrast media, antithyroid drugs, and lithium may influence the thyroid scan. If a scintigraphic examination with ^{99m}Tc- tin complexes [such as Sn^{2+} citrate, diethylenetriamine pentaacetate, pyrophosphate, methylene diphosphonate, etc.] has been performed, this may lead to an accumulation of the tracer in red blood cells with very poor uptake in the thyroid. It is necessary to wait at least 14 days after the administration of tin complexes before performing a thyroid uptake study.

Paravenous injection may lead to thyroid scans of poor quality. In addition, especially in small children, the quality of scans is frequently impaired by motion artifacts. To prevent these, special fixation supports (e.g. vacuum cushions) may be helpful.

Side Effects and Radiation Exposure

Because of the very low mass of ions needed for scintigraphy, pharmacologic side effects do not occur in thyroid scintigraphy with ^{99m}Tc pertechnetate or ^{123}I sodium iodide. The only potential risk which has to be considered in thyroid scintigraphy is radiation exposure. However, the absorbed dose to the thyroid dose is rather low when ^{99m}Tc is used (table 1). For an adult the corresponding effective dose is 1 mSv. An effective dose of 1 mSv corresponds to the lower range of the yearly natural background in Germany. As the radiation exposure with ^{123}I sodium iodide is approximately 4–5 times higher as compared to ^{99m}Tc pertechnetate, the administration of ^{123}I should be reserved for special indications.

Furthermore, because the dose to the thyroid with ^{131}I sodium iodide is 100-fold higher, ^{131}I is acceptable only for the treatment and follow-up of thyroid cancer in children.

Scintigraphy of the Parathyroids

Radiopharmaceuticals
The mainly oxyphilic cells of parathyroid adenomas contain a great number of mitochondria. It is well known that tracers usually applied for scintigraphy of myocardial perfusion are taken up by parathyroid adenomas as well. Today, ^{99m}Tc Sestamibi (MIBI) is used as the tracer of choice. However, the follicular cells of the thyroid epithelium also take up those tracers. Therefore, specific imaging techniques are necessary to differentiate uptake in enlarged parathyroids from uptake in the thyroid [Kettle et al., 2006].

Indications
Scintigraphy of the parathyroids is rarely indicated in children and adolescents [Damiani et al., 1998, Kollars et al., 2005]. Only in patients who have undergone surgery for parathyroid adenomas or in the case of recurrent or permanent disease may scintigraphy be helpful in the localization of ectopic parathyroid tissue.

Investigation Procedure
No special preparation is necessary before scintigraphy of the parathyroids with MIBI. In adults, an activity of approximately 200 MBq ^{99m}Tc MIBI is administered through a peripheral venous line. In children, the activity has to be reduced according to figure 4. Planar scans of the neck have to be acquired 10–15 min p.i. (including the thorax for exclusion of ectopic adenomas). Double-phase scintigraphy of the parathyroids includes late scans 2–3 h after injection [Kettle et al., 2006].

Adenomas of the parathyroids present scintigraphically with increased uptake of ^{99m}Tc MIBI early after injection. The most specific sign, however, is trapping of the activity demonstrated by late scans after 2–3 h. The sensitivity of this diagnostic procedure depends on the volume of the adenoma. It has been shown that tomographic scans in the SPECT technique increases the diagnostic sensitivity for the localization of small adenomas from 72 to 96% [Moka et al., 1997].

Side Effects and Radiation Exposure
No side effects of ^{99m}Tc MIBI need be anticipated. The absorbed dose for adults is 0.05 mGy/MBq for the upper intestine; the effective dose is 0.009 mSv/MBq(ICRP80). If, in rare cases, children or adolescents are to be diagnosed the activity should be modified according to the table given by Piepsz et al. [1990].

Scintigraphy of the Adrenal Medulla

Pathophysiologic Background

In conjunction with biochemical tests, radionuclide scanning provides unique metabolic information, permitting adrenal disease to be localized despite the lack of anatomical detail [Gross and Shapiro, 1989; Sisson et al., 1987].

The synthesis of *m*-iodobenzylguanidine (MIBG), a physiologic norepinephrine analog, was first accomplished by a group from the University of Michigan [Wieland et al., 1981]. Since the first report of the detection of pheochromocytoma with MIBG in humans [Sisson et al., 1981, 1987], there have been several studies on the role of this agent in the diagnosis and treatment of pheochromocytoma [Shapiro et al., 1984; Perel et al., 1997; O'Halloran et al., 2001].

With a sensitivity of about 90% and a specificity of nearly 100% [Shapiro et al., 1984; Gross and Shapiro, 1989; Francis et al., 1992], MIBG has been shown to be a reliable diagnostic tool for the detection of pheochromocytoma.

Pheochromocytoma

Pheochromocytomas can occur in either sex and at any age. Approximately 10% occur in children [Armstrong et al., 2008, Bissada et al., 2008, Havekes et al., 2009]. In a study by Melicow [1977], 11 of 100 patients with pheochromocytoma were children ranging in age between 5 and 15 years.

Some characteristics of pheochromocytoma in children include a multiplicity of tumors, bilaterality, concurrent intra- and extra-adrenal tumors, recurrences, severity of symptoms, and a familial tendency [Stackpole et al., 1963].

Pheochromocytomas are tumors of indolent nature. Evidence of malignancy may occur years after the successful surgical excision of an apparently benign tumor [Bravo, 1994]. Pheochromocytoma arises from the paraganglionic cells anywhere in the autonomic nervous system. Approximately 98% of pheochromocytomas originate in the abdomen, predominantly (90%) in the adrenal medulla [Radin et al., 1986]. Most extra-adrenal pheochromocytomas are associated with the paravertebral sympathetic ganglia or the organ of Zuckerkandl and, infrequently, the urinary bladder. Pheochromocytoma occurs sporadically, but in 10% of cases, it is inherited [Rodriguez-Sanchez et al., 2005] either as an isolated disease or as part of a systemic disorder such as multiple endocrine neoplasia (MEN IIa or IIb). About 10% of pheochromocytomas are malignant, but the occurrence of malignancy is higher in extra-adrenal masses [van Heerden et al., 1982; Proye et al., 1986]. Malignancy can often be defined only by the presence of metastases rather than by histologic appearance. Multiple pheochromocytomas occur in about 10% of sporadic cases [Cryer, 1985], but 30% of cases of multiple occurrence are found to be associated with a systemic disease [Atuk et al., 1979]. A total of 90% of pheochromocytomas are hormonally active [Dunn et al., 1986]. These tumors can secrete parathyroid hormone, calcitonin, gastrin, serotonin, and adrenocorticotropic hormone (ACTH) with or without cat-echolamines [White and Hickson, 1979]. In contrast with sporadic cases, about 50% of pheochromocytomas associated with MEN II are often asymptomatic.

Radiochemistry and Uptake Mechanism of MIBG

MIBG is a radioiodinated aromatic analog of norepinephrine. Wieland et al. [1981] combined the benzyl portion of bretylium with the guanidine group of guanethidine, which led to the radioiodinated aralkylguanidines *o*-, *p*-, and *m*-iodobenzylguanidine. The *m*-isomer was shown to be the most stable form.

MIBG is thought to have uptake and storage mechanisms similar to those of nor-epinephrine. It is concentrated in adrenergic storage vesicles and therefore has a strong affinity for the adrenal medulla and adrenergic nerve tissue.

Unlike norepinephrine, MIBG is not bound to the postsynaptic receptors [Wieland et al., 1981] and, owing to its molecular structure, it cannot be metabolized by either monoamine oxidase (MAO) or catechol-*o*-methyl transferase (COMT).

Indications for MIBG Scanning

MIBG scanning is the most specific test for both preoperative and postoperative evaluation of disease [Hadley et al., 1986, Maurea et al., 1993; Melicow et al., 1977]. Anatomical tumor volumes can be better determined from CT or MRI scans; how-ever, for tumor staging and the assessment of viable tumor tissue, MIBG scintigraphy is superior because of its high specificity related to selective MIBG uptake in adrener-gic tissues [van Gills et al., 1991; Velchik et al., 1989].

Thus, in patients with biochemical evidence for pheochromocytoma, an MIBG scan is the logical pretherapeutic study to confirm the primary diagnosis and exclude coexisting distant metastases. In addition, because of the high specificity and sensitiv-ity of MIBG, this method is useful for identifying undiagnosed disease.

Preparation of Patients

Sodium or potassium perchlorate should be administered orally for at least 5 days at a daily dose of 1,000 mg in adults to block thyroidal uptake of free iodine. In children, the appropriate doses can be estimated according to body weight. The patient's weight should be recorded in order to calculate the correct MIBG dosage. In addition, the patient's medication history must be carefully reviewed to determine whether he or she has taken drugs that may interfere with tracer uptake. Such medications include tricyclic antidepressants, phenylpropanolamine and sympathomimetics.

Investigation Procedure

In adults, the activity of ^{123}I MIBG is administered through a peripheral venous line. The appropriate activity in children based on body weight according to the recom-mendations of the European Association for Nuclear Medicine [Lassmann et al., 2007] can be calculated according to the tables given by Lassmann's group. Selected

Table 4. Activities to be administered and effective doses in MIBG scintigraphy for typical activities of the [123]I- and ^{131}I-labeled tracer depending on weight [International Commission on Radiological Protection 1988, 1998; Lassmann et al., 2007]

	Weight	[123]I MIBG	[131]I MIBG
Recommended activity	3 kg	80 MBq	35 MBq
	10 kg	80 MBq	35 MBq
	20 kg	136 MBq	35 MBq
	55 kg	326 MBq	65 MBq
	adults	400 MBq	80 MBq
Effective dose	3 kg	5.4 mGy	20 mGy
	10 kg	3.0 mGy	15 mGy
	20 kg	3.5 mGy	12 mGy
	55 kg	5.5 mGy	12 mGy
	adults	5.2 mGy	11 mGy

weight dependent activities are listed in table 4. The patient should be adequately hydrated and empty the bladder before scintigraphy.

Anterior and posterior whole-body scans should be performed 24 and 48 h after the injection of ^{123}I MIBG with a gamma camera with a large viewing field and equipped with a low-energy all-purpose (LEAP) or high-resolution collimator.

Additional tomographic SPECT images can be performed to better delineate the location and extent of the tumor.

Interpretation
At 24 h after the injection of MIBG, there is remarkable activity in the urinary bladder, liver, heart, and salivary glands. After adequate thyroidal blockage, the thyroid is usually not visualized. The normal distribution of MIBG frequently includes low to moderate uptake in the spleen and diffuse low uptake in the lower and middle zones of the lung. The extremities show almost the same activity as the background, and the joints appear as photopenic areas.

Side Effects and Radiation Exposure
Slow injection of MIBG is recommended because a postulated competitive displacement of norepinephrine from the storage granules by MIBG could precipitate a hypertensive crisis. Vital signs should be monitored after the injection, although no adverse reactions have been reported since the introduction of MIBG for the diagnosis of neuroendocrine tumors.

The recommended injected activities (table 4) for MIBG labeled with ^{123}I lead to an effective dose of 5.4 mSv in a small child and 5.2 mSv in an adult.

References

Arbeitskreis Jodmangel: Presseinformation: Jod- und Fluoridprophylaxe für Säuglinge und Kleinkinder weiterhin wichtig, 2008.

Armstrong R, Sridhar M, Greenhalgh KL, Howell L, Jones C, Landes C, McPartland JL, Moores C, Losty PD, Didi M: Phaeochromocytoma in children. Arch Dis Child 2008;93:899–904.

Atuk NO, McDonald T, Wood T, Carpenter JT, Walzak MP, Donaldson M, Gillenwater JY: Familial pheochromocytoma, hypercalcaemia und von Hippel-Lindau disease: a ten-year study of a large family. Medicine 1979;58:209–218.

Bissada NK, Safwat AS, Seyam RM, Al Sobhi S, Hanash KA, Jackson RJ, Sakati N, Bissada MA: Pheochromocytoma in children and adolescents: a clinical spectrum. J Pediatr Surg 2008;43:540–543.

Bravo E: Evolving concepts in the pathophysiology, diagnosis, and treatment of pheochromocytoma. Endocr Rev 1994;15:356–368.

Clerc J, Monpeyssen H, Chevalier A, Amegassi F, Rodrigue D, Leger FA, Richard B: Scintigraphic imaging of paediatric thyroid dysfunction. Horm Res 2008;70:1–13.

Corrias A, Einaudi S, Chiorboli E, Weber G, Crinò A, Andreo M, Cesaretti G, de Sanctis L, Messina MF, Segni M, Cicchetti M, Vigone M, Pasquino AM, Spera S, de Luca F, Mussa C, Bona G: Accuracy of fine needle aspiration biopsy of thyroid nodules in detecting malignancy in childhood: comparison with conventional clinical laboratori, and imaging approaches. J Clin Endocrinol Metab 2001;86:4644–4648.

Cryer PE: Pheochromocytoma. Clin Endocrinol Metab 1985;14:203–220.

Dadachova E, Carrasco N: The Na/I symporter (NIS): imaging and therapeutic applications. Semin Nucl Med 2004;34:2–31.

Damiani D, Aguiar CH, Bueno VS, Montenegro FL, Koch VH, Cocozza AM, Cordeiro AC, Dichtchekenian V, Setian N: Primary hyperparathyroidism in children: patient report and review of the literature. J Pediatr Endocrinol Metab 1998;11:83–86.

Dietlein M, Dressler J, Eschner W, Leisner B, Reiners C, Schicha H: Procedure guideline for thyroid scintigraphy. Nuklearmedizin 2007;46:203–205.

Dige-Petersen H: Efficiency of organic binding of trapped iodide in sporadic goiter, evaluated by the decrease of radioiodide clearance. Nucl Med 1997;16:168–173.

Dunn GD, Brown MJ, Sapsford RN, Mansfield AO, Hemingway AP, Sever PS, Alliso DJ: Functioning middle mediastinal paraganglioma associated with intercaroti paraganglioma. Lancet 1986;i:1061–1063.

El-Desouki M, Al-Jurayyan N, Al-Nuaim A, Al-Herbish A, Abo-Bakr A, Al-Mazrou Y, Al-Swailem A: Thyroid scintigraphy and perchlorate discharge test in the diagnosis of congenital hypothyroidism. Nucl Med 1995;22:1005–1008.

Francis IR, Gross MD, Shapiro B, Korobkin M, Quint LE: Integrated imaging of adrenal disease. Radiology 1992;184:1–13.

Franzius C, Dietlein M, Biermann M, Frühwald M, Linden T, Bucsky P, Reiners C, Schober O: Procedure guideline for radioiodine therapy and [131]iodine whole-body scintigraphy in paediatric patients with differentiated thyroid cancer. Nuklearmedizin 2007;46:224–231.

Gross MD, Shapiro BS: Scintigraphic studies in adrenal hypertension. Semin Nucl Med 1989;19:122–143.

Hadley GP, Rabe E: Scanning with ^{131}I-meta-iodobenzylguanidine in children with solid tumors: an initial appraisal. J Nucl Med 1986;27:620–626.

Havekes B, Vomjin JA, Eisenhofer G, Adams K, Pacak K: Update on pediatric pheochromocytoma. Pediatr Nephrol 2009;24:943–950.

Hilditch TE, Horten PW, McCruden DC, Young RE, Alexander WD: Defects in intrathyroidal binding of iodine and the perchlorate discharge test. Acta Endocrinol 1982;100:237–244.

International Commission on Radiological Protection: Biokinetic models, absorbed doses and effective dose equivalents for individual radiopharmaceuticals; in: Annals of the International Commission on Radiological Protection: Radiation Dose to the Patient from Radiopharmaceuticals (Publication 53). London, Pergamon, 1988, pp 329–331.

International Commission on Radiological Protection Radiation dose to patients from radiopharmaceuticals (Publication 80). Annals of ICRP 1998 28:3; Pergamon Press, Oxford.

Kettle AG, O'Doherty MJ: Parathyroid imaging: how good is it and how should it be done? Semin Nucl Med 2006;36:206–211.

Kollars J, Zaaroug AE, van Heerden J, Lteif A, Stavlo P, Suarez L, Moir C, Ishitani M, Rodeberg D: Primary hyperparathyroidism in pediatric patients. Pediatrics 2005;115:974–980.

Lassmann M, Biassoni L, Monsieurs M, Franzius C, Jacobs F: The new EANM pediatric dosage card. Eur J Nucl Med 2007;34:796–798.

Luster M, Handkiewicz-Junak D, Grossi A, Zacharin M, Taieb D, Cruz D, Hithel A, Casa JA, Mäder U, Dottorini ME: Recombinant thyrotropin use in children and adolescents with differentiated thyroid cancer: a multicenter retrospective study. J Clin Endocrinol Metab 2009;94:3948–3953.

Mahlstedt J, Bähre M, Börner W, Joseph K, Montz R, Reiners Chr, Schicha H: Indikationen zur Schilddrüsenszintigraphie: Empfehlungen der Arbeitsgemeinschaft Schilddrüse der Deutschen Gesellschaft für Nuklearmedizin. Nuklearmedizin 1989;12:223–228.

Maurea S, Cuocolo A, Reynolds JC, Tumeh SS, Begley MG, Linehan WM, Norton JA, Walthers MM, Keiser HR, Neumann RD: ^{131}I-MIBG scintigraphy in preoperative and postoperative evaluation of paragangliomas: comparison with CT and MRI. J Nucl Med 1993;34:173–175.

Melicow MM: One hundred cases of pheochromocytoma (107 tumors) at the Columbia-Presbyterian Medical Center. Cancer 1977;40:1987–2004.

Meller J, Zappel H, Conrad M, Roth C, Emrich D, Becker W: Diagnostic value of [123]Iodine scintigraphy and perchlorate discharge test in the diagnosis of congenital hypothyroidism. Exp Clin Endocrinol Diabetes 1997;105:24–27.

Meller J, Zappel H, Conrad M, Roth C, Emrich D, Becker W: [123]Iodine scintigraphy and perchlorate discharge test in the diagnosis of congenital hypothyroidism. Nuklearmedizin 1998;37:1–5.

Moka D, Voth E, Larena-Avellaneda A, Schicha H: Tc-99m MIBI Spect parathyroid scintigraphy for pre-operative localisation of small parathyroid adenomas. Nuklearmedizin 1997;36:240–244.

Nagataki S: Other factors regulating thyroid function; in Bravermann LE, Utiger RD (eds): Werner and Ingbar's the Thyroid. Lippincott, Philadelphia, 1991, pp 306–321.

O'Halloran T, McGreal G, McDermott E, O'Higgins N: 47 years of phaeochromocytomas. Ir Med J 2001; 94:200–203.

Paltiel HJ, Summerville DA, Treves ST: Iodine-123 scintigraphy in the evaluation of pediatric thyroid disorders: a ten-year experience. Pediatr Radiol 1992;22:251–256.

Paltiel HJ, Larsen R, Treves ST: Thyroid; in Treves ST (ed): Pediatric Nuclear Medicine, ed 2. New York, Springer, 1994, pp 135–148.

Perel Y, Schlumberger M, Marguerite G, Alos N, Revillon Y, Sommelet D, De Lumley L, Falamant F, Dyon JF, Lutz P, Heloury H, Lemerle J: Pheochromocytoma and paraganglioma in children: a report of 24 cases of the French Society of Pediatric Oncology. Pediatr Hematol Oncol 1997;14:413–422.

Piepsz A, Hahn K, Rocer I, Ciofetta G, Toth G, Gordon J, Kulinska J, Gwidlet JA: Radiopharmaceutical schedule for imaging in pediatrics. EurJ Nucl Med 1990; 17:127–129.

Pintar JE, Dominique Toran-Allerand C: Normal development of the hypothalamic-pituitary-thyroid axis; in Braverman LE, Utiger RD (eds): Werner and Ingbar's the Thyroid. Philadelphia, Lippincott, 1991, pp 7–21.

Proye C, Fosati P, Fontaine P, Lefevre J, Decoulx M, Wemeau JL, Dewaill D, Rwamasirabo E, Cecat P: Dopamine-secreting pheochromocytoma: an unrecognised entity? Classification of pheochromocytoma according to their type of secretion. Surgery 1986;100:1154–1157.

Radin DR, Ralls PW; Boswell WD, Colletti PM, Lapin SA, Halls HM: Pheochromocytoma detection by unenhanced CT. AJR Am J RoentgenoI 1986;146: 741–744.

Reiners C: Operative Standards in der endokrinen Chirurgie: Präoperative Schilddrüsendiagnostik. Langenbecks Arch Chir 1990;suppl 2:932.

Rodriguez-Sanches A, Lopez-Menchero C, Rodriguez-Arnao MD: Multiple endocrine neoplasia: paediatric perspective. J Pediatr Endocrinol Metab 2005;18: 1237–1244.

Shapiro B, Sisson JC, Lloyd R, Nakajo M, Saterlee W, Beierwaltes WH: Malignant pheochromocytoma: clinical, biochemical and scintigraphic characterisation. Clin EndocrinoI 1984;20:189–203.

Sisson JC, Frager MS, Valk TW; Gross MD, Swanson DP, Wieland DM, Tobes MC, Beierswaltes BH, Thompson NW: Scintigraphic localization of pheochromocytoma. N Engl J Med 1981;305:12–17.

Sisson JC, Wieland DM, Sherman P, Mangner TJ, Tobes TC, Jaques S: Metaiodobenzylguanidine as an index of the adrenergic nervous system integrity and function. J Nucl Med 1987;28:1620–1624.

Stackpole RH, Melicow MM, Uson AC: Pheochromocytoma in children. J Pediatr 1963;63:315–330.

Taurog A: Hormone synthesis: thyroid iodine metabolism; in Bravermann LE, Utiger RD (eds): Werner and Ingbar's the Thyroid. Philadelphia, Lippincott, 1991, pp 51–97.

van Gills AP, Falke THM, van Erkel AR: MR imaging and MIBG scintigraphy o pheochromocytomas and extra-adrenal functioning paragangliomas. Radiographic 1991;11:37–57.

van Heerden JA, Sheps SG, Hamberger B, Sheedy PF, Poston JG, ReMine WH: Pheochromocytoma: current status and changing trends. Surgery 1982;91: 367–373.

Velchik MG, Alavi A, Kressel HY, Engelman K: Localization of pheochromocytoma: MIBG, CT, and MRI correlation. J Nucl Med 1989;30:328–336.

White MC, Hickson BR: Multiple paragangliomas secreting catecholamines and calcitonin with intermittent hypercalcemia. J R Soc Med 1979;72:525–531.

Wieland DM, Brown LE, Tobes MC, Rogers WL, Marsh DD, Mangner TJ, Swanson DP Beierwaltes WH: Imaging the primate adrenal medulla with [123I] and [131I]metaiodobenzylguanidine: concise communication. J Nucl Med 1981;22:358–364.

Prof. Dr. Christoph Reiners
Department of Nuclear Medicine, University of Würzburg
Josef-Schneider-Strasse 2
DE–97080 Würzburg (Germany)
Tel. +49 931 35868, Fax +49 931 35247, E-Mail reiners@nuklearmedizin.uni-wuerzburg.de

Ranke MB, Mullis P-E (eds): Diagnostics of Endocrine Function in Children and Adolescents, ed 4.
Basel, Karger, 2011, pp 85–101

Diagnostic Tests of Thyroid Function in Children and Adolescents

H. Krude · A. Grüters

Institute of Pediatric Endocrinology, University Children's Hospital, Charite, Humboldt-University Berlin, Berlin, Germany

The assessment of thyroid function is the most frequently applied endocrine investigation in children and adolescents. The clinical symptoms of hypothyroidism are diverse, nonspecific and often mild, and therefore the predictive value of a careful clinical diagnosis for hypothyroidism is low and the majority of measurements result in normal values. Nevertheless, in most patients with growth disorders and obesity, thyroid function tests are carried out in order to exclude hypothyroidism as a possible cause. Moreover, in many patients whose development is retarded or who have neurological symptoms such as muscular hypotonia or attention-deficit hyperactivity disorder, thyroid function tests are performed to exclude hypothyroidism or thyroid hormone resistance as causes of these symptoms. The frequent measurement of thyroid function parameters and the low rate of pathological results lead to a high detection rate of mildly elevated values which are in most cases 'normal variants'. The discrimination of these mildly elevated but nonpathologic thyroid function values from those that reflect a disease state is the daily burden of thyroid diagnostics in pediatrics.

In contrast to other endocrine problems, disturbances in thyroid function can be diagnosed easily in the majority of patients by just measuring the basal concentrations of the hormones. The evaluation of the hypothalamic-pituitary axis is usually not a necessary part of the diagnostic work-up for hypo- or hyperthyroidism. In addition, the circadian variation of thyroid hormone profiles are only minor [26] – with a significant increase of TSH during the night phase – so that the time point of blood sampling is less relevant compared to other hormones like growth hormone and cortisol.

Laboratory Workup of Thyroid Function

The diagnostic tests used in the assessment of thyroid function can be divided into two categories and are carried out in the following order: (1) tests to detect or exclude disturbances in thyroid function, and (2) tests to identify the cause of thyroid dysfunction or disturbed thyroid growth.

Tests to Assess Thyroid Function

For the assessment of thyroid function, serum concentrations of thyrotropin (TSH), thyroxine (T4) and triiodothyronine (T3) are used. T4 and T3 are bound by more than 99% to serum proteins like thyroxin-binding globulin (TBG). Since only the free hormone fraction is biologically active and binds to the T3 receptor, measurement of free hormones is important. Assays that discriminate total from free hormones are available and are in clinical use. Instead of a direct measurement of FT4, the concentration of TBG can be determined and the T4/TBG ratio is used to assess the amount of FT4.

In patients with renal failure or protein deficiency of other origin as well as in patients receiving other medications that might compete with the binding of thyroid hormones to transport proteins, FT4 is the method of choice, because decreased total thyroid hormone levels but normal free thyroid hormone levels can be found in patients with low TBG and/or prealbumin concentrations. In some patients with severe nonthyroid illness, FT4 levels are normal although total thyroid hormone levels are in the hypothyroid range. However, in the majority of pediatric patients, in contrast to the adult population which is characterized by multimorbidity and influenced by different pharmacological treatments that potentially influence protein binding, the determination of total thyroid hormones is usually sufficient. Therefore, as long as age-specific reference ranges for total thyroid hormone concentrations are established in a laboratory, there is no need to switch to the determination of free thyroid hormones.

TSH is usually measured by so-called 'third-generation' immunometric assays, which are characterized by a high sensitivity of 0.01–0.05 mU/l and are reliable for more then 10 years [1].

For the determination of thyroid hormones, automated nonradioimmunometric methods, e.g. enzyme immunoassays or chemiluminescence assays, are generally used. For the routine measurement of free thyroid hormones, direct immunometric one-step analogue or two-step assays are used. While the reproducibility is sufficient for FT4, it is less for FT3. Since T3 is bound to TBG to a much lesser extent, measurement of FT3 is usually not necessary.

Some confusion can arise due to the use of traditional rather than SI units. In principle, the total values are 100 times higher compared to the free hormones and the concentration of T4 is 10 times higher compared to T3. An overview of SI units and their conversion factors is given in table 1.

The biologically almost inactive reverse T3 (rT3, 3,3',5'-triiodothyronine) results from monodeiodination of the inner ring of T4 (in contrast to outer ring deiodination which results in bioactive T3) in extrathyroidal tissues, especially in the liver (fig. 1) [6]. An active inner ring monodeiodination has been demonstrated in some hemangiomata. Furthermore, this monodeiodination is used preferentially in preterm

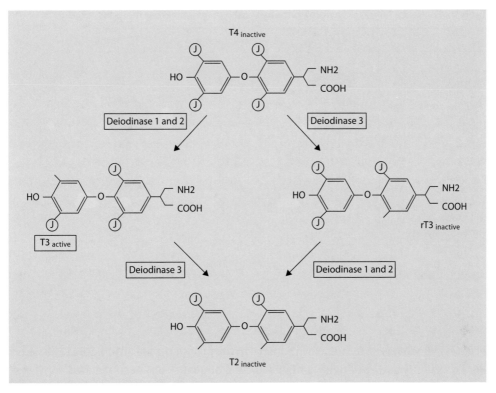

Fig. 1. Molecular composition of thyroid hormone and its derivates. Despite the subtle difference of one iodine atom that distinguishes T4 from T3, immunometric assays have been developed that have a very high specificity for each of the thyroid hormone metabolites.

Table 1. SI units and their conversion factors

	Metric units	SI units	Conversion factor
fT4	ng/dl	pmol/l	× 12,87
T4	µg/dl	nmol/l	× 12,87
T3	ng/dl	nmol/l	× 0,0154

infants and patients with severe nonthyroid illness. This parameter is therefore used in patients with low thyroid hormones and normal TSH concentrations to confirm a suspected case of nonthyroid illness. It is not used as a routine measurement and is therefore provided only by research laboratories.

There are discrepancies between different laboratory methods and it is necessary for each laboratory to elaborate method-specific reference ranges or at least refer their results to the company assay specific reference ranges [30]. With the continuous

Table 2. Reference ranges of thyroid hormones based on two different methods

	T4, nmol/l	fT4, pmol/l	T3, nmol/l
Delfia®			
1st week	137–295	23–67	2.7–5.3
Full-term	114–399	29–79	2.7–8.0
>1 month	130–243	23–54	1.95–4.8
>1 year	106–195	20–31	1.50–3.3
1–5 years	95–165	15–32	1.4–3.3
5–10 years	78–162	12–30	1.3–3.2
>10 years	75–157	12–26	1.7–2.9
Immulite®			
8–15 days	178–534	18–63	2.4–5.1
1 month–3 years	75–155	11–27	1.9–3.4
4–6 years	82–150	13–24.5	1.8–3.2
13 years	72–118	8.5–22.5	1.9–2.7

progress which has been made by industry in the production of automated tests with a high specificity and sensitivity, a high standard of quality has been reached. However, this development also has some disadvantages, because methodological changes are restricted to the manufacturers and therefore methodological competence of the applying laboratories has been lost.

Method-specific variations have to be taken into account when evaluating thyroid function in children, especially during the first years of life. Differences depending on the specific method used can account for up to 30%, especially in the newborn period, but it also has to be taken into account that differences in the iodine supply as well as other unidentified confounders like maternal thyroid disease and iodine contamination may influence the concentrations which are judged as normal. After the first months of life, the reference ranges established with different assays are more comparable. The differences are mostly below 20% and therefore in the range of inter-assay variations (table 2).

Age-Specific Reference Ranges for TSH, Thyroid Hormones
One important aspect of thyroid function is the dynamic change that takes place during development. Therefore, assessment of thyroid function needs to be considered in the context of thyroid ontogeny. Although interpretation of the thyroid function tests is similar to that applied in adults, the reference data differ from adults since they depend on maturation of the hypothalamic-pituitary-thyroid axis. It is therefore essential that age-specific reference ranges are applied and that interpretation is based on a thorough knowledge of thyroid physiology from fetal life to adulthood.

Fetal Development of Thyroid Function

Development of the human thyroid begins as early as in the 3rd week of gestation [7]. In the following weeks of gestation, further organogenesis is characterized by proliferation and differentiation. The TSH receptor, TPO, sodium iodide (NIS) and thyroglobulin genes are expressed starting from the 10th week of gestation. Subsequently, iodide uptake as well as fetal hormone biosynthesis is possible and can be detected in the fetal circulation as well as in fetal organs. TSH synthesis increases from 12 to 30 weeks of gestation and correlates with maturation of the hypothalamic-pituitary axis [7] and is followed by an increase of fetal T4 levels up to term. In contrast, fetal T3 concentrations are low throughout gestation. The low fetal T3 production is caused by a decreased outer ring deiodinase activity in the fetal liver.

The dynamics of fetal thyroid function need to be considered during a diagnostic workup for fetal thyroid pathology and especially for the diagnosis of preterm thyroid function.

Normal values for fetal TSH, T4 and T3 were established using serum taken at cordocentesis [9]. These data can be used to assess fetal thyroid dysfunction in the case of maternal and clinical suspicion of fetal hyperthyroidism and when ultrasound reveals a fetal goiter [21]. In addition, reference intervals for thyroid function were established for amniotic fluid parameters, which are much lower compared to cordocentesis samples [22].

Postnatal cord blood values in preterm neonates correlate with fetal cordocentesis values in that a marked increase of T4 levels occurs during gestation while T3 remains low throughout pregnancy [31]. Postnatally, an increase of T4 and T3 within the first 4 weeks of life occurs in preterm neonates, which is also dependent on gestational week. This increase is more pronounced for T3 with a 2-times increment in the group of 23–27 weeks of gestation and almost 5 times in the term neonate group [31]. The dynamic changes of thyroid values in preterm babies in relation to gestational age (fig. 2) as well as to postnatal age makes interpretation of thyroid function in preterm neonates very difficult and reference data need to be adjusted. Considering the additional interassay variability and the principle need for laboratory-specific normative data, it seems necessary to centralize laboratory diagnostics for neonatal thyroid function in preterms in specialized laboratories.

Postnatal Development of Thyroid Function

Immediately after birth (1–6 h), T4 as well as T3 levels rise due a marked postnatal increase of TSH secretion, which reaches levels up to 100 mU/l [7].

After a period of neonatal hyperthyrotropinemia resulting in increased peripheral thyroid hormones, which differs individually and is not well defined, thyroid hormone (T4 and T3) levels decrease with age. This is accompanied by a decrease in free thyroid hormone levels. In newborns and young infants, normal reference ranges for thyroid hormones are in the adult range of hyperthyroid levels. In addition, the turnover rate of thyroid hormones is higher in young infants also decreasing with age.

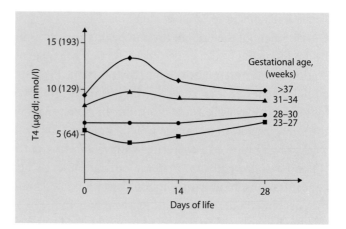

Fig. 2. Based on the published data for postnatal total T4 [31], dynamic changes of thyroid function in correlation to gestational age are illustrated.

Thus, thyroid hormone metabolism during infancy and childhood is characterized by progressively decreasing T4, T3 as well as free thyroid hormone concentrations, while TSH concentrations after the initial phase of hyperthyrotropinemia remain rather stable. There are no differences between male and female individuals except a small increase of total T4 and T3 concentrations in late pubertal stages (Tanner stage >3) and after puberty, which are most likely caused by increased TBG levels [5].

The dynamic neonatal changes in thyroid hormone values are clinically relevant for the diagnosis of congenital thyroid diseases. Confirmation of neonatal screening results is dependent on serum thyroid function tests and due to the complex situation of postnatal changes in thyroid function, the standard of laboratory tests for neonatal thyroid function in association with screening laboratories needs to be very high. One central question is the exact reference application for the postnatal age-range. However, up to now even the most elaborated reference values available for postnatal T4 which are based on the frequently used Immulite® assay [5] and which show a surge of T4 values within the first days of life are not sufficient to define the exact normal values for each day during the critical time period of 14 days that is relevant for screening confirmation diagnosis. Interpretation of thyroid function tests in neonates detected in TSH neonatal screening process is therefore difficult and the decision to treat a child has to be based on exact, postnatal detailed reference values to avoid overtreatment (fig. 3).

Tests to Assess the Cause of a Thyroid Disorder
TRH is a tripeptide secreted by the hypothalamus and stimulates pituitary TSH secretion. A standard intravenous TRH test is performed by a bolus injection of 5–7 µg/kg TRH and measurement of baseline as well as 30-min TSH values. If a hypothalamic disorder is suspected, a further 60-min value is taken. The only indication to use the TRH test in children and adolescents might be for investigation of the hypothalamic-

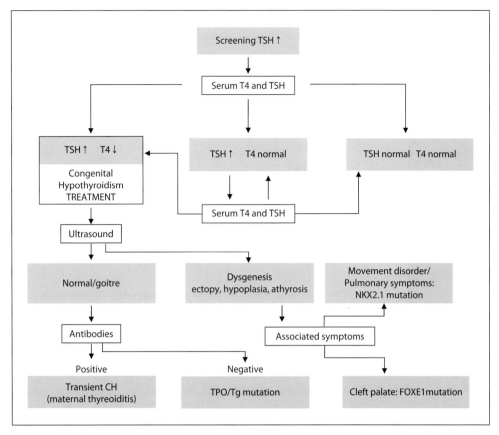

Fig. 3. Algorithm for diagnostic procedures and treatment indication for congenital hypothyroidism in newborn screening for TSH.

pituitary-thyroid axis in central hypothyroidism. However, a comprehensive study in more then 50 patients with central hypothyroidism questions the impact of a TRH test for this diagnostic process because the discrimination of pituitary and hypothalamic central hypothyroidism was not significant [18].

An absent response to TRH is also found in patients with a complete loss of function of the β-TSH gene. However, with the use of a third-generation TSH assay diagnosis can be made without carrying out a TRH test.

In light of the frequent discomfort that occurs like nausea and flushing, TRH testing has today lost its role in routine nonscientific laboratory workup in neonates and children and only the use of sensitive TSH assays are recommended.

Thyroglobulin (Tg) is a high-molecular-weight protein stored in the colloid of the thyroid gland. In the euthyroid state and with intact follicular structures, Tg is not secreted into the circulation. However, it is detectable in a situation of increased TSH stimulation of the thyroid gland, increased proliferation and especially if abnormal (e.g. malignant) thyroid tissue is present. Therefore, it is used as a parameter for the assessment of normal and malignant proliferation. The main indication of its use is in the follow-up of patients with differentiated thyroid carcinoma in order to detect tumor recurrence or differentiated metastasis. A measurable Tg after ablative therapy indicates the presence of residual tissue and an increase after ablative therapy indicates recurrence. Tg can also be used to assess the presence of functional thyroid tissue in patients with congenital hypothyroidism and thyroid dysgenesis [3]. In Tg assays, the interference of anti-Tg antibodies which inhibit the binding of Tg antibodies to the antigen leads to falsely decreased and elevated levels [20]. This can be resolved by recovery tests with long incubation periods of serum with the assay antibody to guarantee a state of equilibrium.

Several antibodies to thyroid-specific antigens are used to investigate the possibility of an autoimmune thyroid disorder as the cause of disturbed thyroid function or goiter. In patients with an echo structure indicative of autoimmune thyroiditis – diffuse echo pattern, small cystic lesions, inhomogeneous structure, hyper- or hypoechogenicity – anti-TPO or anti-Tg antibodies are detectable. In patients with hyperthyroidism, the additional presence of TSH receptor antibodies as measured by competitive binding assays is suggestive of morbus Basedow. To verify these antibodies as stimulating antibodies, bioassays with the measurement of cAMP in cell lines have to be used usually in research laboratories. In contrast, in patients with hypothyroidism, anti-TSH receptor antibodies may be inhibitory and this can also be verified by the use of bioassays [1].

For the detection of anti-TPO and anti-Tg, technologies like immunoluminescence assays using recombinant human TPO should be used because they provide a higher sensitivity. TSH receptor antibodies are determined by so-called 'second-generation' assays, e.g. immunoluminescence assays using labeled recombinant human TSH receptor instead of radioreceptor assay porcine thyroid membranes as antigen. With these methods, a higher sensitivity (>98%) can be achieved [1]. Measurements of anti-TPO and anti-Tg antibody titers are recommended in the further workup of elevated TSH values to exclude thyroid autoimmune disease. However, normal values for anti-TPO and anti-Tg antibody titers are defined in the range below 100 U/ml. Mildly elevated antibody titers alone are not sufficient to confirm the diagnosis of autoimmune thyreoiditis and further information, especially the morphological changes typical for thyroiditis, need to be determined. Typically, in cases with thyreoiditis and manifest hypothyroidism antibody titers are found that are 10 times higher than the upper normal range [16].

Measurement of urinary iodine concentrations is used to evaluate the individual iodine intake. Simple and rapid ammonium persulfate oxidation is a frequently used method for the determination of total urinary iodine content. Sophisticated automated techniques such as the Technicon Autoanalyzer, paired-ion reversed-phase HPLC or iodine ion-selective electrodes are reserved for research purposes or high-throughput laboratories [25]. A rapid semiquantitative colorimetric test has been developed which has sufficient reliability compared to the Sandel-Kolthoff method [17].

The most frequent use of urine iodine determination occurs in the context of epidemiological surveys. However, the individual clinical situation where iodine determination plays an important diagnostic role is during workup of congenital hypothyroidism when contamination with iodine is suspected. Very high values in neonatal urine samples confirm the differential diagnosis of iodine contamination and a transient course of hypothyroidism can be expected.

In order to improve the diagnosis and therapy, molecular genetic testing has been used in patients with different thyroid disorders. For screening missense or nonsense mutations, direct sequencing of PCR products amplified from patient white blood cell DNA is the most established method today revealing a mutation detection sensitivity of >95%. For the exclusion of deletions, FISH or quantitative PCR has to be used.

So far, the clinically most important mutational analysis in the field of thyroid disease in childhood has been established for the ret-protooncogene in patients with a risk of familial MEN 2 or medullary carcinoma (FMTC) [12]. Clinical algorithms have been developed that lead to prophylactic thyreoidectomy in the case of a proven ret-protooncogene mutation in young family members of FMTC patients.

In all other conditions, especially the molecular workup of congenital hypothyroidism, genetic testing does not contribute to a therapeutic decision. However, genetic testing can confirm the clinical diagnosis of thyroid dyshormonogenesis in patients with normal or enlarged thyroid glands, which occurs as recessive traits, and therefore a genetic counseling can be offered (table 3). Among these defects, mutations in the thyroid peroxidase gene are the most frequent and explain almost 50% of the patients in this CH subgroup [27].

In addition, in rare more syndromic forms of congenital hypothyroidism the detection of mutations in some transcription factors like FOXE1 and gene NKX2.1 are clinically relevant to confirm the differential diagnosis. In patients with an associated cleft palate and severe mental retardation, FOXE1 mutations are likely and confirm a recessively transmitted genetic disease [2]. In patients with a movement disorder in addition to congenital hypothyroidism as well as some pulmonary alterations after birth, a dominant inheritance of NKX2.1 gene deficiency can be diagnosed [13].

In patients with inherited central hypothyroidism without detectable TSH, a mutation in the β-TSH gene confirms the isolated form of TSH deficiency and further suspicion of combined pituitary deficiency can be excluded [19].

Clinical Applications

In almost all cases, the clinical suspicion of a thyroid function defect in children, the measurement of basal TSH and T4, either total T4 or free T4 and in some additional cases also of total T3, is sufficient to diagnose hypo- or hyperthyroidism. A

Table 3. Molecular genetic testing in CH

Gene	Thyroid phenotype	Associated problems
	primary hypothyroidism	
Thyroid peroxidase TPO (autosomal-recessive)	normal gland or goiter, pathological perchlorate discharge test	no
Sodium-iodide transporter (NIS) (autosomal-recessive)	normal gland or goiter, absent iodine or technetium uptake	no
Thyroglobulin Tg (autosomal-recessive)	goiter	no
Thox2 (autosomal-recessive)	normal gland	transient hypothyroidism in heterozygous patients
Pendrin (autosomal-recessive)	goiter	sensineuronal haering loss
Thyroid hormone receptor-β (autosomal-recessive or autosomal-dominant)	goiter	sensineuronal hearing loss attention-deficit hyperactivity disorder mental retardation
TSH-receptor (autosomal-recessive)	thyroid hypoplasia ('apparent athyrosis')	no, elevated TSH-1 heterozygous patients
PAX-8 (autosomal-dominant)	thyroid hypoplasia ectopy	renal malformation
FOXE1 (autosomal-recessive)	hypoplasia	cleft palate choanal atresia curly hair developmental delay
NKX 2.1 (autosomal dominant)	athyrosis hypoplasia normal developed gland	choreoathetosis pulmonary problems mental retardation hypothalamic abnormalities
	central hypothyroidism	
β-Thyrotropin gene (autosomal-recessive)	hypoplasia	no

Table 4. Summary of possible laboratory results of thyroid function testing and their differential diagnosis

TSH	fT4	Total T4	Total T3	Differential diagnosis	Confirmation test
↑	↑	↑	↑	T3 resistance	T3 receptor gene
↑	↓	↓	↓	hypothyroidism primary congenital acquired	ultrasound Tg-Ab, TPO-Ab
↓	↓	↓	↓	hypothyroidism secondary/central congenital	TSH-β-gene/ TRH R-gene
n/ (↑)	↓	↓	↓	isolated congenital combined acquired	Pit-/Prop-gene MRI
n	n	n	↓	low T3 syndrome	severe illness, anorexia?
n	n	↓	↓	TBG deficiency	TBG measurement
n	n	↑	↑	increased TBG binding	TBG genetics
n	↑	↑	n	T4-antibodies	T4-Ab
n (↑)	n	n	↑	MCT8 deficiency	MCT8 gene
↓	n	n	↑	mild hyperthyroidism	TSH R-Ab TPO-Ab Tg-Ab
↓	↑	↑	↑	Hyperthyroidism, morbus Basedow/Hashimoto's disease	TSH R-Ab TPO-Ab Tg-Ab

summary of all the relevant pathological constellations of these three parameters is given in table 4.

Hypothyroidism
Hypothyroidism is defined by low thyroid hormone values, which in association with an elevated TSH results from a primary thyroid defect and in the case of low

TSH reflects a central form of hypothyroidism. TSH elevation in the light of normal thyroid hormones is not sufficient for the diagnosis of hypothyroidism. However, an increased TSH level is frequently diagnosed but in most cases it is not a sign of thyroid pathology but rather a normal variant, especially in the childhood population. The term 'hyperthyreotropinemia' is therefore more appropriate compared to 'latent hypothyroidism'. In order to diagnose hypothyroidism in the ambulatory pediatric patient without any other severe illness, it is sufficient to measure TSH and total or free T4.

Neonatal Hypothyroidism

Today, the diagnosis of congenital primary hypothyroidism in Western societies is usually made based on neonatal screening programs. In Europe (with the exception of The Netherlands), TSH is measured on dried filter-paper blood spots; therefore, patients with central hypothyroidism are not picked up by the screening programs. The detection rate depends on the quality control of the screening program and a missed diagnosis is usually not due to laboratory pitfalls but to logistic problems in the pre- or postanalytical period. TSH concentrations are reported as mU/l whole blood. However, a pathological screening result is not sufficient for the diagnosis of congenital hypothyroidism. In order to confirm the diagnosis, neonatal thyroid function needs to be determined in an additional serum sample. Several guidelines for the workup of screening confirmation diagnostics are available [32]. Since hypothyroidism is defined by subnormal thyroid hormone values and because most often T4 is initially low while T3 remains normal, the main parameter for the confirmation diagnosis is a reduced total T4 or free T4. In the majority of cases, severe hypothyroidism is present with very high TSH and low T4 and T3 concentrations and the diagnosis is obvious. However, in those cases with only mild elevation of TSH a more sophisticated laboratory diagnosis is warranted and the definition of the normal range of T4 becomes the central tool for an appropriate confirmation diagnosis. As outlined above, normal reference intervals for total T4 and fT4 are only available for a limited number of methods and are in general not detailed enough to assess normal thyroid function on an exact daily basis. In principle, those cases with mildly elevated TSH and borderline T4 values should be further diagnosed by serial serum investigations at weekly intervals. A constant rise of TSH and decline of T4 values leads to a clear diagnosis of congenital hypothyroidism and needs to be treated (fig. 3). However, neonates with a normal T4 and stable mildly elevated TSH do not fulfill the criteria of congenital hypothyroidism. Based on the available data, it does not seem obligatory to treat those children with isolated TSH elevation. This becomes even more important in those screening programs that are nowadays based on lower TSH cutoff levels [14].

In patients with confirmed primary congenital hypothyroidism and a normal thyroid gland as shown in a subsequent ultrasound investigation, the determination of thyroid autoantibodies and iodine concentration in the urine is performed to predict the possibility of a transitory form of CH in situations of maternal autoimmune thyroid disease or iodine contamination.

In addition, genetic testing for several candidate genes has allowed identification of a molecular cause in a small number of patients with congenital hypothyroidism. To date, molecular genetic testing is clinically relevant in cases with dyshormonogenesis to detect those patients with a recessive basis of disease in the case of thyroid peroxidase gene mutations [27]. In patients with thyroid dysgenesis, associated symptoms should prompt further genetic workup to also perform a precise genetic counseling (fig. 3). In children with associated cleft palate and a 'spiky hair phenotype', mutations in the FOXE1 gene can be identified [2]. Neonates with thyroid dysgenesis and pulmonary problems like respiratory distress and pneumonia as well as in infants with an associated movement disorder like choreoathetosis, the NKX2.1 gene should be investigated to detect a dominant form of congenital hypothyroidism [13].

Acquired Hypothyroidism

The most frequent cause of juvenile-acquired hypothyroidism in populations with a sufficient iodine intake is proliferative autoimmune thyroiditis (Hashimoto's thyroiditis) [10]. In order to investigate the cause of acquired hypothyroidism, thyroid ultrasound and the determination of thyroid autoantibodies is performed. Thyroid ultrasound reveals an enlarged gland with diffuse echo pattern and a reduced echogenicity is suggestive of autoimmune thyreoiditis. The diagnosis is confirmed by measurements of anti-TPO, anti-Tg and TSH receptor-blocking antibodies.

Central Hypothyroidism

In patients with clinical suspicion of hypothyroidism, low T4 and or low T3 values and normal or only mildly elevated TSH, a defect in the central regulation of thyroid function in terms of central hypothyroidism is present. If this constellation occurs during childhood, acquired causes of central disturbance need to be further evaluated and a cranial MRI is obligatory to exclude a pituitary or hypothalamic tumor. In addition, the complete pituitary function need to be tested to exclude combined pituitary deficiency.

The further discrimination of a pituitary or hypothalamic disturbance can be reached by a TRH stimulation test. However, a recent study has shown that most patients with central hypothyroidism cannot be easily categorized within this scheme and the value of performing a TRH stimulation test, especially in the light of significant discomfort like nausea and flushing, is questionable [18]. In this context, the primary question is the clear confirmation of hypothyroidism which cannot be reached by a TRH test but needs to be determined by serial documentation of low T4 values.

In neonates, the very rare condition of central hypothyroidism due to isolated TSH deficiency can be diagnosed by sequencing the β-TSH gene [19].

Hyperthyreotropinemia

The term hyperthyreotropinemia or subclinical describes a condition with elevated TSH concentrations and normal peripheral thyroid hormone levels. In pediatric patients, a negative impact on child health of isolated elevation of TSH has not been demonstrated so far. Moreover, a variety of recent studies with very large numbers of probands have shown that the majority of children with an elevated TSH and normal T4 have a transient course of this laboratory finding. The risk of developing overt hypothyroidism is very low within observation periods up to 5 years [15]. A TSH below 7.5 mU/l was indicative of a negligible risk of overt hypothyroidism during the follow-up period. In the case of normal T4 and T3 values, an elevated TSH value should lead to a control investigation within a 3-month interval. If the constellation maintains a steady level, serial TSH measurements are sufficient and treatment is recommended at least for TSH <10 mU/l. Autoimmune disease as an underlying potential cause of elevated TSH should be ruled out by measuring the levels of thyroid antibodies.

A particular and still growing subgroup of children with hyperthyreotropinemia is found in the obese childhood population. Typically, these children are severely obese and TSH values are below 10 mU/l. It has been shown that in these cohorts T3 values are within the normal range but significantly higher compared to normal-weight control groups. This constellation suggests a central activation of thyroid function, which can be interpreted as a counterregulation to overcome the obese state. A study has recently shown that elevated TSH levels decline when body weight is significantly reduced [24]. This finding further argues that hyperthyreotropinemia is more a consequence rather then the cause of obesity in these children and that thyroid hormone treatment is not indicated.

Hyperthyroidism

The most frequent cause of hyperthyroidism in children and adolescents is morbus Basedow. In contrast to hypothyroidism where the measurement of TSH and T4 is sufficient, the first step towards the diagnosis of hyperthyroidism is determination of serum TSH, T4 as well as T3 because in some milder cases hyperthyroidism is associated with elevated T3 while T4 remains initially normal.

If TSH is suppressed and total and/or free thyroid hormones are increased, an ultrasound study is performed. If the echogenicity is in favor of an autoimmune thyroid disease, thyroid autoantibodies are measured. A hyperthyroid phase of autoimmune thyroiditis is assumed if no TSH receptor antibodies but significant titers of anti-TPO and anti-Tg antibodies are found. In contrast, in morbus Basedow characteristically significant titers of TSH receptor antibodies are measured, but usually anti-TPO antibodies are also found.

If the echogenicity is normal and no thyroid antibodies are found in the presence of a clinically and biochemically clearly hyperthyroid condition, mutational analysis of the TSH receptor is indicated to investigate the possibility of an activating mutation of the TSH receptor [4]. Radionuclide imaging is performed only if a nodule is detected by ultrasound to diagnose a thyroid adenoma, which is a rare condition in children and adolescents. Diffuse thyroid enlargement in a hyperthyroid patient with antithyroid autoantibodies is not an indication for scintigraphy.

Thyroid Hormone Resistance

If TSH is not suppressed in the presence of elevated thyroid hormone levels, the main differential diagnosis is resistance to thyroid hormones. Sequencing of the thyroid hormone receptor beta gene can confirm the diagnosis in these cases [23]. Treatment indication is difficult because of the combined occurrence of hypothyroid symptoms due to the mutant beta receptor and hyperthyroid symptoms via the intact alpha receptor which is expressed in the heart and the brain.

Elevated total thyroid hormone levels in the presence of measurable TSH concentrations can also be due to an increased binding capacity (e.g. familial increased TBG or dysalbuminemia) or an increase of TBG due to the administration of estrogens, conditions which need to be further evaluated in the differential diagnosis of thyroid hormone resistance.

Thyroid Hormone Transport Defect

A more recently defined disease of thyroid function is caused by the x-chromosomal inheritance of mutations in the thyroid hormone transporter gene MCT8. The disease has been described initially as a variant of x-chromosomal mental retardation with movement disorders like ataxia or severe muscular hypotonia called Allan-Herndon-Dudley disease [8]. In patients with a MCT8 defect, a pathognomonic thyroid hormone constellation is present that is characterized by an elevated T3, normal or borderline low T4 and normal or mildly elevated TSH. The high T3 and normal / low T4 seems to result from a particular organ-specific expression of the MCT8 gene that influences the peripheral metabolism of thyroid hormones favoring deiodination of available T4 into T3. A treatment option to improve the poor clinical condition of these patients does not exist so far.

References

1 Ajjan RA, Weetman AP: Techniques to quantify TSH receptor antibodies. Nat Clin Pract Endocrinol Metab 2008;4:461–468.

2 Castanet M, Polak M: Spectrum of human Foxe1/TTF2 mutations. Horm Res Paediatr 2010;73:423–430.

3 Czernichow P, Schlumberger M, Pomarède R, Fragu P: Plasma thyroglobulin measurements help determine the type of thyroid defect in congenital hypothyroidism. J Clin Endocrinol Metab 1983;56:242–245.

4 Davies TF, Ando T, Lin RY, Tomer Y, Latif R: Thyrotropin receptor-associated diseases: from adenomata to Graves' disease. J Clin Invest 2005;115:1972–1983.

5 Elmlinger MW, Kühnel W, Lambrecht HG, Ranke MB: Reference intervals from birth to adulthood for serum thyroxine (T4), triiodothyronine (T3), free T3, free T4, thyroxine-binding globulin (TBG) and thyrotropin (TSH). Clin Chem Lab Med 2001;39:973–979.

6 Engler D, Burger AG: The deiodination of iodothy-ronines and their derivatives in man. Endocr Rev 1984;5:151.

7 Fisher DA, Klein AH: Thyroid development and disorders of thyroid function in the newborn. N Engl J Med 1981;304:702–712.

8 Friesema EC, Grueters A, Biebermann H, Krude H, von Moers A, Reeser M, Barrett TG, Mancilla EE, Svensson J, Kester MH, Kuiper GG, Balkassmi S, Uitterlinden AG, Koehrle J, Rodien P, Halestrap AP, Visser TJ: Association between mutations in a thyroid hormone transporter and severe X-linked psychomotor retardation. Lancet 2004;364:1435–1437.

9 Guibourdenche J, Noël M, Chevenne D, Vuillard E, Voluménie JL, Polak M, Boissinot C, Porquet D, Luton D: Biochemical investigation of foetal and neonatal thyroid function using the ACS-180SE analyser: clinical application. Ann Clin Biochem 2001;38:520–526.

10 Hunter I, Greene SA, MacDonald TM, Morris AD: Prevalence and aetiology of hypothyroidism in the young. Arch Dis Child 2000;83:207–210.

11 Inherit J: Newborn screening strategies for congenital hypothyroidism: an update. Metab Dis 2010.

12 Jhiang SM: The RET proto-oncogene in human cancers. Oncogene 2000;20:5590–5597.

13 Krude H, Schütz B, Biebermann H, von Moers A, Schnabel D, Neitzel H, Tönnies H, Weise D, Lafferty A, Schwarz S, DeFelice M, von Deimling A, van Landeghem F, DiLauro R, Grüters A: Choreoathetosis, hypothyroidism, and pulmonary alterations due to human NKX2-1 haploinsufficiency. J Clin Invest 2002;109:475–480.

14 Krude H, Blankenstein O: Treating patients not numbers: the benefit and burden of lowering TSH newborn screening cut-offs. Arch Dis Child 2010.

15 Lazar L, Frumkin RB, Battat E, Lebenthal Y, Phillip M, Meyerovitch J: Natural history of thyroid function tests over 5 years in a large pediatric cohort. J Clin Endocrinol Metab 2009;94:1678–1682.

16 Lorini R, Gastaldi R, Traggiai C, Perucchin PP: Hashimoto's thyroiditis. Pediatr Endocrinol Rev 2003;(suppl 2):205–211.

17 Markou KB, Georgopoulos NA, Anastasiou E, Vlasopoulou B, Lazarou N, Vagenakis GA, Sakellaropoulos GC, Vagenakis AG, Makri M: Identification of iodine deficiency in the field by the rapid urinary iodide test: comparison with the classic Sandell-Kolthoff reaction method. Thyroid 2002;5:407–410.

18 Metha A, Hindmarsh PC, Stanhope RG, Brain CE, Preece MA, Dattani MT: Is the thyrotropin-releasing hormone test necessary in the diagnosis of central hypothyroidism in children. J Clin Endocrinology Metab 2003;88:5696–5703.

19 Miyai K: Congenital thyrotropin deficiency: from discovery to molecular biology, postgenome and preventive medicine. Endocr J 2007;54:191–203.

20 Penny R, Spencer CA, Frasier SD, Nicoloff JT: Thyroid-stimulating hormone and thyroglobulin levels decrease with chronological age in children and adolescents. J Clin Endocrinol Metab 1983;56:177–180.

21 Polak M, Le Gac I, Vuillard E, Guibourdenche J, Leger J, Toubert ME, Madec AM, Oury JF, Czernichow P, Luton D: Fetal and neonatal thyroid function in relation to maternal Graves' disease. Best Pract Res Clin Endocrinol Metab 2004;18:289–302.

22 Pratima KS, Parvin CA, Gronowski AM: Establishment of reference intervals for markers of fetal thyroid status in amniotic fluid. J Clin Endocrinol Metab 1988;4175–4179.

23 Refetoff S, Dumitrescu AM: Syndromes of reduced sensitivity to thyroid hormone: genetic defects in hormone receptors, cell transporters and deiodination. Best Pract Res Clin Endocrinol Metab 2007;21:277–305.

24 Reinehr T, de Sousa G, Andler W: Hyperthyrotropinemia in obese children is reversible after weight loss and is not related to lipids. J Clin Endocrinol Metab 2006;91:3088–3091.

25 Rendl J, Bier D, Reiners C: Methods for measuring iodine in urine and serum. Exp Clin Endocrinol Diabetes 1998;106:34–41.

26 Reselfsema F, Pereira AM, Veldhuis, JD, Adriaanse R, Endert E, Fliers E, Romijn JA: Thyrotropin secretion profiles are not different in men an women. J Clin Endocrinol Metab 2009;94:3964–3967.

27 Ris-Stalpers C, Bikker H: Genetics and phenomics of hypothyroidism and goiter due to TPO mutations. Mol Cell Endocrinol 2010;322:38–43.

28 Spencer CA, Takeuchi M, Kazarosyan M: Current status and performance goals for serum thyrotropin assays. Clin Chem 1996;42:140.

29 Thorpe-Beeston JG, Nicolaides KH, McGregor AM: Fetal thyroid function. Thyroid 1992;2:207–217.

30 Veitl M, Hamwi A, Huber A, Flores J, Dudczak R, Bieglmayer C: Methodenvergleich von Immunoassays für Sexual- und Schilddrüsenhormone von Fünf Routineanalysern: ARCHITECT, AxSYM, Centaur, Elecsys 2010 und IMMULITE 200. J Lab Med 2002;26:191–202.

Krude · Grüters

31 Williams Fl, Simpson J, Delahunty C, Ogston SA, Bongers-Schokking JJ, Murphy N, van Toor H, Wu SY, Visser TJ, Hume R: Developmental trends in cord and postpartum serum thyroid hormones in preterms infants. J Clin Endocrinol Metab 2004;89: 5314–5320.

32 American Academy of Pediatrics, Rose SR: Section on Endocrinology and Committee on Genetics, American Thyroid Association, Brown RS; Public Health Committee, Lawson Wilkins Pediatric Endocrine Society, Foley T, Kaplowitz PB, Kaye CI, Sundararajan S, Varma SK: Update of newborn screening and therapy for congenital hypothyroidism. Pediatrics 2006;117:2290–2303.

Prof. Dr. Heiko Krude
Institute of Pediatric Endocrinology, University Children's Hospital, Charite
Humboldt-University Berlin, Augustenburgerplatz 1
DE–13353 Berlin (Germany)
Tel. +49 30 450 666 039, Fax +49 30 450 566 926, E-Mail heiko.krude@charite.de

Ranke MB, Mullis P-E (eds): Diagnostics of Endocrine Function in Children and Adolescents, ed 4.
Basel, Karger, 2011, pp 102–137

Growth Hormone Deficiency: Diagnostic Principles and Practice

Michael B. Ranke

University Children's Hospital, Tübingen, Germany

Growth hormone deficiency (GHD) by and large involves a wide range of disorders, including an impairment in GH secretion and/or a reduced impact of GH (table 1) [1]. It has been proposed that GH and IGF-1 are analogous to other endocrine systems in that they are interconnected, with GH being the regulatory hormone and IGF-1 the hormone acting primarily. A distinction is thus made between 'primary IGF deficiency', which involves IGF-1 impairment but normal GH secretion and action, whereas 'secondary IGF deficiency' is a state in which IGF-1 is impaired due to irregularities in GH secretion [2]. These disorders are diagnosed via a combination of diagnostic tools [see also chapters by Blum and Albertsson-Wikland, this vol.]. In addition, imaging techniques and molecular genetic methods [see chapter by Pandey and Mullis, this vol.] can be applied to confirm and/or specify the diagnosis.

More specifically, GHD is characterized by GH secretion levels that are below those for age- and sex-matched norms. In a broader sense, GHD is the clinical disorder resulting from the impaired secretion or action of GH in an individual. The first task in the diagnostic procedure should thus be to establish whether or not the clinical presentation of an individual corresponds with the situation of impaired GH secretion or action. If this is plausible, evidence must be sought, in a second step, for an impairment in GH secretion (or action). The difficulty in associating an individual's anthropometrical and biochemical phenotype with GH impairment is partly related to the fact that the phenotype may vary, depending on age and severity, as well as according to the duration of GH impairment at the time the patient presents. Moreover, certain signs or symptoms typical for GHD are also attributable to other causes. A combination of typical signs could thus be more helpful than a single characteristic specific to GH impairment. Finally, it must be mentioned that the empirical basis used to make a causal association between the quantitative deviation of anthropometrical/biochemical signs and a measurable degree of GH impairment is very narrow.

Table 1. Disorders of the GH-IGF axis (Wit et al. [1])

ESPE code		Diagnosis
1B.3		growth hormone deficiency (secondary IGF deficiency)
1B.3a		congenital GHD
1B.3a.1		associated with other complex syndromes
1B.3a.2		known genetic defects
	1B.3a.2a	-HESX1
	1B.3a.2b	-LHX3
	1B.3a.2c	-LHX4
	1B.3a.2d	-PROP1
	1B.3a.2e	-POU1F1
	1B.3a.2f	-GHRHR
	1B.3a.2g	-GH
	1B.3a.2y	-other specified genetic defects
1B.3a.3		associated with cerebral or facial malformations (e.g. SOD, empty sella syndrome, solitary central maxillary incisor syndrome, mid-line palatal cleft syndrome, arachnoidal cyst, congenital hydrocephalus, HME = hypoplastic anterior pituitary+missing stalk+ectopic posterior pituitary)
1B.3a.4		associated with prenatal infections
1B.3a.9		Idiopathic GHD
	1B.3a.9a	'classical' idiopathic GHD
	1B.3a.9b	GH neurosecretory dysfunction
1B.3b		acquired GHD
	1B.3b.1	-craniopharyngioma
	1B.3b.2	-other pituitary tumors
	1B.3b.3	-cranial tumors distant to pituitary
	1B.3b.4	-tumors outside the cranium
	1B.3b.5	-head trauma
	1B.3b.6	-CNS infection
	1B.3b.7	-granulomatous disease
	1B.3b.8	-vascular anomaly

Table 1. Continued

ESPE code		Diagnosis
1B.4		other disorders of GH-IGF axis (primary IGF-1 deficiency and resistance)
	1B.4a	bio-inactive GH
	1B.4b	anomalies of GH receptor
	1B.4c	anomalies of GH signal transduction
	1B.4d	ALS deficiency
	1B.4e	IGF-1 deficiency
	1B.4f	IGF-1 resistance (IGF-1R defect, postreceptor defect)
	1B.4z	other disorders
		other causes of disorders of the GH-IGF axis
1B.5		endocrine disorders
1B.6		metabolic disorders
1B.7		psychosocial disorders
1B.8		iatrogenic

The problem faced by the clinician in diagnosing GHD has been examined from different levels [3–8].

1 The first difficulty is in defining the diagnostic entrance criteria in such a way that the secondary diagnostic steps can thereby be justified and not excluded. If very stringent criteria (e.g. cut-offs) are a constituent part of the initial diagnostic steps, some individuals may possibly be excluded from the further work-up. This is an error of the first order (although the patient is affected, she/he is defined as healthy). On the other hand, the criteria must be chosen in such a way as to avoid an error of the second order (the individual is considered sick, and therefore subjected to further – possibly unnecessary – diagnostic procedures; however, she/he is in fact healthy).

2 In a second step, proof of an impairment in GH secretion must be obtained. The strain on the patient, arising from the scope of the diagnostic procedure, should be limited and errors of the first or second order should be minimized.

3 In a third step, techniques to define the causes of impaired GH secretion need to be applied.

4 Finally, there is the question about whether the altered signs and symptoms resulting from the normalization of GH through replacement therapy can be used to confirm or refute the diagnosis of GH impairment, and thus become part of a 'secondary' diagnostic step [9, 10].

Table 2. Criteria for estimating the likelihood of GHD before GH testing

	Congenital GHD infancy		Congenital GHD childhood		Acquired GHD	
	likely	less likely	likely	less likely	likely	less likely
Perinatal history	hypoglycemia ikterus prolonged traumatic birth family history of GHD		hypoglycemia ikterus prolonged traumatic birth family history of GHD		head trauma postmalignancy neurosurgery meningitis	
Phenotype	doll-like		n.r.		n.r.	
Age, years	n.r.			m > 12 f > 10	n.r.	
Ht	n.r.		<-2.5 SDS	>-2.0 SDS	n.r.	
Ht - MPH	n.r.		>-1.3 SDS	<-1.3 SDS	n.r.	
Wt		Wt SDS < < Ht SDS	Wt SDS - Ht SDS > + 1.0	Wt SDS < < Ht SDS		Wt SDS < < Ht SDS
Ht velocity	<-1.0 SDS	>-1.0 SDS	<-1.0 SDS	>0.0 SDS	<-1.0 SDS	>0.0 SDS
Bone age, years	n.r.		CA-BA >> 1 .0	BA > = CA	n.r.	
Head circumference (HC)		<-2.0 SDS	n.r	Ht SDS – HC SDS	n.r.	
Body proportions	n.r.			SH SDS > > Ht SDS	n.r	
Other pituitary deficit	yes	n.r.	yes	n.r.	yes	no
IGF-1	<-1.0 SDS	>-1.0 SDS	<-2.0 SDS	>-1.0 SDS	<-2.0 SDS	>-1.0 SDS
IGFBP-3	<-2.0 SDS	>-1.0 SDS	<-2.0 SDS	>0.0 SDS	<-2.0 SDS	>0.0 SDS

BA = Bone age; CA = chronological age; GHD = growth hormone deficiency; HC = head circumference; Ht = height; MPH = mid-parental height; n.r. = not relevant; SDS = standard deviation score for CA; Wt = weight.

Considerations before GH Testing

Entrance Criteria

It is important to ensure that a combination of various anamnestic, auxological and biochemical information is available before GH testing is done in infants, children and adolescents with GHD, as this is crucial to establishing the diagnosis of GHD firmly (table 2). The proper classification of a disorder on the GH-IGF axis must be based on biochemical analyses (table 3).

Table 3. Pattern of biochemical findings in varying disorders of growth hormone deficiency (GHD) syndrome

Diagnosis (level of disorder)	GH (standard tests)	GH (GHRH test)	GH (spontaneous secretion)	IGF-1	IGFBP-3	Comment
Primary disorders of GH-IGF axis						
Disorders related to GH deficiency						
GH insufficiency (GH gene deletion)	↓	↓	↓	↓	↓	potentially growth-inhibiting GH-ABs to GH treatment
GH insufficiency (pituitary level)	↓	↓/n	↓	↓	↓	growth response to GH therapy
GH insufficiency (hypothalamic level)	↓	n	↓/n	↓	↓	therapy with GHRH possible
GH insufficiency (bioinactive GH)	n	n	n	↓	↓	growth response to GH therapy
GH insufficiency (neurosecretory dysfunction)	n	↓/n	↓	↓	↓/n	growth response to GH therapy
Disorders related to impaired action of GH or IGF						
GHBP excess/ antiGH ABs	↑	↑	↑	n/↓	n/↓	GHBP measurement, IGF generation test growth improves with exogenous GH
States of congenital GH impaired IGF-1 generation (primary IGF deficiency)	↑	↑	↑	↓	↓	therapy with IGF-1 possible
Primary IGF resistance (IGF receptor/post-receptor defect)	↑	↑	↑	↑	↑	no therapy known to date
Secondary disorders of GH-IGF axis						
Acquired inhibition of IGF-1 action (e.g. IGFBP excess in chronic renal failure) (CRF)	↑/n	↑/n	↑/n	↓/n	↑	growth improves with exogenous GH
Hyperalimentation	↓n	↓	↓	n/?	n	tall stature

Table 3. Continued

Diagnosis (level of disorder)	GH (standard tests)	GH (GHRH test)	GH (spontaneous secretion)	IGF-1	IGFBP-3	Comment
Hypercortisolism, hypothyroidism	↓	↓	↓	↓/n	n	no therapy with GH
Diabetes mellitus, fasting, hepatopathy	↑	↑	↑	↓	↓	

n = Normal; ↑ = increased; ↓ = diminished.

History

Genetic forms of isolated or combined GHD are rare and only occur in about 3% of cases [11, 12]. Thus, in addition to measuring height in both parents, a detailed family history needs to be recorded. Other historical events, such as head trauma [13] or treatment for malignancies [14, 15] are also strong indicators of GHD in a short child.

Perinatal History and Signs

In the early years of research on GHD, it was observed that a high proportion of affected children were delivered vaginally and in a breech position [16]. Whether GHD is caused by a trauma possibly occurring during such a delivery has yet to be clarified. Evidence has also to be found for pituitary defects in the fetus which possibly led to a breech position. It is standard practice to perform a caesarean section in most cases in which an unfavorable presentation at birth is apparent. Nevertheless, a head trauma during delivery may cause pituitary damage similar to postnatal head trauma [13].

A small penis and bilateral undescended testes can be an indication of insufficient fetal exposure to gonadotrophins/testosterone in males. This may be associated with GHD. Prolonged jaundice may also be a symptom of GHD combined with hypocortisolism [17]. Hypoglycemia may occur in congenital GHD [18]; however, it is not clear whether this is possibly the result of isolated GHD or, instead, of GHD combined with other pituitary defects. In these instances GHD can be suspected even if small body size (length) is not a presenting symptom.

Phenotypic Appearance

Children with severe GHD have a relatively large neurocranium in relation to the mid-facial region. This gives them a typical 'doll-like' appearance. Head circumference is about 2 SDS above height SDS [19]; thus, microcephaly is a very unlikely feature of GHD. Typical characteristics include small hands and feet and a less mature voice, and the overall appearance does not correspond with age. Frequently, however, the appearance of children with GH is not conspicuous.

Anthropometric Symptoms at Presentation

The most frequent sign of GHD in a child is height development [20, 21]. Short stature is defined as height/length below the 3rd centile for age. Children with GHD are less likely to present with a height of >–2.5 SDS [22]. In addition, the child's height/length needs to be examined in relation to parental height [23]. It is uncommon for a child's height to be within the range of the reference population but outside the target range for the parents (roughly: height SDS minus MPH SDS <–1.3 SDS), and further diagnostics are required to identify GHD. Since shortness in children with GHD is proportional (sitting height and arm span deviate to the same degree as does height), these anthropometrical parameters need to be documented and compared with appropriate references.

Another important aspect to consider is height within the context of delayed puberty [24], as this is an explicit indicator of GHD. The height of children with pubertal age but prepubertal stage may be compared with extrapolated references based on the ICP model devised previously [25–27].

Since growth is not static, like height, but takes place in a dynamic process, height velocity is considered the more appropriate parameter for defining abnormal growth. Duche et al. [8] observed a sensitivity of 92%, with a specificity of 72%, in diagnosing GHD by combining a height velocity of <–1.0 SDS with an IGF-1 SDS of <–2.0 SDS. However, the difficulty in applying height velocity is that two measurements must be taken at appropriate intervals in order to obtain an exact calculation. The time frame for the two measurements must include a stage of height velocity (the lower, the longer) and the calculation depends on the precision of the measuring device. Usually, data relating to 6 (infancy) to 12 (childhood) consecutive months are needed to establish accurate height velocity. If the diagnosis of GHD is likely in a given child, the diagnostic (therapeutic) process should not be delayed for the sake of height velocity, whereas a delay would be justified if the diagnosis of GHD is less likely. The question about which limits should be considered as abnormal in a short child is still controversial. A child with normal size at birth, who however grows slowly, will obviously have short stature. It is not clear what height velocity can be expected once height is below the normal range. If growth dynamics are expressed in terms of delta height (SDS), then a value below –0.5 SDS is congruent with normal variation. If growth dynamics are expressed in terms of height velocity (cm/year), then a value above the 25th centile for age (equal to approximately –1.0 SDS) is not very likely in a child with GHD, and a value above the 50th centile for age (approximately –0.0 SDS) is highly unlikely in GHD. In children at pubertal age but delayed puberty, special references need to be considered [28].

It is a common assumption that bone age (BA) is delayed and BA progression is retarded in GHD. However, there is considerable overlap in normal or short non-

GHD children [29]. This may be due to the following reasons: (1) bone age determinations are prone to subjective error, (2) appropriate, contemporary references are usually not available, (3) there is a natural variation in BA at a given chronological age, and (4) bone age is not completely independent of height, with smaller children in an age cohort presenting with lower BA. Nevertheless, a bone age equivalent to or higher than chronological age is not likely in GHD.

In GHD, weight is typically not diminished to the same degree as is height [30] (weight SDS minus height SDS > +1.0 SDS). The children look relatively well-nourished. However, overt obesity is the exception in congenital GHD. Although the deficit in muscle mass and the relative abundance of subcutaneous fat can be documented in GHD by means of special techniques [31], body composition assessment is at present not considered to be a standard component in the diagnostics of short stature. The same is true for bone mass determinations [32]. Since these aspects are significant in treating patients with permanent GHD during the transition to adult age, it is probable that pediatric practices relating to diagnosis and follow-up will be adapted for adult care in future.

Biochemical Markers of GHD

It is a well-known fact that various circulating biochemical compounds depend on GH secretion. Indicators of bone growth (e.g. alkaline phosphatase) and collagen metabolism are low in GHD patients, but normalize during GH therapy [see also article by Crofton, this vol.]. Particular mention must be made of the GH-dependent factors in the IGF system (e.g. IGF-1, IGFBP-3) whose role in the diagnostics of GHD in children and adults has been a controversial matter for the past few decades. The main issues pertain to the partial effects of both GH and IGF-1 at the sites of growth as well as to the relevance of circulating IGF-1 during growth [33–35]. A more specific discussion focused on the diagnostic role of IGF-1 (and IGFBP-3) blood levels in GHD. IGF measurements are advantageous because they can easily be obtained from a single sample; in addition, reference levels for children and adolescents are available [see chapter by Blum]. It must be remembered that this debate on the diagnostic role of IGFs is related to the fact that a 'golden standard' for establishing the diagnosis of GHD does not exist. Authors have associated the diagnosis of GHD with the degree of sensitivity and specificity of IGF-1 (IGFBP-3) by means of their own definitions and diagnostic settings [36]. Interim conclusions show that low levels (in relation to age and sex) of IGF-1 (IGFBP-3) support the diagnosis of GHD, whereas normal levels (e.g. IGF-1 > –1.0 SDS; IGFBP-3 > 0.0 SDS) do not [37, 38] (table 2). Thus, IGF measurements have become an essential part of the work-up for GHD.

Pituitary Imaging

Special cerebral imaging techniques, such as computed tomography (CT) and magnetic resonance imaging (MRI) were conventionally done after the diagnosis of GHD was established, with the aim of ascertaining the cause of GHD. A high frequency of abnormalities in the hypothalamus-pituitary region was documented by means of MRI in children with GHD [39]. A strong but not definite indicator of GHD could be an impairment in the size of the anterior pituitary, if MRI shows no evidence of a structural abnormality in the pituitary region [40]. The ready accessibility of imaging tools has led to a growing demand for techniques providing immediate results; however, although these methods are non-invasive, they are not necessarily suitable for examining younger children. In addition, operating the equipment and interpreting the results require considerable skill. A simple X-ray may often be more helpful in the further diagnostics of short stature in a child; e.g. calcifications in the pituitary region have explained 90% of craniopharyngioma cases.

Growth Hormone

Natural Variation of GH Molecules
GH is the gene product of the GH-N gene which is primarily expressed in the somatotrophs of the pituitary but also, to a lesser degree, in other tissues [41, 42]. The major gene product (approximately 80–90%) is a peptide hormone of 191 amino acids (size 22 kDa); however, due to alternative splicing, a shorter form (lacking amino acids 32–46; size 20 kDa) is also produced, which accounts for 10–20%. Shorter and larger forms are also formed in the circulation, either by means of proteolytic fragmentation or as a result of an association of forms of GH. Thus, there is not only one natural GH, and the circulating amount of the different components may depend on their production, metabolic circumstances and varying degrees of degradation [43]. In the human placenta, a GH-variant gene (GH-V) is expressed. Since three different variants of the GH receptor exist, which, through conformational changes during GH binding, transmit signals to the target cell [44], it is conceivable that the different forms of circulating GH exert different effects [45]. GH forms also vary, depending on GH-secretory stimuli [46].

GH-Binding Protein
There is an additional level of complexity arising from the fact that the external part of the GH receptor can be cleaved into the circulation by proteolysis and can bind GH [47]. It is assumed that up to 50% of circulating GH is complexed to this GH-binding protein (GHBP) [48, 49]. GHBP prolongs the half-life of GH by protecting it from degradation. The GH-GHBP complex is a hormone reservoir. Several reports refer to immunometrical assays used to determine GHBP [50–53]. The assays have not been standardized, and there is no international reference preparation available for GHBP. However, measurements in normal adults show that serum GHBP are relatively constant (ranging between approximately 0.5 to 3.8 nmol/l) and correlate positively with BMI and negatively with age.

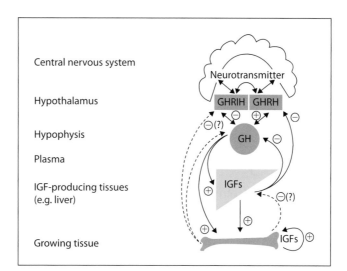

Fig. 1. Model of the GH regulatory system.

GHBP levels are low during fetal life, rise in the first years after birth and thereafter achieve adult levels [54–57]. The levels also correlate with BMI and are thought to reflect the individual sensitivity to GH [54]. In patients with primary IGF deficiency, GHBP is absent/diminished in serum [58] due to a defect in the extracellular domain of the GH receptor (GH resistance of the Laron syndrome type). On the other hand, GH action can be demonstrated by the excess of GHBP [59, 60]. It is probably relevant to measure GH if GHBP is absent [61] in these and other specific situations.

Both GHBP and human antibodies (AB) to GH in the circulation may affect the reading of GH in an immunoassay. Human anti-GH AB bind part of the labeled GH within the assay, and the amount of label bound to the non-human AB of the assay will be low. Falsely high or low GH levels are a result of AB being label-free or bound to non-human AB, e.g. excess GHBP in a RIA or the presence of high-affinity human anti-GH AB would cause inappropriately high GH readings [62].

Regulation of GH Secretion

The mechanisms of GH release are complex. The interested reader is referred to reviews of this rapidly evolving field for more details [63–66]. A brief summary of the mechanisms involved will be given here. The major components of GH regulation are growth hormone-releasing hormone (GHRH), which is stimulatory, and growth hormone release-inhibiting hormone (GHRIH), also referred to as somatostatin, which inhibits the pituitary somatotrophs (fig. 1). The site of GHRH production is predominantly in the arcuate nucleus. GHRH binds to a G-protein-coupled receptor at the surface of the somatotrophs. The production of GHRIH occurs predominantly in the paraventricular nucleus of the hypothalamus. Recently, another peptide, ghrelin, which is produced in the stomach as well as in the hypothalamus, was recognized to affect GH release. It acts via the growth hormone secretagogue receptor 1a (GHSR1a) located on the somatotrophs and serves as a link between food intake, GH secretion and energy metabolism [67].

The secretion of both hypothalamic hormones is regulated via a neuronal network involving complex, short and long loop feedback regulation at the neuroendocrine levels. A variety of neurotransmitter substances interact with specific receptors, exerting positive or negative effects at the sites of hypothalamic hormone production. The major receptor sites have binding properties for adrenergic, dopaminergic, serotoninergic, and cholinergic transmitter substances. A multitude of substances interact with these (and other) receptors in an agonistic or antagonistic mode. These events subsequently mediate the effects of GH secretion by changing the secretory levels of GHRH and/or GHRIH. There are also substances which act directly at the level of the somatotrophs. The pulsatile secretion of GH occurs as the consequence of all these interactions [68]. The neurotransmitter-modulated effects of a number of substances affecting GH release are listed in table 4. There are also other factors modulating GH secretion, of which sex steroids and – via feedback – IGF-1 are particularly significant [66, 69].

GH Measurement

Preanalytical Aspects
It is standard practice to measure GH in serum or plasma; however, urine [70] or dried full blood [71] may also be used. The stability of GH in vitro is considered to be quite good. Blood samples should be kept cool (refrigerated, not frozen!) until serum/plasma is separated (within a few hours). Serum samples remain stable for at least 24 h at room temperature [72, 73]. Frozen (<–20 °C) hGH remains stable over several months (or years).

GH Analyses/Methods
GH can be measured by means of various methods. In order to selectively measure the biologically relevant part of circulating GH, a radioreceptor assay (RRA) [74] and bioassay methods have been developed [75–79]. Although these technically sophisticated and exact methods are valuable research tools, they are not relevant to common clinical problems.

GH determinations in a clinical setting are done through immunoassays. The assay systems may differ according to three essential components: the antibodies against GH, the GH preparation used as a reference, and the indicator system. Antibodies determine the specificity and sensitivity of the assay, whereas the reference preparation determines the degree of quantitative agreement, and the indicator system may affect the sensitivity and practical aspects (e.g. speed plus automation equal 'high throughput') of the measurement.

Table 4. GH release as modulated by neurotransmitter systems

Stimulates GH release	Inhibits GH release
α-Receptor agonists	α-Receptor antagonists
Clonidine	Phentolamine
Arginine	
Ornithine	
Vasopressin	
Stress	
Exercise	
Hypoglycemia	
Glucagon	
Galanine	
L-Dopa	
β-Receptor antagonists	β-Receptor agonists
Propranolol	Salbutamol
Aminophylline	
Amphetamines	
Dopaminergic agonists	Dopaminergic antagonists
L-Dopa	Pimazide
Pyridostigmine	
Bromocriptine	
Apomorphine	
Serotoninergic agonists	Serotoninergic antagonists
L-Tryptophan	Methysergide
Sleep	Cyproheptadine

(a) Antibodies may be directed against multiple epitopes (polyclonal) or only one epitope (monoclonal) and may be directed against epitopes interacting with the GH receptor or against epitopes in other regions of the GH molecule. Historically, GH antibodies were generated by exposing animals (e.g. rabbits) with pituitary GH, thus the antibodies were polyclonal and directed against a number of epitopes. Subsequently, more specific polyclonal antibodies were developed by exposing animals only to 22 kDa hGH. More recently, however, monoclonal antibodies against specific epitopes have been generated. In addition to recognizing the full complement of hGH epitopes, polyclonal antibodies – despite lacking epitope specificity – often have the advantage of high affinity. Assays employing polyclonal antibodies result in higher readings of GH than assays employing monoclonal antibodies.

(b) Reference preparations have undergone considerable changes over the past decades. Initially, pituitary-derived hGH preparations were introduced (IRP 66/217; HS2243 E) which had a specific activity of 2 IU/mg. This was followed by pituitary hGH material (IRP 80/505) with a specific activity of 2.6 IU/mg. Subsequently, recombinant hGH with a specific activity of 3.0 IU/mg was employed in standard material (IRP 88/624; IRP 98/574). The results of GH measurements should be expressed in terms of μg/l.

(c) In the standard assays, GH in the sample or standard was labeled (e.g. with radioactive isotopes as in a radioimmunoassay; RIA) and competed with an antibody in the solution for binding sites. After reaching equilibrium (after >24 h), the bound and free label were separated and measured. The measured signal was inversely correlated to the amount of measured GH. In the modern, noncompetitive type of assay there is one fixed antibody for 'catching' hGH while a second antibody attaches to an indicator system. Such 'sandwich' systems allow higher sensitivity in determining hGH. The measured signal is also directly related to the amount of hormone in the sample. These assays are, however, not often in equilibrium, and are thus more sensitive to external influences (e.g. temperature, time). These novel assays enable automated and rapid measurement (within hours/minutes); they are not necessarily more economical than other assays but are possibly significant from a clinical perspective (e.g. intra-operative monitoring during neurosurgery). An 'immunofunctional' assay (IFA), i.e. an immunoassay with functional characteristics, can be developed by means of a selection of antibodies against epitopes which bind to the GH receptor [80, 81].

To date there is no definite consensus on how to measure hGH; however, several reports and recommendations are available in the literature [82–88]. The quality of commercially available assays varies widely, to the extent that the same assay sold in two different market areas by the same manufacturer could produce widely dissimilar results [88]. The minimum requirement recommended for achieving more uniform measurements involves the calibration of the assays against recombinant 22 kDa hGH (e.g. IRP 98/574) and the use of antibodies specifically directed against the 22 kDa form of hGH. Most assays are chosen by central laboratories on grounds of cost and technical aspects, and the treating physician or pediatrician cannot usually make decisions relating to this important diagnostic tool. Despite this, however, the treating physician must be knowledgeable about the chosen assay and its current components (e.g. change in antibodies, reference). In addition, it is essential to be updated regularly on quality schemes and their outcome. Pertinent information must also be forwarded by the laboratory carrying out the assay.

It is unlikely that a uniform methodology will develop in a competitive market, which makes it important to establish systems to (re-)measure hGH in relevant samples or calculate mathematical algorithms to equalize the differences between assays. Specimens of relevant samples should also be kept for a certain period of time to ensure that a central re-assessment can be done later, which may allow for more accurate classification of short children [89].

Testing for Impaired GH Secretion

Some researchers have argued against conducting GH tests for establishing the diagnosis of impaired GH secretion [90], and offer reasons ranging from the dangers involved to the lack of reproducibility and accuracy. They propose that, in addition to auxology, newer diagnostic tools, such as high-resolution neuroimaging, determinations of IGF parameters, and genetic tests, are making GH testing obsolete. It must be emphasized, however, that GHD is a diagnosis based on GH secretion and thus requires biochemical evidence that can only be gained by means of GH testing [5, 91–93].

Testing for impaired growth hormone secretion is mostly done in slowly growing children and/or children with short stature. Therefore, very little is known about GH responsiveness to stimulatory procedures in normal children during the course of normal development. Considerable intraindividual variation was found in the magnitude of the GH response to various stimuli among tested individuals. With regard to the approach in which two test procedures are done [94], there is general consensus on how the diagnosis of impaired GH secretion is established, namely, that both tests must provide evidence of subnormal GH secretion. See 'Appendix B' for recommendations on the diagnostic work-up.

It is a fundamental principle in medical diagnostics to confirm abnormal observations by conducting repeated investigations. Clearly, a single-test procedure to establish a diagnosis is a questionable approach. Usually, single tests are done after the diagnosis has been established and data on the patient's growth response to GH therapy has been documented.

The test results depend on the cut-off point set for the maximum GH level, which is chosen a priori, and the diagnosis of GHD may thus be confirmed or even incorrectly rejected. In fact, an approach using a fixed cut-off level is in itself incorrect because GHD is perceived as a continuum with a blurred upper border. This limit may vary, depending on specific patient characteristics (e.g. age, sex or puberty) and the GH stimulatory strength of the agent employed. It must also be noted that damage to the GH secretory system may lead to progressive deterioration in the GH secretory capacity of patients. This, in turn, may lead to abnormal test results even if prior tests proved normal. Despite these constraints, testing for GHD continues to be good medical practice in the hands of experienced physicians.

Preparation for Testing

Possible external influences on the results can be reduced by standardizing the test conditions. Interpretation of results in a given clinical unit is probably best done by adhering to standard procedures and we and many others carry out standard tests only in the morning (08:30–10:00 a.m.) after overnight fasting (water ad libitum).

The patient is kept in a supine position and a plastic cannula is inserted into a vein at least 30 min before the test. The vein is kept open by means of a saline (never glucose!) solution. Stress should be kept to a minimum in order to avoid premature GH release, since this may deter the response to the test substance. Even if prior GH measurements exceeded the cut-off levels, it is still possible to carry out tests with the aim of excluding GHD. We are convinced that standardization cannot be achieved if the patient arrives on the morning of the test instead of on the previous evening, during which time s/he can become familiar with the facilities and the cannula can be inserted. The sequential application of two standard tests within 24 h is also not advisable* since stimulation may effect the hypothalamus-pituitary regulation and the composition of GH isoforms [9].

Test Procedures

A number of procedures have been described for testing GH stimulation. The results of a recent pharmaco-epidemiological survey [95] based on 87,000 tests showed the following distribution: arginine (24.1%), insulin (24.1%), clonidine (13.3%); L-dopa (9.5%), GHRH (4.5%), glucagon (3.9%), ornithine (3.0%), propranolol-glucagon (2.5%) and others (4.2%). Spontaneous GH secretion was tested in 9.9% to evaluate the GH secretory capacity [see chapter by Albertsson-Wikland, this vol.]. It is interesting to note that the frequency of tests varied according to countries, e.g. a US survey [96] showed that the most widely used tests were (in order of frequency): clonidine, L-dopa, arginine, and insulin-induced hypoglycemia, whereas spontaneous GH secretion was the most common procedure in Sweden and is considered equivalent to a standard GH test. In order to create an optimal setting and conduct two tests within a short time, the author hospitalized patients (accompanied by parent(s) if age <10 years) in the afternoon, and did an overnight analysis of spontaneous GH secretion followed by a standard stimulation test in the morning. As mentioned above, two GH tests are recommended for confirming the diagnosis of GHD. In a published analysis of an international survey of 3,896 children with GHD [97], it was reported that 36 different test combinations were used, among them arginine plus insulin (21%); insulin plus arginine (10%), arginine plus clonidine (4%); arginine plus sleep (4%); insulin plus clonidine (4%); and clonidine plus insulin (4%). However, to the knowledge of the author there is no reason not to repeat the same test on another occasion.

The response variable for interpreting the test results is usually the maximum GH level recorded. Over the past decades, the cut-off limit indicating impaired GH secretion has been raised from 5 to 10 µg/l. At present, some investigators use the term 'severe' GHD to refer to GH levels below 5 µg/l and 'less severe' GHD if the levels range between 5 and 10 µg/l. The author is unaware of empirical evidence to support such categorization. It can be speculated that the present cut-off of 10 µg/l resulted from translating 20 mIU/l – which corresponded to 10 µg/l at a time when GH was measured by means of a RIA calibrated against pituitary GH – into present times, although more specific sandwich assays, calibrated against 22 kD rhGH, are currently used to determine GH. Thus, a case can be made for a cut-off limit below 10 µg/l (e.g. 8.0 µg/l [98] for standard GH provocation tests – spontaneous GH secretion and GHRH tests excluded). It needs to be remembered, however, that an absolute limit to differentiate adequate from inadequate GHD in a single sample does not exist since several factors could affect the test results, e.g. the patient's age, sex, weight, pubertal status, the pulsatility of spontaneous GH secretion, the stimulatory potency of the test substances and the method of measurement. The list of tests described in this chapter is therefore not exhaustive.

Specific (Standard) Test Procedures
Physical Exercise
Exercise has long been shown to stimulate GH release. Systematic studies in both adults and children have shown that physical exercise is a suitable physiological method for testing GH secretion capacity [99–101]. The mechanisms involved in provoking GH secretion are not fully understood [102]. It is assumed that adrenergic mechanisms play a role, since exercise-induced GH release can be enhanced by pre-treatment with a β-receptor antagonist and, conversely, diminished by an α-receptor antagonist. The degree of physical fitness affects GH release induced through exercise in adults. Whether this also applies to children has yet to be clarified. Table 5 lists the recommended test procedures. Various approaches are taken by investigators to exert the necessary submaximal physical stress, since strenuous exercise in young children may involve practical problems.

The latency between exercise start and the peaking of GH depended on the patient's fitness level. Most frequently, the peak was observed 15–20 min after the test began. In about 70% of non-GHD patients, GH levels of >10 µg/l were observed. In a comparison of 47 small children with normal growth versus 30 children with GHD, in which a treadmill exhausting test was carried out, Donaubauer et al. [103] observed a sensitivity of 90%, with a specificity of only 11%. Although the exercise test has low positive predictive value, it is a safe and inexpensive screening procedure. The exercise test was re-evaluated in children with normal stature [104, 105] and normative data are listed in tables 4 and 5.

Arginine Tolerance Test/Ornithine Tolerance Test
The injection of various amino acids (e.g. ornithine, arginine) is followed by an increase in circulating GH levels. Merimee et al. [106] and Parker et al. [107] were the first to formally investigate the effects of arginine on GH release in children. Arginine stimulates GH secretion via α-adrenergic receptors and subsequent GHRH release.

Table 5. GH stimulation tests

Stimulus	Dosage and procedure	Sampling for GH (min)
Exercise	forced climbing of steps cycle ergometer, 2 W/kg BW (10 min)	0, 15–20 after start
Arginine HCl	0.5 g/kg BW (max. 30 g) (infused i.v. 10% arginine HCl in 0.9% NaCl at a constant rate over 30 min)	−30, 0, 15, 30, 45, 60, 90, 120
Ornithine HCl	12 g/m^2 BSA (infused i.v. 6.25% ornithine HCl in 0.9% NaCl at a constant rate over 30 min)	−30, 0, 15, 30, 45, 60, 90, 120
Insulin (regular)	0.1–0.05 IU/kg BW i.v.	−30, 0 15, 30, 45, 60, 90, 120
Arginine-HCl -insulin	see arginine test (insulin is injected (see above) 60 min after administration of arginine)	−30, 0, 15, 30, 45, 60, 80, 90, 105, 120, 150
Clonidine (2-[2.6-dichlorphenyl]-amino-2-imidazoline)	0.15 mg/m^2 BSA orally	−30, 0, 30, 60, 90, 120, 150
Glucagon	0.1 mg/kg BW (i.m. or s.c.) (may be combined with propranolol, 0.75 mg/kg BW orally 2 h before glucagon)	−30, 0, 60, 90, 120, 150, 180
L-Dopa (L-3,4-dihydroxyphenylalanine)	<15 kg BW: 125 mg <35 kg BW: 250 mg >35 kg BW: 500 mg (taken orally)	−30, 0, 30, 60, 90, 120
GHRH (1-40) (1-44) (1-29)NH$_2$	1 µg/kg BW i.v. bolus	−30, 0, 15, 30, 45, 60, 90, 120

BW = Body weight; BSA = body surface area.

The test procedure is listed in table 5. Usually, the peak GH level is reached about 60 min after the arginine infusion starts. Some authors doubt that sampling exceeding 90 min is meaningful as no further essential data is thereby gained [108, 109]. The mean peak GH levels observed in arginine tests of healthy subjects range from 14 to 26 µg/l. The arginine test was re-evaluated in children with normal stature [104, 105, 110], and normative data are listed in tables 6 and 7. The accuracy of a single test in positively predicting GHD ranges between 86% (at a cut-off level of 3 µg/l) and 75% (at a cut-off level of 10 µg/l). The test has practically no side-effects and also allows an assessment of the secretory capacity of insulin and glucagon.

Insulin Tolerance Test (ITT)

Insulin-induced hypoglycemia induces GH release [111]. The effects are complex and involve both the suppression of GHRIH as well as mechanisms that can be suppressed by blocking α-adrenergic receptors (e.g. a phentolamine). A decrease of at least 30 mg/dl (1.7 mmol/l) from basal glucose levels is required to provoke GH release. It is generally recommended that a 50% decline from the basal glucose level be taken as the prerequisite for a proper stimulus. The test methods are listed in table 5.

While the nadir of glucose is usually observed after 15–30 min, maximal GH levels are seen after about 60 min in the majority of cases [112]. In normal children, mean peak levels of GH, ranging between 12 and 20 µg/l, were observed and there is a trend toward higher levels during puberty. The test is sensitive to weight, and lower levels are recorded in obese children [113]. Data on the GH response to insulin-induced hypoglycemia in children with normal stature are still limited [110, 114, 115] (table 6). The accuracy of a single test in positively predicting GHD ranges between 100% (at a cut-off level of 3 µg/l) and 85% (at a cut-off level of 10 µg/l). The test also allows evaluation of the secretory capacity of cortisol, glucagon and epinephrine. However, its value in assessing adrenal function has been questioned. The glucagon test (see below) could be used as a substitute for the ITT in evaluating adrenal function [116].

The ITT may induce hypoglycemia and hypocaliemia with a clear clinical correlate. However, particularly in children with GHD, hypoglycemia may occur without any symptoms. Due to its potentially life-threatening risk [117, 118] the ITT has been prohibited in some countries. On the other hand, the ITT is used as the main reference method in adults and has also been considered safe in children [119]. Therefore, the test should only be performed when continuous observation by trained medical staff is guaranteed, including bedside monitoring of blood glucose, and emergency treatment with glucose solution (10–20%). The author applies the ITT only in adolescents (see Transition below). The measuring of GH levels after glucose rescue from hypoglycemia may be continued.

Combined Arginine and Insulin Tolerance Test (AITT)

It is possible to combine the ATT and the ITT and administer them sequentially [120] (table 5). The mean peak levels of the combined test range between 12 and 28 µg/l in normal children, and the accuracy of the test in positively predicting GHD is 100% at the cut-off level of 10 µg/l. The results are evidently equivalent to those of the two tests when performed separately. Any risks posed by the combined test are presumably the same as in an isolated ITT.

Clonidine Test

Clonidine, a selective α-receptor agonist, causes GH release via GHRH secretion. It has been widely used to test for GHD [121, 122]. The test procedures are listed in

Table 6. Maximum GH levels (µg/l) in children of normal height

Test	Pubertal stage	n	Mean ± SD	95% CI limit(upper-lower)
Exercise[a]	1	18	5.7 ± 4.1	23.1–0.7
	2	16	7.6 ± 4.6	24.1–1.6
	3	18	15.9 ± 8.5	49.3–3.5
	4	14	11.3 ± 7.5	33.7–7.5
	5	18	17.2 ± 14.7	91.0–1.4
Arginine-insulin[a]	1	18	4.3 ± 4.5	16.7–0.7
	2	16	7.2 ± 4.6	27.5–1.1
	3	18	10.5 ± 4.5	24.5–3.7
	4	14	19.6 ± 12.2	65.0–3.9
	5	18	26.2 ± 13.0	59.0–9.4
Clonidine[b]	all stages	66	21.0 ± 10.7	3.0–43
Male	1	12	16.9 ± 6.7	
Female	1	13	12.8 ± 5.1	
Male	2–3	10	17.8 ± 7.7	
Female	2–3	10	18.3 ± 9.0	
Male	4–5	10	26.5 ± 12.0	
Female	4–5	11	35.5 ± 5.1	
Arginine[b]	all stages	23	13.1 ± 6.1	2.6–27.0
Insulin[b]	all stages	19	14.2 ± 6.3	3.6–27.0

[a]Marin et al. [104]; RIA, polyclonal antibody to GH (Hazelton Biotechnologies, Vienna, Va., USA); standard?
[b]Zadik et al. [110]; RIA, polyclonal antibody; standard?

table 5. The GH response is dose dependent, and standard doses given to control groups of children showed mean maximum GH levels between 23 and 37 µg/l. The GH response is considerably higher than in tests with other stimuli, and each investigator should empirically determine the cut-off level for normal values.

The clonidine test was re-evaluated in children with normal stature [104, 105, 110] and normative data are listed in tables 6 and 7. The accuracy of a single test in positively predicting GHD is reportedly 80%, at a cut-off level of 10 µg/l. Since the known side effects include tiredness and a decrease in blood pressure, it is advisable to monitor blood pressure up to 30 min after it normalizes.

Table 7. Peak GH response of children with normal stature to various stimuli [105]

	Exercise	IIH	Arginine	Clonidine
n (M/F)	33 (20/13)	59 (42/17)	79 (46/23)	69 (46/23)
Peak GH, μg/l, mean (SEM)	12.7 (1.1)	13.2 (1.2)	16.7 (1.2)	13.1 (1.8)
2.5–97.5th centile	3.8–23.7	4.1–42.1	4.4–45.5	4.5–56.5
	L-dopa	glucagon	pyridostigmine	
n (M/F)	55 (36/19)	40 (25/15)	53 (37/16)	
Peak GH, μg/l, mean (SEM)	13.0 (1.1)	16.9 (1.9)	13.5 (1.0)	
2.5–97.5th centile	2.8–34.6	3.1–39.0	3.7–33.5	
	GHRH	PD+GHRH	ARG+GHRH	
n (M/F)	134 (93/41)	94 (63/31)	81 (53/28)	
Peak GH, μg/l, mean (SEM)	28.8 (2.0)	47.8 (1.9)	61.8 (2.8)	
2.5–97.5th centile	4.2–89.3	22.6–90.0	22.4–107.8	

ARG = Arginine; PD = pyridostigmine; GHRH = GH-releasing hormone (hGH method: noncompetitive type IRMA (HGH-CPK, Sorin, Saluggia, Italy).

Glucagon Test

Glucagon exerts GH-stimulatory effects via α-adrenergic receptors, which can be further augmented by blocking β-receptors with propranolol [123, 124]. Sampling beyond 150 min does not lead to a gain in further information [125]. The test procedures are summarized in table 5. The highest GH levels observed in the majority of children in control groups occurred at about 120 min, and the mean response to glucagon appears to be somewhat higher than to arginine or insulin-induced hypoglycemia [105]. Intramuscular administration of glucagon could lead to nausea, vomiting, and abdominal pain.

L-Dopa Stimulation Test

The capacity of L-dopa to release GH was first observed in patients with Parkinson's disease. Weldon et al. [126] established L-dopa as part of the diagnostics of GHD. It stimulates GHRH release via an α-adrenergic mechanism and also inhibits the GH secretion mediated by β-adrenergic receptors, an effect which can be blocked by propranolol. The peak response of GH varies widely (30–120 min), with mean peak levels in control groups of children ranging from 11 to 21 μg/l. Normative data are listed in table 7 [105]. Detailed studies on the influence of age and sex on test results are not available. The accuracy of a single test in positively predicting GHD ranges between 81% (cut-off = 6 µg/l) and 56% (cut-off = 7 µg/l). In about one-third of the patients, nausea was reported, and, less frequently, vomiting, vertigo, fatigue and headache.

Testing with GHRH

The availability of biosynthetic GHRH had led to this hormone being extensively used as a test agent (for a review, see Ranke et al. [127]). Three different analogues of GHRH are marketed: GHRH (1–40), GHRH (1–44) and GHRH (1–29) NH_2, and tests containing these peptides have shown equivalent stimulatory potency (table 7). The magnitude of the acute response of GH to GHRH is dose dependent. Although the dosages differ with respect to the molar amounts, if given on an identical weight basis, the maximum response is probably reached at a dosage of 1 µg/kg BW i.v. given as a bolus (within 1 min).

The timing of the test – morning versus afternoon – is possibly relevant to the magnitude of the observed response; however, many investigators carry out the test in the morning, following overnight fasting. The chosen response variable is usually the maximum GH level at any time point. The magnitude of the GH response to GHRH appears to be influenced by sex differences and pubertal development, but to a lesser degree than in tests using other stimulators (e.g. arginine). In normal children, the maximum is generally reached within 30 min. after the injection, while in GHD patients it is reached later (approximately 45+ min). Normative data are given in table 7 [105]. We tested 86 children without GHD by applying GHRH (1–29) NH_2 and the GH peaks exceeded 10 µg/l, whereas in 45 children with GHD the levels were below 20 µg/l.

Depending on the chosen cut-off limit for normal values as well as the cohorts tested in comparison, a single GHRH test can confirm or refute the diagnosis of GHD established by other methods (table 7). Brook et al. [128] suggest that it is easier to differentiate between normal subjects and those with GHD if the blood sampling is done within minutes after GHRH is administered. In general, less-pronounced results are found in children with organic causes of GHD affecting the pituitary in comparison to those with idiopathic GHD of potentially hypothalamic origin. If a maximum GH level of 7–10 ng/ml is used as the cut-off limit, the specificity of the GHRH test is >95%, while the sensitivity is about 30%. Thus, a subnormal response is likely to indicate GHD, while a 'normal' (10–20 µg/l) response does not exclude GHD. Since the predictive value of GHRH testing, i.e. to correctly identify patients with GHD, is low, according to most investigators, the test is primarily used to determine the cause of GHD (pituitary versus hypothalamic), rather than as a diagnostic test. If GHD is established by other methods and GHRH is administered over a period of time, the diagnosis of hypothalamic GHD is assumed when the response to a single bolus of GHRH exceeds normal levels (cut-offs). Whether the GHRH test or a normal growth response to long-term treatment with GHRH should be taken to define hypothalamic GHD still remains an unresolved issue.

Combined Arginine plus GHRH Test

The combination of arginine and GHRH to provoke GH secretion is based on their synergic action on somatotrophs. Arginine potentiates the effect of GHRH by reducing the inhibitory effect of somatostatin [129, 130]. In cases in which GHD of pituitary origin is suspected, the arginine GHRH test is now a standard procedure like the ITT [131]. The lower limit for normal values in healthy adults was reported to be 16 µg/l [132]. The diagnostic value is similar to the ITT, provided different cut-offs are chosen [133]. Since GHRH is not available in the USA, some investigators have made a case for glucagon as an alternative [134].

The combination of a GHRH bolus with an infusion of arginine HCl was evaluated [105] and the conclusion was reached that it was a potent and safe means to test GH secretion in children. The test is based on the somewhat different pathogenic mechanisms of both secretagogues (table 4) which lead to a higher GH peak than in traditional tests using a single agent (table 7). A study of normal, tall children by Ghigo et al. [105] showed that the lower limit of peak GH levels was 20 µg/l. Keller et al. [135] retested 30 children with proven GHD (maximum GH < 8.0 µg/l) by applying the arginine, ITT and arginine-GHRH test. The highest observed peaks were between 0.5 and 7.7 mg/l in the ITT; 1.0 and 7.8 mg/l in the arginine test and between 4.3 and 84.5 µg/l in the combined test. It was concluded that the arginine-GHRH test was an unsuitable primary diagnostic tool in children. Further investigations are necessary to re-assess the value of this test in children.

Combined Pyridostigmine plus GHRH Test

Since the anticholinesterase, pyridostigmine (PD), suppresses somatostatin, its combination with GHRH appears to be a very powerful means of testing the GH secretory capacity of the pituitary. Indeed, this combination has been exploited as a test in adults and in children [105, 129, 136–141]. Pyridostigmine is given orally in a dose of 60 mg, 60 min before administering GHRH (table 5). The lower limit of normal values in children is about 20 µg/l, which is similar to the combined arginine-GHRH test. Reference levels are listed in table 7. PD may cause nausea and longer-lasting atonia of the intestine, bladder and bronchial spasms. Anticholinergic substances (atropine) act as antidotes. The test has not gained much popularity in the work-up of children with short stature.

Growth Hormone-Releasing Peptides (GHRPs) and Ghrelin

Through the innovative work of Cyril Bowers and collaborators [142], it was discovered that a group of peptides – comprising the heptapeptide GHRP-1 and hexapeptides GHRP-2, GHRP-6, and hexarelin – have a high potency to release GH in human beings [143]. In addition, nonpeptidal substances were developed which elicit a GH-releasing effect through the specific receptor. Very recently [144], the natural ligand of the receptor for GH secretagogues – ghrelin – was isolated from the gut. These substances are highly potent in releasing GH from the pituitary [145]. This effect is partly mediated through GHRH and inhibited by somatostatin [146], with Ghrelin and GHRH acting synergistically. In adults with GH, Ghrelin has been effective in defining GHD of childhood onset. Its relevance as a diagnostic substance in paediatrics has not yet been established.

Special Diagnostic Situations

Priming with Sex Steroids before GH Testing
In a large proportion of prepubertal children with slow growth, subnormal GH levels (GH levels below cut-offs) were found during stimulation, even though they could not be diagnosed with GHD (GH levels above cut-offs) either by means of repeated testing or upon retesting at the time of puberty [147]. Since sex steroids (estrogens directly, testosterone by conversion to estrogen) cause an increase in GH secretion during puberty, it can be assumed that, by exposing prepubertal children with (near normal) pubertal age to sex steroids ('priming') GH release would be facilitated among non-GHD children. In these cases, a retesting would be unnecessary or a false classification would be avoided. In recent years, 'priming' in peri-pubertal children suspected of GHD has been conducted more frequently [148–153].

Several procedures have been suggested for 'priming': most common in boys is a testosterone depot preparation (e.g. 100 mg of testosterone depot), which is injected i.m. about a week (5–8 days) before a standard provocation test is done; in girls, estrogen is given in a less uniform mode, usually 3 days prior to testing. The type of estrogen may vary (e.g. 17β-estradiol, estradiol valerate, ethinyl estradial) as may the mode of application (orally, transdermally). The recommended doses tend to be equivalent to adult replacement doses. Estrogen may also be used for priming in prepubertal boys in the same way as in girls.

Marin et al. [104] compared the response to exercise and/or the arginine-insulin test, in 11 prepubertal children (both girls and boys) who had orally received 40 μg/m² BSA ethinyl estradiol 2 days prior to testing, with the response of 18 children who had received a placebo. They observed peak GH levels of 6.9 μg/l (95% CI limits, 20.3–1.9 μg/l) in the controls versus 18.7 μg/l (95% CI limits, 40.5–7.2 μg/l) in the treated group. Martinez et al. [154] gave micronized E2 (1 or 2 mg) or placebo, for 3 days to 15 children with GHD and 44 children with non-GHD short stature before a sequential arginine-clonidine test. After placebo, a cut-off limit of 3.7 μg/l (the lower 95% CI limit) resulted in 73% sensitivity, 95% specificity, and an overall 90% diagnostic efficiency. After estrogen, a cut-off limit of 8.3 μg/l resulted in a sensitivity of 87%, a specificity of 98%, and a diagnostic efficiency of 95%. Molina et al. [153] tested 8 females and 31 boys (aged 8–15 years) who had responded inadequately to a clonidine challenge after 3 days on estradiol valerate at a dose of 1 mg daily or testosterone enanthate (males) at 100 mg i.m. 5–8 days prior to GH stimulation. The GH response was higher in 21 out of 39 children (53.8%), rising to a level of >10 μg/l following priming with gonadal steroids. Coutant et al. [151] conducted a combined arginine-insulin test in 14 peri-pubertal boys, seven days after a single i.m. injection of testosterone (100 mg) and in 14 peri-pubertal girls after oral 17β-estradiol (2 mg once daily) for 3 days and observed an increase from about 10 to 20 μg/l in both sexes. Mueller et al. [150] conducted an arginine test in 26 boys with short stature who only showed early signs of puberty; and the findings failed to show an adequate response of serum GH in the first test after testosterone. In 77% (20/26 patients) the GH peak exceeded 10 μg/l.

Even though the rationale of this approach is beyond question, it should be remembered that, in the presence of sex steroids, higher cut-off levels than during prepuberty may have to be used to avoid misclassification (i.e. false non-GHD) in prepubertal children with GHD. However, since these procedures lacked general acceptance, they were not incorporated into the GRC recommendations [5]. In a recent study, Gonc et al. [155] showed that all 50 peri-pubertal boys, who showed sub cut-off GH levels before priming but levels higher than cut-offs after priming, spontaneously achieved normal height in the adult range. Thus, in short peri-pubertal children in whom isolated idiopathic GHD is suspected, priming with sex steroids is probably a proper method to avoid unnecessary treatment.

Transition from Adolescence to Adult Life

In recent years it has become evident that childhood-onset GHD may continue during adult life. This may not only occur in cases with organic GHD but also in 'idiopathic' GHD. At the same time, it is recognized that GH secretion follows a distinct pattern during the human life span: high GH levels but low GH sensitivity are found during neonatal life and infancy, low GH secretion but high GH sensitivity during childhood, high GH secretion with moderate GH sensitivity during puberty, and a continual decrease in GH secretion with steady GH sensitivity from early adulthood to senescence. Whereas impaired height growth is the leading symptom of GHD during childhood, completion and maintenance of normal body composition and functioning are the aims of GH treatment during adult life. Thus, when adult height is reached through pediatric GH treatment, the diagnosis of GHD must be confirmed before a decision to continue GH replacement in adulthood is made [95].

The biochemical definition of GHD during childhood and adult differs: a GH level of 7–10 μg/l during an ITT is an accepted cut-off in children; however, the cut-off limit in adult life is 3 μg/l [131]. It is a known fact that GH secretion during the late teens and the thirties is higher than in adult life but lower than in childhood and adolescence. Recommendations for appropriate ways of confirming GHD for the purpose of continuing GH replacement have been published [156]. The diagnostic algorithms are based on (a) information related to the likelihood of permanent GHD, (b) IGF-1 levels after discontinuation of GH, and finally (c) GH testing (table 8). A high likelihood of permanent GHD is assumed in young adults with: (a) severe GHD in childhood with or without two or three additional hormonal deficiencies, which may

Table 8. Diagnostic algorithm for confirmation of GHD during transition from adolescence to adult life (adapted from Clayton et al. [105])

GHD diagnosed in childhood; patient at end of growth and puberty			
Discontinue GH treatment for at least 4 weeks			
A priori likelihood of GHD	Serum IGF-1 measurement	GH test	Interpretation
High	<-2.0 SDS	no GH testing	GHD confirmed
High	>-2.0 SDS	GH low	GHD confirmed
High	>-2.0 SDS	GH normal	GHD unlikely
Low	<-2.0 SDS	GH low	GHD confirmed
Low	<-2.0 SDS	GH normal	follow-up
Low	>-2.0 SDS	GH low	follow-up
Low	>-2.0 SDS	GH normal	GHD unlikely

be due to a defined genetic cause, (b) severe GHD due to structural hypothalamic-pituitary abnormalities, (c) central nervous system (CNS) tumors, or (d) a history of high-dose cranial irradiation. Less likelihood is assumed in the remaining patients, including those with idiopathic GHD, either isolated or with one additional hormonal deficiency.

In the event that re-testing is required, it is recommended that GH replacement is interrupted for at least 4 weeks. Additional pituitary deficits should be treated (as in childhood, e.g. thyroxin 100 $\mu g/m^2$ day; hydrocortisone 8–12 mg/m^2 day). The GH tests suitable for this transitional phase is still a matter of debate as is the question about who should do the testing and evaluation. Structured strategies should be established for ensuring the proper transition of care from pediatric to adult endocrinologists. Most experts favor tests that are relevant to the diagnosis of GHD during adult life as against those commonly done in pediatrics [157]. If the ITT is chosen, 5–6 $\mu g/l$ is considered an appropriate cut-off level [158, 159]. In the case of an arginine-GHRH test, the cut-off limit of 19 $\mu g/l$ is considered appropriate [160, 161].

The decision to re-confirm the diagnosis may also be made at the time of puberty in patients less likely to have permanent GHD. Zucchini et al. [162] re-evaluated 69 subjects (40 male, 29 female) who were diagnosed with isolated GHD before puberty, by means of arginine and L-dopa tests; and the same tests were repeated after at least 2 years of therapy and following puberty onset. If the re-tested peak GH levels were higher than 10 $\mu g/l$, therapy was discontinued. The termination of GH therapy after re-testing these patients did not lead to catch-down growth, and the adult height they achieved was similar to that in GHD subjects treated up to adult height.

GHD after Treatment for Malignancies

GHD in combination with other pituitary hormonal defects are very likely in children who grow poorly after undergoing surgery in the pituitary region on grounds of a malignancy or a nonmalignant disorder such as craniopharyngioma. In some cases, however, normal growth without GH treatment has been observed. After surgical treatment for craniopharyngioma, GHD can be expected in >90% of the patients [163]; however, diagnostic procedures must be done with caution in these patients.

Poor growth is also not an uncommon symptom in children treated for malignancies outside or inside the cranium but not directly involving the pituitary [15, 164]. Therapies for malignancies are complex and challenging and are often a combination of chemotherapy and X-ray therapy. Poor growth may thus result from the negative effects of therapy on the GH-IGF-axis, on the growing tissue, on nutrition and emotions – or from a combination of these factors. The negative effect of X-ray exposure on the hypothalamus-pituitary region depends on the dose and increases with time [165–167]. The mechanisms of functional and anatomical impairment involve damage to the GHRH-secreting neuron, the pituitary somatotrophs and the vascular system interconnecting the hypothalamus and pituitary. In order to distinguish the level(s) of a defect in its progression, several test methods may have to be applied in these patients [167–170] and there is controversy about which test to use [171]. The complexity of the situation can be seen in adults: in some patients, near-maximum compensatory overdrive of the partially-damaged somatotroph axis may result in near-normal quantitative restoration of spontaneous GH secretion, thus limiting further stimulation by means of the ITT, to the extent that impaired GH responses can be seen even before spontaneous GH secretion starts to decline [172].

After a defect in the complex neuroregulatory control of GH secretion was observed in CNS-irradiated humans and animals, it was hypothesized that a disorder in neurosecretion, GHND, caused short stature [173]; however, this situation is found when GH secretion to pharmacological stimuli is normal, but spontaneous GH secretion is not [174]. In addition to a history of CNS irradiation and poor growth, low IGF levels also indicate GHND. Apart from the poor growth following treatment for malignancies, the concept of GHND has been well accepted, and 'idiopathic' GHND is now diagnosed frequently. Although 'idiopathic' GHND may be 'overdiagnosed' [175], the author considers GHND as a truly existing form of GHD which can be confirmed by carefully done clinical and biochemical investigations.

Neonatal Period – Infancy

The criteria applicable to the diagnostics of GHD during the neonatal phase and in infancy are different from those applied during childhood (table 2). The levels of growth hormone and IGF parameters have been studied in normal children at birth and also during the neonatal period [176–178] [see also the chapters by Ogilvy-Stuart and Blum]. After birth, IGF-1 and IGFBP-3 levels are low and correlated positively with birth weight, while GH levels are higher at this time in comparison to later phases of life. GH levels fluctuate between about 5 and 50 μg/l on the first day of life, and, during the first week, between about 5 and 30 μg/l. Pulsatile GH secretion is observable during the first days of life; and a distinct increase of GH occurs after feeding, with a maximum being reached after about 60 min. There is also a sexual dimorphism, with the levels of IGF-1, IGFBP-3 and GH being slightly, but significantly higher in female neonates.

Even though GHD is congenital in a large number of children, the diagnosis is usually not made during infancy [179]. The reason for this is related to the fact that, unlike in the case of primary hypothyroidism or CAH, systematic screening for GHD is not done. Hypoglycemia, prolonged icterus and micropenis in boys are typical symptoms of congenital GHD. Serum levels of IGF-1 and IGFBP-3 below –2.0 SDS have been observed in most infants with GHD [180]. In the case of neonatal hypoglycemia, a counter-regulatory increase of GH would be expected in a healthy newborn. GH levels below 20 μg/l at the time of hypoglycemia are considered insufficient. In cases with suspected GHD, we carry out several GH (and blood glucose) measurements before and about 60 min after meals. GH levels that remain below 10 μg/l (with blood glucose in the normal range) indicate the likelihood of GHD. Although tests involving GHRH or glucagons can be carried out in newborns [181], the accurate interpretation of results remains unresolved. An ITT is not an appropriate method for determining GHD in infants.

Combined Pituitary Tests
It is obviously practical and economical to consider carrying out as many combined tests as possible when several pituitary hormonal deficiencies are suspected. On the other hand, it must be remembered that each test could possibly influence the other and thus confound the interpretation. It is probably most advisable to test each hormonal axis separately. Agents which negatively influence the release of GH should not be combined with GH stimulatory tests, e.g. ACTH, synacten or CRH should not be combined with a test of GH release. On the other hand, a test combining GnRH and/or TRH with arginine (ornithine) is common practice in the diagnostics of children and adolescents.

Conclusion

The measurement of GH in stimulatory tests continues to be a diagnostic cornerstone when it comes to establishing impaired GH secretion in a clinical setting. This is remarkable in view of the number of difficulties associated with GH testing. The practical advantages of such testing, however, will ensure that this course of action will continue in future, which is why it is important to keep the following aspects in mind before arriving at conclusions based on the findings:

1 Test procedures are, in general, not physiological.
2 The stimulatory potency of secretagogues varies.
3 The responsiveness to tests may be influenced by the age, sex, and pubertal stage of the patient.
4 The reproducibility of tests in the same patient is not very good (coefficients of variation between two tests may be less than 50%).
5 Truly normative data hardly exist.
6 The normal range of responses to stimuli is relatively broad.
7 Using a fixed GH level – cut-off point – to distinguish a normal from a subnormal response is, to a certain extent, arbitrary. In the light of new assay methods and reference preparations (see above), the general level of 10 μg/l is consider a standard cut-off (but not in tests involving GHRH!), but is probably too high and should, therefore, be re-evaluated.

Considering the complexity of the situation and the difficulties involved, it is very important that the investigator acquires as much experience as possible with a reasonable number of test procedures. Other methods [see Albertsson-Wikland and Rosberg, Blum, Mullis, this vol.] should also be considered, particularly when abnormalities on the GH axis are suspected on clinical and auxological grounds.

References

1 Wit JM, Ranke MB, Kelnar CJH: ESPE classification of pediatric endocrine diagnoses. Horm Res 2007;68 (suppl 2):1–120.

2 Rosenfeld RG: The IGF system: new developments relevant to pediatric practice. Endocr Dev 2005;9:1–10.

3 Rosenfeld RG, Albertsson-Wikland K, Cassorla F, Fraisier SD, Hasegawa, Y, Hintz RL, Lafranchi S, Lippe B, Loriaux L, Melmed S, Preece MA, Ranke MB, Reiter EO, Rogol AD, Underwood LE, Werther GA: Diagnostic controversy: the diagnosis of childhood growth hormone deficiency revisited. J Clin Endocrinol Metab 1995;80:1532–1540.

4 Shalet SM, Toogood A, Rahim A, Brennan BM: The diagnosis of growth hormone deficiency in children and adults. Endocr Rev 1998;19:203–223.

5 Growth Hormone Research Society: Consensus guidelines for the diagnosis and treatment of adults with growth hormone deficiency: summary statement of the Growth Hormone Research Society Workshop on adult growth hormone deficiency. J Clin Endocrinol Metab 1997;83:379–381.

6 Wilson DM, Frane J: A brief review of the use and utility of growth hormone stimulation testing in the NCGS: do we need to do provocative GH testing? Growth Horm IGF Res 2005;15(suppl A):S21–S25.

7 Richmond EJ, Rogol AD: Growth hormone deficiency in children. Pituitary 2008;11:115–120.

8 Duché L, Trivin C, Chemaitilly W, Souberbielle JC, Bréart G, Brauner R, Chalumeau M: Selecting short-statured children needing growth hormone testing: derivation and validation of a clinical decision rule. BMC Pediatr 2008;8:29.

9 Cole TJ, Hindmarsh PC, Dunger DB: Growth hormone (GH) provocation tests and the response to GH treatment in GH deficiency. Arch Dis Child 2004;89:1024–1027.

10 Chaler EA, Rivarola MA, Guerci B, Ciaccio M, Costanzo M, Travaglino P, Maceiras M, Pagani S, Meazza C, Bozzola E, Barberi S, Bozzola M, Belgorosky A: Differences in serum GH cut-off values for pharmacological tests of GH secretion depend on the serum GH method: clinical validation from the growth velocity score during the first year of treatment. Horm Res 2006;66:231–235.

11 Alatzoglou KS, Dattani MT: Genetic forms of hypopituitarism and their manifestation in the neonatal period. Early Hum Dev 2009;85:705–712.

12 Alatzoglou KS, Turton JP, Kelberman D, Clayton PE, Mehta A, Buchanan C, Aylwin S, Crowne EC, Christesen HT, Hertel NT, Trainer PJ, Savage MO, Raza J, Banerjee K, Sinha SK, Ten S, Mushtaq T, Brauner R, Cheetham TD, Hindmarsh PC, Mullis PE, Dattani MT: Expanding the spectrum of mutations in GH1 and GHRHR: genetic screening in a large cohort of patients with congenital isolated growth hormone deficiency. J Clin Endocrinol Metab 2009;94:3191–3199.

13 McDonald A, Lindell M, Dunger DB, Acerini CL: Traumatic brain injury is a rarely reported cause of growth hormone deficiency. J Pediatr 2008;152:590–593.

14 Mulder RL, Kremer LC, van Santen HM, Ket JL, van Trotsenburg AS, Koning CC, Schouten-van Meeteren AY, Caron HN, Neggers SJ, van Dalen EC: Prevalence and risk factors of radiation-induced growth hormone deficiency in childhood cancer survivors: a systematic review. Cancer Treat Rev 2009;35:616–632.

15 Haddy TB, Mosher RB, Nunez SB, Reaman GH: Growth hormone deficiency after chemotherapy for acute lymphoblastic leukemia in children who have not received cranial radiation. Pediatr Blood Cancer. 2006;46:258–261.

16 Bierich JR: Aetiology and pathogenesis of growth hormone deficiency. Baillieres Clin Endocrinol Metab 1992;6:491–511.

17 Binder G, Martin DD, Kanther I, Schwarze CP, Ranke MB: The course of neonatal cholestasis in congenital combined pituitary hormone deficiency. J Pediatr Endocrinol Metab 2007;20:695–702.

18 Bell JJ, August GP, Blethen SL, Baptista J: Neonatal hypoglycemia in a growth hormone registry: incidence and pathogenesis. J Pediatr Endocrinol Metab 2004;17:629–635.

19 Darendeliler F, Baş F, Gökçe M, Poyrazoğlu S, Sükür M, Bundak R, Saka N, Günöz H: The effect of growth hormone treatment on head circumference in growth hormone-deficient children. Turk J Pediatr 2008;50:331–335.

20 Grote FK, van Dommelen P, Oostdijk W, de Muinck Keizer-Schrama SM, Verkerk PH, Wit JM, van Buuren S: Developing evidence-based guidelines for referral for short stature. Arch Dis Child. 2008;93:212–217.

21 Grote FK, Oostdijk W, De Muinck Keizer-Schrama SM, van Dommelen P, van Buuren S, Dekker FW, Ketel AG, Moll HA, Wit JM: The diagnostic work up of growth failure in secondary health care; an evaluation of consensus guidelines. BMC Pediatr. 2008;8:21.

22 van Buuren S, van Dommelen P, Zandwijken GR, Grote FK, Wit JM, Verkerk PH: Towards evidence based referral criteria for growth monitoring. Arch Dis Child 2004;89:336–341.

23 Hermanussen M, Cole J: The calculation of target height reconsidered. Horm Res 2003;59:180–183.

24 Molinari L, Hermanussen M: The effect of variability in maturational tempo and midparent height on variability in linear body measurements. Ann Hum Biol 2005;32:679–682.

25 Karlberg J, Engström I, Karlberg P, Fryer JG: Analysis of linear growth using a mathematical model. I. From birth to three years. Acta Paediatr Scand 1987;76:478–488.

26 Ranke MB, Price DA, Albertsson-Wikland K, Maes M, Lindberg A: Factors determining pubertal growth and final height in growth hormone treatment of idiopathic growth hormone deficiency. Analysis of 195 Patients of the Kabi Pharmacia International Growth Study. Horm Res. 1997;48:62–71.

27 Lindberg A, Ranke MB: Data analysis within KIGS; in Ranke M, Price A, Reiter E (eds): Growth Hormone Therapy in Pediatrics – 20 Years of KIGS. Basel, Karger, 2007, pp 23–28.

28 Rikken B, Wit J: Prepubertal height velocity references over a wide age range. Arch Dis Child 1992;67:1277–1280.

29 Darendeliler F, Ranke MB, Bakker B, Lindberg A, Cowell CT, Albertsson-Wikland K, Reiter EO, Price DA: Bone age progression during the first year of growth hormone therapy in pre-pubertal children with idiopathic growth hormone deficiency, Turner syndrome or idiopathic short stature, and in short children born small for gestational age: analysis of data from KIGS (Pfizer International Growth Database). Horm Res 2005;63:40–47.

30 Ranke MB, Reiter EO, Price DA: Idiopathic growth hormone deficiency in KIGS: Selected aspects; in: Ranke MB, Reiter EO, Price DA (eds): Growth Hormone Therapy in Pediatrics – 20 Years of KIGS. Basel, Karger, 2007, pp 116–135.

31 Schweizer R, Martin DD, Haase M, Roth J, Trebar B, Binder G, Schwarze CP, Ranke MB: Similar effects of long-term exogenous growth hormone (GH) on bone and muscle parameters: a pQCT study of GH-deficient and small-for-gestational-age (SGA) children. Bone 2007;41:875–881.

32 Högler W, Briody J, Moore B, Lu PW, Cowell CT: Effect of growth hormone therapy and puberty on bone and body composition in children with idiopathic short stature and growth hormone deficiency. Bone 2005;37:642–650.

33 Yakar S, Pennisi P, Wu Y, Zhao H, LeRoith DJ: Clinical relevance of systemic and local IGF-I. Endocr Dev 2005a;9:11–16.

34 Yakar S, Pennisi P, Kim CH, Zhao H, Toyoshima Y, Gavrilova O, LeRoith DJ: Studies involving the GH-IGF axis: Lessons from IGF-I and IGF-I receptor gene targeting mouse models. J Endocrinol Invest 2005;28(5 suppl):19–22.

35 LeRoith D: Clinical relevance of systemic and local IGF-I: lessons from animal models. Pediatr Endocrinol Rev 2008;5(suppl 2):739–743.

36 Ranke MB, Schweizer R, Lindberg A, Price DA, Reiter EO, Albertsson-Wikland K, Darendeliler F: Insulin-like growth factors as diagnostic tools in growth hormone deficiency during childhood and adolescence: the KIGS experience. Horm Res 2004;62(suppl 1):17–25.

37 Ranke MB, Schweizer R, Elmlinger ME, Weber K, Binder G, Schwarze CP, Wollmann HA: Significance of basal IGF-I, IGFBP-3 and IGFBP-2 measurements in the diagnostics of short stature in children. Horm Res 2000;54:60–68.

38 Federico G, Street ME, Maghnie M, Caruso-Nicoletti M, Loche S, Bertelloni S, Cianfarani S, Study Group on Physiopathology of Growth Processes, Council of ISPED: Assessment of serum IGF-I concentrations in the diagnosis of isolated childhood-onset GH deficiency: a proposal of the Italian Society for Pediatric Endocrinology and Diabetes (SIEDP/ISPED). J Endocrinol Invest 2006;29:732–737.

39 Maghnie M, Ghirardello S, Genovese E: Magnetic resonance imaging of the hypothalamus-pituitary unit in children suspected of hypopituitarism: who, how and when to investigate. J Endocrinol Invest 2004;27:496–509.

40 Argyropoulou M, Perignon F, Brunelle F, Brauner R, Rappaport R: Height of normal pituitary gland as a function of age evaluated by magnetic resonance imaging in children. Pediatr Radiol 1991;21:247–249.

41 Chawla RK, Parks S, Rudman D: Structural variants of human growth hormone. Ann Rev Med 1983;34:519–547.

42 Baumann G: Growth hormone heterogeneity: genes, isohormones, variants and binding protein. Endocr Rev 1991;12:424–449.

43 De Palo EF, De Filippis V, Gatti R, Spinella P: Growth hormone isoforms and segments/fragments: molecular structure and laboratory measurement. Clin Chim Acta 2006;364:67–76.

44 Brooks AJ, Wooh JW, Tunny KA, Waters MJ: Growth hormone receptor: mechanism of action. Int J Biochem Cell Biol 2008;40:1984–1989.

45 Vickers MH, Gilmour S, Gertler A, Breier BH, Tunny K, Waters MJ, Gluckman PD: 20-kDa placental hGH-V has diminished diabetogenic and lactogenic activities compared with 22-kDa hGH-N while retaining antilipogenic activity. Am J Physiol Endocrinol Metab 2009;297:E629–E637.

-46 Pagani S, Cappa M, Meazza C, Ubertini G, Travaglino P, Bozzola E, Bozzola M: Growth hormone isoforms release in response to physiological and pharmacological stimuli. J Endocrinol Invest 2008;31:520–524.

47 Leung DW, Spencer SA, Cachianes G, Hammonds RG, Collins C, Henzel WJ, Barnard R, Waters MJ, Wood WI: Growth hormone receptor and serum binding protein: purification, cloning and expression. Nature 1987;330:537–543.

48 Baumann G: Growth hormone binding to a circulating receptor fragment – the concept of receptor shedding and receptor splicing. Exp Clin Endocrinol Diabetes 1995;103:2–6.

49 Baumann G: Growth hormone binding protein 2001. J Pediatr Endocrinol Metab 2001;14:355–375.

50 Mercado M, Carlsson L, Vitangcol R, Baumann G: Growth hormone-binding protein determination in plasma: a comparison of immunofunctional and growth hormone-binding assays. J Clin Endocrinol Metab 1993;76:1291–1294.

51 Carlsson L, Mercado M, Baumann G, Stene M, Attie K, Reichert M, Albertsson-Wikland K, Dawson K, Wong WL: Assay systems for the growth hormone-binding protein. Proc Soc Exp Biol Med 1994;206:312–315.

52 Rajkovic IA, Valiontis E, Ho KK: Direct quantitation of growth hormone binding protein in human serum by a ligand immunofunctional assay: comparison with immunoprecipitation and chromatographic methods. J Clin Endocrinol Metab. 1994;78:772–777.

53 Fisker S, Frystyk J, Skriver L, Vestbo H, Ho KK, Orskov H: A simple, rapid immunometric assay for determination of functional and growth hormone-occupied growth hormone-binding protein in human serum. Eur J Clin Invest 1996;26:779–785.

54 Gelander L, Bjarnason R, Carlsson LM, Albertsson-Wikland K: Growth hormone-binding protein levels over one year in healthy prepubertal children: intraindividual variation and correlation with height velocity. Pediatr Res 1998;43:256–261.

55 Juul A, Fisker S, Scheike T, Hertel T, Müller J, Orskov H, Skakkebaek NE: Serum levels of growth hormone binding protein in children with normal and precocious puberty: relation to age, gender, body composition and gonadal steroids. Clin Endocrinol (Oxf) 2000;52:165–172.

56 Salazar TE, Méricq MV, Espinoza M, Iñiguez G, de Carvallo P, Cassorla F: Reference values of growth hormone binding protein (GHBP) for a normal pediatric population. Rev Med Chil 2001;129:382–389.

57 Ong KK, Elmlinger M, Jones R, Emmett P; ALSPAC Study Team, Holly J, Ranke MB, Dunger DB: Growth hormone binding protein levels in children are associated with birth weight, postnatal weight gain, and insulin secretion. Metabolism 2007;56: 1412–1417.

58 Burren CP, Woods KA, Rose SJ, Tauber M, Price DA, Heinrich U, Gilli G, Razzaghy-Azar M, Al-Ashwal A, Crock PA, Rochiccioli P, Yordam N, Ranke MB, Chatelain PG, Preece MA, Rosenfeld RG, Savage MO: Clinical and endocrine characteristics in atypical and classical growth hormone insensitivity syndrome. Horm Res 2001;55:125–130.

59 Iida K, Takahashi Y, Kaji H, Nose O, Okimura Y, Abe H, Chihara K: Growth hormone (GH) insensitivity syndrome with high serum GH-binding protein levels caused by a heterozygous splice site mutation of the GH receptor gene producing a lack of intracellular domain. J Clin Endocrinol Metab 1998;83:531–537.

60 Aalbers AM, Chin D, Pratt KL, Little BM, Frank SJ, Hwa V, Rosenfeld RG: Extreme elevation of serum growth hormone-binding protein concentrations resulting from a novel heterozygous splice site mutation of the growth hormone receptor gene. Horm Res 2009;71:276–284.

61 Frystyk J, Andreasen CM, Fisker S: Determination of free growth hormone. J Clin Endocrinol Metab 2008;93:3008–3014.

62 Ebdrup L, Fisker S, Sorensen HH, Ranke MB, Orskov H: Variety in growth horomne determinations due to use of different immunoassays and to the interference of growth hormone-binding protein. Horm Res 1999;1(suppl):20–26.

63 Berthelier C, Bertrand P, Bluet-Pajo MT, Clauser H, Durand D, Enjalbert A, Epelbaum J, Rerat E, Kordon C: Multifactorial regulation of growth hormone; in Müller EE, Cocchi D, Locatelli V (eds): Advances in Growth Hormone and Growth Factor Research. Berlin, Springer, 1989, pp 231–245.

64 Camanni F, Ghigo E, Mazza E, Imperiale E, Goffi S, Martina V, De Gennaro Colonna V, Cella SG, Cocchi D, Locatelli V, Massara F, Müller EE: Aspects of neurotransmitter control of GH secretion: basic and clinical studies; in Müller EE, Cocchi D, Locatelli V (eds): Advances in Growth Hormone and Growth Factor Research. Berlin, Springer, 1989, pp 263–281.

65 Pombo M, Pombo CM, Garcia A, Caminos E, Gualillo O, Alvarez CV, Casanueva F, Dieguez C: Hormonal control of growth hormone secretion. Horm Res 2001;55(suppl):11–16.

66 Gahete MD, Durán-Prado M, Luque RM, Martínez-Fuentes AJ, Quintero A, Gutiérrez-Pascual E, Córdoba-Chacón J, Malagón MM, Gracia-Navarro F, Castaño JP: Understanding the multifactorial control of growth hormone release by somatotropes: lessons from comparative endocrinology. Ann NY Acad Sci 2009;1163:137–153.

67 Castañeda TR, Tong J, Datta R, Culler M, Tschöp MH: Ghrelin in the regulation of body weight and metabolism. Front Neuroendocrinol 2010;31:44–60.

68 Veldhuis JD, Bowers CY: Human GH pulsatility: an ensemble property regulated by age and gender. J Endocrinol Invest 2003;26:799–813.

69 Chowen JA, Frago LM, Argente J: The regulation of GH secretion by sex steroids. Eur J Endocrinol 2004; 151(suppl 3):U95–U100.

70 Girard J, Fischer-Wasels T: Measurement of urinary growth hormone: a noninvasive method to assess the 'growth hormone status'. Horm Res 1990;33(suppl 4):12–18.

71 Langkamp M, Weber K, Ranke MB: Human growth hormone measurement by means of a sensitive ELISA of whole blood spots on filter paper. Growth Horm IGF Res 2008;18:526–532.

72 Evans MJ, Livesey JH, Ellis MJ, Yandle TG: Effect of anticoagulants and storage temperatures on stability of plasma and serum hormones. Clin Biochem 2001;34:107–112.

73 Derr RL, Cameron SJ, Golden SH: Pre-analytic considerations for the proper assessment of hormones of the hypothalamic-pituitary axis in epidemiological research. Eur J Epidemiol 2006;21:217–226.

74 Gavin Jr III, Trivedi B, Daughaday WH: Homologous IM-9 lymphocyte radio-receptor assay and receptor modulation assays for human serum growth hormone. J Clin Endocrinol Metab 1982;58:133–139.

75 Tanaka T, Shiu RPC, Gout PW, Beer CT, Noble RL, Friesen HG: A new sensitive and specific bioassay for lactogenetic hormones: measurement of prolactin and growth hormone in human serum. J Clin Endocrinol Metab 1980;51:1058–1063.

76 Dattani MT, Ealey PA, Pringle PJ, Hindmarsh PC, Brook CG, Marshall NJ: An investigation into the lability of the bioactivity of human growth hormone using the ESTA bioassay. Horm Res 1996;46:64–73.

77 Rowland JE, Marshall NJ, Leung KC, Ho KKY, Cotterill AM, Rowlinson SW, Waters MJ: A novel bioassay for human somatogenic activity in serum samples supports the clinical reliability of immunoassays. Clin Endocrinol (Oxf) 2002;56:475–485.

78 Rowlinson SW, Behncken SN, Rowland JE, Clarkson RW, Strasburger CJ, Wu Z, Baumbach W, Waters MJ: Activation of chimeric and full-length growth hormone receptors by growth hormone receptor monoclonal antibodies. A specific conformational change may be required for full-length receptor signaling. J Biol Chem 1998;273:5307–5314.

79 Ikeda M, Wada M, Fujita Y, Takahashi S, Maekawa K, Honjo M: A novel bioassay based on human growth hormone (hGH) receptor mediated cell proliferation: measurement of 20K-hGH and its modified forms. Growth Horm IGF Res 2000;10:248–255.

80 Strasburger CJ, Wu Z, Pflaum CD, Dressendorfer RA: Immunofunctional assay of human growth hormone (hGH) in serum: a possible consensus for quantitative hGH measurement. J Clin Endocrinol Metab 1996;81:2613–2620.

81 Strasburger CJ, Dattani MT: New growth hormone assays: potential benefits. Acta Paediatr (Suppl) 1997;432:5–11.

82 Ranke MB, Orskov H, Bristow AF, Seth J, Baumann G: Consensus on how to measure growth hormone in serum. Horm Res 1999;51(suppl):27–29.

83 Bayle M, Chevenne D, Dousset B, Lahlou N, Le Bouc Y, Massart C, Noel M, Porquet D, Salles JP, Sault C, Souberbielle JC: SFBC de la section 'Evaluation des dosages des paramètres de l'axe somatotrope': Recommendations for the standardization of growth hormone assays. Ann Biol Clin (Paris). 2004;62:155–163.

84 Trainer PJ, Barth J, Sturgeon C, Wieringaon G: Consensus statement on the standardization of GH assays. Eur J Endocrinol 2006;155:1–2.

85 Wieringa GE, Trainer PJ: Commentary: harmonizing growth hormone measurements: learning lessons for the future. J Clin Endocrinol Metab 2007; 92:2874–2875.

86 Bidlingmaier M, Strasburger CJ: Growth hormone assays: current methodologies and their limitations. Pituitary 2007;10:115–119.

87 Amed S, Delvin E, Hamilton J: Variation in growth hormone immunoassays in clinical practice in Canada. Horm Res 2008;69:290–294.

88 Bidlingmaier M, Freda PU: Measurement of human growth hormone by immunoassays: current status, unsolved problems and clinical consequences. Growth Horm IGF Res 2009;20:19–25.

89 Hauffa BP, Lehmann N, Bettendorf M, Mehls O, Dörr HG, Partsch CJ, Schwarz HP, Stahnke N, Steinkamp H, Said E, Sander S, Ranke MB, German KIGS/IGLU Study Group: Central reassessment of GH concentrations measured at local treatment centers in children with impaired growth: consequences for patient management. Eur J Endocrinol 2004;150:291–297.

90 Badaru A, Wilson DM: Alternatives to growth hormone stimulation testing in children. Trends Endocrinol Metab 2004;15:252–258.

91 Hindmarsh PC, Swift PG: An assessment of growth hormone provocation tests. Arch Dis Child 1995; 72:362–367.

92 Guyda HJ: Growth hormone testing and the short child. Pediatr Res 2000;48:579–580.

93 Sizonenko PC, Clayton PE, Cohen P, Hintz RL, Tanaka T, Laron Z: Diagnosis and management of growth hormone deficiency in childhood and adolescence. 1. Diagnosis of growth hormone deficiency. Growth Horm IGF Res 2001;11:137–165.

94 Tassoni P, Cacciari E, Cau M, Colli C, Tosi M, Zucchini S, Cicognani A, Pirazolli P, Salardi S, Balsamo A, Frejaville E, Cassio A, Zappulla F: Variability of growth hormone response to pharmacological and sleep tests performed twice in short children. J Clin Endocrinol Metab 1990;71:230–234.

95 Tauber M, Moulin P, Pienkowski C, Jouret B, Rochiccioli P: Growth hormone retesting and auxological data in 131 GH-deficient patients after completion of treatment. J Clin Endocrinol Metab 1997; 82:353–356.

96 Wyatt DT, Mark D, Slyper A: Survey of growth hormone treatment practices by 251 pediatric endocrinologists. J Clin Endocrinol Metab 1995;80:3292–3297.

97 Rochiccioli P, Tauber M: Growth hormone deficiency: establishment of the diagnosis by means of growth hormone secretion tests in the Kabi International Growth Study; in Ranke MB, Gunnarsson R (eds): Progress in Growth Hormone Therapy – 5 Years of KIGS. Mannheim, J&J Verlag, 1994, pp 68–76.

98 Binder G, Braemswig JH, Kratsch J, Pfaeffle R, Woelfle J: Guidelines on the diagnosis of growth hormone deficiency in children and adolescents. Monatschr Kinderheilk 2009;157:997–1028.

99 Buckler JMH: Exercise as a screening test for growth hormone release. Acta Endocrinol (Copenh) 1972; 69:219–229.

100 Keenan BS, Killmer LB, Sode J: Growth hormone response to exercise: a test of pituitary function in children. Pediatrics 1972;50:760–764.

101 Eliakim A, Nemet D: Exercise provocation test for growth hormone secretion: methodologic considerations. Pediatr Exerc Sci 2008;20:370–378.

102 Cappa M, Bizzarri C, Martinez C, Porzio O, Giannone G, Turchetta A, Calzolari A: Neuroregulation of growth hormone during exercise in children. Int J Sports Med 2000;21(Suppl 2):S125–128.

103 Donaubauer J, Kratzsch J, Fritzsch C, Stach B, Kiess W, Keller E: The treadmill exhausting test is not suitable for screening of growth hormone deficiency! Horm Res 2001;55:137–140.

104 Marin G, Domené HM, Barnes KM, Blackwell BJ, Cassorla FG, Cutler GB Jr: The effect of estrogen priming in puberty on the growth hormone response to standardised treadmill exercise and arginine-insulin in normal girls and boys. J Clin Endocrinol Metab 1994;79:537–541.

105 Ghigo E, Bellone J, Aimaretti G, Bellone S, Loche S, Cappa M, Bartolotta E, Dammacco F, Camanni F: Reliability of provocative tests to assess growth hormone secretory status: study in 472 normally growing children. J Clin Endocrinol Metab 1996;81:3323–3327.

106 Merimee TJ, Lilicrap DA, Rabinowitz D: Effect of arginine on serum levels of human growth hormone. Lancet 1965;ii:668–670.

107 Parker ML, Hammond JM, Daughaday WH: The arginine provocation test: an aid in the diagnosis of hyposomatotropism. J Clin Endocrinol Metab 1967;27:1129–1136.

108 Galluzzi F, Quaranta MR, Salti R, Stagi S, Nanni L, Seminara S: Diagnosis of growth hormone deficiency by using the arginine provocative test: is it possible to shorten testing time without altering validity? Horm Res 2009;72:142–145.

109 Muster L, Zangen DH, Nesher R, Hirsch HJ, Muster Z, Gillis D: Arginine and clonidine stimulation tests for growth hormone deficiency revisited – do we really need so many samples? J Pediatr Endocrinol Metab 2009;22:215–223.

110 Zadik Z, Chale SA, Kowarski A: Assessment of growth hormone secretion in normal stature children using 24-hour integrated concentration of GH and pharmacological stimulation. J Clin Endocrinol Metab 1990;71:932–936.

111 Roth J, Glick SM, Yallow RS, Berson SA: Hypoglycemia: a potent stimulus to secretion of growth hormone. Science 1963;140:987.

112 Muzsnai A, Sólyom J, Ilyés I, Kovács J, Sólyom E, Niederland T, Péter F: Appropriate sampling times for growth hormone (GH) measurement during insulin tolerance testing (ITT) in children. Horm Res 2007;68(suppl 5):205–206.

113 Stanley TL, Levitsky LL, Grinspoon SK, Misra M: Effect of body mass index on peak growth hormone response to provocative testing in children with short stature. J Clin Endocrinol Metab 2009;94:4875–4881.

114 Frasier SD, Hilburn JM, Smith FG Jr: Effect of adolescence on the serum growth hormone response to hypoglycemia. J Pediatr 1977;77:465–467.

115 Gelato MC, Malozowski S, Caruso-Nocoletti M, Ross JL, Pescovitz OH, Rose S, Loriaux DL, Cassorla F, Merriam GR: Growth hormone (GH) response to GH-releasing hormone during pubertal development in normal boys and girls: comparison to idiopathic short stature and GH deficiency. J Clin Endocrinol Metab 1986;63:174–179.

116 Böttner A, Kratzsch J, Liebermann S, Keller A, Pfaffle RW, Kiess W, Keller E: Comparison of adrenal function tests in children – the glucagon stimulation test allows the simultaneous assessment of adrenal function and growth hormone response in children. J Pediatr Endocrinol Metab 2005;18:433–442.

117 Shah A, Stanhope R, Matthew D: Hazards of pharmacological tests of growth hormone secretion in childhood. Br Med J 1992;304:173–174.

118 Binder G, Bosk A, Gass M, Ranke MB, Heidemann PH: Insulin tolerance test causes hypokalaemia and can provoke cardiac arrhythmias. Horm Res 2004;62:84–87.

119 Galloway PJ, McNeill E, Paterson WF, Donaldson MD: Safety of the insulin tolerance test. Arch Dis Child 2002;87:354–356.

120 Penny R, Blizzard RM, Davis WT: Sequential arginine and insulin tolerance test on the same day. J Clin Endocrinol Metab 1968;29:1499–1501.

121 Gil-Ad I, Topper E, Laron Z: Oral clonidine as a growth hormone stimulation test. Lancet 1979;ii:278–280.

122 Milner RDG: Comparison of the intravenous insulin and oral clonidine tolerance test for growth hormone secretion. Arch Dis Child 1981;56:852–854.

123 Mitchell ML, Suvunrungsi P, Sawin CT: Effect of propranolol on the response of serum growth hormone to glucagon. J Clin Endocrinol Metab 1971;32:470–475.

124 Parks JS, Amrhein JA, Vaidya V, Moshang T Jr, Bongiovanni AM: Growth hormone responses to propranolol-glucagon stimulation: a comparison with other tests of growth hormone reserve. J Clin Endocrinol Metab 1973;37:85–92.

125 Strich D, Terespolsky N, Gillis D: Glucagon stimulation test for childhood growth hormone deficiency: timing of the peak is important. J Pediatr 2009;154:415–419.

126 Weldon VV, Gupta SK, Haymond MW, Pagliari AS, Jacobs LS, Daughaday WH: The use of L-dopa in the diagnosis of hyposomatotropism in children. J Clin Endocrinol Metab 1973;36:42–46.

127 Ranke MB, Gruhler M, Rosskamp R, Brügmann G, Attanasio A, Blum WF, Bierich JR: Testing with growth hormone-releasing factor (GRF(1–29)NH2) and somatomedin C measurements for the evaluation of growth hormone deficiency. Eur J Pediatr 1986;145:485–492.

128 Brook CGD, Hindmarsh PC, Smith PJ, Stanhope R: Therapeutic application of hypothalamic hormones; in Brook CGD (ed): Clinical Pediatric Endocrinology, ed 2. Oxford, Blackwell, 1989, p 245.

129 Ghigo E, Bellone J, Mazza E, Imperiale E, Procopio M, Valente F, Lala R, De Sanctis C, Camanni F: Arginine potentiates the GHRH- but not the pyridostigmine-induced GH secretion in normal short children. Further evidence for a somatostatin suppressing effect of arginine. Clin Endocrinol (Oxf) 1990;32:763–767.

130 Ghigo E, Imperiale E, Boffano GM, Mazza E, Bellone J, Arvat E, Procopio M, Goffi S, Barreca A, Chiabotto P, Lala R, DeSanctis C, Boghen MF, Müller EE, Camanni F: A new test for the diagnosis of growth hormone deficiency due to primary pituitary impairment: combined administration of pyridostigmine and growth hormone-releasing hormone. J Endocrinol Invest 1990;13:307–316.

131 Ho KK: GH Deficiency Consensus Workshop Participants: Consensus guidelines for the diagnosis and treatment of adults with GH deficiency. II. A statement of the GH Research Society in association with the European Society for Pediatric Endocrinology, Lawson Wilkins Society, European Society of Endocrinology, Japan Endocrine Society, and Endocrine Society of Australia. Eur J Endocrinol 2007;157:695–700.

132 Ghigo E, Aimaretti G, Gianotti L, Bellone J, Arvat E, Camanni F: New approach to the diagnosis of growth hormone deficiency in adults. Eur J Endocrinol 1996;134:352–356.

133 Aimaretti G, Corneli G, Razzore P, Bellone S, Baffoni C, Arvat E, Camanni F, Ghigo E: Comparison between insulin-induced hypoglycemia and growth hormone (GH)-releasing hormone + arginine as provocative tests for the diagnosis of GH deficiency in adults. J Clin Endocrinol Metab 1998;83:1615–1618.

134 Yuen KC, Biller BM, Molitch ME, Cook DM: Clinical review: Is lack of recombinant growth hormone (GH)-releasing hormone in the United States a setback or time to consider glucagon testing for adult GH deficiency? J Clin Endocrinol Metab 2009;94:702–207.

135 Keller A, Donaubauer J, Kratzsch J, Pfaeffle R, Hirsch W, Kiess W, Keller E: Administration of arginine plus growth hormone releasing hormone to evaluate growth hormone (GH) secretory status in children with GH deficiency. J Pediatr Endocrinol Metab 2007;20:1307–1314.

136 Aimaretti G, Baffoni C, DiVito L, Bellone S, Grottoli S, Maccario M, Arvat E, Camanni F, Ghigo E: Comparisons among old and new provacative tests of GH secretion in 178 normal adults. Eur J Endocrinol 2000b;142:347–352.

137 Arvat E, Cappa M, Casanueva FF, Diguez C, Ghigo E, Nicolosi M, Valcavi R, Zini M: Pyridostigmine potentiates growth hormone (GH)-releasing hormone-induced release in both men and women. J Clin Endocrinol Metab 1993;76:374–377.

138 Hoeck HC, Vestergaard P, Jakobsen PE, Falhof J, Laurberg P: Diagnosis of growth hormone (GH) deficiency in adults with hypothalamic-pituitary disorders: comparison of test results using pyridostigmine plus GH-releasing hormone (GHRH), clonidine plus GHRH, and insulin-induced hypoglycemia as GH secretagogues. J Clin Endocrinol Metab 2000;85:1467–1472.

139 Ghigo E, Mazza E, Imperiale E, Rizzi G, Benso L, Müller EE, Camanni F, Massara F: Enhancement of cholinergic tone by pyridostigmine promotes both basal and growth hormone (GH)-releasing hormone-induced GH secretion in children of short stature. J Clin Endocrinol Metab 1987;65:452–456.

140 Ghigo E, Aimaretti G, Gianotti L, Bellone J, Arvat E, Camanni F: New approach to the diagnosis of growth hormone deficiency in adults. Eur J Endocrinol 1996;134:352–356.

141 Ghigo E, Aimaretti G, Corneli G, Bellone J, Arvat E, Maccario M, Camanni F: Diagnosis of GH deficiency in adults. Growth Horm IGF Res 1998; 8(suppl):55–58.

142 Tannenbaum GS, Bowers CY: Interactions of growth hormone secretagogues and growth hormone-releasing hormone/somatostatin. Endocrine 2001; 14:21–27.

143 Camanni F, Ghigo E, Arvat E: Growth hormone-releasing peptides and their analogues. Fron Neuroendocrinol 1998;19:47–72.

144 Kojima M, Hosoda H, Date Y, Nakazato M, Matsuo H, Kangawa K: Ghrelin is a growth-hormone-releasing acylated peptide from stomach. Nature 1999;402:656–660.

145 Aimaretti G, Baffoni C, Broglio F, Janssen JAM, Corneli G, Deghenghi R, Van der Lely AJ, Ghigo E, Arvat E: Endocrine responses to ghrelin in adult patients with isolated childhood-onset growth hormone deficiency. Clin Endocrinol (Oxf) 2002;56:765–771.

146 Di Vito L, Broglio F, Benso A, Gottero, C, Prodam F, Papotti M, Muccioli G, Dieguez C, Casanueva FF, Deghenghi R, Ghigo E, Arvat E: The GH-releasing effect of ghrelin, a natural GH secretagogue, is only blunted by the infusion of exogenous somatostatin in humans. Clin Endocrinol (Oxf) 2002;56:643–648.

147 Illig R, Bucher H: Testosterone priming of growth hormone release; in Laron Z, Butenandt O (eds): Evaluation of Growth Hormone Secretion. Basel, Karger, 1983, pp 75–85.

148 Gonc EN, Yordam N, Kandemir N, Alikasifoglu A: Comparison of stimulated growth hormone levels in primed versus unprimed provocative tests: effect of various testosterone doses on growth hormone levels. Horm Res. 2001;56:32–37.

149 Chemaitilly W, Trivin C, Souberbielle JC, Brauner R: Assessing short-statured children for growth hormone deficiency. Horm Res 2003;60:34–42.

150 Müller G, Keller A, Reich A, Hoepffner W, Kratzsch J, Buckler JM, Kiess W, Keller E: Priming with testosterone enhances stimulated growth hormone secretion in boys with delayed puberty. J Pediatr Endocrinol Metab 2004;17:77–83.

151 Coutant R, de Casson FB, Rouleau S, Douay O, Mathieu E, Gatelais F, Bouhours-Nouet N, Voinot C, Audran M, Limal JM: Divergent effect of endogenous and exogenous sex steroids on the insulin-like growth factor I response to growth hormone in short normal adolescents. J Clin Endocrinol Metab. 2004;89:6185–6192.

152 Borghi MM, Longui CA, Calliari LE, Faria CD, Kochi C, Monte O: Transdermal estradiol priming during clonidine stimulation test in non-growth hormone deficient children with short stature: a pilot study. J Pediatr Endocrinol Metab. 2006;19:223–237.

153 Molina S, Paoli M, Camacho N, Arata-Bellabarba G, Lanes R: Is testosterone and estrogen priming prior to clonidine useful in the evaluation of the growth hormone status of short peripubertal children? J Pediatr Endocrinol Metab. 2008;21:257–266.

154 Martinez AS, Domene HM, Ropelato MG, Jasper HG, Pennisi PA, Escobar ME, Heinrich JJ: Estrogen priming effect on growth hormone (GH) provocative test: a useful tool for the diagnosis of GH deficiency. J Clin Endocrinol Metab 2000;85:4168–4172.

155 Gonc EN, Kandemir N, Ozon A, Alikasifoglu A: Final heights of boys with normal growth hormone responses to provocative tests following priming. J Pediatr Endocrinol Metab. 2008;21:963–971.

156 Clayton PE, Cuneo RC, Juul A, Monson JP, Shalet SM, Tauber M, European Society for Paediatric Endocrinology: Consensus statement on the management of the GH-treated adolescent in the transition to adult care. Eur J Endocrinol 2005;152:165–170.

157 Styne DM: A practical approach to the diagnosis of growth hormone (GH) deficiency in patients transitioning to adulthood using GH stimulation testing. J Pediatr Endocrinol Metab 2003;16(suppl 3):637–643.

158 Gasco V, Corneli G, Beccuti G, Prodam F, Rovere S, Bellone J, Grottoli S, Aimaretti G, Ghigo E: Retesting the childhood-onset GH-deficient patient. Eur J Endocrinol 2008;159(suppl 1):S45–52.

159 Bonfig W, Bechtold S, Bachmann S, Putzker S, Fuchs O, Pagel P, Schwarz HP: Reassessment of the optimal growth hormone cut-off level in insulin tolerance testing for growth hormone secretion in patients with childhood-onset growth hormone deficiency during transition to adulthood. J Pediatr Endocrinol Metab 2008;21:1049–1056.

160 Aimaretti G, Baffoni C, Bellone S, Di Vito L, Corneli G, Arvat E, Benso L, Camanni F, Ghigo E: Retesting young adults with childhood-onset growth hormone (GH) deficiency with GH-releasing-hormone-plus-arginine test. J Clin Endocrinol Metab 2000;85:3693–3699.

161 Corneli G, Di Somma C, Prodam F, Bellone J, Bellone S, Gasco V, Baldelli R, Rovere S, Schneider HJ, Gargantini L, Gastaldi R, Ghizzoni L, Valle D, Salerno M, Colao A, Bona G, Ghigo E, Maghnie M, Aimaretti G: Cut-off limits of the GH response to GHRH plus arginine test and IGF-I levels for the diagnosis of GH deficiency in late adolescents and young adults. Eur J Endocrinol. 2007;157:701–708.

162 Zucchini S, Pirazzoli P, Baronio F, Gennari M, Bal MO, Balsamo A, Gualandi S, Cicognani A: Effect on adult height of pubertal growth hormone retesting and withdrawal of therapy in patients with previously diagnosed growth hormone deficiency. J Clin Endocrinol Metab 2006;91:4271–4276.

163 Karavitaki N, Brufani C, Warner JT, Adams CB, Richards P, Ansorge O, Shine B, Turner HE, Wass JA: Craniopharyngiomas in children and adults: systematic analysis of 121 cases with long-term follow-up. Clin Endocrinol (Oxf) 2005;62:397–409.

164 Taskinen M, Lipsanen-Nyman M, Tiitinen A, Hovi L, Saarinen-Pihkala UM: Insufficient growth hormone secretion is associated with metabolic syndrome after allogeneic stem cell transplantation in childhood. J Pediatr Hematol Oncol 2007;29:529–534.

165 Merchant TE, Goloubeva O, Pritchard DL, Gaber MW, Xiong X, Danish RK, Lustig RH: Radiation dose-volume effects on growth hormone secretion. Int J Radiat Oncol Biol Phys 2002;52:1264–1270.

166 Darzy KH, Pezzoli SS, Thorner MO, Shalet SM: Cranial irradiation and growth hormone neurosecretory dysfunction: a critical appraisal. J Clin Endocrinol Metab 2007;92:1666–1672.

167 Darzy KH, Shalet SM: Hypopituitarism following radiotherapy revisited. Endocr Dev 2009;15:1–24.

168 Schmiegelow M, Lassen S, Poulsen HS, Feldt-Rasmussen U, Schmiegelow K, Hertz H, Müller J: Growth hormone response to a growth hormone-releasing hormone stimulation test in a population-based study following cranial irradiation of childhood brain tumors. Horm Res 2000;54:53–59.

169 Lissett CA, Saleem S, Rahim A, Brennan BM, Shalet SM: The impact of irradiation on growth hormone responsiveness to provocative agents is stimulus dependent: results in 161 individuals with radiation damage to the somatotropic axis. J Clin Endocrinol Metab. 2001;86:663–668.

170 Bakker B, Oostdijk W, Geskus RB, Stokvis-Brantsma WH, Vossen JM, Wit JM: Growth hormone (GH) secretion and response to GH therapy after total body irradiation and haematopoietic stem cell transplantation during childhood. Clin Endocrinol (Oxf) 2007;67:589–597.

171 Björk J, Link K, Erfurth EM: The utility of the growth hormone (GH) releasing hormone-arginine test for diagnosing GH deficiency in adults with childhood acute lymphoblastic leukemia treated with cranial irradiation. J Clin Endocrinol Metab 2005;90:6048–6054.

172 Darzy KH, Thorner MO, Shalet SM: Cranially irradiated adult cancer survivors may have normal spontaneous GH secretion in the presence of discordant peak GH responses to stimulation tests (compensated GH deficiency). Clin Endocrinol (Oxf) 2009;70:287–293.

173 Bercu BB, Diamond FB Jr: Growth hormone neurosecretory dysfunction. Clin Endocrinol Metab 1986;15:537–590.

174 Bercu BB, Shulman D, Root AW, Spiliotis BE: Growth hormone (GH) provocative testing frequently does not reflect endogenous GH secretion. J Clin Endocrinol Metab 1986;63:709–716.

175 Zadik Z: The lost honor of neurosecretory growth hormone dysfunction. J Pediatr Endocrinol Metab 2009;22:767–768.

176 Miller JD, Esparza A, Wright NM, Garimella V, Lai J, Lester SE, Mosier HD Jr: Spontaneous growth hormone release in term infants: changes during the first four days of life. J Clin Endocrinol Metab 1993;76:1058–1062.

177 Ogilvy-Stuart AL, Hands SJ, Adcock CJ, Holly JM, Matthews DR, Mohamed-Ali V, Yudkin JS, Wilkinson AR, Dunger DB: Insulin, insulin-like growth factor I (IGF-I), IGF-binding protein-1, growth hormone, and feeding in the newborn. J Clin Endocrinol Metab 1998;83:3550–3557.

178 Binder G, Weidenkeller M, Blumenstock G, Langkamp M, Weber K, Franz AR: Rational approach to the diagnosis of severe growth hormone deficiency in the newborn. J Clin Endocrinol Metab 2010;95:2219–2226.

179 Geary MP, Pringle PJ, Rodeck CH, Kingdom JC, Hindmarsh PC: Sexual dimorphism in the growth hormone and insulin-like growth factor axis at birth. J Clin Endocrinol Metab 2003;88:3708–3714.

180 Jensen RB, Jeppesen KA, Vielwerth S, Michaelsen KF, Main KM, Skakkebaek NE, Juul A: Insulin-like growth factor I (IGF-I) and IGF-binding protein 3 as diagnostic markers of growth hormone deficiency in infancy. Horm Res 2005;63:15–21.

181 Hughes IA: Handbook of Endocrine Testing in Children. Bristol, Wright, 1986.

Prof. Dr. Michael B. Ranke
University Children's Hospital
Hoppe-Seyler-Strasse 1
DE–72076 Tübingen (Germany)
Tel. +49 7071 298 3417, Fax +49 7071 294157, E-Mail michael.ranke@gmx.de

Ranke MB, Mullis P-E (eds): Diagnostics of Endocrine Function in Children and Adolescents, ed 4.
Basel, Karger, 2011, pp 138–156

Methods of Evaluating Spontaneous Growth Hormone Secretion

Kerstin Albertsson-Wikland · Sten Rosberg

GP-GRC, Queen Silvia Children's Hospital, Göteborg, Sweden

Growth hormone (GH) is secreted in pulses 24 h/day [1], the result of a large-scale network organization of GH-secreting cells [2]. These GH pulses will lead to organ-specific and effector specific actions since the signaling pattern coveys distinct information to different cells as brain, skeleton, muscle, fat and liver. Because GH secretion is pulsatile, a single measurement of GH concentrations in blood does not adequately reflect endogenous GH secretion. Therefore, both physiologic and pharmacologic test procedures have been developed to estimate GH secretion. The motivations and methods for analyzing pulsatile hormone secretion was reviewed recently [3].

The advantage of pharmacologic tests (such as the administration of arginine, insulin, clonidine, glucagon, or levodopa) is that the intensity of the stimulus is easily controlled. The tests are therefore presumed to be reproducible. For clinical purposes, a cut-off value of the GH response to such tests has become accepted clinical practice for deciding when to treat a patient or not with GH. However, there are several major drawbacks with such a clinical approach [4, 5]. The episodic pattern of GH release from the hypophysis is the result of an interplay between two hypothalamic neuro-peptides, the stimulatory GH-releasing hormone (GHRH) and the inhibitory hormone, somatostatin [6, 7]. Both these peptides are secreted in a pulsatile manner. The status of this balance at the precise moment the pharmacologic stimulus is introduced accounts for both the degree of GH response and the variation in response [8]. The reproducibility of the GH response to the tests in individual children is therefore not very good. In fact, this problem has today increased in clinical settings, due to that more children with some endogenous GH secretion are investigated. More children are falsely diagnosed as GH deficient. During the 1980s, it became clear that there is a biological correlation between height and height velocity and the rate of pulsatile GH secretion [9, 10]; later confirmed by [11]. The growth rate is mainly determined by the amplitude of the pulses of GH secretion. Like growth, GH secretion is a

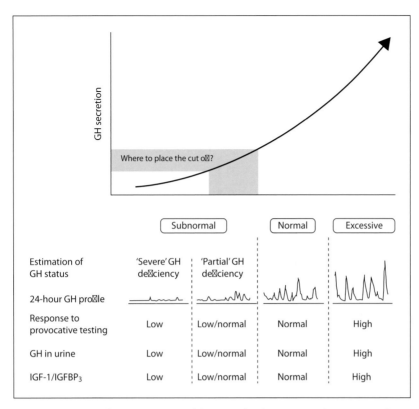

Fig. 1. Spectrum of GH secretion and direct and indirect ways of estimating the GH status.

continuous variable (fig. 1). Therefore, the idea of a cut-off value that strictly defines normality is misleading. Finally, several reports have shown that provocative GH testing frequently does not reflect endogenous GH secretion [12–14]. In a recent clinical trial we could show that about 50% of children diagnosed as GHD according to usual criteria, showed high values during spontaneous secretion profile and thus were rediagnosed as ISS [15]. Moreover, the accuracy of models predicting growth response to GH are highly improved when the actual GH_{max} from spontaneous secretion is added to growth data in comparison to GH_{max} from provocation tests [16, 17].

At the same time, however, the goal of investigation is sometimes not simply to estimate GH secretion, but also to study the pulsatile pattern of GH secretion. The reason for interest in pulsatile GH secretion has arisen from the results of animal studies. It has been shown that the pulsatile pattern of GH secretion can work as a biological signal for optimizing growth and differentiating other effects both within a single organ and between different organs [1]. This is in line with the general assumption of biological implications of pulsatile hormone signals [18, 19].

In animals, this pulsatile secretion may act as a biological signal for tissue specific responses [20]. It has been shown that the production of mRNA for insulin-like growth factor 1 (IGF-1) differs in muscle and liver, in response to the pattern of GH secretion [21, 22]. Moreover, the enzymes in liver differ in male and female rats owing to different patterns of GH secretion [23, 24]. A pattern of GH secretion with several high peaks separated by low troughs is observed in rats with the highest growth rate [25–27]. The impact of frequency has also been reported in man: for example, GH-deficient children on substitution therapy were found to grow about 2 cm more per year if the same weekly amount of GH were divided among daily injections instead of being given in two to three injections per week [28, 29]. In contrast, depot preparations of GH, assuming even GH level, will give less growth for given amount of GH. Recently, Veldhuis et al. [3] summarized that GH pulses are optimal for CNS-negative feedback and skeletal and muscle growth, whereas continuous GH stimulation is favored for hepatic expression of IGF-1, GH-binding protein, and low density lipoprotein receptor. GH pulses induce nuclear signaling via STAT5b and HNF4i, both activating anabolic (male-like) patterns of gene transcription.

Direct Estimation of Spontaneous GH Secretion

The plasma GH level at any particular moment is the result of GH secretion from the somatotrophs in the pituitary, distribution in various body fluids, and elimination. Therefore, it is not accurate to consider a GH concentration profile as directly equivalent to the secretion rate. In order to estimate the secretion rate from measured 24-hour plasma concentrations, it is necessary to use a numerical deconvolution method and basic kinetic parameters of GH [3, 7]. Measurements of endogenous secretion of GH are expensive and time-consuming. Repeated sampling of blood throughout a 24-hour period is also very taxing for the child. It is therefore of the utmost importance to ensure that the test procedure implemented is well tolerated and as simple to perform as possible.

Pulsatile Pattern of GH Secretion versus GH Secretion Rate
It is important to be aware of what one is aiming to accomplish with the test, i.e. whether the goal is to obtain a reliable estimate not only of the overall GH secretion rate, but also to describe the pulsatile pattern of GH secretion. When the aim is to determine the pulsatile pattern of GH secretion, it is important to take blood samples at intervals short enough not to miss any peaks but long enough to permit characterization of possible circadian or ultradian rhythms. In order to establish the sampling interval, it is necessary to know the half-life of GH.

There are different approaches toward estimating the half-life ($t\frac{1}{2}$) of GH. The basic kinetic parameters of GH can be obtained from intravenous single injection studies on GH-deficient children. A slow component with a $t\frac{1}{2}$ of 20 min and a fast component with a $t\frac{1}{2}$ of 4 min were observed [30]. It is possible to question whether the basal kinetic parameters found in this sample group of GH-deficient children are representative. However, the very same value for t½ for both the fast and the slow components were found both in a group of healthy men [31] and in a study of both men and women [32]. In these studies, the kinetics of endogenous GH disappearance were estimated in vivo in man after stimulation of GH secretion by GHRH and suppression with somatostatin [31], a potential method for obtaining patient-specific estimates of kinetic parameters by this method the t½ for the slow component was several minutes shorter in the morning than in the evening. Another way to obtain patient specific estimates is to give an injection of GH in combination with a somatostatin infusion [33–35]. With such a study, obesity was found with increased GH clearance [36, 37]. Also so called blind deconvolution methods, that simultaneously measure GH half-live and secretion rate are now in use [3]. The mechanisms by which GH are eliminated are largely unknown. Probably, the first step is binding of GH to the GH receptors and GH-binding proteins (GHBP). Recent studies of GHBP have shown that, in plasma, there is only a slight day-night variation in concentration of GHBP [38] and exogenous GH will only to a minor degree influence the serum levels of GHBP [39].

Practical Considerations

Sampling Interval. The number of GH peaks detected remains fairly constant during a sampling interval of between 10 and 30 min [40]. A shorter sampling period (5 min) also reveals the fine structure of the major GH peaks, i.e. the additional pulses recognizable with the more intensive sampling were always found within the major secretory peaks [40–42]. Therefore, in our opinion, a sampling interval of 20–30 min can serve as a practical approach (fig. 2) for most clinical and research purposes [43]. If longer interval are used, the GH secretion pattern will be blunted and neither basal GH secretion nor GH_{max} values can be evaluated.

Integrated versus Discrete Sampling

GH concentrations measured in blood drawn through an intravenous catheter at discrete intervals permit an accurate estimate of the concentration at that particular moment. However, with this method the child is disturbed at every sampling. Discrete sampling performed at short intervals also means that the supervising nurse is kept completely occupied. An automated microsampling system has been developed for use in newborns that permits the measurements of hormones in small prediluted samples of blood (40 μl) taken at 10-min intervals over 12 h [44]. With 'modern' techniques for continuous withdrawal in children and adolescents, a thin heparinized catheter (Carmeda AB, Stockholm, Sweden) is inserted through an intravenous needle and connected to a constant withdrawal pump (Swemed AB, Göteborg, Sweden). The rate of withdrawal can range from 0.5 to 6 ml/h and the volume of the tube is 0.1–0.2 ml. With such a system, the child and/or the parents can easily change the tube at indicated times themselves. This makes it possible for the child to move around 'freely' in the hospital area, and the nurse's attention is required

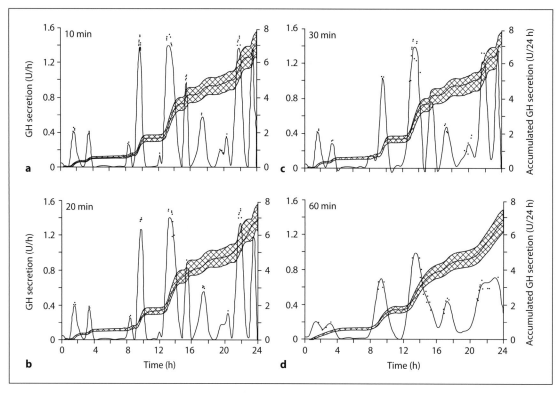

Fig. 2. Analysis of a simulated set of plasma GH profiles with continuous blood specimen collection at intervals of 10 (**a**), 20 (**b**), 30 (**c**) or 60 min (**d**). Note the drastic change in peak pattern with increasing time interval as contrasted to the virtually unchanged GH secretion rate (hatched area).

only when problems arise. Such a system is not very stressful for the child. This is important, since GH secretion is affected by stress. However, continuous withdrawal yields an integrated value for the interval chosen between tube changes. When not only the rate of secretion but also the pulsatile pattern of GH secretion is to be studied, it is important to ensure that the interval between tube changes is short enough. Previously, we showed that no obvious blunting or widening of the peaks was found with an integrated sampling technique of 20- to 30-min intervals (fig. 3) [9]. With longer sampling intervals, however, the pulsatile pattern is not characterized (fig. 2) [43]. As a result, we recommend a sampling interval of 20 min for determining the pattern of secretion. When the investigation focuses on the secretion rate alone, longer sampling intervals are sufficient.

Sampling Period

The sampling period has to be prolonged over a whole 24-hour interval in order to detect not only short-term frequencies, but also possible circadian rhythms. In children with severe GH deficiency, GH secretion is more or less blunted both during

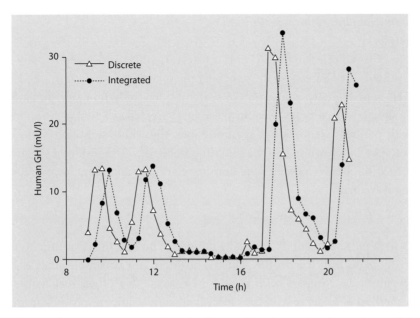

Fig. 3. Plasma GH concentrations in discrete blood samples drawn in parallel with integrated samples in one child. The discrete samples (o) were drawn every 20 min through an indwelling intravenous catheter and the integrated samples (D) were collected for the same period as described. These samples were collected between 09.00 and 21.00 h in a prepubertal 12.5-year-old boy with a height of +0.6 SD. The integrated curve has not been corrected for the time delay in the tubing system.

the day and at night. To assess whether periods shorter than 24 h would yield the same information as obtained from the whole 24-hour GH profile, the 24-hour GH profiles of a large group of healthy children were subdivided into segments of shorter duration. However, in children of both short and normal stature, GH secretion during the day was less than during the night period [9, 45–48]. This difference was more marked in the short children, among whom a subgroup of short children had detectable GH secretion only at night. However, if the goal is limited to evaluate the occurrence of any peaks at all, nocturnal secretion is more often maintained and is therefore the period of choice. In fact, the spontaneous GH_{max} value has a very high predictive value for the growth response to GH treatment, when used together with auxological variables in prediction models. For the vast majority of the children (97%), GH serum concentrations obtained during only 12 h of night-time GH sampling was by far a better predictor than the GH response to provocative testing, even though a GH peak lower than the 'true' GH_{max} was used [17]. If the sampling period is further shortened, a further loss in prediction power is found. However, it can still be evaluated to be clinically relevant with only a 6-hour sampling period [49]. Today, if starting at bed time, this is the optimal way for evaluating GH secretion in a clinical setting.

Analysis of Data in Evaluating Hormone Pulsatility

Time Series Analysis

Classical methods of time series analysis (Fourier transformation and spectral analysis [50, 51]) are suitable for analyses of the generally distinct circadian pattern of GH secretion [52–54]. Fourier analysis is a way of searching for underlying rhythmical components in a signal. Any complex waveform can be expressed as a sum of sine and cosine terms, with periods (frequencies) spanning over the whole sampling period (24 h for a 24-hour profile) down to half the sampling frequency. The resultant amplitude (power) at each frequency indicates the dominant and subdominant harmonics in the underlying waveform.

Pulse Detection

Two main goals with pulse detections are easily defined. The first one is to uncover the true underlying pattern in the profile. This is, however, not so simple since the underlying true pattern to compare with is seldom known. The other goal with a pulse detection method is to serve as a tool to evaluate and compare profiles from different groups of patients.

The considerable interest in defining endocrine pulse signals has resulted in the development of several computerized peak detection algorithms, a comparative study of which was performed [55–58]. This interest remains and there are recent publications of new pulse identification methods [59]. In our opinion, it is important always to use a peak detection algorithm for comparison purposes, even if none of them are entirely 'true'. In this way, it is at least possible to keep the same 'eyes' for a complete study [9]. For characterization of GH secretion, two algorithms are widely used: the Pulsar [60] and the Cluster [61] programs. The Pulsar program identifies secretory peaks by height and duration from a smoothed baseline, using the assay standard deviation as a scale factor. Investigators must then establish the G values themselves [9]. The G values represent the different criteria for cut-off levels for peaks of different widths. The Cluster program defines a pulse as a statistically significant increase in a cluster of hormone values, followed by a statistically significant decrease in a second cluster of values. Again, each investigator must then specify the number of points to be used in testing pre- and postpeak nadirs, as well as certain other settings of the program [62]. Comparisons between these two methods have shown that they give virtually the same results, with similar high peak detection efficacies [63, 64]. The Pulsar algorithm, however, appears to be more robust when GH series with lower sampling intensities are analyzed [63]. The results from these pulse algorithms can be used for further analyzes, e.g. in terms of changes in pulse amplitudes versus different factors, such as puberty [65, 66], GH status [67] or size at birth [68]. Complementary to these pulse detection methods is the method of approximate entropy (ApEn) to quantitate sequential irregularity [66].

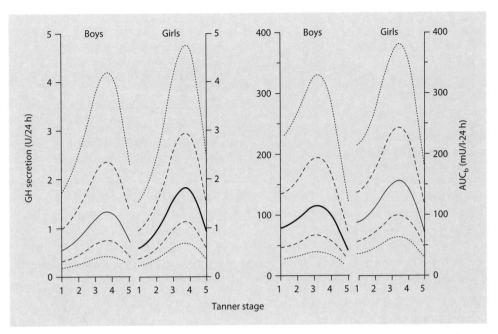

Fig. 4. GH secretion (left) and area under the plasma concentration curve above the baseline (AUC$_b$, right) for normal boys and girls at different stages of puberty. The figures show mean values (solid lines), ± 1 SD (dashed lines) and ± 2 SD (dotted lines). GH was assessed with a polyclonal assay (Pharmacia) with the IRP 66/217 reference preparation as reference [65].

Distribution Methods

With distribution methods, the log-transformed GH concentration values are sorted in ascending order regardless of their temporal attribute. The distribution of these values can then be plotted and compared between patient groups. With this method the through concentration can also be defined, as the threshold below which the GH concentrations are assessed to be 5% of the time [69].

Deconvolution Techniques

As previously stated, the plasma concentration measured during any interval represents the result of GH secretion into and elimination from the blood. Therefore, deconvolution procedures have been used for assessing the properties of the underlying secretory signal. In general, deconvolution (i.e. a process of uncoiling or unrolling) procedures remove mathematically the impact of clearance kinetics on plasma GH concentrations. As a result, the underlying secretion profiles are exposed. There are different deconvolution methods in use for GH secretion [30, 33, 70–72]. The estimated GH secretion rates for healthy children of normal height has previously been reported [65, 73] (fig. 4). A fully automated deconvolution procedure, AutoDecon, have recently been developed for LH [74], and 'translated to GH' [75]. However,

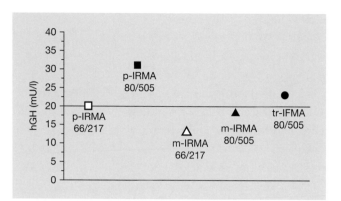

Fig. 5. Change in the calculated numerical value of GH plasma concentration due to a change of standard (reference preparation) and/or changes of antibodies.

sensitivity and specificity of pulse detection was estimated in simulated models with a new deconvolution method [76].

GH Measurements

Recent reports [4, 77] have emphasized that various radioimmunoassays or immunoradiometric assays differ in their measurements of concentrations of circulating GH [78–83]. Partly, these differences (up to 250%) are due to the use of polyclonal or monoclonal antibodies. All assays detect the 22-kDa form, but to a variable degree other forms of GH, e.g. the 20-, 17.5- and 5-kDa forms [84, 85]. Today, mainly assays with monoclonal antibodies are available. Furthermore, the influence of GH-binding protein(s) in the assay cannot be ruled out, even if some assays do not show any interference with the binding protein(s) for GH [4, 86]. The sensitivity of most of the radioimmunoassays in the low range detection limit (DL 0.5–1.0 µg/l) has earlier not been sufficient to evaluate plasma GH concentrations in the lower range. New methods, mainly immunoassays with higher sensitivities, are available (DL ~0.2 µg/l) [78, 82, 87–91] and even down to DL 0.002 µg/l [92]. Moreover, a shift in the reference preparation also contributes to different absolute levels (fig. 5) [93]. Furthermore, a change from international units-based to a weight-based reference preparation, in combination with a shift from pituitary-derived (66/217 and 80/505) to recombinant GH (88/624 and 98/574) in the reference, was agreed upon in 1994 by the Expert Committee on Biological Standardization. However, this has not been implemented fully, since some commercially available assays still not have shifted to recombinant GH references. Such a shift in the reference preparation will also influence the absolute levels. These differences must be kept in mind when comparing data from different groups and must also be considered when discussing 'cut-off levels' for normality [89, 94–96]. Moreover, GH immunoreactivity does not completely reflect bioactivity [97–99]. At present, a bioassay capable of confirming the results of various immunoassays on each sample of a 24-hour GH profile is not available, even if promising candidates have been developed [100, 101].

Reproducibility

For group data, there is a high degree of reproducibility for both GH secretion and GH patterns. However, intraindividual reproducibility is somewhat less pronounced, with a range of about 30% and a mean intraindividual coefficient of variation about 10–20%. This produces a sound skepticism when biological phenomena are related to a single GH profile of an individual child [102, 103]. When repeated GH profiles were determined for the nocturnal period only, greater variability was found for GH plasma concentrations [104–107]. We conclude that the reproducibility of repeated 24-hour profiles is nearly as low as the reproducibility of GH response to repeated pharmacologic tests to an individual child. If there are any differences, they are less pronounced for 24-hour integrated concentrations than for GH response to pharmacologic tests [14, 108, 109].

Biological Effects of Spontaneous GH Secretion

For an overview of studies relating to spontaneous GH secretion see our previous publication [110]. The studies included reflect different practical settings, such as mode of sampling, type of GH assay, and mode of analysis of data. All these parameters have to be taken into consideration when data of different studies are compared. Furthermore, before comparisons between different studies can be made, a careful characterization of the children investigated will be needed regarding height, weight, body composition and pubertal development.

The normal postnatal growth pattern can be divided into different phases: infancy, childhood, juvenility and puberty. The entire process is governed by many factors which operate during the different developmental stages. Growth during the fetal and the early postnatal periods is mainly nutrition dependent and not regarded as being entirely dependent on the secretion of hypophyseal GH [44], but GH originating from the placenta may also influence fetal growth. The transition from the infancy growth phase to the childhood growth phase is supposed to be due to the onset of the GH-IGF-1 axis action for growth [111]. In early childhood, the GH secretory pattern can be described with higher basal levels and lower peak amplitudes compared to later in childhood [68, 112, 113]. During childhood there is a relationship between GH secretion and growth [9, 10, 114–118], as well as during puberty [65, 66]. Excess of GH is known to cause gigantism, while GH deficiency leads to markedly short stature. Growth rates between these extremes, which are reflected in children's height, are principally determined by the amount of pulsatile GH secreted. This amount of GH can be expressed as the integrated area under the 24-hour GH concentration curve (AUC) or as the sum of the amplitudes of the individual peaks during a 24-hour period. Transforming the 24-hour plasma concentration profiles by deconvolution analysis into GH secretory rates in children further strengthens the correlation between height and GH secretion in healthy children [30, 65, 119].

A marked (2- to 4-fold) increase in GH secretion during puberty (fig. 4) [30, 45, 62, 65, 66, 119–123] parallels the growth spurt, which occurs earlier in girls than in boys. This increase in GH secretion seems to be an effect of sex steroid hormones, not least estrogens, and results from increased pulse amplitude during the day and at night without any change in pulse frequency [119, 124–126]. Time series analysis can be used to evaluate differences in rhythmicity between groups, e.g. in girls with Turner syndrome [127] and in patients with acute lymphatic leukemia [128].

Age-related changes in GH levels were described already in 1972 [129]. In adulthood, GH continues to be secreted in a pulsatile fashion [55]. Fasting [54] and exercise are well-known triggers of GH secretion, owing to increased pulse amplitudes and frequency [130, 131]. In contrast, GH concentrations is low in obesity due to an increased rate of degradation of GH [3, 7, 36, 37, 132–134]. Overall secretion decreases with age [135–138]. With use of accurate reference groups, GH secretion has been shown to be increased in children with diabetes [139].

Conclusions

In our opinion, direct measurements in blood of spontaneous GH secretion has markedly increased our knowledge of regulation of GH secretion in both normal and pathophysiologic states. For group data, reproducibility has proven to be high both regarding secretion rate and the pulsatile pattern. Therefore, we can conclude that for both clinical and scientific purposes 24-hour profiles will continue to be useful tools in future investigations as well. In a clinical setting, we propose a 6h sampling starting at bedtime or preferably 12 h, for diagnostic decision for growth and for selecting the GH dose for eventual treatment.

When evaluating the biological effects of GH, estimations of GH secretion (however precise they might be) can never account for more than 'half of the coin' (fig. 6). Such measurement will only be able to estimate the complexity of events leading to GH synthesis and pulsatile release from the somatotrophes to the bloodstream. Therefore, different studies in short children of heterogeneous etiology can give different results [46, 140–142]. The other 'half of the coin' consists of peripheral responsiveness to the GH molecule, i.e. the existence of functioning GH receptor(s), normal binding to the extracellular domain of the receptor (the so-called binding protein), and normal activation of intracellular postreceptor events, and more insights into that cascade of events are gathering [100, 101, 143–145].

Since variation in GH secretion is a gradual phenomenon, there will never be one single test that can provide us with an easily defined cut-off level by which abnormality may be separated from normality not least due to assay diversities. Of course, this is true also for 24-hour secretory profiles, although the variation for spontaneous GH secretion seems to be lower than for repeated provocative tests.

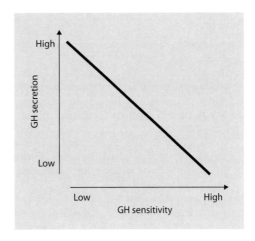

Fig. 6. Continuum in GH secretion and sensitivity.

Patients with severe GH deficiency can always be identified. For a proper diagnosis, the patients within the gray zone of GH insufficiency will certainly need a multivariate diagnostic approach, since the accepted diagnostic procedure only predicts 33% of the variation in growth response to GH treatment [146]. More information is needed for selecting the children with functional GH insufficiency who will benefit from GH treatment [147–150].

Today, several excellent prediction models have been developed in order to accurately estimate the individual growth response to GH treatment, at start of treatment for children with GHD [95], for children with isolated GHD or ISS [16], and for girls with Turner syndrome [151] and children born SGA [152, 153] and with use of 1st year growth that could replace early growth and 24 hGH$_{max}$ [154]. With use of these models both a better functional diagnosis can be made and a tailor-made treatment regimen for each individual to ensure that the treatment goal will be reached. In fact, when individual dosing was based on estimated responsiveness from use of prediction model, a more narrow range around a predefined height goal was obtained as well as reduced range of insulin levels and HOMA [15, 155].

References

1 Robinson I: Chronopharmacology of growth hormone and related peptides. Adv Drug Deliv Rev 1991;6:57–82.

2 Bonnefont X, Lacampagne A, Sanchez-Hormigo A, Fino E, Creff A, Mathieu MN, Smallwood S, Carmignac D, Fontanaud P, Travo P, Alonso G, Courtois-Coutry N, Pincus SM, Robinson IC, Mollard P: Revealing the large-scale network organization of growth hormone-secreting cells. Proc Natl Acad Sci USA 2005;102:16880–16885.

3 Veldhuis JD, Keenan DM, Pincus SM: Motivations and methods for analyzing pulsatile hormone secretion. Endocr Rev 2008;29:823–864.

4 Bidlingmaier M, Freda PU: Measurement of human growth hormone by immunoassays: current status, unsolved problems and clinical consequences. Growth Horm IGF Res 2010;20:19–25.

5 Rosenfeld RG, Albertsson-Wikland K, Cassorla F, et al: Diagnostic controversy: the diagnosis of childhood growth hormone deficiency revisited. J Clinl Endocrinol Metabol 1995;80:1532–1540.

6 Tannenbaum GS, Painson JC, Lapointe M, Gurd W, McCarthy GF: Interplay of somatostatin and growth hormone-releasing hormone in genesis of episodic growth hormone secretion. Metabolism 1990;39(9 suppl 2):35–39.

7 Veldhuis JD, Roemmich JN, Richmond EJ, Bowers CY: Somatotropic and gonadotropic axes linkages in infancy, childhood, and the puberty-adult transition. Endocrine reviews 2006;27:101–140.

8 Gelander L, Albertsson-Wikland K: Growth hormone (GH) release after administration of GH-releasing hormone in relation to endogenous 24-h GH secretion in short children. J Endocrinol 1989;122:61–68.

9 Albertsson-Wikland K, Rosberg S: Analyses of 24-hour growth hormone profiles in children: relation to growth. J Clin Endocrinol Metab 1988;67:493–500.

10 Hindmarsh P, Smith PJ, Brook CG, Matthews DR: The relationship between height velocity and growth hormone secretion in short prepubertal children. Clin Endocrinol (Oxf) 1987;27:581–591.

11 Diamond FB, Jorgensen EV, Root AW, Shulman DI, Sy JP, Blethen SL, Bercu BB: The role of serial sampling in the diagnosis of growth hormone deficiency. Pediatrics 1998;102:521–524.

12 Bercu BB, Shulman D, Root AW, Spiliotis BE: Growth hormone (GH) provocative testing frequently does not reflect endogenous GH secretion. J Clin Endocrinol Metab 1986;63:709–716.

13 Garner P, Raynaud F, Job J: Growth hormone secretion during sleep. I. Comparison with GH responses to conventional pharmacologic stimuli in pubertal and early pubertal short subjects: effects of treatment with human GH in patients with discrepant measurements of GH secretion. Horm Res 1988;29:133–139.

14 Zadik Z, Chalew SA, Gilula Z, Kowarski AA: Reproducibility of growth hormone testing procedures: a comparison between 24-hour integrated concentration and pharmacological stimulation. J Clin Endocrinol Metab 1990;71:1127–1130.

15 Kriström B, Aronson AS, Dahlgren J, Gustafsson J, Halldin M, Ivarsson SA, Nilsson NO, Svensson J, Tuvemo T, Albertsson-Wikland K: Growth hormone (GH) dosing during catch-up growth guided by individual responsiveness decreases growth response variability in prepubertal children with GH deficiency or idiopathic short stature. J Clin Endocrinol Metab 2009;94:483–490.

16 Albertsson-Wikland K, Kristrom B, Rosberg S, Svensson B, Nierop AF: Validated multivariate models predicting the growth response to GH treatment in individual short children with a broad range in GH secretion capacities. Pediatr Res 2000;48:475–484.

17 Kriström B, Löfqvist C, Rosberg S, Albertsson-Wikland K: Effect of spontaneous GH secretion and the GH sampling period on the accuracy of models for predicting growth responses to GH treatment. J Clin Endocrinol Metab 2001;86:4963–4964.

18 Albers N: Overview of pulse actions in the human. Growth Horm IGF Res 2001;11(suppl A):S39–S42.

19 Hauffa BP: Clinical implications of pulsatile hormone signals. Growth Horm IGF Res 2001;11(suppl A):S1–S8.

20 Oscarsson J: Growth Hormone Regulation of Serum Lipoproteins in the Rat. Göteborg, University of Göteborg, 1990.

21 Isgaard J, Carlsson L, Isaksson OG, Jansson JO: Pulsatile intravenous growth hormone (GH) infusion to hypophysectomized rats increases insulin-like growth factor I messenger ribonucleic acid in skeletal tissues more effectively than continuous GH infusion. Endocrinology 1988;123:2605–2610.

22 Maiter D, Underwood LE, Maes M, Davenport ML, Ketelslegers JM: Different effects of intermittent and continuous growth hormone (GH) administration on serum somatomedin-C/insulin-like growth factor I and liver GH receptors in hypophysectomized rats. Endocrinology 1988;123:1053–1059.

23 Dhir RN, Shapiro BH: Interpulse growth hormone secretion in the episodic plasma profile causes the sex reversal of cytochrome P450s in senescent male rats. Proc Natl Acad Sci USA 2003;100:15224–15228.

24 Mode A, Norstedt G, Simic B, Eneroth P, Gustafsson JA: Continuous infusion of growth hormone feminizes hepatic steroid metabolism in the rat. Endocrinology 1981;108:2103–2108.

25 Clark RG, Jansson JO, Isaksson O, Robinson IC: Intravenous growth hormone: growth responses to patterned infusions in hypophysectomized rats. J Endocrinol 1985;104:53–61.

26 Jansson JO, Albertsson-Wikland K, Eden S, Thorngren KG, Isaksson O: Effect of frequency of growth hormone administration on longitudinal bone growth and body weight in hypophysectomized rats. Acta Physiol Scand 1982;114:261–265.

27 Jansson JO, Albertsson-Wikland K, Eden S, Thorngren KG, Isaksson O: Circumstantial evidence for a role of the secretory pattern of growth hormone in control of body growth. Acta Endocrinol (Copenh) 1982;99:24–30.

28 Albertsson-Wikland K, Westphal O, Westgren U: Daily subcutaneous administration of human growth hormone in growth hormone deficient children. Acta Paediatr Scand 1986;75:89–97.

29 Ranke MB, Guilbaud O: Growth response in prepubertal children with idiopathic growth hormone deficiency during the first year of treatment with human growth hormone: analysis of the Kabi International Growth Study. Acta Paediatr Scand 1990;370:122–130.

30 Albertsson-Wikland K, Rosberg S, Libre E, Lundberg LO, Groth T: Growth hormone secretory rates in children as estimated by deconvolution analysis of 24-h plasma concentration profiles. Am J Physiol 1989;257:E809–E814.

31 Faria AC, Veldhuis JD, Thorner MO, Vance ML: Half-time of endogenous growth hormone (GH) disappearance in normal man after stimulation of GH secretion by GH-releasing hormone and suppression with somatostatin. J Clin Endocrinol Metab 1989;68:535–541.

32 Bright GM, Veldhuis JD, Iranmanesh A, Baumann G, Maheshwari H, Lima J: Appraisal of growth hormone (GH) secretion: evaluation of a composite pharmacokinetic model that discriminates multiple components of GH input. J Clin Endocrinol Metab 1999;84:3301–3308.

33 Hindmarsh PC, Matthews DR, Brain C, Pringle PJ, Brook CG: The application of deconvolution analysis to elucidate the pulsatile nature of growth hormone secretion using a variable half-life of growth hormone. Clin Endocrinol (Oxf) 1990;32:739–747.

34 Hindmarsh PC, Matthews DR, Brain CE, Pringle PJ, di Silvio L, Kurtz AB, Brook CG: The half-life of exogenous growth hormone after suppression of endogenous growth hormone secretion with somatostatin. Clin Endocrinol (Oxf) 1989;30:443–450.

35 Holl RW, Schwarz U, Schauwecker P, Benz R, Veldhuis JD, Heinze E: Diurnal variation in the elimination rate of human growth hormone (GH): the half-life of serum GH is prolonged in the evening, and affected by the source of the hormone, as well as by body size and serum estradiol. J Clin Endocrinol Metab 1993;77:216–220.

36 Langendonk JG, Meinders AE, Burggraaf J, Frolich M, Roelen CA, Schoemaker RC, Cohen AF, Pijl H: Influence of obesity and body fat distribution on growth hormone kinetics in humans. Am J Physiol 1999;277:E824–E829.

37 Langendonk JG, Veldhuis JD, Burggraaf J, Schoemaker RC, Cohen AF, Meinders AE, Pijl H: Estimation of growth hormone secretion rate: impact of kinetic assumptions intrinsic to the analytical approach. Am J Physiol Regul Integr Comp Physiol 2001;280:R225–R232.

38 Carlsson LM, Rosberg S, Vitangcol RV, Wong WL, Albertsson-Wikland K: Analysis of 24-hour plasma profiles of growth hormone (GH)-binding protein, GH/GH-binding protein-complex, and GH in healthy children. J Clin Endocrinol Metab 1993;77:356–361.

39 Bjarnason R, Albertsson-Wikland K, Carlsson LM. Acute and chronic effects of subcutaneous growth hormone (GH) injections on plasma levels of GH binding protein in short children. J Clin Endocrinol Metab 1995;80:2756–2760.

40 Evans WS, Faria AC, Christiansen E, Ho KY, Weiss J, Rogol AD, Johnson ML, Blizzard RM, Veldhuis JD, Thorner MO: Impact of intensive venous sampling on characterization of pulsatile GH release. Am J Physiol 1987;252(4 Pt 1):E549– E556.

41 Hartman ML, Iranmesh A, Thorner MO, Veldhuis JD: Evaluation of pulsatile patterns of growth hormone release in humans: a brief review. Am J Hum Biol 1993;5:603–614.

42 Holl RW, Hartman ML, Veldhuis JD, Taylor WM, Thorner MO: Thirty-second sampling of plasma growth hormone in man: correlation with sleep stages. J Clin Endocrinol Metab 1991;72:854–861.

43 Groth T, Rosberg S, Albertsson-Wikland K: Estimation of growth hormone secretory patterns in children with use of a numerical deconvolution technique: experimental design with use of computer simulation. Horm Res 1994;42:245–252.

44 Adcock CJ, Ogilvy-Stuart AL, Robinson IC, Lewin JE, Holly JM, Harris DA, Watts AP, Doyle KL, Matthews DR, Wilkinson AR, Dunger DB: The use of an automated microsampling system for the characterization of growth hormone pulsatility in newborn babies. Pediatr Res 1997;42:66–71.

45 Delemarre-Van De Waal HA, Wennink JM, Odink RJ: Gonadotrophin and growth hormone secretion throughout puberty. Acta Paediatr Scand Suppl 1991;372:26–31; discussion 2.

46 Rose SR: Overnight studies of growth hormone for the diagnosis of growth hormone deficiency. Endocrinologist 1991;1:25–32.

47 Rose SR, Ross JL, Uriarte M, Barnes KM, Cassorla FG, Cutler GB Jr: The advantage of measuring stimulated as compared with spontaneous growth hormone levels in the diagnosis of growth hormone deficiency. N Engl J Med 1988 28;319:201–207.

48 Saggese G, Cesaretti G, Cinquanta L, Giannessi N, Bracaloni C, Di Spigno G, Cioni C: Evaluation of 24-hour growth hormone spontaneous secretion: comparison with a nocturnal and diurnal 12-hour study. Horm Res 1991;35:25–29.

49 Rose SR, Municchi G: Six-hour and four-hour nocturnal sampling for growth hormone. J Pediatr Endocrinol Metab 1999;12:167–173.

50 Chatfield C: The Analysis of Time Series. London, Chapman & Hall, 1989.

51 Matthews DR: Time series analysis in endocrinology. Acta Paediatr Scand Suppl 1988;347:55–62.

52 Dunger DB, Matthews DR, Edge JA, Jones J, Preece MA: Evidence for temporal coupling of growth hormone, prolactin, LH and FSH pulsatility overnight during normal puberty. J Endocrinol 1991;130:141–149.

53 Hindmarsh PC, Matthews DR, Brook CG: Growth hormone secretion in children determined by time series analysis. Clin Endocrinol (Oxf) 1988;29:35–44.

54 Ho KY, Veldhuis JD, Johnson ML, Furlanetto R, Evans WS, Alberti KG, Thorner MO: Fasting enhances growth hormone secretion and amplifies the complex rhythms of growth hormone secretion in man. J Clin Invest 1988;81:968–975.

55 Hartman ML, Faria AC, Vance ML, Johnson ML, Thorner MO, Veldhuis JD: Temporal structure of in vivo growth hormone secretory events in humans. Am J Physiol 1991;260:E101–E110.

56 Kushler RH, Brown MB: A model for the identification of hormone pulses. Stat Med 1991;10:329–340.

57 Randall J, Kaiser D, van Cauter E, Johnson M, Veldhuis J: Comparative assessments of objective peak-detection algorithms. II. Studies in men. Am J Physiol 1988;254:E113–E119.

58 Veldhuis JD, Faria A, Vance ML, Evans WS, Thorner MO, Johnson ML: Contemporary tools for the analysis of episodic growth hormone secretion and clearance in vivo. Acta Paediatr Scand Suppl 1988;347:63–82.

59 Vis DJ, Westerhuis JA, Hoefsloot HC, Pijl H, Roelfsema F, van der Greef J, Smilde AK: Endocrine pulse identification using penalized methods and a minimum set of assumptions. Am J Physiol 2010;298:E145–E155.

60 Merriam GR, Wachter KW: Algorithms for the study of episodic hormone secretion. Am J Physiol 1982;243:E310–E318.

61 Veldhuis JD, Johnson ML: Cluster analysis: a simple, versatile, and robust algorithm for endocrine pulse detection. Am J Physiol 1986;250(4 Pt 1):E486–E493.

62 Mauras N, Blizzard RM, Link K, Johnson ML, Rogol AD, Veldhuis JD: Augmentation of growth hormone secretion during puberty: evidence for a pulse amplitude-modulated phenomenon. J Clin Endocrinol Metab 1987;64:596–601.

63 Hauffa BP, Stolecke H: Receiver-operated characteristic curve analysis of two algorithms assessing human growth hormone pulsatile secretion (PULSAR, CLUSTER): comparison of peak detection efficacy. Horm Res 1994;41:169–176.

64 Partsch CJ, Abrahams S, Herholz N, Peter M, Veldhuis JD, Sippell WG: Variability of pulsatile luteinizing hormone secretion in young male volunteers. Eur J Endocrinol 1994;131:263–272.

65 Albertsson-Wikland K, Rosberg S, Karlberg J, Groth T. Analysis of 24-hour growth hormone profiles in healthy boys and girls of normal stature: relation to puberty. J Clin Endocrinol Metab 1994;78:1195–1201.

66 Pincus SM, Veldhuis JD, Rogol AD. Longitudinal changes in growth hormone secretory process irregularity assessed transpubertally in healthy boys. Am J Physiol 2000;279:E417–E424.

67 Zadik Z, Chalew SA, Kowarski A: The definition of a spontaneous growth hormone (GH) peak: studies in normally growing and GH-deficient children. J Clin Endocrinol Metab 1992;74:801–805.

68 Boguszewski M, Rosberg S, Albertsson-Wikland K: Spontaneous 24-hour growth hormone profiles in prepubertal small for gestational age children. J Clin Endocrinol Metab 1995;80:2599–2606.

69 Matthews DR, Hindmarsh PC, Pringle PJ, Brook CG: A distribution method for analysing the baseline of pulsatile endocrine signals as exemplified by 24-hour growth hormone profiles. Clin Endocrinol (Oxf) 1991;35:245–252.

70 Groth TL: Conversion of diurnal plasma hormone concentration profiles into secretion rates. Acta Paediatr Scand Suppl 1991;372:57–61, discussion 2.

71 Oerter KE, Guardabasso V, Rodbard D: Detection and characterization of peaks and estimation of instantaneous secretory rate for episodic pulsatile hormone secretion. Comput Biomed Res 1986;19:170–191.

72 Veldhuis JD, Carlson ML, Johnson ML: The pituitary gland secretes in bursts: appraising the nature of glandular secretory impulses by simultaneous multiple-parameter deconvolution of plasma hormone concentrations. Proc Natl Acad Sci USA 1987;84:7686–7690.

73 Martha PM Jr, Gorman KM, Blizzard RM, Rogol AD, Veldhuis JD: Endogenous growth hormone secretion and clearance rates in normal boys, as determined by deconvolution analysis: relationship to age, pubertal status, and body mass. J Clin Endocrinol Metab 1992;74:336–344.

74 Johnson ML, Pipes L, Veldhuis PP, Farhy LS, Boyd DG, Evans WS: AutoDecon, a deconvolution algorithm for identification and characterization of luteinizing hormone secretory bursts: description and validation using synthetic data. Analyt Biochem 2008;381:8–17.

75 Johnson ML, Pipes L, Veldhuis PP, Farhy LS, Nass R, Thorner MO, Evans WS: AutoDecon: a robust numerical method for the quantification of pulsatile events. Methods Enzymol 2009;454:367–404.

76   Liu PY, Keenan DM, Kok P, Padmanabhan V, O'Byrne KT, Veldhuis JD: Sensitivity and specificity of pulse detection using a new deconvolution method. Am J Physiol 2009;297:E538–E544.

77   Popii V, Baumann G: Laboratory measurement of growth hormone. Clin Chim Acta 2004;350:1–16.

78   Albertsson-Wikland K, Jansson C, Rosberg S, Novamo A: Time-resolved immunofluorometric assay of human growth hormone. Clin Chem 1993; 39:1620–1625.

79   Albertsson-Wikland K, Rosberg S: Pattern of spontaneous growth hormone secretion in Turner syndrome. Excerpta Medica ICS 1991;924:89–94.

80   Andersson AM, Orskov H, Ranke MB, Shalet S, Skakkebaek NE: Interpretation of growth hormone provocative tests: comparison of cut-off values in four European laboratories. Eur J Endocrinol 1995;132:340–343.

81   Boguszewski CL, Hynsjo L, Johannsson G, Bengtsson BA, Carlsson LM: 22-kD growth hormone exclusion assay: a new approach to measurement of non-22-kD growth hormone isoforms in human blood. Eur J Endocrinol 1996;135:573–582.

82   Jansson C, Boguszewski C, Rosberg S, Carlsson L, Albertsson-Wikland K: Growth hormone (GH) assays: influence of standard preparations, GH isoforms, assay characteristics, and GH-binding protein. Clin Chem 1997;43:950–956.

83   Strasburger CJ: Laboratory assessment of GH. Growth Horm IGF Res 1998;8(suppl A):41–46.

84   Jeffcoate SL: Analytical and clinical significance of peptide hormone heterogeneity with particular reference to growth hormone and luteinizing hormone in serum. Clin Endocrinol (Oxf) 1993;38:113–121.

85   Jonsdottir I, Luthman M, Ekre HP, Skoog B, Brostedt P, Roos P, Werner S, Perlmann P: High molecular weight growth hormone (>160 kD) in human serum characterized with monoclonal antibodies. Horm Res 1994;41:197–204.

86   Celniker AC, Chen AB, Wert RM Jr, Sherman BM: Variability in the quantitation of circulating growth hormone using commercial immunoassays. J Clin Endocrinol Metab 1989;68:469–476.

87   Goji K: Pulsatile characteristics of spontaneous growth hormone (GH) concentration profiles in boys evaluated by an ultrasensitive immunoradiometric assay: evidence for ultradian periodicity of GH secretion. J Clin Endocrinol Metab 1993;76:667–670.

88   Iranmanesh A, Grisso B, Veldhuis JD: Low basal and persistent pulsatile growth hormone secretion are revealed in normal and hyposomatotropic men studied with a new ultrasensitive chemiluminescence assay. J Clin Endocrinol Metab 1994;78:526–535.

89   Mauras N, Walton P, Nicar M, Welch S, Rogol AD: Growth hormone stimulation testing in both short and normal statured children: use of an immunofunctional assay. Pediatr Res 2000;48:614–618.

90   Pringle PJ, Di Silvio L, Hindmarsh PC, Matthews DR, Kurtz AB, Brook CG: Analysis of trough serum growth hormone concentrations: comparison of an immunoradiometric assay and a sensitive ELISA for growth hormone. Clin Endocrinol (Oxf) 1992;37:169–174.

91   Reutens AT, Hoffman DM, Leung KC, Ho KK: Evaluation and application of a highly sensitive assay for serum growth hormone (GH) in the study of adult GH deficiency. J Clin Endocrinol Metab 1995;80:480–485.

92   Chapman IM, Hartman ML, Straume M, Johnson ML, Veldhuis JD, Thorner MO: Enhanced sensitivity growth hormone (GH) chemiluminescence assay reveals lower postglucose nadir GH concentrations in men than women. J Clin Endocrinol Metab 1994; 78:1312–1319.

93   Löfqvist C: GH Secretion in Children: Methodological Aspects of Determining Immunoreactive and Bioactive Isoforms. Göteborg, Göteborg University, 2000.

94   Chaler E, Belgorosky A, Maceiras M, Mendioroz M, Rivarola MA: Between-assay differences in serum growth hormone (GH) measurements: importance in the diagnosis of GH deficiency in childhood. Clin Chem 2001;47:1735–1738.

95   Ranke MB, Lindberg A, Chatelain P, Wilton P, Cutfield W, Albertsson-Wikland K, Price DA: Derivation and validation of a mathematical model for predicting the response to exogenous recombinant human growth hormone (GH) in prepubertal children with idiopathic GH deficiency. KIGS International Board. Kabi Pharmacia International Growth Study. J Clin Endocrinol Metab 1999;84: 1174–1183.

96   Schmidt H, Dorr HG, Butenandt O, Galli-Tsinopoulou A, Kiess W: Measurement of spontaneous, 12-hour sleep-associated GH secretion in prepubertal children with short stature: clinical relevance and practicability? Horm Res 1996;46:33–37.

97   Ikeda M, Wada M, Fujita Y, Takahashi S, Maekawa K, Honjo M: A novel bioassay based on human growth hormone (hGH) receptor mediated cell proliferation: measurement of 20K-hGH and its modified forms. Growth Horm IGF Res 2000;10: 248–255.

98   Ishikawa M, Nimura A, Horikawa R, Katsumata N, Arisaka O, Wada M, Honjo M, Tanaka T: A novel specific bioassay for serum human growth hormone. J Clin Endocrinol Metab 2000;85:4274–4279.

99 Radetti G, Bozzola M, Pagani S, Street ME, Ghizzoni L: Growth hormone immunoreactivity does not reflect bioactivity. Pediatr Res 2000;48:619–622.

100 Strasburger CJ: Antigenic epitope mapping of the human growth hormone molecule: a strategy to standardize growth hormone immunoassays. Acta Paediatr Scand Suppl 1990;370:82–86.

101 Strasburger CJ: Implications of investigating the structure-function relationship of human growth hormone in clinical diagnosis and therapy. Horm Res 1994;41(suppl 2):113–119, discussion 20.

102 Albertsson-Wikland K, Rosberg S: Reproducibility of 24-h growth hormone profiles in children. Acta Endocrinol (Copenh) 1992;126:109–112.

103 Barton J, Saini S, Hindmarsh P, Matthews D, Pringle P, Jones J, Preece M, Brook C: Reproducibility of 24 hour serum growth hormone profiles in man. 29th Ann Meet Eur Socr Paediatric Endocrinology (ESPE), Vienna, 1990.

104 Donaldson DL, Hollowell JG, Pan FP, Gifford RA, Moore WV: Growth hormone secretory profiles: variation on consecutive nights. J Pediatr 1989;115:51–56.

105 Lanes R: Diagnostic limitations of spontaneous growth hormone measurements in normally growing prepubertal children. Am J Dis Child 1989;143:1284–1286.

106 Spadoni GL, Cianfarani S, Bernardini S, Vaccaro F, Galasso C, Manca Bitti ML, Costa F, Boscherini B: Twelve-hour spontaneous nocturnal growth hormone secretion in growth retarded patients. Clin Pediatr (Phila) 1988;27:473–478.

107 Tassoni P, Cacciari E, Cau M, et al: Variability of growth hormone response to pharmacological and sleep tests performed twice in short children. J Clin Endocrinol Metab 1990;71:230–234.

108 Ropelato MG, Martinez A, Heinrich JJ, Bergada C: Reproducibility and comparison of growth hormone secretion tests. J Pediatr Endocrinol Metab 1996;9:41–50.

109 Saini S, Hindmarsh PC, Matthews DR, Pringle PJ, Jones J, Preece MA, Brook CG: Reproducibility of 24-hour serum growth hormone profiles in man. Clin Endocrinol (Oxf) 1991;34:455–462.

110 Albertsson-Wikland K, Rosberg S: Methods of evaluating spontaneous growth hormone secretion; in Ranke M (ed): Functional Endocrinologic Diagnostics in Children and Adolescents, ed 3. Mannheim, J&J Verlag, 2003, pp 129–159.

111 Hochberg Z, Albertsson-Wikland K: Evo-devo of infantile and childhood growth. Pediatr Res 2008;64:2–7.

112 de Waal WJ, Hokken-Koelega AC, Stijnen T, de Muinck Keizer-Schrama SM, Drop SL: Endogenous and stimulated GH secretion, urinary GH excretion, and plasma IGF-I and IGF-II levels in prepubertal children with short stature after intrauterine growth retardation. The Dutch Working Group on Growth Hormone. Clin Endocrinol (Oxf) 1994;41:621–630.

113 Miller JD, Tannenbaum GS, Colle E, Guyda HJ: Daytime pulsatile growth hormone secretion during childhood and adolescence. J Clin Endocrinol Metab 1982;55:989–994.

114 Bierich JR, Brugmann G, Kiessling E: Spontaneous secretion of growth hormone in deep nocturnal sleep. II. Studies on hypophyseal dwarfism and constitutional developmental delay. Monatsschr Kinderheilkd 1989;137:80–85.

115 Bierich JR, Brugmann G, Schippert R: Spontaneous secretion of growth hormone in deep nocturnal sleep. I. Measurement, calculation and normal values in childhood. Monatsschr Kinderheilkd 1985;133:342–346.

116 Gill MS, Thalange NK, Foster PJ, Tillmann V, Price DA, Diggle PJ, Clayton PE: Regular fluctuations in growth hormone (GH) release determine normal human growth. Growth Horm IGF Res 1999;9:114–122.

117 Gill MS, Tillmann V, Veldhuis JD, Clayton PE: Patterns of GH output and their synchrony with short-term height increments influence stature and growth performance in normal children. J Clin Endocrinol Metab 2001;86:5860–5863.

118 Weill J, Duhamel A, Dherbomez M, Beuscart R, Ponte C: Pulsatility of growth hormone secretion and its relation to growth. Horm Res 1992;38:134–139.

119 Veldhuis JD, Roemmich JN, Rogol AD: Gender and sexual maturation-dependent contrasts in the neuroregulation of growth hormone secretion in prepubertal and late adolescent males and females–a general clinical research center-based study. J Clin Endocrinol Metab 2000;85:2385–2394.

120 Martha PM, Jr., Rogol AD, Veldhuis JD, Kerrigan JR, Goodman DW, Blizzard RM: Alterations in the pulsatile properties of circulating growth hormone concentrations during puberty in boys. J Clin Endocrinol Metab 1989;69:563–570.

121 Rose SR, Municchi G, Barnes KM, Kamp GA, Uriarte MM, Ross JL, Cassorla F, Cutler GB Jr: Spontaneous growth hormone secretion increases during puberty in normal girls and boys. J Clin Endocrinol Metab 1991;73:428–435.

122 Wennink JM, Delemarre-van de Waal HA, Schoemaker R, Blaauw G, van den Braken C, Schoemaker J: Growth hormone secretion patterns in relation to LH and testosterone secretion throughout normal male puberty. Acta Endocrinol (Copenh) 1990;123:263–270.

123 Wennink JM, Delemarre-van de Waal HA, Schoemaker R, Blaauw G, van den Braken C, Schoemaker J: Growth hormone secretion patterns in relation to LH and estradiol secretion throughout normal female puberty. Acta Endocrinol (Copenh) 1991;124:129–135.

124 Link K, Blizzard RM, Evans WS, Kaiser DL, Parker MW, Rogol AD: The effect of androgens on the pulsatile release and the twenty-four-hour mean concentration of growth hormone in peripubertal males. J Clin Endocrinol Metab 1986;62:159–164.

125 Ross JL, Pescovitz OH, Barnes K, Loriaux DL, Cutler GB Jr: Growth hormone secretory dynamics in children with precocious puberty. J Pediatr 1987;110:369–372.

126 Ulloa-Aguirre A, Blizzard RM, Garcia-Rubi E, Rogol AD, Link K, Christie CM, Johnson ML, Veldhuis JD: Testosterone and oxandrolone, a non-aromatizable androgen, specifically amplify the mass and rate of growth hormone (GH) secreted per burst without altering GH secretory burst duration or frequency or the GH half-life. J Clin Endocrinol Metab 1990;71:846–854.

127 Wit JM, Massarano AA, Kamp GA, Hindmarsh PC, van Es A, Brook CG, Preece MA, Matthews DR: Growth hormone secretion in patients with Turner's syndrome as determined by time series analysis. Acta Endocrinol (Copenh) 1992;127:7–12.

128 Lannering B, Rosberg S, Marky I, Moell C, Albertsson-Wikland K: Reduced growth hormone secretion with maintained periodicity following cranial irradiation in children with acute lymphoblastic leukaemia. Clin Endocrinol (Oxf) 1995;42:153–159.

129 Finkelstein JW, Roffwarg HP, Boyar RM, Kream J, Hellman L: Age-related change in the twenty-four-hour spontaneous secretion of growth hormone. J Clin Endocrinol Metab 1972;35:665–670.

130 Hartman ML, Veldhuis JD, Johnson ML, Lee MM, Alberti KG, Samojlik E, Thorner MO: Augmented growth hormone (GH) secretory burst frequency and amplitude mediate enhanced GH secretion during a two-day fast in normal men. J Clin Endocrinol Metab 1992;74:757–765.

131 Roemmich JN, Clark PA, Mai V, Berr SS, Weltman A, Veldhuis JD, Rogol AD: Alterations in growth and body composition during puberty: III. Influence of maturation, gender, body composition, fat distribution, aerobic fitness, and energy expenditure on nocturnal growth hormone release. J Clin Endocrinol Metab 1998;83:1440–1447.

132 Abdenur JE, Solans CV, Smith MM, Carman C, Pugliese MT, Lifshitz F: Body composition and spontaneous growth hormone secretion in normal short stature children. J Clin Endocrinol Metab 1994;78:277–282.

133 Iranmanesh A, Lizarralde G, Veldhuis JD: Age and relative adiposity are specific negative determinants of the frequency and amplitude of growth hormone (GH) secretory bursts and the half-life of endogenous GH in healthy men. J Clin Endocrinol Metab 1991;73:1081–1088.

134 Veldhuis JD, Iranmanesh A, Ho KK, Waters MJ, Johnson ML, Lizarralde G: Dual defects in pulsatile growth hormone secretion and clearance subserve the hyposomatotropism of obesity in man. J Clin Endocrinol Metab 1991;72:51–59.

135 Ho KY, Evans WS, Blizzard RM, Veldhuis JD, Merriam GR, Samojlik E, Furlanetto R, Rogol AD, Kaiser DL, Thorner MO. Effects of sex and age on the 24-hour profile of growth hormone secretion in man: importance of endogenous estradiol concentrations. J Clin Endocrinol Metab 1987;64:51–58.

136 Marchesi G, Morosini P, Nardi B, Santone G, Arnaldi G: Age-related modifications of the human growth hormone circadian secretory pattern studied with a new statistical method in healthy adults. Med Sci Res 1989;17:697–698.

137 Minuto F, Barreca A, Ferrini S, Mazzocchi G, Del Monte P, Giordano G: Growth hormone secretion in pubertal and adult subjects. Acta Endocrinol (Copenh) 1982;99:161–165.

138 Zadik Z, Chalew SA, McCarter RJ, Jr., Meistas M, Kowarski AA: The influence of age on the 24-hour integrated concentration of growth hormone in normal individuals. J Clin Endocrinol Metab 1985;60:513–516.

139 Edge JA, Dunger DB, Matthews DR, Gilbert JP, Smith CP: Increased overnight growth hormone concentrations in diabetic compared with normal adolescents. J Clin Endocrinol Metab 1990;71:1356–1362.

140 Costin G, Kaufman FR: Growth hormone secretory patterns in children with short stature. J Pediatr 1987;110:362–368.

141 Pozo J, Argente J, Barrios V, Gonzalez-Parra S, Munoz MT, Hernandez H: Growth hormone secretion in children with normal variants of short stature. Horm Res 1994;41:185–192.

142 Zadik Z, Chalew SA, Raiti S, Kowarski AA: Do short children secrete insufficient growth hormone? Pediatrics 1985;76:355–360.

143 Beattie J: Structural and functional aspects of the interaction between growth hormone and its receptor. Biochim Biophys Acta 1993;1203:1–10.

144 Cunningham BC, Jhurani P, Ng P, Wells JA: Receptor and antibody epitopes in human growth hormone identified by homolog-scanning mutagenesis. Science 1989;243:1330–1336.

145 Roupas P, Herington AC: Cellular mechanisms in the processing of growth hormone and its receptor. Mol Cell Endocrinol 1989;61:1–12.

146 Kristrom B, Karlberg J, Albertsson-Wikland K: Prediction of the growth response of short prepubertal children treated with growth hormone. Swedish Paediatric Study Group for GH treatment. Acta Paediatr 1995;84:51–57.

147 Consensus guidelines for the diagnosis and treatment of growth hormone (GH) deficiency in childhood and adolescence: summary statement of the GH Research Society. GH Research Society. J Clin Endocrinol Metab 2000;85:3990–3993.

148 Cohen P, Rogol AD, Deal CL, Saenger P, Reiter EO, Ross JL, Chernausek SD, Savage MO, Wit JM: Consensus statement on the diagnosis and treatment of children with idiopathic short stature: a summary of the Growth Hormone Research Society, the Lawson Wilkins Pediatric Endocrine Society, and the European Society for Paediatric Endocrinology Workshop. J Clin Endocrinol Metab 2008;93:4210–4217.

149 Wit JM, Clayton PE, Rogol AD, Savage MO, Saenger PH, Cohen P: Idiopathic short stature: definition, epidemiology, and diagnostic evaluation. Growth Horm IGF Res 2008;18:89–110.

150 Wit JM, Reiter EO, Ross JL, Saenger PH, Savage MO, Rogol AD, Cohen P: Idiopathic short stature: management and growth hormone treatment. Growth Horm IGF Res 2008;18:111–135.

151 Ranke MB, Lindberg A, Chatelain P, Wilton P, Cutfield W, Albertsson-Wikland K, Price DA: Prediction of long-term response to recombinant human growth hormone in Turner syndrome: development and validation of mathematical models. KIGS International Board. Kabi International Growth Study. J Clin Endocrinol Metab 2000;85:4212–4218.

152 Dahlgren J, Kriström B, Niklasson A, Nierop AF, Rosberg S, Albertsson-Wikland K: Models predicting the growth response to growth hormone treatment in short children independent of GH status, birth size and gestational age. BMC Med Informatics Decision Making 2007;7:40.

153 Ranke MB, Cutfield WS, Lindberg A, Cowell CT, Albertsson-Wikland K, Reiter EO, Wilton P, Price DA: A growth prediction model for short children born small for gestational age. J Pediatr Endocrinol Metab 2002;15(suppl 5):1273.

154 Kriström B, Dahlgren J, Niklasson A, Nierop AF, Albertsson-Wikland K: The first-year growth response to growth hormone treatment predicts the long-term prepubertal growth response in children. BMC Med Informatics Decision Making 2009;9:1.

155 Decker R, Albertsson-Wikland K, Kriström B, Nierop AF, Gustafsson J, Bosaeus I, Fors H, Hochberg Z, Dahlgren J: Metabolic outcome of GH treatment in prepubertal short children with and without classical GH-deficiency. Clin Endocrinol (Oxf) 2010 accepted.

Kerstin Albertsson-Wikland
GP-GRC
Queen Silvia Children's Hospital
SE–41685 Göteborg (Sweden)
Tel. +46 31 343 5165, Fax +46 31 84 8952 , E-Mail kerstin.albertsson-wikland@pediat.gu.se

Ranke MB, Mullis P-E (eds): Diagnostics of Endocrine Function in Children and Adolescents, ed 4.
Basel, Karger, 2011, pp 157–182

Insulin-Like Growth Factors and Their Binding Proteins

Werner F. Blum[a] · Claudia Böttcher[b] · Stefan A. Wudy[b]

[a]Eli Lilly and Company, Bad Homburg, and [b]Center of Child and Adolescent Medicine, Justus Liebig University, Giessen, Germany

The insulin-like growth factors (IGF) and their binding proteins (IGFBP) have a wide variety of physiological actions that are still being revealed. Both IGF and IGFBP have effects that are independent as well as interdependent in controlling cellular growth and functions. Although they are commonly considered to be indicators of growth hormone (GH) secretion or action, their regulation is multifactorial and complex. The determination of IGF and IGFBP concentrations has become a widely used tool in the diagnostic evaluation of growth disorders. However, in order to fully exploit their potential for diagnostic purposes, the various factors that influence IGF and IGFBP levels must be taken into account. Generally speaking, abnormal serum levels of these peptides indicate a disturbance proximal to the growing tissue, suggesting disturbed growth regulation such as GH deficiency (GHD) or insufficient nutrient supply rather than, for instance, a skeletal defect. This chapter focuses on IGF-1 and IGFBP-3 and provides guidelines for the appropriate interpretation of IGF-1 and IGFBP-3 measurements.

Biochemistry

Insulin-like growth factors 1 and 2 (IGF-1 and IGF-2) are well-characterized peptides with molecular weights of 7,649 and 7,471, respectively, which exhibit a high sequence homology to proinsulin [Rinderknecht and Humbel, 1978a, b]. In contrast to many other polypeptide hormones and growth factors, IGFs are bound to specific IGFBPs with high affinity (dissociation constants approximately 10^{-11} mol/l). It has been estimated that less than 1% of circulating IGF is present in its free form [Frystyk et al., 2010]. At least six classes of IGFBP can be distinguished on the basis of their primary structure, showing a high degree of sequence homology. The recommended

Table 1. Biochemical characteristics of human IGFBPs

	Amino acids n	Cysteine residues n	Mass kDa	RGD sequence	Glycosylation[a]	Phos-phoryl-ation	Proteo-lysis	IGF affinity	Chromo-some
IGFBP-1	234	18	28.1	+	O	+	−	I ≥ II	7p
IGFBP-2	289	18	31.3	+	−	−	+	I < II	2q
IGFBP-3	264	18	28.7	−	N	+	+	I ≤ II	7p
IGFBP-4	237	20	26.3	−	N	−	+	I = II	17q
IGFBP-5	252	18	28.6	−	O	+	+	I < II	2q
IGFBP-6	216	16	22.8	−	O	?	+	I << II	12

RGD = Arginine-glycine-asparagine. [a]The glycosylated forms of IGFBP-3, IGFBP-4, and IGFBP-6 have higher molecular weights by sodium dodecylsulfate polyacrylamide gel electrophoresis (SDS-PAGE): doublet around 42, 30 and 34 kDa, respectively. O = Carbohydrate moiety attached to serine; N = carbohydrate moiety attached to asparagine. The carbohydrate chains of these two types are different and have different functions.

designation is as IGFBP-1 through to IGFBP-6. Some biochemical characteristics of the IGFBPs are given in table 1 [reviewed in Firth and Baxter, 2002; Bach, 2004; Jogie-Brahim et al., 2009].

The most abundant IGFBP in the circulation after the first few weeks of life is IGFBP-3. It binds IGF-1 and IGF-2 with similar affinities (K_a for IGF-1 is 2.1×10^{10} l/mol and for IGF-2, 3.3×10^{10} l/mol) [Martin and Baxter, 1986]. Its peptide core (M_r 28.7 kDa) is substantially glycosylated, which results in a total estimated molecular weight of approximately 42 kDa, and shows heterogeneity by various biochemical techniques. After binding of either IGF-1 or IGF-2, it is able to associate with an acid-labile subunit (ALS) to constitute a high-molecular-weight ternary complex (120–150 kDa) [Baxter, 1988]. This complex is retained within the intravascular space and is considered to be a circulating reservoir of IGFs.

Physiological Aspects

IGFs and IGFBPs are synthesized and secreted by a multitude of cell types. The fact that these peptides are produced locally in many organs led to the concept of an autocrine/paracrine mechanism of action [reviewed in Kaplan and Cohen, 2007]. With respect to circulating IGF-1, IGF-2 and IGFBP-3, there is strong evidence that the liver is the major source [Chin et al., 1994] and levels are significantly decreased with impaired liver function [Holt et al., 1996]. However, the liver possesses few IGF-1

Blum · Böttcher · Wudy

receptors and therefore cannot be a target organ, which lends support to the endocrine concept and is highly pertinent from a diagnostic point of view.

The appropriate use of these parameters for diagnostic purposes requires some understanding of their physiological roles. The classic concept of the role of IGF-1 – the 'somatomedin hypothesis' – considers this peptide as a mediator of GH action on longitudinal growth. This view, however, is too narrow because it implies a sequential mode of action; a large body of experimental and clinical findings support a rather synergistic mode of action of GH and IGF-1: (1) the 'dual effector theory' [Green et al., 1985]; (2) two important target tissues for GH, the liver and adipose tissue, possess few functional IGF-1 receptors [LeRoith et al., 1995], and (3) IGFs have important insulin-like metabolic effects in peripheral tissues. These metabolic effects are mostly opposite to GH effects, e.g. the inhibiting effect of GH on insulin sensitivity is counteracted by a stimulatory effect of IGFs.

In addition to GH, a number of other regulators control IGF-1, among which nutrition and the immune system are the most potent. On the other hand, IGF-1 not only stimulates the epiphyseal growth plate, which is important for longitudinal growth, but almost every cell able to perform certain specific actions, such as proliferation, differentiation, or particular cellular functions like the synthesis of extracellular matrix by chondrocytes or steroid synthesis by gonadal cells. Overall, IGF-1 action appears then as a synergistic potentiation of the stimulation of cellular functions by cell-specific signals. Moreover, IGF-1 inhibits programmed cell death (apoptosis), which has been recognized as an important mechanism for tissue growth and developmental sculpting.

Therefore, IGF-1 should no longer be regarded as a link in a linear chain of hormonal signals – the GH-IGF axis – but rather as a node within an informational network. Chronic nutritional deprivation causes suppression of IGF-1, as does insufficient GH secretion [Zapf et al., 1981; Rosenfeld et al., 1986]. GH secretion itself is regulated by endogenous signals coming from the central nervous system (e.g., the increase in GH during puberty) or by chronic psychosocial or physical distress (e.g., psychosocial growth retardation or extreme training load in high-performance athletes). In addition, the immune system may be involved and, when activated, it causes suppression of IGF-1 (e.g. in sepsis, systemic inflammatory disease, or malignancies) [Juul, 2003]. In the event that one of these major regulators is missing (GH or nutrients) or activated (immune system), there is resistance against the other factors with respect to IGF-1 production. That is, IGF-1 transmits integrated information at the cellular level on the nutritional status, the GH secretory status, and the immune status of the organism. Generally speaking, IGF-1 provides information to the cells on the well-being of the organism. Thus, the rate of cellular activities such as proliferation, differentiation, or the synthesis of cell-specific products is adapted to the situation. Evidently, this kind of signal is of the utmost importance to the growing organism.

Many of the actions of IGF-2 are similar to those of IGF-1. They occur, however, through the IGF-1 receptor [LeRoith et al., 1995] and possibly the insulin receptor [Morrione et al., 1997] but require higher concentrations to elicit the response. Although IGF-2 was shown to be an important fetal growth factor, its true physiological role is still unclear.

Historically, it was thought that the role of IGFBPs was to transport IGFs in the circulation, to facilitate transport from the circulation to the target tissue and to modulate IGF action locally. However, this picture needs to be expanded and revised. IGFBPs were shown to exert IGF-1-independent actions on cells thereby acting as hormones per se [reviewed in Firth and Baxter, 2002; Jogie-Brahim et al., 2009]. The existence of membrane-bound receptors for IGFBP-3 and IGFBP-5 has been demonstrated. Further, IGFBP-3 and IGFBP-5 have been shown to be transferred to the cell nucleus by an importin-β-dependent mechanism. Once inside the nucleus, IGFBP-3 has been shown to interact with the retinoid X receptor-α (RXRα) and is directly involved in forming transcription units and starting gene transcription. It has now been established that IGFBP-3 independently stimulates apoptosis in cells that are triggered accordingly and this effect may be shared by IGFBP-5. The apoptotic effects of IGFBP-3 are opposite to the cell proliferation effects of IGFs and are abrogated by binding of IGFs [reviewed in Firth and Baxter, 2002; Jogie-Brahim et al., 2009].

A revised concept of IGFs and IGFBPs (in particular IGFBP-3) may therefore be delineated as follows: there are two classes of hormones, IGFs and IGFBPs. Generally speaking, IGFs stimulate cell proliferation, differentiation and specific cellular actions, and they inhibit apoptosis. In contrast, IGFBP-3, and possibly other IGFBPs, inhibits cell proliferation and stimulates apoptosis. The binding of IGFBP-3 to IGFs neutralizes the effect of either component. Overall, it appears that the fine-tuned balance of IGFs and IGFBPs is important to direct cells in their tissue-specific environment either towards proliferation or apoptosis.

IGFBP-3 is primarily regulated by GH, being high in acromegaly [Jørgensen et al., 1994] and low in GHD [Blum et al., 1990]. However, many other factors such as glucocorticoids, parathyroid hormone, transforming growth factor-β1 (TGF-β1), tumor necrosis factor-α (TNF-α), retinoic acid, vitamin D, estradiol and p53 affect IGFBP-3 production [reviewed in Jogie-Brahim et al., 2009].

Relationship between IGF and IGFBP-3

IGF-1, IGF-2 and IGFBP-3 levels are not independent of each other. Owing to the short metabolic half-life of free serum IGFs (approximately 10 min), the total serum concentration of either IGF peptide is primarily determined by the concentration of IGFBP-3. Other IGFBPs play only a minor role quantitatively in normal and most pathologic situations, as shown by a close linear correlation of the sum of total IGF-1 and IGF-2 levels and IGFBP-3 concentrations, even in extreme situations such as Laron syndrome [Blum and Ranke, 1991].

With respect to diagnostic purposes, therefore, it may be questioned whether the measurement of both IGFs – normally IGF-1 – and IGFBP-3 is meaningful or whether the information is redundant. The answer implies two aspects: firstly, the correlation between IGF-1 and IGFBP-3 is not linear, but rather exponential [Blum and Ranke, 1991], and, secondly, the determination of both parameters can serve as an internal control. Gross discrepancies between the results should alert the investigator to consider a laboratory error. The nonlinearity of serum IGF-1 versus IGFBP-3 means that the ratio of IGF-1 to IGFBP-3 is variable [Löfqvist et al., 2005]. Although the regulation of either parameter by various factors is qualitatively the same, the magnitude of the variation of IGF-1 is always much greater than that of IGFBP-3.

Methodological Aspects

Measurement of IGF-1 and IGF-2
The development of immunoassays, radioimmunoassays (RIA), and later also immunoradiometric assays (IRMA), enzyme immunoassays (EIA) and fluorescence immunoassays (FIA) made IGFs interesting parameters for clinical practice, in particular IGF-1 due to its GH-dependent regulation. These assays measure total immunoreactive IGF-1 (or IGF-2) in the circulation. More recently assays for the measurement of complex-associated IGF-1, free IGF-1 and bioactive IGF-1 have been developed. However, they do not appear to provide additional value in the diagnosis and management of GH disorders, although they are of interest for specific scientific questions [Frystyk et al., 2010].

Interference of IGFBP
Although, historically, IGF-1 was measured in unprocessed plasma samples by RIA, there is now general agreement that the separation of IGFs from their binding proteins – whether physically or functionally – is required in order to obtain reliable results [Blum and Breier, 1994; Frystyk et al., 2010]. In a RIA system, the tracer binds both to anti-IGF immunoglobulin and to IGFBP. Thus, at a low IGF concentration, i.e. a high ratio of ^{125}I-labeled IGF to unlabeled IGF, less tracer is available for binding to the antibody in chemical equilibrium. As a consequence, the radioactive signal of the precipitate obtained by a second antibody technique will be decreased. This would be interpreted as indicating the presence of unlabeled hormone and IGF levels will be overestimated. At a high IGF concentration, i.e. a low ratio of ^{125}I-labeled IGF to unlabeled IGF, relatively more unlabeled IGF will bind to the IGFBP, and IGF concentrations will be underestimated [Blum and Breier, 1994].

This interference becomes worse (a) the higher the affinity of the IGFBPs, (b) the lower the affinity of the antibody, and (c) the higher the IGFBP concentration in the assay mixture [Blum and Breier, 1994]. The latter two variables can be influenced by the design of the assay: first, the IGFBP concentration can be reduced by appropriate sample preparation (e.g. extraction of IGFBPs), and secondly, high-affinity antibodies must be used (half-maximal displacement should occur at <2 µg/l).

The dissociation rate of IGFs from IGFBP-3, the major IGFBP in blood, is extremely slow. The half-time at 37°C is in the range of 17 h. At 4°C, it will take about 6 days until half of the IGF has dissociated from IGFBP-3 and is able to participate in the equilibrium reaction with the antibody. Sample preparation, therefore, requires a step which rapidly dissociates IGFs from IGFBPs. This can be achieved by acidification to pH < 3.4 for IGF-1 and to pH < 2.8 for IGF-2. At these low pH values, dissociation occurs within minutes.

Physical Separation of IGFs from Their Binding Proteins
Size Exclusion Chromatography (SEC). Complete separation can be achieved by SEC under acidic conditions (pH <3) [Zapf et al., 1981]. The major disadvantage of this technique is that it is laborious and time-consuming and excludes the processing of a large number of samples for routine purposes. Although SEC is still regarded as the 'gold standard', its importance lies mainly in validating other assay systems.

Acid-Ethanol Extraction. The most widely used technique for separation is an acid-ethanol extraction procedure [Daughaday et al., 1980]. It includes only pipetting and centrifugation steps, thereby allowing the processing of a large number of samples at one time. The major disadvantage is that considerable amounts of IGFBP (most of IGFBP-1 and IGFBP-2) remain in the extract and may interfere in the IGF assay system. Further, the reported high recoveries of more than 95% are valid only for added free IGF. The recovery of IGFBP-bound IGFs, however, is rather in the range of 70–80% [Blum and Breier, 1994]. Therefore, IGF determinations after acid-ethanol extraction underestimate the true concentrations. Also, the extraction step causes a predilution of the sample, which reduces the sensitivity of the assay significantly. Even though extraction procedures suffice in most clinical situations, extremely low levels as, for example, in severe GHD or in GH receptor defect (Laron syndrome), require more sensitive methods (see below). Further, acid-ethanol extraction removes mainly IGFBP-3 bound in the ternary complex which makes it unsuitable for other specimens such as cerebrospinal fluid, milk, or conditioned cell culture media [Blum and Breier, 1994].

Functional Separation of IGFs from IGFBPs
The classic extraction procedures share a number of disadvantages which can be circumvented by blocking the IGFBP-binding sites through an excess of non-measured IGF, i.e. IGF-2 in the IGF-1 assay and IGF-1 in the IGF-2 assay ('functional separation') [Blum and Breier, 1994]. A prerequisite is that the antibody must be highly specific and have high affinity, i.e. the assay should have a high sensitivity resulting in a substantial reduction of the amount of IGFBPs in the assay mixture through dilution. The assay system can then be composed in such a manner that the sample is diluted

in an acidic buffer to dissociate IGFs from IGFBPs. The first antibody together with an excess of non-measured IGF is dissolved in a buffer which is able to re-neutralize the diluted sample. Upon adding this solution, the excess of nonmeasured IGF will then occupy the IGF-binding sites of IGFBPs. Extensive validation of this approach has shown that this third generation of IGF assays offers a number of advantages over assays using extraction procedures: they are (a) more simple, (b) more precise, (c) markedly more sensitive, and (d) particularly useful in samples other than blood.

IGF-1 Measurement

Numerous immunoassay systems have been developed by various laboratories and are commercially available. Most important is the quality of the antibody. Polyclonal or monoclonal antibodies against the complete IGF-1 molecule or partial sequences of it may be used. However, they should be of high specificity (cross-reactivity with IGF-2 <1%) and high affinity (half-maximal displacement at <2 μg/l). Although an international reference preparation is available [Frystyk et al., 2010], different antibodies may give different results owing to the presence of components with mismatched disulfide bridges. Also, different antibodies may detect IGF-1 variants [Blum and Breier, 1994] in blood differently. Therefore, the comparability of absolute values obtained with different assay systems is limited. Results may be expressed as either micrograms per liter (or nanograms per milliliter) or, alternatively, as nanomoles per liter. The conversion factor for nmol/l to μg/l is 7.649. The expression as 'units' referring to the potency of a standard plasma pool is obsolete and should be abandoned.

Measurement of IGFBP-3

For the determination of IGFBP-3, commercial RIA, IRMA and EIA kits are available which are based on either authentic or recombinant IGFBP-3. From a technical point of view, their major advantage is that no extraction step is required. The assays are unaffected by the presence of IGF, and they quantitatively recognize the complete IGFBP-3 complex. Standards have been prepared from pure authentic or recombinant IGFBP-3 or calibrated serum or plasma. The preparation used should preferably be glycosylated IGFBP-3. Unglycosylated IGFBP-3 as a standard must be carefully validated, since nonparallelism with serum dilutions is frequently observed. In general, the absolute values of different assays are not comparable, mainly for two reasons: (1) the use of different standards may give different results, and (2) in certain clinical situations, e.g., pregnancy or severe illness, IGFBP-3 is substantially proteolysed, and the various fragments, which may still be functional [reviewed in Firth and Baxter, 2002; Jogie-Brahim et al., 2009], are detected differently by different antibodies.

If a heterogeneous mixture of complete IGFBP-3 and IGFBP-3-derived fragments is suspected, calculated molar concentrations of IGFBP-3 can only be, at best, a rough estimate. The only scientifically sound solution to this problem is to express concentrations as nanograms per milliliter or milligrams per liter of the pure substance and to state what assay has been used.

Stability of IGFs and IGFBP-3

IGF-1, IGF-2 and IGFBP-3 in serum or plasma are quite stable. In our laboratories, incubation of samples at 37°C for several days had no effect on their levels as measured by RIA. However, it must be kept in mind that high activities of IGFBP-3 proteases are present in certain clinical conditions [Firth and Baxter, 2002; Juul, 2003; Jogie-Brahim et al., 2009]. They produce fragments which may be recognized differently by different antibodies. Sample stability should therefore be tested for each assay. From long-standing experience over years, however, it can be stated that sample preparation and shipping of samples for diagnostic purposes by ordinary mail is unproblematic. Shipping of full blood should be avoided as the stability of the analytes in such samples is limited [reviewed in Frystyk et al., 2010].

Normal Ranges of IGF-1, IGF-2 and IGFBP-3

A variety of factors influence IGF and IGFBP-3 levels (see below). The most important factors, however, that have an impact in a healthy normal population are gender and age. It is recommended, therefore, to establish reference ranges according to age as a continuous variable and to stratify for gender.

Although absolute values of the normal ranges of IGF-1 and IGFBP-3 levels vary among different studies, they show a common age-dependent pattern [Ranke et al., 2000; Juul, 2003]. Serum IGF-1 levels are very low at birth and increase slowly during early childhood. At puberty, there is a marked increase, which is followed by a constant and significant decline with age (table 2; fig. 1). The pubertal peak occurs about 1 year earlier in girls than in boys, following the normal course of sexual development. IGF-2 levels, in contrast, are low at birth and rise rapidly during the first weeks of life. They show only a slight further increase thereafter and lack a pubertal peak. IGFBP-3 levels exhibit a pattern which falls between the age-dependence of IGF-1 and IGF-2 (table 3; fig. 2). Not surprisingly, an abnormal tempo of maturation influences IGF-1 and IGFBP-3 levels. In precocious puberty, serum IGF-1 and IGFBP-3 are elevated as compared with age-matched controls. Therefore, in accelerated or delayed puberty, bone age should be taken into consideration for a critical interpretation of IGF-1 and IGFBP-3 levels.

The differences of results among assays are probably due to methodological differences, different standards and different study cohorts. They make direct comparisons difficult; often, however, regressions between the results of different assays are very good, which allows conversion of results with sufficient precision so that data from different assays can be compared or pooled.

To interpret serum IGF and IGFBP-3 levels appropriately, their age and gender dependence need to be taken into account. This can be achieved by comparing measured values to graphs or tables providing age- and gender-dependent percentiles

Table 2. Serum levels (µg/l) of IGF-1 in healthy subjects at various ages[a]

Age group	Percentile					
	0.1	5	10	50	90	95
0–2 years	13	28	34	66	128	156
2–4 years	20	40	48	87	159	189
4–6 years	26	50	59	108	196	233
6–7 years	34	62	72	124	212	248
7–8 years	45	78	90	148	243	281
8–9 years						
Female	55	99	115	193	324	376
Male	54	90	102	160	250	284
9–10 years						
Female	68	114	130	205	323	369
Male	63	102	115	176	269	304
10–11 years						
Female	81	134	153	239	374	426
Male	77	117	130	189	274	305
11–12 years						
Female	91	160	185	305	503	581
Male	85	129	144	209	304	339
12–13 years						
Female	116	201	231	377	614	707
Male	88	141	159	243	371	419
13–14 years						
Female	163	256	287	428	637	716
Male	111	179	203	311	477	540
14–15 years						
Female	193	284	314	443	625	691
Male	140	229	260	404	628	713
15– years						
Female	187	279	309	442	632	700
Male	176	269	299	433	626	697

Table 2. Continued

Age group	Percentile					
16–17 years						
Female	183	270	298	422	597	660
Male	178	267	296	424	607	673
17–18 years						
Female	176	246	268	362	488	533
Male	173	243	265	358	484	527
18–19 years						
Female	167	233	254	341	458	499
Male	167	235	256	347	469	512
19–20 years	158	220	240	322	433	471
20–30 years	72	115	130	198	302	340
30–40 years	68	109	123	188	287	324
40–50 years	64	103	116	178	272	310
50–60 years	60	97	110	169	260	292
60–70 years	55	91	103	161	251	292
70–80 years	25	47	55	98	173	207
>80 years	21	40	47	85	153	184

[a]Measurements by an IGFBP-blocked RIA without acid-ethanol extraction [Blum and Breier, 1994].

(tables 2, 3). An alternative and elegant approach is to convert absolute IGF-1 and IGFBP-3 levels to standard deviation scores (SDS), thus adjusting for age and gender. SDS values immediately show any deviation from the corresponding age-related mean. Normal reference ranges of IGF-1 and IGFBP-3 are log-normally distributed. This requires logarithmic transformation of measured values before making any further calculations. The formula for computation of SDS is as follows:

SDS = [log(measured value) – mean of reference at patient's age(log-transformed)]/ SD of reference range(log-transformed) at patient's age.

Means and standard deviation (SD) of log-transformed reference ranges may be provided for defined age groups, e.g. boys 10–11 years. Even though mathematically simple, this approach has the disadvantage that SDS values 'jump' when the patient crosses the age-group boundary, especially with IGF-1 during the pubertal surge. A more elegant approach is to fit regression curves to the logarithmic means (age) and

Blum · Böttcher · Wudy

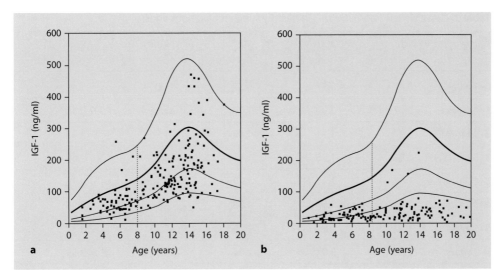

Fig. 1. Serum IGF-1 levels in (**a**) short-stature children and adolescents without GHD (n = 219) and (**b**) patients with GHD (n = 155). The age-dependent normal range is given by the 0.1st, 5th, 50th and 95th percentiles. Note: Measurements were performed after acid-ethanol extraction in contrast to the values given in table 2.

SD (age) and use these equations to calculate 'continuous' SDS values. Because such an approach is mathematically more demanding, computer software has been developed that makes SDS calculations easy (e.g. 'SDS Easy', Mediagnost GmbH, Reutlingen, Germany; referring to the normal ranges given in tables 2 and 3).

Reporting IGF-1 and IGFBP-3 levels as SDS has a number of advantages: (1) Comparison of a patient's serum level with the general population is straightforward. For instance, an IGF-1 SDS value of 0 means that the patient has a totally normal IGF-1 level for his age and gender (mean of normal population), whereas an SDS value of –3 means that he has an IGF-1 level clearly below the population's average, outside the normal range. (2) Patient data from different age groups and genders can be directly compared or pooled. (3) Data from different assays using different reference ranges can be compared or pooled. In this context, however, it needs to be mentioned that the same deviation from the reference mean may result in different SDS values, if SD (age) values differ between assays and reference ranges.

Besides these advantages, however, caution needs to be exercised regarding SDS: (1) Converting absolute values in SDS introduces a new source of error. Therefore, if age and gender differences do not really require adjustment, one should keep to the absolute values. (2) Calculation of SDS requires reliable reference ranges with sufficiently large cohorts. (3) Due to the log transformation, very low IGF or IGFBP-3 levels transform to extremely low (negative) SDS values. This is especially the case with IGF-1 at the age of puberty.

Table 3. Serum levels (mg/l) IGFBP-3 in healthy subjects at various ages[a]

Age group	5th percentile	20th percentile	50th percentile	80th percentile	95th percentile
0–1 week	0.42	0.57	0.77	1.05	1.41
1–4 weeks	0.77	0.99	1.29	1.68	2.16
1–3 months	0.87	1.13	1.48	1.94	2.52
3–6 months	0.98	1,25	1.61	2.07	2.65
6–12 months	1.07	1.35	1.72	2.19	2.76
1–3 years	1.41	1.69	2.05	2.48	2.98
3–5 years	1.52	1.84	2.25	2.75	3.33
5–7 years	1.66	2.01	2.44	2.97	3.59
7–9 years					
Female	1.88	2.25	2.72	3.28	3.94
Male	1.73	2.07	2.50	3.02	3.61
9–11 years					
Female	2.20	2.62	3.13	3.75	4.45
Male	1.99	2.36	2.81	3.35	3.97
11–13 years					
Female	2.24	2.74	3.38	4.17	5.10
Male	2.19	2.63	3.18	3.84	4.62
13–15 years					
Female	2.39	2.91	3.56	4.36	5.30
Male	2.24	2.76	3.42	4.24	5.22
15–17 years					
Female	2.26	2.73	3.31	4.02	4,85
Male	2.36	2.84	3.44	4.17	5.01
17–20 years	2.24	2.72	3.33	4.07	4.95
20–30 years	2.20	2.68	3.29	4.04	4.92
30–40 years	2.08	2.56	3.18	3.95	4.86
40–50 years	2.01	2.48	3.08	3.83	4.72
50–60 years	1.96	2.42	3.02	3.76	4.65
60–70 years	1.90	2.37	2.98	3.75	4.67

[a]Measurements by RIA [Blum et al., 1990].

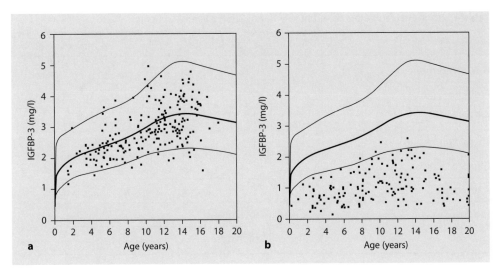

Fig. 2. Serum IGFBP-3 levels in short-statured patients (**a**) without (n = 219) or (**b**) with (n = 155) GHD. The normal range is given by the 5th, 50th and 95th percentiles.

Factors Influencing Serum IGF-1 and IGFBP-3 Concentrations

Although IGF-1 and IGFBP-3 measurements are mainly used in the diagnostic work-up of suspected GHD, their serum levels are under the control of a multitude of other factors which have to be considered for the appropriate interpretation of results. In general, total IGF-1 and IGFBP-3 concentrations in blood are regulated by the same factors, which cause qualitatively similar changes (table 4). This is not surprising in the light of their inter-dependence (see above). However, the variations of IGF-1 are always much more pronounced than those of IGFBP-3, a phenomenon which causes variations in the ratio of IGF-1 to IGFBP-3 [Juul et al., 1995; Löfqvist et al., 2005]. This means that, phenomenologically, IGF-1 responds more sensitively to regulators than IGFBP-3. For diagnostic purposes, this can be an advantage, but it can also be a disadvantage because modulating factors have a greater influence.

Circadian Levels
Twenty-four-hour profiles of IGF-1 show a moderate fluctuation, whereas IGFBP-3 is more or less constant [Jørgensen et al., 1990; Juul, 2003]. In the individual case, variations of about 20% can be observed, which is within the variance of the methods under routine conditions. This means that a single determination at any time of the day is informative, in contrast to GH determinations. This point in particular makes the diagnostic use of these parameters for out-clinic patients so attractive.

Table 4. Hormonal regulators of serum IGF-1 and IGFBP-3 levels[a]

Hormone	Effect
Growth hormone	↑↑↑
Prolactin	↑?
Insulin	↑
Thyroid hormones	↑
Glucocorticoids	↑
Androgens	↑
Estrogens	low dose ↑
	high dose ↓

↑↑↑ = Very strong stimulation; ↑ = stimulation; ↑? = possible stimulation; ↓ = inhibition. [a]Gonadotropins, thyroid-stimulating hormone (TSH), adrenocorticotropic hormone (ACTH), or parathyroid hormone have no direct effect on IGF and IGFBP-3 serum levels, although they stimulate IGF-1 production in their target tissues.

Growth Hormone

For clinical purposes, the most important regulator of serum IGF-1 and IGFBP-3 levels is GH. Serum levels clearly depend on the GH status and show a significant correlation with integrated GH secretion [Blum et al., 1993]. Their rates of change are slow; this is particularly true for IGFBP-3 [Blum et al., 1990; Jørgensen et al., 1991]. A rise in serum IGFBP-3 after intravenous GH administration is not observed until 16–20 h later [Jørgensen et al., 1991]. The kinetics of IGF-1 under these conditions is faster and more pronounced; after a GH bolus, IGF-1 may have already returned to basal levels by the next day. This is important with respect to the IGF generation test or the use of these parameters for monitoring GH therapy and explains why IGFBP-3 measurements give more robust results in these situations. Normal levels of IGF-1 and IGFBP-3 in patients with GHD are reached within 4–7 days after the start of therapy. A corresponding time course is observed after GH treatment ends.

The pulsatility of GH secretion or daily GH administration in patients with GHD is not reflected in fluctuations of IGFBP-3 levels. Therefore, a single measurement is sufficient and provides information on the GH secretory status in terms of days rather than hours. In fact, this aspect is the principal basis for the diagnostic determination of IGF-1 and IGFBP-3 in the evaluation of abnormal GH secretion (see diagnostic algorithm in 'Appendix B, Chart 3').

Other Hormones

Insulin has a permissive effect on the production of IGF-1 and IGFBP-3. Their serum levels are therefore decreased in untreated diabetes mellitus and normalize during appropriate therapy [reviewed in Juul, 2003; Bach, 2004].

The increase in serum IGF-1 and IGFBP-3 during normal or precocious puberty suggests a stimulatory effect of sex steroids. Even though this may be partially mediated through stimulated GH secretion, there is evidence for a direct effect [Rosenfeld et al., 1994]. Glucocorticoids induce a marked increase in serum IGF-1 and a minor increase in IGFBP-3 [Miell et al., 1993]. Corresponding changes are observed in Cushing syndrome [Bang et al., 1993]. These findings can be explained as the result of a stimulation of hepatic gene expression.

In hypothyroidism, IGF-1 and IGFBP-3 levels are somewhat diminished [reviewed in Juul, 2003]. However, levels were unchanged in patients with thyroid eye disease associated with euthyroid Grave's disease and in hyperthyroidism [Krassas et al., 2003].

Nutrition

Serum IGF-1 levels decline rapidly with fasting and show an observable decrease after 24 h. In contrast, the decrease in IGFBP-3 levels as a result of fasting is less rapid and negligible within a 24-hour period [reviewed in Juul, 2003]. However, long-term fasting, as well as states of malnutrition or malabsorption, must be considered in order to avoid misinterpretations of the measured levels of these peptides. In this context, it should be mentioned that there is a relative insensitivity to GH during fasting. Low IGF-1 and IGFBP-3 values contrast with high GH secretion. The opposite is found in obesity due to hypernutrition, where high-normal IGF and IGFBP-3 levels contrast with low GH secretion. This situation should not mislead the investigator to diagnose GHD.

Liver Function

The major source of circulating IGF-1, IGF-2 and IGFBP-3 is the liver, and serum levels of all three peptides show a highly significant correlation with conventional indicators of hepatic function (cholinesterase, thromboplastin time, serum albumin) in various liver diseases [Kratzsch et al., 1995; Juul, 2003].

Postaggression Syndrome and Severe Illness

After polytrauma or severe surgical trauma, during massive activation of the immune system, e.g., in sepsis, systemic autoimmune disease, or malignant disease, or in cachexia, IGF-1 and IGFBP-3 levels are significantly diminished [reviewed in Juul, 2003]. Although the exact mechanisms of this down-regulation are as yet unknown, cytokines such as interleukins 1 and 6 or tumor necrosis factor may be involved.

Kidney Function

In chronic renal failure, serum IGF-1 levels are low normal to normal, while IGF-2 levels are normal to high normal. In contrast, IGFBP-3 levels are considerably elevated, owing to the accumulation of low-molecular-weight forms [Blum et al., 1991]. There is an inverse correlation between the glomerular filtration rate (GFR) and IGFBP levels [Tönshoff et al., 1995]. A decrease in the GFR by 50% causes an average increase in IGFBP-3 of approximately 1 mg/l, while serum creatinine values may well remain in the normal range. Therefore, IGF and IGFBP determinations have to be interpreted with caution when impaired renal function is suspected, even in the presence of normal creatinine values.

Clinical Applications

The major relevance of IGF-1 and IGFBP-3 levels as clinical indicators is in the evaluation of insufficient or excessive GH secretion. The underlying rationale for this clinical application is the fact that GH is the predominant regulator of these peptides.

GH Deficiency
GHD, or GHD syndrome, causes a number of disturbances depending on the time of onset and duration. In pediatric patients, the most prominent symptom is growth retardation. The differential diagnosis of short stature, however, can be quite extensive (see diagnostic algorithm in 'Appendix B, Chart 3'). Although the patient's history, clinical findings and specific biochemical findings will normally guide the investigator to make the correct diagnosis in case of a dysmorphic syndrome or a metabolic disease, the question quite frequently continues to be a particular diagnostic challenge of whether there is a disturbance of the GH-IGF system.

The evaluation of the GH secretory capacity, however, must overcome a number of pitfalls, which are not always appropriately acknowledged in clinical practice. The most severe problem concerns the poor diagnostic sensitivity and specificity of pharmacological and physiological GH tests. The diagnostic specificity of a single GH stimulation test is in the range of about 0.5–0.7, i.e. 50–30% of the tests give a false-positive answer with respect to GHD [Tassoni et al., 1990; Rochiccioli et al., 1991; Cacciari et al., 1994], and, therefore, at least two tests are required. It should be noted, however, that even the combination of two tests with a specificity of, for example, 0.6 will give a false-positive result in 16% ($0.4 \times 0.4 = 0.16$) of the cases. Therefore, additional parameters such as IGF-1 and IGFBP-3 which reflect GH secretion should be included in the diagnostic evaluation of suspected GHD.

During the past 25 years, numerous studies have shown that IGF-1 levels are low in GHD and can therefore be used as a diagnostic parameter for this condition (table 5) [Rosenfeld et al., 1986; Blum et al., 1990; Lee et al., 1990; Smith et al., 1993; Nunez et al., 1996; Juul and Skakkebæk, 1997; Tillmann et al., 1997; Mitchell et al., 1999; Ranke et al., 2000]. However, some limitations of using IGF-1 levels have become obvious: (1) Because normal IGF-1 levels in young children are already low, the discrimination

Table 5. Sensitivity and specificity of serum IGF-1 and IGFBP-3 measurements for the diagnosis of GHD in pediatric patients in various studies

Author	Patients with ISS n	Patients with GHD n	Assay	GH peak (cut-off)	Cut-off	Sensitivity %	Specificity %
IGF-1							
Rosenfeld et al., 1986	44	68	RIA	7 µg/l	5th centile	82	68
Blum et al., 1990	130	132	RIA	10 µg/l	5th centile	96	54
Lee et al., 1990	153	19	RIA	7 µg/l	–2 SDS	81	53
Smith et al., 1993	23	57	RIA	10 µg/l	–2 SDS	86	70
Hasegawa et al., 1994	103	108	RIA	10 µg/l	5th centile	66	77
Nunez et al., 1996	74	16	RIA	7 µg/l	5th centile	69	76
Juul, Skakkebaek, 1997	0–10 years 48 10–20 years 94	0–10 years 15 10–20 years 46	RIA	10 µg/l	–2 SDS	53 74	98 67
Tillmann et al., 1997	109	58	RIA	clinical features	–2 SDS	34	72
Mitchell et al., 1999	158	148	RIA		–2 SDS	62	47
Ranke et al., 2000	76	187	RIA	10 µg/l	5th centile	75	32
IGFBP-3							
Blum et al., 1990	130	132	RIA	10 µg/l	5th centile	97	95
Smith et al., 1993	23	57	RIA	10 µg/l	–2 SDS	93	57
Hasegawa et al., 1994	103	59 49	RIA	<5 µg/l 5–10 µg/l	5th centile	92 39	69
Nunez et al., 1996	74	16	RIA	7 µg/l	5th centile	50	69
Juul, Skakkebaek, 1997	0–10 years 48 10–20 years 94	0–10 years 15 10–20 years 46	RIA	10 µg/l	–2 SDS	60 57	98 79

Table 5. Continued

Author	Patients with ISS n	Patients with GHD n	Assay	GH peak (cut-off)	Cut-off	Sensitivity %	Specificity %
Tillmann et al., 1997	109	58	RIA	clinical features	–2 SDS	22	92
Mitchell et al., 1999	158	148	IRMA		–2 SDS	15	98
Ranke et al., 2000	76	187	RIA	10 µg/l	5th centile	67	50

of subnormal IGF-1 levels is difficult in this age group. (2) This problem is further aggravated by methodological problems. Owing to the interference of IGFBPs in RIA, there is a tendency to overestimate low IGF concentrations, even if high-affinity antisera are used. (3) A substantive proportion (40–50%) of children with idiopathic short stature (ISS), but without GHD, have subnormal IGF-1 levels, if the limit to normality is set at the 5th percentile or at –2 SDS.

In addition, IGFBP-3 levels have also been advocated as a parameter for the diagnosis of GHD (table 5) [Blum et al., 1990; Smith et al., 1993; Hasegawa et al., 1994; Juul and Skakkebæk, 1997; Tillmann et al., 1997; Rikken et al., 1998; Mitchell et al., 1999; Ranke et al., 2000; GH Research Society, 2000]. However, in studies where the selection of patients was probably not strictly limited to severe GHD, results were not always clear-cut (table 5). Because of the relatively high normal serum concentration of IGFBP-3 in young children, determination of IGFBP-3 is superior to IGF-1 as a diagnostic parameter in children of less than 8 years of age (fig. 2). In short children without 'classic' GHD, there is some clustering of IGFBP-3 and, even more obviously, of IGF-1 in the low-normal range (fig. 2, 3). This finding is not surprising in the light of a significant correlation between height SDS and the IGF-1 and IGFBP-3 levels adjusted for age and gender [Blum et al., 1993].

If GH secretion in a given population is distributed continuously [see Albertsson-Wikland and Rosberg, this vol.], the question of whether GHD is present becomes irrelevant in borderline cases, and there is no reason to assume that IGF measurements could ever introduce discontinuity where continuity exists. The key question, therefore, is not whether a particular child with short stature has GHD, but rather, whether he or she will benefit from GH treatment. In this respect, IGF-1 and IGFBP-3 measurements can be useful. Basal IGF-1 and IGFBP-3 levels were shown to correlate significantly with the gain in height velocity and explain about 30–35% of its variance [Hasegawa et al., 1994; Kristrom et al., 1997], i.e. the lower

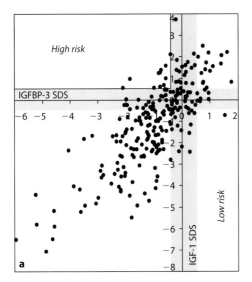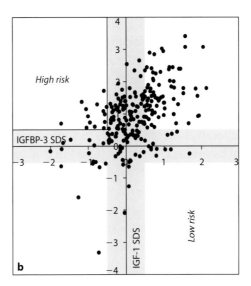

Fig. 3. IGF-1 SDS vs. IGFBP-3 SDS in GH-treated patients with (**a**) and without (**b**) GH deficiency. The high-risk area is defined by IGF-1 SDS in the upper tertile (>+0.5 SDS) and IGFBP-3 SDS in the lower tertile (<−0.5 SDS) of the general population.

these values are, the better the response to GH treatment will be. However, as a word of caution, the precision of IGF-1 or IGFBP-3 as predictors of height velocity is insufficient in the individual patient. Other variables need to be included in multiple regression models to obtain acceptably precise predictions [Schoenau et al., 2001].

Patients with GH insensitivity (Laron-type dwarfism) have markedly decreased IGF-1 and IGFBP-3 levels [Savage et al., 1993; Rosenfeld et al., 1994]. Therefore, in such cases, measurements of IGF-1 and IGFBP-3 are obligatory in the evaluation of the GH-IGF system, particularly if the clinical presentation and auxological data contrast with normal GH secretion [see paper by Ranke this vol., p 102–137].

In other clinical situations with severe growth retardation where the defect is rather at the target tissue level, e.g. Ullrich-Turner syndrome, Silver-Russell syndrome and hypochondroplasia, IGF-1 and IGFBP-3 levels are normal, reflecting normal GH secretion.

Recommendations

Using appropriate limits, the diagnostic accuracy of IGF-1 and IGFBP-3 measurements as a test for GHD is comparable to that of any single pharmacological or physiological GH test. Moreover, because of the rather constant circadian levels of serum IGF-1 and IGFPB-3, determination in a single blood sample is sufficient. The ease with which IGF-1 and IGFBP-3 levels can be determined makes them particularly ideal parameters for endocrinological outpatient clinics.

Therefore, in order to evaluate growth disorders, the diagnostic algorithm shown in 'Appendix B, Chart 3' should be used. If the patient's history, clinical presentation and auxological data do not a priori exclude insufficient GH secretion as a cause of growth retardation, determination of IGF-1 and IGFBP-3 levels should be the first laboratory screening test. In some cases, especially in adults, they can take the place of laborious GH testing [Clayton et al., 2005; Ho et al., 2007].

In the majority of short-statured children, both IGF-1 and IGFBP-3 will be (clearly) above the 10th percentile of the normal range. In these cases, GHD is extremely unlikely, and no further testing is required. If no dysmorphic features are present, the diagnoses may be constitutional delay of growth and adolescence, familial SS, intra-uterine growth retardation, or a combination of them. In a small number of patients, IGF-1 may be below the 1st percentile and IGFBP-3 below the 5th percentile. This finding must alert the investigator: something is possibly wrong with the patient, but it may not necessarily be associated with GH secretion or GH effectiveness. In these cases, further diagnostic measures are obligatory. IGF-1 levels below the 10th percentile and IGFBP-3 levels below the 20th percentile call for caution. A disturbance of the GH-IGF-axis, e.g., partial GHD, cannot be excluded. However, in addition to GH there are a variety of other hormonal and non-hormonal regulators of IGF-1 and IGFBP-3.

Although disorders underlying these causes of suppressed IGF-1 and IGFBP-3 levels (tables 6, 7) are commonly detected by specific clinical and biochemical criteria at an early diagnostic stage, this may not always be the case. If extended diagnostics provide no evidence for other causes of low IGF-1 and IGFBP-3, GH tests must be performed. If GH secretion is clearly normal, GH insensitivity syndrome (GHIS) has to be assumed and an IGF generation test must be performed. If IGF-1 increases by >15 µg/l and IGFBP-3 by >0.4 mg/l, then severe GHIS is unlikely [Blum et al., 1994]. Theoretically, the diagnosis 'bioinactive GH' is possible; this, however, is certainly a rarity. If the increases in IGF-1 and IGFBP-3 are below these values, a GH receptor defect may be considered, and serum growth hormone-binding protein (GHBP) should be determined by a functional assay. Even though partial GH receptor defects may be more frequent than commonly believed [Goddard et al., 1995], it is worthwhile to search again for causes of secondary GH insensitivity such as liver disease, malnutrition, malabsorption, or a severe systemic disease (table 6).

As a word of caution, it must be emphasized that IGF-1 and IGFBP-3 measurements alone can never prove GHD. There is a multitude of other factors besides GH that influence IGF-1 and IGFBP-3 levels. The proof of impaired GH secretion requires measurements of GH, either overnight or in response to stimulation. Low IGF-1 and IGFBP-3 levels are a necessary, but not sufficient proof for diagnosing GHD in children. Their value lies mainly in guiding the investigator to consider specific diagnostic possibilities.

Blum · Böttcher · Wudy

Table 6. Clinical situations with abnormal IGF-1 and IGFBP-3 serum levels

Significantly diminished	GHD, including neurosecretory dysfunction and psychosocial growth retardation
	Bioinactive GH
	GH receptor defect (Laron syndrome) Defects in post-GH receptor signal transmission
	Significant titer of GH antibodies
	Malnutrition, malabsorption
	Liver insufficiency
	Severe illness (e.g. systemic inflammatory disease, malignant disease, sepsis, cachexia)
	Severe trauma, including surgical trauma
	IGF-2-producing tumors
Moderately diminished	Diabetes mellitus
	Hypothyroidism
	GH insufficiency (partial GHD)
	GHD in the presence of severe obesity (e.g. Prader-Willi syndrome)
	GHD after treatment for malignancy
	Partial GH receptor deficiency
	Constitutional delay of growth and adolescence (low IGF-1, normal IGFBP-3) Sex steroid deficiency (e.g. Turner syndrome at the age of puberty)
Significantly elevated	Acromegaly, pituitary gigantism
	Chronic renal failure (normal IGF-1, increased IGFBP-3)
	Precocious puberty
Moderately elevated	Premature adrenarche
	Cushing syndrome, glucocorticoid excess
	Severe obesity
	Constitutional tall stature
	Renal disease other than chronic renal failure (increased IGFBP-3)

GH Excess

In acromegaly and in children with pituitary gigantism, IGF-1 levels are elevated as a consequence of excessive GH secretion and may be used for diagnostic purposes [Duncan and Wass, 1999]. Additionally, IGFBP-3 measurements may also be used

Table 7. Potential causes of discrepancies between IGF-1 and IGFBP-3 serum levels and results of GH stimulation tests

Low IGF-1 and IGFBP-3, but normal GH	Laboratory error
	Neurosecretory dysfunction
	Transient increase in GH secretion
	Bioinactive GH
	Primary GH insensitivity (partial)
	Secondary GH insensitivity (e.g. due to malnutrition, liver disease)
Normal IGF-1 and IGFBP-3, but low GH	Laboratory error
	False low stimulation test (frequent, particularly just before onset of puberty)
	Obesity
Normal IGF-1, high IGFBP-3, normal GH	Renal disease

for this purpose [Jørgensen et al., 1994; Duncan and Wass, 1999; Juul, 2003]. These parameters have been shown to correlate positively with mean GH levels. Although the elevation of IGFBP-3 in acromegaly is not as marked as the increase in IGF-1, its levels appear to be less variable upon repeated testing. Occasionally, discrepant results may be obtained when either IGF-1 or IGFBP-3 levels are still normal. Therefore, the measurement of both these parameters may complement each other and will provide enhanced sensitivity to excessive GH secretion.

In summary, therefore, the typical constellation suggesting abnormally high GH secretion is characterized by very high IGF-1 and high IGFBP-3 levels. So far, only plasma IGF-1 has been firmly established as a diagnostic parameter in this clinical situation, and also in the monitoring of therapeutic efficacy [Duncan and Wass, 1999; Juul, 2003].

Monitoring of GH Treatment

Measurements of IGF-1 and IGFBP-3 during GH therapy should be performed mainly for three purposes: (1) guidance for dose adjustments, (2) safety reasons, and (3) monitoring of compliance [Ranke et al., 2001]. Care has to be taken that GH has been administered appropriately during the days before blood collection otherwise levels may be falsely low.

It has been suggested that the GH dosage should be increased (or decreased) to titrate IGF-1 levels so that they are around the mean of the normal age-dependent

Blum · Böttcher · Wudy

range [Ho et al., 2007]. However, in this context it ought to be mentioned that very low IGF-1 levels in patients with severe GHD rarely increase to the normal range, even though they usually rise substantially when expressed as a percentage of the baseline concentration. Nevertheless, a low substitution dose is effective in such cases with good increases in the growth of pediatric patients. Titration of IGF-1 to the normal range as a method for GH dose adjustment should therefore be used with caution. On the other hand, excessive IGF-1 levels due to high GH doses should be avoided.

Epidemiologic studies have suggested that high IGF-1 levels are associated with a higher risk of developing certain cancers later in life. On the other hand, high IGFBP-3 levels had a protective effect. However, findings in more recent studies are controversial [reviewed in Juul, 2003; Bach, 2004; Jogie-Brahim et al., 2009]. A hypothesis that may explain these findings relates to the anti-apoptotic action of IGF-1 and the opposing apoptotic action of IGFBP-3 [Firth and Baxter, 2002; Jogie-Brahim et al., 2009], with the effects of each counterbalancing the other. Since GH stimulates both, the potential risk of developing cancer due to changes in the IGF-1GFBP system may be abrogated. This hypothetical conclusion is consistent with a large body of empirical data on GH treatment and the risk of developing neoplasias. However, GH treatment always increases the IGF-1/IGFBP-3 ratio and, therefore, some safety concerns remain. Based on the epidemiological data showing the opposite effects of IGF-1 and IGFBP-3, it is evident that the monitoring of IGF-1 alone to avoid supra-physiological levels is insufficient. The authors therefore propose a two-dimensional approach: IGF-1 SDS is plotted versus IGFBP-3 SDS. Based on published literature, where risk groups were classified according to tertiles, a high-risk area can be defined: IGF-1 SDS above +0.5 and IGFBP-3 SDS below –0.5 (fig. 3). In patients whose IGF-1/IGFBP-3 values fall within this area, a GH dose reduction should be considered.

While high IGF-1 and low IGFBP-3 levels may theoretically increase the risk of developing cancer later in life, the opposite has been reported regarding the risks of ischemic heart disease and of developing type 2 diabetes mellitus [reviewed in Juul, 2003]. Therefore, adjusting IGF-1 and IGFBP-3 properly during GH therapy is like traveling between Scylla and Charybdis. Monitoring both parameters and interpreting them appropriately is warranted and should become part of standard patient management.

Because GH therapy is expensive and misuse by athletes has created a black market, it is the physician's responsibility to ensure the compliance of the patient. If a pediatric patient does not grow appropriately during GH treatment, GH injections should be given under supervision for 1 week and IGF-1 and IGFBP-3 should be tested before and 1 day after the last injection.

References

Bach LA: The insulin-like growth factors system: towards clinical applications. Clin Biochem Rev 2004;25:155–164.

Bang P, Degerblad M, Thorén M, Schwander J, Blum WF, Hall K: Insulin-like growth factor (IGF)-I and -II and IGF-binding protein (IGFBP) 1, 2 and 3 in serum from patients with Cushing's syndrome. Acta Endocrinol (Copenh) 1993;128:397–404.

Baxter RC: Characterization of the acid-labile subunit of the growth hormone-dependent insulin-like growth factor binding protein complex. J Clin Endocrinol Metab 1988;67:265–272.

Blum WF, Breier BH: Radioimmunoassays for IGFs and IGFBPs. Growth Regul 1994;4(suppl 1):11–19.

Blum WF, Ranke MB: Plasma IGFBP-3 levels as clinical indicators; in Spencer EM (ed): Modern Concepts of Insulin-Like Growth Factors. New York, Elsevier, 1991, pp 381–393.

Blum WF, Ranke MB, Kietzmann K, Gauggel E, Zeisel HJ, Bierich JR: A specific radioimmunoassay for the growth hormone (GH)-dependent somatomedin-binding protein: Its use for diagnosis of GH deficiency. J Clin Endocrinol Metab 1990;70:1292–1298.

Blum WF, Ranke MB, Kietzmann K, Tönshoff B, Mehls O: Growth hormone resistance and inhibition of somatomedin activity by excess of insulin-like growth factor binding protein in uremia. Pediatr Nephrol 1991;5:539–544.

Blum WF, Albertsson-Wikland K, Rosberg S, Ranke MB: Serum levels of insulin-like growth factor I (IGF-1) and IGF-binding protein 3 (IGFBP-3) reflect spontaneous growth hormone secretion. J Clin Endocrinol Metab 1993;76:1610–1616.

Blum WF, Cotterill AM, Postel-Vinay MC, Ranke MB, Savage MO, Wilton P: Improvement of diagnostic criteria in growth hormone insensitivity syndrome: solutions and pitfalls. Acta Paediatr 1994;(suppl 399):117–124.

Cacciari E, Tassoni P, Cicognani A, Pirazzoli P, Salardi S, Balsamo A, Cassio A, Zucchini S, Colli C, Tassinari D, Tani G, Gualandi S: Value and limits of pharmacological and physiological tests to diagnose growth hormone (GH) deficiency and predict therapy response: first and second retesting during replacement therapy of patients defined as GH deficient. J Clin Endocrinol Metab 1994;79:1663–1669.

Chin E, Zhou J, Dai J, Baxter RC, Bondy CA: Cellular localization and regulation of gene expression for components of the insulin-like growth factor ternary binding protein complex. Endocrinology 1994;134:2498–2504.

Clayton PE, Cuneo RC, Juul A, Monson JP, Shalet SM, Tauber M: Consensus statement on the management of the GH-treated adolescent in the transition to adult care. Eur J Endocrinol 2005;152:165–170.

Daughaday WH, Mariz IK, Blethen SL: Inhibition of access of bound somatomedin to membrane receptor and immunobinding sites: a comparison of radioreceptor and radioimmunoassay of somatomedin in native and acid-ethanol-extracted serum. J Clin Endocrinol Metab 1980;51:781–788.

Duncan E, Wass JAH: Investigation protocol: acromegaly and its investigation. Clin Endocrinol 1999;50:285–293.

Firth SM, Baxter RC: Cellular actions of the insulin-like growth factor binding proteins. Endocr Rev 2002;23:824–854.

Frystyk J, Freda P, Clemmons DR: The current status of IGF-1 assays: a 2009 update. GH IGF Res 2010;20:8–18.

Goddard AD, Covello R, Luoh SM, Clackson T, Attie KM, Gesundheit N, Rundle AC, Wells JA, Carlsson LMS: Mutations of the growth hormone receptor in children with idiopathic short stature. N Engl J Med 1995;333:1093–1098.

Green H, Morikawa M, Nixon T: A dual effector theory of growth hormone action. Differentiation 1985;29:195–198.

Grinspoon S, Clemmons D, Swearingen B, Klibanski A: Serum insulin-like growth factor-binding protein-3 levels in the diagnosis of acromegaly. J Clin Endocrinol Metab 1995;80:927–932.

Growth Hormone Research Society: Consensus guidelines for the diagnosis and treatment of growth hormone deficiency in childhood and adolescence: summary statement of the Growth Hormone Research Society. J Clin Endocrinol Metab 2000;85:3990–3993.

Hasegawa Y, Hasegawa T, Aso T, Kotoh S, Nose O, Ohyama Y, Araki K, Tanaka T, Saisyo S, Yokoya S, Nishi Y, Miyamoto S, Sasaki N, Kurimoto F, Stene M, Tsuchiya Y: Clinical utility of insulin-like growth factor binding protein-3 in the evaluation and treatment of short children with suspected growth hormone deficiency. Eur J Endocrinol 1994;131:27–32.

Ho KKY, the 2007 GH Deficiency Workshop Consensus Participants: Consensus guidelines for the diagnosis and treatment of adults with GH deficiency. II. A statement of the GH Research Society in association with the European Society for Pediatric Endocrinology, Lawson Wilkins Society, European Society of Endocrinology, Japan Endocrine Society and Endocrine Society of Australia. Eur J Endocrinol 2007;157:695–700.

Holt RI, Jones JS, Stone NM, Baker AJ, Miell JP: Sequential changes in insulin-like growth factor (IGF)-I and IGF-binding proteins in children with end-stage liver disease before and after successful orthotopic liver transplantation. J Clin Endocrinol Metab 1996;81:160–168.

Jogie-Brahim S, Feldman D, Oh Y: Unraveling insulin-like growth factor binding protein-3 actions in human disease. Endocr Rev 2009;30:417–437.

Jørgensen JOL, Blum WF, Møller N, Ranke MB, Christiansen JS: Circadian patterns of serum insulin-like growth factor (IGF)-II and IGF-binding protein 3 in growth hormone deficient patients and age- and sex-matched normal subjects. Acta Endocrinol (Copenh) 1990b;123:257–262.

Jørgensen JOL, Blum WF, Møller N, Ranke MB, Christiansen JS: Short-term changes in serum insulin-like growth factors (IGF) and IGF-binding protein 3 after different modes of intravenous growth hormone (GH) exposure in GH-deficient patients. J Clin Endocrinol Metab 1991;72:582–587.

Jørgensen JOL, Møller N, Møller J, Weeke J, Blum WF: Insulin-like growth factors (IGF)-I and -II and IGF-binding protein-1, -2 and -3 in patients with acromegaly before and after adenomectomy. Metabolism 1994;43:579–583.

Juul A: Serum levels of insulin-like growth factor I and its binding proteins in health and disease. GH IGF Res 2003;13:113–117.

Juul A, Skakkebæk NE: Prediction of the outcome of growth hormone provocative testing in short children by measurement of serum levels of insulin-like growth factor I and insulin-like growth factor binding protein 3. J Pediatr 1997;130:197–204.

Juul A, Dalgaard P, Blum WF, Bang P, Hall K, Michaelsen KF, Muller J, Skakkebæk NE: Serum levels of insulin-like growth factor (IGF)-binding protein-3 (IGFBP-3) in healthy infants, children and adolescents: the relation to IGF-1, IGF-2, IGFBP-1, IGFBP-2, age, sex, body mass index and pubertal maturation. J Clin Endocrinol Metab 1995;80:2534–2542.

Kaplan AS, Cohen P: The somatomedin hypothesis 2007: 50 years later. J Clin Endocrinol Metab 2007;92:4529–4535.

Krassas GE, Pontikides N, Kaltsas T, Dumas A, Frystyk J, Chen JW, Flyvbjerg A: Free and total insulin-like growth factor (IGF)-I, -II and IGF-binding protein-1, -2 and -3 serum levels in patients with active thyroid eye disease. J Clin Endocrinol Metab 2003;88:132–135.

Kratzsch J, Blum WF, Schenker E, Keller E: Regulation of growth hormone (GH), insulin-like growth factor (IGF)-I, IGF-binding proteins-1, -2, -3 and GH-binding protein during progression of liver cirrhosis. Exp Clin Endocrinol 1995;103:285–291.

Kristrom B, Jansson C, Rosberg S, Albertsson-Wikland K: Growth response to growth hormone (GH) treatment relates to serum insulin-like growth factor I (IGF-1) and IGF-binding protein-3 in short children with various GH secretion capacities. Swedish Study Group for Growth Hormone Treatment. J Clin Endocrinol Metab 1997;82:2889–2898.

Lee PD, Wilson DM, Rountree L, Hintz RL, Rosenfeld RG: Efficacy of insulin-like growth factor I levels in predicting the response to provocative growth hormone testing. Pediatr Res 1990;27:45–51.

LeRoith D, Werner H, Beitner-Johnson D, Roberts CT Jr: Molecular and cellular aspects of the insulin-like growth factor I receptor. Endocr Rev 1995;16:143–163.

Löfqvist C, Andersson E, Gelander L, Rosberg S, Hulthen L, Blum WF, Albertsson Wikland K: Reference values for insulin-like growth factor-binding protein-3 (IGFBP-3) and the ratio of insulin-like growth factor-I to IGFBP-3 throughout childhood and adolescence. J Clin Endocrinol Metab 2005;90:1420–1427.

Martin JL, Baxter RC: Insulin-like growth factor-binding protein from human plasma: purification and characterization. J Biol Chem 1986;261:8754–8760.

Miell JP, Taylor AM, Jones J, Holly JMP, Gaillard RC, Pralong FP, Ross RJM, Blum WF: The effect of dexamethasone treatment on immunoreactive and bioactive insulin-like growth factors (IGFs) and IGF-binding proteins in normal male volunteers. J Endocrinol 1993;136:525–533.

Mitchell H, Dattani MT, Nanduri V, Hindmarsh PC, Preece MA, Brook CGD: Failure of IGF-1 and IGFBP-3 to diagnose growth hormone insufficiency. Arch Dis Childh 1999;80:443–447.

Morrione A, Valentinis B, Xu SQ, Yumet G, Louvi A, Efstratiadis A, Baserga R: Insulin-like growth factor II stimulates cell proliferation through the insulin receptor. Proc Natl Acad Sci USA 1997;94:3777–3782.

Nunez SB, Municchi G, Barnes KM, Rose SR: Insulin-like growth factor (IGF)- I and IGF-binding protein-3 concentrations compared to stimulated and night growth hormone in the evaluation of short children: a clinical research center study. J Clin Endocrinol Metab 1996;81:1927–1932.

Ranke MB, Schweizer R, Elmlinger MW, Weber K, Binder G, Schwarze CP, Wollmann HA: Significance of basal IGF-1, IGFBP-3 and IGFBP-2 measurements in the diagnostics of short stature in children. Horm Res 2000;54:60–68.

Ranke MB, Schweizer R, Elmlinger MW, Weber K, Binder G, Schwarze CP, Wollmann HA: Relevance of IGF-1, IGFBP-3 and IGFBP-2 measurements during GH treatment of GH-deficient and non-GH-deficient children and adolescents. Horm Res 2001;55:115–124.

Rikken B, van Doorn J, Ringeling A, Van den Brande JL, Massa G, Wit JM: Plasma levels of insulin-like growth factor (IGF)-I, IGF-2 and IGF-binding protein-3 in the evaluation of childhood growth hormone deficiency. Horm Res 1998;50:166–176.

Rinderknecht E, Humbel RE: The amino acid sequence of human insulin-like growth factor I and its structural homology with proinsulin. J Biol Chem 1978a; 253:2769–2776.

Rinderknecht E, Humbel RE: Primary structure of human insulin-like growth factor II. FEBS Lett 1978b;89:283–286.

Rochiccioli P, Pienkowski C, Tauber MT, Uboldi F, Enjaume C: Association of pharmacological tests and study of 24-hour growth hormone secretion in the investigation of growth retardation in children: analysis of 257 cases. Horm Res 1991;35:70–75.

Rosenfeld RG, Wilson DM, Lee PDK, Hintz RL: Insulin-like growth factors I and II in evaluation of growth retardation. J Pediatr 1986;109:428–433.

Rosenfeld RG, Rosenbloom AL, Guevara-Aguirre J: Growth hormone (GH) insensitivity due to primary GH receptor deficiency. Endocr Rev 1994;15:369–390.

Savage MO, Blum WF, Ranke MB, Postel-Vinay MC, Cotterill AM, Hall K, Chatelain PG, Preece MA, Rosenfeld RG, Danielson K, Wilton P: Clinical features and endocrine status in patients with growth hormone insensitivity (Laron syndrome). J Clin Endocrinol Metab 1993;77:1465–1471.

Schoenau E, Westermann F, Rauch F, Stabrey A, Wassmer G, Keller E, Braemswig J, Blum WF: A new and accurate prediction model for growth response to growth hormone treatment in children with growth hormone deficiency. Eur J Endocrinol 2001;144:13–20.

Smith WJ, Taek JN, Underwood LE, Busby WH, Celnicker A, Clemmons DR: Use of insulin-like growth factor-binding protein (IGFBP)-2, IGFBP-3 and IGF-1 for assessing growth hormone status in short children. J Clin Endocrinol Metab 1993;77:1294–1299.

Tassoni P, Cacciari E, Cau M, Colli C, Tosi M, Zucchini S, Cicognani A, Pirazzoli P, Salard S, Balsamo A, Frejaville E, Cassio A, Zappulla F: Variability of growth hormone response to pharmacological and sleep tests performed twice in short children. J Clin Endocrinol Metab 1990;71:230–234.

Tillmann V, Buckler JM, Kibirige MS, Price DA, Shalet SM, Wales JK, Addison MG, Gill MS, Whatmore AJ, Clayton PE: Biochemical tests in the diagnosis of childhood growth hormone deficiency. J Clin Endocrinol Metab 1997;82:531–535.

Tönshoff B, Blum WF, Wingen AM, Mehls O: Serum insulin-like growth factors (IGFs) and IGF-binding proteins 1, 2 and 3 in children with chronic renal failure: Relationship to height and glomerular filtration rate. J Clin Endocrinol Metab 1995;80:2684–2691.

Zapf J, Walter H, Froesch ER: Radioimmunological determination of insulin-like growth factors I and II in normal subjects and in patients with growth disorders and extrapancreatic tumor hypoglycemia. J Clin Invest 1981;68:1321–1330.

Werner F. Blum, MD, PhD
Eli Lilly and Company
Werner-Reimers-Strasse 2–4
DE–61352 Bad Homburg (Germany)
Tel. +49 6172 273 2248, Fax +49 6172 273 2358, E-Mail blum_werner@lilly.com

Ranke MB, Mullis P-E (eds): Diagnostics of Endocrine Function in Children and Adolescents, ed 4.
Basel, Karger, 2011, pp 183–193

Diagnosis of Growth Hormone Excess and Hyperprolactinemia

Stefan Riedl · Herwig Frisch

Pediatric Department, Medical University of Vienna, Vienna, Austria

Pathophysiology of Acromegaly and Hyperprolactinemia

Acromegaly is a relatively rare disease that is caused by long-standing growth hormone (GH) hypersecretion. The estimated prevalence of the disease is 60 cases per million with 3–4 new cases per million per year [1]. In exceptional cases, the disease is diagnosed prior to epiphyseal fusion, leading to pituitary gigantism. After completion of growth, the clinical symptoms become more similar to those in acromegalic adults like coarse facial features, acral changes, hyperhydrosis, headaches and visceromegaly.

In most cases, acromegaly is caused by pituitary adenomas, but it has become evident that lesions of hypothalamic, pituitary, or extracranial origin may be responsible for GH excess. Hypersecretion of GH-releasing hormone (GHRH) may be the result of a hypothalamic tumor, for example, hamartoma or ganglioneuroma, which either directly secretes GHRH or, alternatively, may stimulate hypothalamic GHRH production or impair the secretion of somatostatin. More frequently, GHRH secretion occurs from an ectopic GHRH-producing tumor like carcinoid tumors, pancreatic cell tumors, small cell lung cancer, and adrenal tumors [2]. GHRH may lead to GH hypersecretion and eventually pituitary acromegaly. GHRH is a potent mitogenic factor, and transgenic mice expressing the GHRH gene may develop somatotropic adenomas, which shows that GHRH is a direct tropic stimulus for the somatotropic cell [3]. Similarly, in McCune-Albright syndrome, constitutive activation of the GHRH-cAMP signaling pathway caused by an activating *GNAS* mutation leads to GH hypersecretion and pituitary adenoma formation in up to one third of patients [4, 5]. GHRH may also stimulate prolactin (PRL) secretion in acromegalic subjects, and about one third of such patients have hyperprolactinemia [1].

Several aspects favor the 'pituitary' hypothesis underlying acromegaly. In 90% of acromegalics, a pituitary tumor can be found, and these tumors can be plurihormonal, which implies that the hypersecretory cells must originate from a common stem cell. Furthermore, in nearly all cases the somatotropic tissue surrounding the tumor is not hyperplastic. This indicates that the primary disorder arises from a pituitary disorder. In addition, the high cure rate after selective adenomectomy and the low recurrence rate militate against a primary hypothalamic defect. The pituitary tumors may be pure GH cell adenomas, or they may be composed of two different cell types and secrete GH and PRL. The adenoma may also derive from the common GH and PRL stem cell and express both hormones. Plurihormonal tumors may express GH in combination with various other hormones such as ACTH or, rarely, TSH [5].

Still little is known about the genetic causes of common pituitary tumors. Nevertheless, the molecular basis of pituitary tumorigenesis in familial acromegaly and sporadic pituitary tumors has been elucidated during the last decade [6]: The occurrence of isolated familial somatotropinomas (IFS) was reported in 20 families and usually affects younger patients [7]. In familial isolated pituitary adenoma (FIPA), 50% of the adenomas are prolactinomas, with GH-secreting and mixed GH- and PRL-secreting adenomas accounting for the remainder [8]. Moreover, mammosomatotroph pituitary adenomas may occur in MEN-1 [9] and the Carney complex [10].

Hyperprolactinemia is more frequent in females and leads to hypogonadism by impairing pulsatile gonadotropin release causing delayed menarche or menstrual irregularities/amenorrhea in girls and pubertal arrest in boys. In postpubertal subjects, symptoms of estrogen/testosterone deficiency like decreased libido, apathy and decreased bone mineral density predominate. In both sexes, rarely in boys, galactorrhea may occur. However, prolactin does not play a direct role in gynecomastia since it does not act as a growth hormone for the breast.

Hyperprolactinemia may be caused by a prolactinoma, which is the most frequent hormone-secreting pituitary tumor. Concordantly, a total of 45% of pituitary adenomas found in autopsy material were positive for PRL immunostaining. The age distribution of patients with these tumors was equal throughout the age range of 16–86 years [11]. Depending on the size of the tumor, symptoms of a pituitary mass like visual abnormalities – most frequently bitemporal hemianopsia, opththalmoplegia or headache may occur. Another possible pathomechanism of elevated PRL levels is pituitary stalk compression by a tumor, leading to a decrease of PRL inhibition by dopamine. Besides mass effects, symptoms from pituitary insufficiency by compression of normal pituitary tissue may prevail in this case. Moderately elevated PRL levels may also result from interfering macroprolactin which can be differentiated by using polyethylene glycol precipitation.

Regulation of Growth Hormone Secretion

The secretion of GH is under the hypothalamic control of GHRH, which stimulates the synthesis and secretion of both GH and somatostatin. The latter acts to suppress the secretion of GH. The episodic pattern of GH secretion is predominantly regulated by fluctuations in somatostatin secretion [12]. Episodic secretion is also preserved in the presence of tonically elevated levels of circulating GHRH that results from an ectopic tumor [13].

Most of the growth-promoting effects of GH are mediated by insulin-like growth factor 1 (IGF-1), which exerts a negative feedback action on GH secretion and suppresses the pituitary synthesis of GH messenger ribonucleic acid (mRNA) [14]. IGF-1 is a GH-dependent peptide that is secreted mainly by the liver, but in addition, synthesis of IGF-1 also occurs in many tissues in an autocrine/paracrine manner. IGF-1 is age- and sex-dependent, but shows virtually no diurnal variation because it circulates in combination with a binding protein (BP). More than 95% of IGF-1 is bound to insulin-like growth factor-binding protein 3 (IGFBP-3), a 150-kDa complex which acts as a carrier for IGF and regulates its bioavailability. IGFBP-3 is predominantly regulated by GH and reflects GH secretory status [see chapter by Blum et al., this vol.].

Regulation of Prolactin Secretion

PRL is secreted in a pulsatile manner, and there is diurnal variation with an increase in pulse amplitude after the onset of sleep. PRL is predominantly under an inhibitory influence of hypothalamic dopamine, whereas thyrotropin-releasing hormone (TRH), among other substances, is the main PRL-releasing factor. This explains why a mass lesion in the hypothalamic or pituitary stalk area, resulting in a decrease of anterior pituitary hormones, causes the elevation in PRL concentrations and why hyperprolactinemia is found in primary hypothyroidism, respectively. Other factors (e.g. vasoactive intestinal polypeptide (VIP), serotonin, opioid peptides, or GHRH) can stimulate PRL release; increased levels are also found during pregnancy and in chronic renal failure [15].

Tests of Growth Hormone Secretion

Basal Serum GH Levels
Increased GH secretion is the most prominent biochemical finding in acromegaly (see diagnostic algorithm, 'Appendix B, Chart 6'). The predictive value of random GH samples in identifying acromegaly varies with the selected threshold levels; however, elevated basal GH levels may occur in physiological or pathological conditions like stress (caused by the insertion of the cannula), pubertal growth spurt, exercise, diabetes, malnutrition, or chronic renal failure. Moreover, the spontaneous pulsatility of GH has to be taken into account. In addition, basal levels may be low in about 5% of acromegalic subjects. Nevertheless, acromegaly can be excluded if

the GH level is less than 0.04 µg/l using newer, highly sensitive immunoradiometric assays [5].

Test Procedure. Several random blood samples should be taken from an inserted cannula over an extended period in order to avoid influences of stress, meals, etc. GH concentrations are then determined by immunoassay [see chapter by Ranke, this vol.].

Spontaneous GH Pulses

GH secretion shows a pulsatile pattern, and the secretory pulses are consequent to hypothalamic secretory bursts. The evaluation of GH pulsatility may thus make it possible to obtain information about hypothalamic GHRH secretion. In prepubertal children, a high correlation exists between relative height and the amount of GH secreted during a 24-hour period. In acromegalic patients, integrated 24-hour GH concentrations are significantly increased, and the pattern of spontaneous GH secretion is typically altered: the extent of pulsatile excursions is blunted, GH concentrations do not fall below the limit of detection, and the circadian pattern is abnormal, suggesting a defect in the neuroendocrine mechanisms regulating spontaneous GH secretion [5].

Test Procedure. Blood samples are collected for 24 h (or a defined shorter period) from an intravenous (i.v.) cannula, which permits undisturbed sampling while the subject is asleep. GH samples are taken every 20 min, either by a continuously working withdrawal pump or by discrete samples. The total blood volume taken has to be considered, especially in younger subjects. Various parameters such as mean GH levels, pulse frequency, pulse amplitude, or area under the curve, can be calculated [see chapter by Albertsson-Wikland and Rosberg, this vol.]. Since GH secretion is age-dependent, it is important to compare the results with age-related reference values [see chapter by Albertsson-Wikland and Rosberg, this vol.]. This is a tedious method, which, however, gives reliable information about GH secretory status.

Urinary GH Excretion

Evaluation of urinary GH excretion has been developed as a noninvasive method for screening of GH status [16] However, this method is rarely used any more since great variation of GH excretion on a day-to-day basis exists. Moreover, methodological difficulties add to the low sensitivity and specificity of this test.

GH Stimulation Tests

Insulin Tolerance Test, Arginine Tolerance Test, and GHRH Test
The GH response to the classic GH provocation tests such as the insulin tolerance test (ITT) and the arginine tolerance test (ATT) in acromegalic patients may vary and can comprise a normal increase, no response, or a paradoxical decrease [17]. The stimuli act via the hypothalamic axis, but the tests are of no diagnostic or prognostic value.

Similarly, stimulation with GHRH or GH-releasing peptide does not add to diagnostic information [18].

Dopamine Stimulation Test
In contrast to normal subjects, GH levels decrease by more than 50% in the majority of acromegalic individuals after the administration of dopamine agonists. The reason for this paradoxical reaction is a possible alteration of the somatotropic dopamine receptors. The function of this test is rather to identify possible responders to chronic therapy with a dopamine agonist.

Stimulation with TRH and Luteinizing Hormone-Releasing Hormone
In a large proportion of acromegalic subjects, nonspecific GH release can be provoked by hypothalamic releasing hormones such as TRH or, less frequently, luteinizing hormone-releasing hormone (LHRH) [17]. The abnormal GH response disappears after successful therapy. These tests are of no special value for the diagnosis of acromegaly.

GH Suppression

Oral Glucose Tolerance Test
The oral glucose tolerance test (OGTT) is the most important test for confirming the diagnosis of acromegaly [5, 19, 20]. After oral glucose administration, GH levels decrease to levels <1 μg/l in normal individuals. In acromegalic patients, GH levels are either not suppressible, or they demonstrate a paradoxical increase. In more than 90% of acromegalic subjects, GH does not decrease to <1 μg/l. Thus, the OGTT is a good screening procedure for acromegaly, although its sensitivity is limited by the fact that 7–10% of patients may nonetheless demonstrate suppression of GH levels to <1 μg/l. Moreover, other pathologic conditions such as diabetes, chronic renal failure, or severe malnutrition may be associated with elevated basal GH concentrations and prevent suppression of GH levels after the OGTT, thus limiting the specificity of the test. In addition, in tall children without pituitary disease, nonsuppression of GH after OGTT was found in a considerable percentage [21].

Test Procedure. The patients should be in a fasting and resting state for 12 h prior to commencement of the test. An oral glucose solution (1.75 g/kg body weight) is ingested in the first 5 min of the test (ready-to-drink containers of glucose solution are commercially available). Blood samples for the determination of glucose and GH levels are collected at –30, 0, 30, 60, 90, 120 and 180 min. It is important to carry out the test procedure for the entire 180-min duration. The test results are evaluated by taking into account the fact that normally GH levels decrease to <1 μg/l within 60–120 min after the glucose load. High GH levels which do not decrease or which even display paradoxical increase are characteristic of acromegaly.

IGF-1 and IGFBP-3

IGF-1

Patients with untreated acromegaly consistently have significantly elevated IGF-1 levels that show no overlap with normal individuals [22]. It has been shown that increased IGF-1 levels are able to predict abnormal GH secretion early in the course of acromegaly, when GH levels are relatively low or decrease to 5 µg/l or less after glucose administration. Moreover, IGF-1 concentrations were significantly correlated to various parameters of disease severity such as clinical signs or blood glucose concentrations during the OGTT [23]. Thus, IGF-1 concentrations offer a highly accurate reflection of daily 24-hour GH secretion [5, 19]. In acromegalic individuals, a linear relation exists between IGF-1 and GH levels <20 µg/l. With higher GH levels, IGF-1 concentrations reach a plateau. IGF-1 is thus a sensitive indicator of GH hypersecretion. Even mildly elevated GH concentrations (5–10 µg/l) are associated with IGF-1 elevation. A single measurement of IGF-1 provides reliable information.

Test procedure. In order to determine the serum level of IGF-1, a random blood sample is drawn. After separation of the hormone from its BP by chromatography or extraction, the IGF-1 concentration is determined by immunoassay [see chapter by Blum et al., this vol.]. The test results are then compared with age- and sex-related reference data.

IGFBP-3

Serum IGFBP-3 levels are clearly elevated in untreated patients with acromegaly, and there is no overlap with the normal range. IGFBP-3 correlates significantly with the results of spontaneous GH secretion. In a large sample of untreated acromegalics with confirmed adenomas, IGFBP-3 was elevated even in those cases with normal or only slightly increased IGF-1 concentrations or in patients who showed GH suppression after a glucose load [24]. However, there is consensus that estimation of IGFBP-3 usually offers no advantage to IGF-1 in the assessment of disease activity [19].

Test procedure. IGFBP-3 is determined by immunoassay from a random blood sample. It is important to compare the results with age-related reference values [see chapter by Blum et al., this vol.].

Other Diagnostic Tests in Acromegaly

PRL

Basal PRL levels are elevated in 20–60% of patients with acromegaly [25]. Immunohistochemical studies have shown that all tumors contain PRL- and GH-reactive cells [26]. Elevated PRL may also occur as a consequence of a pituitary stalk lesion resulting in an insufficient dopamine supply. Furthermore, hyperprolactinemia may be the consequence of augmented hypothalamic GHRH secretion, as it is frequently found in patients with ectopic GHRH secretion. GHRH injection also resulted in an increase in PRL [13]. The response of PRL to the administration of TRH in acromegalic patients may be normal, decreased or exaggerated and is therefore of no diagnostic help. Although clinical signs of GH excess already exist before hyperprolactinemia occurs, galactorrhea may be an early symptom in acromegaly. Likewise, any patient with hyperprolactinemia should have an evaluation of GH status.

TSH and Gonadotropins

10–15% of pituitary adenomas in acromegaly show a plurihormonal character, producing also glycoproteinic hormones apart from GH and PRL. Plurihormonal adenomas occur more frequently in childhood and adolescence, and most of them (80%) are macroadenomas [27]. In this context, basal TSH may be increased, but the TSH response to TRH may be impaired by elevated GH levels. If a deficiency of pituitary hormones also develops, gonadotropins are most frequently affected.

Tests of Prolactin Secretion

In general, PRL circulates in human plasma in 3 major variants: monomeric PRL (monoPRL; 23 kDa), dimeric PRL (bigPRL; 48–56 kDa); and polymeric forms (macroPRL; 150–204 kDa). MonoPRL is biologically active and accounts for the majority of immunoreactive PRL. MacroPRL results from an antigen-antibody complex of monoPRL and IgG and accumulates in serum due to its longer renal clearance. MacroPRLemia has been identified in 15–46% of hyperprolactinemic samples [28, 29]. Controversy exists as to biological effects of macroPRL, however, it is recommended to consider its occurrence if PRL levels and the clinical condition do not match, in order to avoid unnecessary radiological investigations or inappropriate treatment with dopamine agonists. Gel filtration chromatography (GFC) is the gold standard method for quantification of monoPRL, bigPRL and macroPRL, but too labor-intensive and expensive for use in clinical practice. In contrast, polyethylene glycol precipitation (PEG), a nonquantitative method, is easy to perform. It is therefore commonly used as a screening test since results correlate well with GFC [28].

For correct interpretation of PRL levels, it is essential to rule out hypothyroidism, chronic renal failure, pregnancy, and medication with neuroleptics, antihypertensive drugs, or calcium channel blockers. In general, normal basal PRL levels range from 5 to 15–25 ng/ml (upper limit range; higher in females). After TRH stimulation, the mean PRL level increases to 22.3 ± 0.5 ng/ml (mean $\pm$ SE) [30]. Slightly elevated basal PRL levels (25–40 ng/ml) may be idiopathic or result from emotional stress. Patients with PRL-secreting macroadenomas consistently exhibit markedly elevated PRL levels (>250 ng/ml, often >1,000 ng/ml). Using immunoradiometric methods, excessive PRL levels may sometimes lead to a 'hook' effect by saturation of antibody capacities and loss of labeled antibody, causing falsely low PRL values [28]. This effect can be overcome by serial dilutions. PRL levels up to 200 ng/ml may also be seen in acromegaly, since pituitary tumors

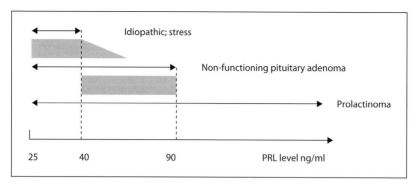

Fig. 1. Interpretation of elevated PRL levels. The overlap (shaded areas) between idiopathic/stress-induced hyperprolactinemia (PRL 25–40 ng/ml) or non-functioning pituitary adenoma (PRL <94 ng/ml) and PRL elevation caused by interfering macroPRL may be differentiated by PEG precipitation. Prolactinoma usually leads to much higher PRL levels. Data compiled from refrences 28 and 31.

may co-secrete GH and PRL. Pituitary tumors causing compression of the stalk show only moderate elevation of PRL (<94 ng/ml) [31]. Since there is a considerable overlap with 'false' hyperprolactinemia caused by macroPRL in that PRL range, it is essential to rule out the occurrence of macroPRL in such patients (fig. 1). The PRL response to TRH is characteristically blunted in patients with prolactinoma, but the response may be normal. Therefore, dynamic tests are not useful for the diagnosis [11].

Test Procedure. PRL tests are usually performed using two site immunoradiometric and chemiluminometric assays. Methods should be calibrated against the 3rd IRP WHO standard 84/500 (1 µg/l is equivalent to 21.2 mIU/l). To identify macroPRL, PEG dissolved in phosphate puffer saline (PBS) is added, before the sample is processed and the supernatant removed. Recovery is calculated by dividing the post-PEG PRL result by the PRL result obtained from the untreated sample. A PRL recovery of >60% after PEG is found if monoPRL is present whereas a PRL recovery of <40% is in line with macroprolactinemia [29]. PRL concentrations are usually reported in nanograms per milliliter.

For TRH test, see chapter by Krude and Grüters, this vol.

Imaging Procedures

Pituitary GH-producing tumors are the cause of more than 98% of acromegaly. High-resolution magnetic resonance imaging (MRI) of the pituitary-hypothalamic region is the method of choice for the detection of a possible tumor in this region. A resolution below 3 mm can be obtained when equipment with a high field strength (1.5–3 Tesla) is used. Spin-echo sequences, half-dose gadolinium injection, delayed sequence, and dynamic imaging add to diagnostic accuracy in small pituitary adenomas [32].

Riedl · Frisch

Evaluation of somatostatin receptors by scintigraphic imaging using radiolabeled somatostatin analogues may help to get information on the function of the tumor [33]. Dopamine antagonist binding to dopamine D2 receptors using PET or SPECT for visualization may discriminate prolactinomas and some GH secreting adenomas from nonfunctioning tumors; in addition, response to dopaminergic treatment may be predicted [34, 35].

Special Aspects

Ectopic Origin of Acromegaly

A rare cause of acromegaly is ectopic hormone secretion, which may be expected when elevated GH and GHRH levels are found in the absence of a primary lesion of the pituitary gland on MRI. Several types of extrapituitary tumors, such as carcinoid tumors, pancreatic cell tumors, small cell lung cancer, endometrial tumors, adrenal adenomas, and pheochromozytomas show positive GHRH immunostaining. Nevertheless, acromegaly in these patients is uncommon. If present, GH and IGF-1 concentrations are elevated, and GH fails to decrease after a glucose load. The response of GH to GHRH, TRH, or LHRH is of no help in distinguishing the central and the ectopic forms of acromegaly. The most useful discrimination parameter is the demonstration of elevated GHRH levels, which warrants further investigation for a peripheral tumor by abdominal and chest imaging. Furthermore, symptoms directly caused by the underlying tumor or unexpected clinical features like dyspnea, facial flushing, or peptic ulcers due to cosecretion of other substances may point at an ectopic origin of acromegaly [2].

PRL Deficiency

Occurrence of PRL deficiency (PRL <5 ng/ml) is generally rare. The incidence of acquired PRL deficiency rises with the number of other pituitary deficiencies and is usually seen in patients with craniopharyngioma, large nonfunctioning adenomas, pituitary apoplexy, and after pituitary surgery [36]. Congenital hypopituitarism including PRL deficiency may be caused by mutations in transcription factors and signaling molecules involved in pituitary development. If early developmental genes are affected, syndromic hypopituitarism may arise (HESX1: + septo-optic dysplasia; LHX3: + short cervical spine; limited neck rotation; sensorineural deafness; SOX3: + mental retardation; OTX2: + bilateral micro- or anophthalmia). The most prevalent monogenetic cause of non-syndromic combined pituitary hormone deficiencies is a PROP1 defect (GH, TSH, LH, FSH, PRL; evolving ACTH deficiency) and may cause pituitary enlargement on MRI. Mutations in POU1F1, which depends on temporal regression of PROP1 and is expressed throughout life, lead to GH, TSH and PRL deficiency, whereas corticotrophic and gonadotrophic functions are preserved [37].

Conclusion

Acromegaly is an extremely rare disorder before epiphyseal closure. The origin of GH hypersecretion may result from primary pituitary disease (approximately 98% of cases), hypothalamic GHRH secretion, or ectopic tumors. GH stimulates IGF-1 production, which in turn promotes the growth of multiple organs and tissues. A pragmatic approach to the diagnosis of acromegaly includes the detection of increased basal levels of GH, IGF-1 and IGFBP-3: this constitutes a simple screening method (see diagnostic algorithm 6). IGF-1 serum concentrations are always elevated in acromegaly. The OGTT represents the most important test in confirming the diagnosis of acromegaly. MRI is essential for detection of a pituitary tumor. Only the rare cases of ectopic hormone production will require further investigations.

Hyperprolactinemia may either result from a prolactinoma or from loss of dopamine-driven PRL suppression by pituitary stalk compression. PEG precipitation is used to overcome interference of macroPRL, causing elevated PRL levels without obvious clinical relevance.

References

1 Holdaway IM, Rajasoorya C: Epidemiology of acromegaly. Pituitary 1999;2:29.

2 Gola M, Doga M, Bonadonna S, Mazziotti G, Vescovi PP, Giustina A: Neuroendocrine tumors secreting growth hormone-releasing hormone: pathophysiological and clinical aspects. Pituitary 2006;9:221.

3 Asa SL, Kovacs K, Stefaneanu L, Horvath E, Billestrup N, Gonzalez-Manchon C, Vale W: Pituitary adenomas in mice transgenic for growth hormone-releasing hormone. Endocrinology 1992;131:2083.

4 Akintoye SO, Chebli C, Booher S, Feuillan P, Kushner H, Leroith D, Cherman N, Bianco P, Wientroub S, Robey PG, Collins MT: Characterization of gsp-mediated growth hormone excess in the context of McCune-Albright syndrome. J Clin Endocrinol Metab 2002;87:5104.

5 Melmed S: Acromegaly pathogenesis and treatment. J Clin Invest 2009;119:3189.

6 Horvath A, Stratakis CA: Clinical and molecular genetics of acromegaly: MEN1, Carney complex, McCune-Albright syndrome, familial acromegaly and genetic defects in sporadic tumors. Rev Endocr Metab Disord 2008;9:1.

7 Gadelha MR, Prezant TR, Une KN, Glick RP, Moskal SF 2nd, Vaisman M, Melmed S, Kineman RD, Frohman LA: Loss of heterozygosity on chromosome 11q13 in two families with acromegaly/gigantism is independent of mutations of the multiple endocrine neoplasia type I gene. J Clin Endocrinol Metab 1999;84:249.

8 Beckers A, Daly AF: The clinical, pathological, and genetic features of familial isolated pituitary adenomas. Eur J Endocrinol 2007;157:371.

9 Agarwal SK, Ozawa A, Mateo CM, Marx SJ: The MEN1 gene and pituitary tumours. Horm Res 2009; 71(suppl 2):131.

10 Boikos SA, Stratakis CA: Carney complex: the first 20 years. Curr Opin Oncol 2007;19:24.

11 Molitch ME: Prolactinoma; in Melmed S (ed): The Pituitary. Oxford, Blackwell Science, 1995, p443.

12 Tannenbaum GS, Ling N: The interrelationship of growth hormone (GH)-releasing factor and somatostatin in generation of the ultradian rhythm of GH secretion. Endocrinology 1984;115:1952.

13 Barkan AL, Shenker Y, Grekin RJ, Vale WW, Lloyd RV, Beals TF: Acromegaly due to ectopic growth hormone (GH)-releasing hormone (GHRH) production: dynamic studies of GH and ectopic GHRH secretion. J Clin Endocrinol Metab 1986;63:1057.

14 Yamashita S, Weiss M, Melmed S: Insulin-like growth factor I regulates growth hormone secretion and messenger ribonucleic acid levels in human pituitary tumor cells. J Clin Endocrinol Metab 1986;63:730.

15 Freeman ME, Kanyicska B, Lerant A, Nagy G: Prolactin: structure, function, and regulation of secretion. Physiol Rev 2000;80:1523.

16 Girard J, Erb T, Pampalone A, Eberle AN, Baumann JB: Growth hormone in urine: development of an ultrasensitive assay applicable to plasma and urine. Horm Res 1987;28:71.

17 Chang-DeMoranville BM, Jackson IM: Diagnosis and endocrine testing in acromegaly. Endocrinol Metab Clin North Am 1992;21:649.

18 Alster DK, Bowers CY, Jaffe CA, Ho PJ, Barkan AL: The growth hormone (GH) response to GH-releasing peptide (His-DTrp-Ala-Trp-DPhe-Lys-NH2), GH-releasing hormone, and thyrotropin-releasing hormone in acromegaly. J Clin Endocrinol Metab 1993;77:842.

19 Growth Hormone Research Society; Pituitary Society: Biochemical assessment and long-term monitoring in patients with acromegaly: statement from a joint consensus conference of the Growth Hormone Research Society and the Pituitary Society. J Clin Endocrinol Metab 2004;89:3099.

20 Carmichael JD, Bonert VS, Mirocha JM, Melmed S: The utility of oral glucose tolerance testing for diagnosis and assessment of treatment outcomes in 166 patients with acromegaly. J Clin Endocrinol Metab 2009;94:523.

21 Holl RW, Bucher P, Sorgo W, Heinze E, Homoki J, Debatin KM: Suppression of growth hormone by oral glucose in the evaluation of tall stature. Horm Res 1999;51:20.

22 Brooke AM, Drake WM: Serum IGF-1 levels in the diagnosis and monitoring of acromegaly. Pituitary 2007;10:173.

23 Chen HS, Lin HD: Serum IGF-1 and IGFBP-3 levels for the assessment of disease activity of acromegaly. J Endocrinol Invest 1999;22:98.

24 Grinspoon S, Clemmons D, Swearingen B, Klibanski A: Serum insulin-like growth factor-binding protein-3 levels in the diagnosis of acromegaly. J Clin Endocrinol Metab 1995;80:927.

25 de Pablo F, Eastman RC, Roth J, Gorden P: Plasma prolactin in acromegaly before and after treatment. J Clin Endocrinol Metab 1981;53:344.

26 Furuhata S, Kameya T, Otani M, Toya S: Prolactin presents in all pituitary tumors of acromegalic patients. Hum Pathol 1993;24:10.

27 Scheithauer BW, Kovacs K, Randall RV, Horvath E, Laws ER Jr: Pathology of excessive production of growth hormone. Clin Endocrinol Metab 1986;15:655.

28 Chahal J, Schlechte J: Hyperprolactinemia. Pituitary 2008;11:141.

29 McCudden C, Sharpless JL, Grenache DG: Comparison of multiple methods for identification of hyperprolactinemia in the presence of macroprolactin. Clin Chim Acta 2010;411:155.

30 Frisch H, Herkner K, Schober E, Stögmann W, Waldhauser F, Weissel M: Prolactin and thyrotrophin response to thyrotrophin-releasing hormone in growth hormone deficiency. Arch Dis Child 1982;57:769.

31 Karavitaki N, Thanabalasingham G, Shore HC, Trifanescu R, Ansorge O, Meston N, Turner HE, Wass JA: Do the limits of serum prolactin in disconnection hyperprolactinaemia need re-definition? A study of 226 patients with histologically verified non-functioning pituitary macroadenoma. Clin Endocrinol 2006;65:524.

32 Bonneville JF, Bonneville F, Cattin F: Magnetic resonance imaging of pituitary adenomas. Eur Radiol 2005;15:543.

33 de Herder WW, Kwekkeboom DJ, Feelders RA, van Aken MO, Lamberts SW, van der Lely AJ, Krenning EP: Somatostatin receptor imaging for neuroendocrine tumors. Pituitary 2006;9:243.

34 Muhr C: Positron emission tomography in acromegaly and other pituitary adenoma patients. Neuroendocrinology 2006;83:205.

35 de Herder WW, Reijs AE, Feelders RA, van Aken MO, Krenning EP, van der Lely AJ, Kwekkeboom DJ: Diagnostic imaging of dopamine receptors in pituitary adenomas. Eur J Endocrinol 2007;156(suppl 1):S53.

36 Toledano Y, Lubetsky A, Shimon I: Acquired prolactin deficiency in patients with disorders of the hypothalamic-pituitary axis. J Endocrinol Invest 2007;30:268.

37 Alatzoglou KS, Dattani MT: Genetic forms of hypopituitarism and their manifestation in the neonatal period. Early Hum Dev 2009;85:705.

Stefan Riedl, MD
St Anna Children's Hospital
Kinderspitalgasse 6
AT–1090 Vienna (Austria)
Tel. +43 1 40400 2800, Fax +43 1 40400 7280, E-Mail stefan.riedl@meduniwien.ac.at

Ranke MB, Mullis P-E (eds): Diagnostics of Endocrine Function in Children and Adolescents, ed 4.
Basel, Karger, 2011, pp 194–209

Testing Water Regulation

Paul Czernichow · Michel Polak

Pediatric Endocrinology, Reference Center for Rare Endocrine Disorders of Growth, Hôpital Necker Enfants
Malades, AP-HP, Université Paris Descartes, Paris, France

A complex regulatory system keeps plasma osmolality stable despite large variations in water consumption or water loss. This osmoregulatory system is controlled by the hypothalamic neurohypophyseal axis, which includes the organs responsible for sensing variations in plasma osmolality or volume, and those responsible for the synthesis, storage, and secretion of the antidiuretic hormone arginine vasopressin (AVP). The osmoregulatory system also includes osmoreceptors of thirst, which control drinking behavior. The osmoreceptors are also stimulated by osmotic changes in plasma.

The second component of the osmoregulatory system involves the kidney. The renal collecting duct is sensitive to the action of AVP. In response to AVP, the functional units of the kidney, through modulation of the aquaporin 2 system, allow dramatic variations in urinary flow in order to maintain water balance.

In order to test water regulation, it is therefore necessary to evaluate not only AVP secretion and kidney sensitivity to AVP, but also thirst.

In this chapter, we will cover diabetes insipidus and the syndrome of inappropriate secretion of antidiuretic hormone. Other aspects of sodium regulation will be covered in the chapter by Ferrari and Bianchetti [this vol.].

Normal Physiology

Release of Vasopressin
AVP is synthesized in neurons located in two bilateral cell clusters in the hypothalamus, the paraventricular nuclei (PVN) and the supraoptic nuclei (SON). The tracts proceeding from these two nuclei on either side of the hypothalamus converge into a single supraopticohypophyseal tract which runs through the pituitary stalk to the posterior pituitary (fig. 1).

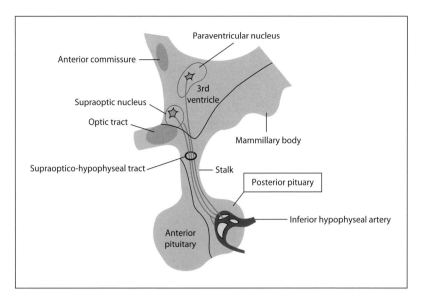

Fig. 1. Anatomy of the hypothalamic neurohypophyseal system.

Osmoreceptor

In recent years, it has been recognized that nausea, glucopenia, and angiotensin may stimulate the release of AVP. However, the physiology and pathophysiology of AVP can be adequately understood in terms of the traditional regulatory system consisting of the osmoreceptor and the volume receptor. The osmoreceptor is exquisitely sensitive to changes in osmolality, and a plasma osmolality increase as small as 1% is sufficient to increase plasma AVP levels [1]. In normal subjects, the 'osmotic threshold' for AVP release is considered to be approximately 280 mosm/kg H_2O. AVP levels increase linearly when osmolality increases from 280 to more than 300 mosm/kg H_2O (fig. 2).

Volume

The main input to the hypothalamus for volume recognition originates in the high-pressure baroreceptors of the carotid sinus and aortic arch and reaches the SON and PVN via the ninth and tenth cranial nerves. The baroreceptor system is much less sensitive than the osmoreceptor, since a change in blood volume of 5–10% is necessary to induce AVP release. However, once the blood volume threshold is exceeded, AVP release may increase exponentially, reaching levels ten times higher than those reached after osmotic stimulation.

Thirst

Thirst has not been studied in great detail in humans. It was first suggested that thirst in humans may not be sensed until plasma osmolality reaches 295 mosm/kg H_2O [2].

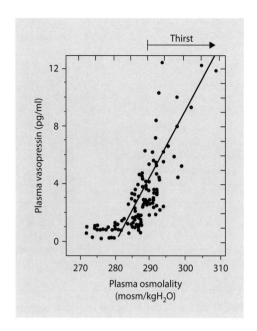

Fig. 2. Relationship between plasma osmolality and plasma AVP in normal subjects [1]. The threshold for AVP secretion is close to, but somewhat lower than that for thirst sensation.

Subsequent data showed that thirst occurred at lower levels of plasma osmolality, i.e. at the same threshold as AVP release [3]. Because most adults drink sufficient water by habit and social custom, intense thirst is rarely experienced.

Role of the Kidney in Water Regulation

Variations in urinary concentration and volume are a function of the spatial arrangement of the renal tubules and AVP effects on the collecting tubules.

The interstitial fluid is isosmolal to plasma in the renal cortex and becomes progressively hyperosmolal toward the papillary tips in the medulla. This corticomedullary gradient is maintained by the countercurrent multiplication system of the loops of Henle. In the collecting ducts, which extend across the hyperosmolal medullary interstitium, the water permeability of the luminal membrane is regulated by AVP. In the absence of AVP, permeability is low and the urine remains dilute. With rising AVP concentrations, permeability increases steeply. The resulting reabsorption of water improves the balance between the tubular urine and interstitial fluid. This results in a sharp rise in urinary osmolality (fig. 3).

The action of AVP on the collecting duct is mediated by displacement of an AVP-regulated water-channel protein to the apical membrane of the duct cells. The aquaporins are a family of membrane proteins present in many water-transporting tissues. Aquaporin-2 is specific of the collecting duct and is responsible for transferring water to the interstitial fluid. Aquaporin-2 is present in urine and its concentration increases during antidiuresis [4].

Czernichow · Polak

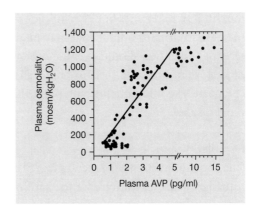

Fig. 3. Relationship between AVP level and urine osmolality [1].

Functional Physiologic Relationships

The exquisite physiologic regulation of the water balance is due to the high sensitivity of the kidney to minute changes in AVP levels. This relationship is illustrated in figure 3. As shown in this figure, the lower limit of urine osmolality occurs in the absence of AVP and corresponds to the maximal capacity of the kidney to excrete free water. The higher limit of urine osmolality corresponds to the maximal ability of the kidney to concentrate the urine in response to increased AVP levels.

Diabetes Insipidus

The term 'diabetes insipidus' designates several water regulation disorders due to AVP deficiency or AVP insensitivity. As a rule, they manifest as polyuria and polydipsia with varying degrees of plasma hypertonicity if the patient does not have free access to beverages or if the thirst threshold is altered. When caused by AVP deficiency, the disorder is called central diabetes insipidus. Insensitivity to AVP is referred to as nephrogenic diabetes insipidus. Usually, polydipsia is secondary to polyuria. Primary polydipsia due to a specific disorder of thirst regulation may be seen in pediatric practice, especially in young children still using the bottle. Usually, polyuria is defined as water excretion in excess of 5 ml/kg/h in infants and 1,500 ml/m^2/day (i.e. 50 ml/kg/day) in children.

Diagnostic Procedures

Basic Parameters

Urine Volume

At first glance, urine volume measurement may seem the simplest and easiest diagnostic procedure. However, precise and reliable urine volume measurement requires either hospitalization or, in the home setting, a certain amount of skill, particularly for children in nappies but also for older children. In addition, there may be a modest increase in urinary output that may be difficult to distinguish from normal. The differential diagnosis should exclude other causes of polyuria, such as osmotic diuresis of glucose or urea and intrinsic renal disease, as well as hypercalcemia. Routine biochemical tests should eliminate polyuria resulting from osmotic diuresis or chronic renal disease.

Osmolality

The most important parameters are plasma and urine osmolality, which are determined by using an osmometer to examine freshly collected, unfrozen specimens. The apparatus should be well calibrated. For plasma, simultaneous sodium measurement is helpful to establish a control for the plasma osmolality level. One can also estimate osmolality using a formula based on blood concentrations: (sodium + potassium) × 2 + urea + glucose (all in mmol/l). This formula is useful, as the equipment needed for direct osmolality measurement is less and less widely available. Urine density measurement is no longer frequently performed, although a good correlation has been reported between urinary osmolality and density. Urinary density is easy and inexpensive to calculate, and this procedure can be performed at the bedside during a dehydration test to obtain information quickly.

AVP Measurement

AVP is measured by radioimmunoassay (RIA) on 1 ml of plasma. A 2-ml blood sample is collected in a chilled, heparinized tube and centrifuged immediately in a refrigerated centrifuge. Platelets contain a certain amount of AVP. Therefore, the blood should be centrifuged for 20 min at 2,000 rpm, and care should be taken when collecting the supernatant to leave the pellet intact. The assay sensitivity is 0.5 pg/ml plasma. Normal values vary according to the technique used. In our laboratory, the average AVP value for normal children is 1.9 ± 0.2 (pg/ml ± SD) for a plasma osmolality of 283 ± 1 (mosm/kg H_2O ± SD). Since the AVP level varies according to osmotic stimulation, it should be compared with plasma osmolality measured at the same time [5].

Test Procedures

Dehydration Test
Purpose
The dehydration test evaluates plasma AVP secretion and action by inducing a certain degree of hypertonicity and volume contraction. These two physiologic inputs work additively to stimulate the release of AVP. Measurement of plasma and urine osmolality at the end of the test is usually sufficient to establish a diagnosis of diabetes insipidus [6–8]. The usual 14-hour test should be reserved for situations where the diagnosis cannot be made easily by stopping oral fluid intake for a few hours then

obtaining sodium and osmolality measurements, which show increases in sodium concentration and plasma osmolality with a urine osmolality lower than the plasma osmolality. The dehydration test is not well accepted by the children and their families. Usually this test follows a period of observation of the drinking habits of the child; if the child drinks more than 4 liters during the day, the test is usually not indicated. The test should always be tailored to the drinking behavior of the child as observed before the test is scheduled.

Protocol
For patients who need this diagnostic procedure (see above), the test is started postprandially at 6 p.m. and finished at 8 a.m. In very young children or in patients with massive polyuria (urine volume >4 liters/24 h); however, the test is started in the morning when medical staff are present and then usually lasts two to 4 h, after which the answer is most often obtained. No food or drink is allowed during the test. The patient must be kept under close surveillance throughout the test, for two reasons: (1) some children drink water surreptitiously, and (2) blood pressure and weight should be measured hourly and signs of dehydration looked for.

The test should be terminated (a) if ≥5% of body weight is lost, and (b) tachycardia is present. The finding of 5% weight loss can be misleading if the patient is clinically well and in stable cardiovascular condition. This test requires a physician to be present on the ward to evaluate the clinical status of the child on a regular basis, as well as trained and experienced nursing staff. During the test, usually on a hourly basis from 6 a.m. over the 14-hour test, spot urine and blood specimens are collected to determine urine and plasma osmolality. These specimens should be processed rapidly by the laboratory so that the test can be stopped as soon as the result is positive (sodium level above 145 mEq/l with higher osmolality in plasma than in urine). At the end of the test, spot urine and blood specimens are collected to determine urine and plasma osmolality and the AVP concentration. Thirst sensation should be recorded throughout the test.

Results
During a test involving 14 h of water deprivation, normal children show almost no variation in plasma osmolality, whereas urine osmolality increases (fig. 4, 5). In patients with polydipsia of about 2–4 liters per day, the test often fails to give an answer within 2–4 h and usually lasts 7 or 8 h. It can be prolonged if the patient is clinically and biochemically stable but has not yet reached a urinary osmolality >800 mosm/kg H_2O for children older than 2 years of age or >600 mosm/kg H_2O for toddlers, with no change between two consecutive determinations.

All patients with diabetes insipidus become hypernatremic and maintain hypo-osmolal urine. Patients with partial AVP deficiency are clearly distinguishable from those with total AVP deficiency, in that the former show moderate elevations in plasma and urine osmolality (fig. 5, 6).

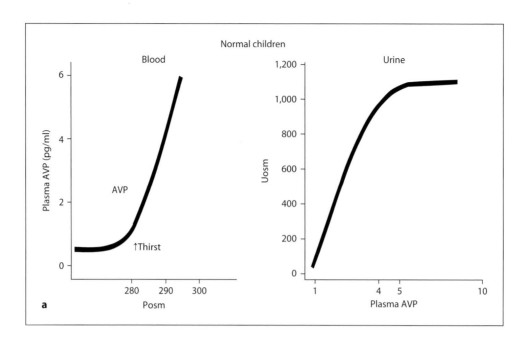

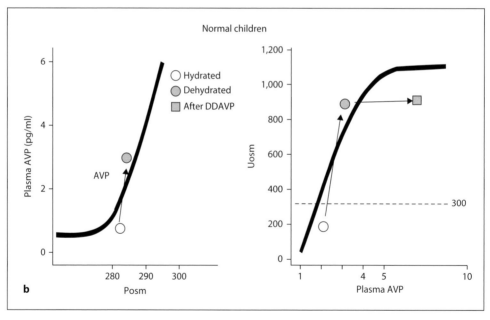

Fig. 4. Results obtained during the dehydration test. **a, b** Normal response, without DDAVP infusion (**a**) and with DDAVP infusion (**b**).

Czernichow · Polak

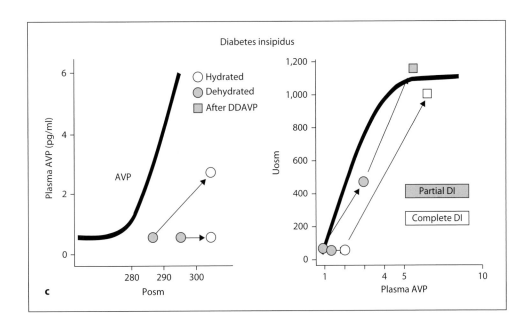

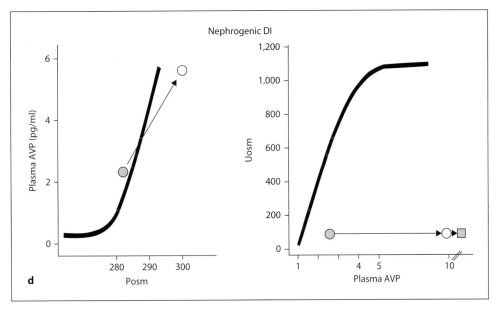

Fig. 4. Results obtained during the dehydration test. **c** Results in a case of central diabetes insipidus (total or partial). **d** Results in a case of nephrogenic diabetes insipidus.

Comments

When the initial evaluation shows elevated plasma osmolality (usually above 300 mosm/kg H_2O) due to hypernatremia (above 145 mEq/l) and inappropriately low urine osmolality (less than the plasma osmolality), a diagnosis of some form of diabetes insipidus can be given without further testing (fig. 4, 5; see also diagnostic algorithm, 'Appendix B: Chart 8'). If the diagnosis is not immediately obvious, a dehydration test must be performed. Patients who are completely unable to secrete AVP have no measurable plasma AVP and show low urine concentration. Urine osmolality in these patients is either <100 mosmol/kg H_2O or, during dehydration with serum sodium elevation (above 145 mEq/l), <300 mosmol/kg H_2O. All three other diagnostic categories, i.e. partial hypothalamic diabetes insipidus, nephrogenic diabetes insipidus, and primary polydipsia, are characterized by some elevation of urine osmolality, which may not attain levels as high as 800 mosm/kg H_2O at maximal urinary concentration. AVP measurement (unfortunately not widely available) should identify patients with nephrogenic diabetes insipidus, in whom AVP levels are high [8]. This is one of the most reliable and clinically useful indications of AVP measurement.

It has also been suggested that AVP measurement during the dehydration test not only identifies nephrogenic diabetes insipidus, but also helps to differentiate between partial central diabetes insipidus and primary polydipsia [9, 10]. In these two disorders, the maximal urinary concentration may be decreased due to washout of the renal medulla. In some patients with partial central diabetes insipidus, the AVP deficiency may be so limited that maximal urinary concentration is achieved, even with the abnormally low levels of AVP secreted in response to hypernatremia. Such cases are indistinguishable from primary polydipsia. To differentiate these two disorders, an extremely sensitive AVP assay is necessary to distinguish very low levels from complete absence of AVP.

In our experience, the water deprivation test as outlined above rarely leads to erroneous diagnoses. An exception to this is nephrogenic diabetes insipidus, in which AVP measurement is required to confirm the diagnosis. However, with nephrogenic diabetes, even a relatively insensitive AVP assay should detect elevated levels.

Short Desmopressin Test

Purpose

Administration of a test dose of desmopressin (DDAVP) is useful in evaluating the maximal renal concentration capacity and in distinguishing nephrogenic from central diabetes insipidus [11].

Protocol

The test is performed with DDAVP, a very potent AVP analog now widely used in the treatment of central diabetes insipidus. It can also be performed with aqueous AVP injected subcutaneously. The test is performed either in the morning after an

Czernichow · Polak

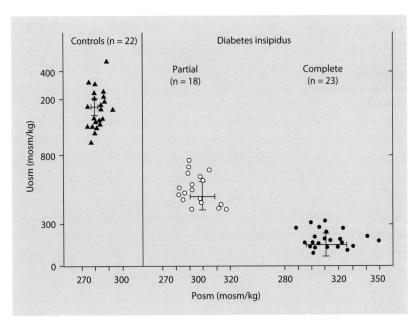

Fig. 5. Urinary osmolality (Uosm) in relation to plasma osmolality (Posm) in normal children and in patients with partial and complete diabetes insipidus. In many patients with massive polyuria, water deprivation for a few hours is enough to demonstrate elevated Posm and inadequate Uosm. Several patients with partial diabetes insipidus have Uosm close to normal at the end of the test. All have elevated Posm at that time.

overnight fast or at the end of the dehydration test. It is important to maintain fluid restriction after the DDAVP dose, i.e. patients are allowed to drink only as much water in ml as their urine output over the last hour. This is the only means of preventing symptomatic hyponatremia in patients with psychogenic polydipsia. DDAVP is insufflated intranasally in a dosage of 20 µg for children and 10 µg for infants. Alternatively, in infants, a DDAVP dose of 0.5 µg/m² body surface area (BSA) may be administered intravenously or subcutaneously. After emptying the bladder at 8 a.m., the patient receives the appropriate dose of DDAVP and the urine is then collected, hourly if possible, for 4 h. Osmolality is measured in each specimen.

Results

The maximal concentration is approximately 1,000 mosm/kg H$_2$O (at least 800) in normal children and close to 500 mosm/kg H$_2$O in infants. The osmolalities achieved by normal children correlate well with the results of the DDAVP test and dehydration test. A subnormal result indicates resistance to AVP. In some protocols, DDAVP is given intramuscularly in a dosage of 1.0 µg in infants (<2 years age) and 2.0 µg in children >2 years. After 4 h, if the urine:plasma osmolality ratio is >1.5, the patient demonstrates normal urine concentration following DDAVP administration.

Fig. 6. Dehydration test lasting 14 h in children. Plasma vasopressin (AVP), plasma osmolality (Posm), and urine osmolality (Uosm) in control subjects (hatched bars), patients with severe central diabetes insipidus (dark circles), patients with partial central diabetes insipidus (open circles), and patients with nephrogenic diabetes insipidus (triangles). Patients with severe central diabetes insipidus have elevated plasma osmolality with markedly dilute urine, while patients with partial diabetes insipidus have moderate plasma osmolality elevation and moderate inability to maximally concentrate urine [8]. Note that patients with polyuria of renal origin show either partial or complete insensitivity to AVP. In this situation, AVP measurement readily establishes the diagnosis.

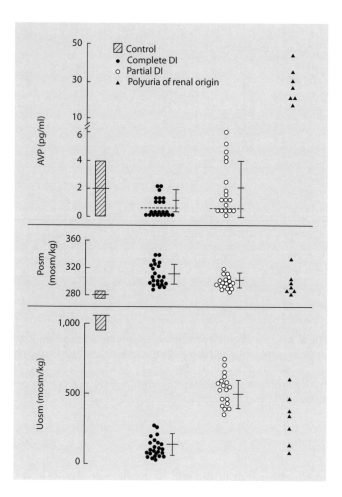

Comments

As originally described [1], patients with complete or partial diabetes insipidus show an increase in urine osmolality during the DDAVP test. Patients with nephrogenic diabetes insipidus show no increase in urinary osmolality. However, these patients may occasionally respond to exogenous AVP, because the dose given is within the pharmacological range. This result suggests that the deficiency in these patients represents only a partial inability to respond to AVP, since pharmacological amounts of this hormone cause further concentration of urine. Patients with primary polydipsia show an increase in urine osmolality during the dehydration test that is close to normal values, and they respond to DDAVP by a urine osmolality increase of less than 10%. This demonstrates that such individuals respond normally to dehydration. The test results can be abnormal after prolonged polyuria related to central diabetes insipidus [12]. This is a rare situation which is explained by a 'wash-out' effect. The renal medulla is hypotonic, which diminishes the concentrating ability of exogenous AVP. In this situation, the test should be repeated after 2–3 days of DDAVP treatment.

An increase in the urinary excretion of aquaporin-2 occurs in response to AVP in patients with central diabetes insipidus but not in those with nephrogenic diabetes insipidus [4]. These results may help, theoretically, to differentiate nephrogenic diabetes insipidus from central diabetes insipidus.

Special Diagnostic Considerations

Central Diabetes Insipidus, Tumors, and Histiocytosis
When a definitive diagnosis of central diabetes insipidus is established, additional investigations should be considered. Nuclear magnetic resonance (NMR) imaging of the hypothalamic-pituitary region should be performed. The multiplanar capabilities of NMR imaging produce three-dimensional images that are superior over CT scans. On T1-weighted images, the posterior lobe has a characteristic high-signal intensity similar to fatty tissue and distinct from the anterior lobe. Thus, the normal posterior lobe is seen clearly. In central diabetes insipidus, the posterior lobe is not visible [13]. Anterior pituitary function should be evaluated. Growth hormone deficiency is frequently associated with an anterior pituitary tumor or Langerhans cell histiocytosis [14]. In the event of adrenocorticotropic hormone deficiency, polyuria may be masked by the glucocorticoid deficiency. Patients should be investigated for diabetes insipidus after 3 days of hydrocortisone replacement therapy (20 mg/m^2 BSA) [5].

NMR imaging visualizes tumors in the hypothalamopituitary region, which can be clearly identified based on specific criteria. In some cases, NMR imaging shows pituitary stalk thickening, which requires regular follow-up. About 20% of cases of pituitary stalk thickening may be related to dysgerminoma [15]. Langerhans cell histiocytosis is another possible cause. When no specific cause is identified, close follow-up should be offered, as evidence of histiocytosis such as pulmonary, skin, or bone lesions may develop up to 10 years later [Polak et al., unpubl. data]. When the stalk is severely enlarged (>8 mm thick), a biopsy has been suggested to establish the correct diagnosis and allow treatment. In patients with histiocytosis, diabetes insipidus is a risk factor for the development of neurodegenerative histiocytosis lesion and therefore warrants brain NMR imaging every 3–5 years, as this modality ensures lesion detection before the onset of clinical manifestations [16]. It should be remembered that most children and young adults with acquired central diabetes insipidus have abnormal brain NMR imaging findings, which may change over time. In a case series of 79 patients, at least half had anterior pituitary hormone deficiencies during follow-up [17].

Infants and Young Children
Central diabetes insipidus is rare in young children and infants. Most cases of nephrogenic diabetes insipidus are observed at this age. One should remember the danger

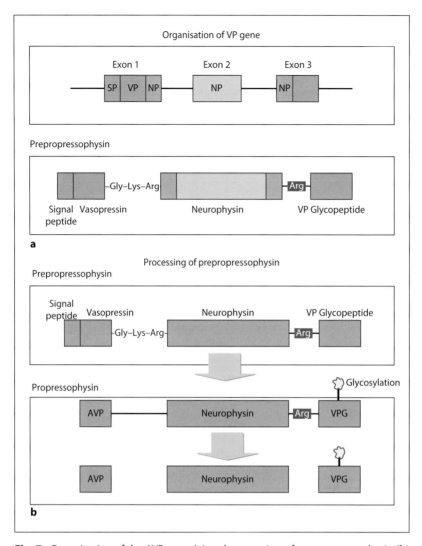

Fig. 7. Organization of the AVP gene (**a**) and processing of prepropressophysin (**b**).

of dehydration at this age, which mandates close monitoring during the dehydration test. Urinary osmolality varies with age in young children. Age should therefore be taken into account when evaluating the results of the DDAVP test (see above, 'Short desmopressin test').

Genetics

Anomalies at the molecular level have been identified in rare cases of familial diabetes insipidus. The affected gene was the AVP gene in familial central diabetes insipidus (fig. 7) and the AVP receptor gene or aquaporin-2 gene in familial nephrogenic diabetes insipidus. Precise identification of the genetic abnormalities will improve the classification of the multiple forms of familial or idiopathic diabetes insipidus. To date, this has not substantially impacted the treatment strategy [18].

Syndrome of Inappropriate Secretion of Antidiuretic Hormone

Pathophysiology
In adults, the syndrome of inappropriate secretion of antidiuretic hormone (SIADH) is often associated with ectopic AVP production related to lung cancer. In other cases in adults and less often in children, the disorder is due to inappropriate secretion of AVP by the posterior pituitary. This excess production may occur because of loss of inhibitory input from the baroreceptor system. A variety of lesions that interfere with this pathway may decrease the inhibitory input to the neurohypophysis, thereby resulting in increased AVP release. In children, SIADH has been observed in association with pulmonary disease (usually viral or bacterial infections) and with infectious and metabolic diseases of the central nervous system.

The importance of volume receptors in this syndrome [12] is demonstrated by reports of SIADH in premature infants treated with mechanical ventilation [9, 19]. Infants receiving assisted ventilation had significantly higher plasma AVP levels and higher urine osmolality. The mechanism by which AVP release is stimulated during mechanical ventilation has been studied in dogs and may involve either hypoxic ischemia or decreased venous return, together with decreased cardiac output and baroreceptor stimulation. Premature infants are particularly likely to develop hypoxic ischemia as a result of either pulmonary disease or cerebral injury. SIADH may be less common in infants than in adults exposed to similar insults, as maximal urine concentration is lower in infants. A variety of drugs may also cause SIADH. In children, cases related to vincristine therapy have been reported.

Recently reported mechanisms include the so-called 'nephrogenic syndrome of inappropriate antidiuresis'. In this syndrome, a gain-of-function mutation in the V2 AVP receptor gene causes constitutive activation of the receptor with an SIADH-like clinical picture and undetectable plasma AVP levels [20].

Diagnostic Procedure

Before investigating SIADH, it is important to rule out other conditions such as renal failure, nephrotic syndrome, or heart failure in the case of hypervolemic hyponatremia. Hypocortisolism and hypothyroidism should be excluded in the case of normovolemic hyponatremia. Cerebral salt-wasting syndrome is an endocrine condition featuring hyponatremia and dehydration in response to trauma/injury or to tumors in or surrounding the brain. This form of hyponatremia is due to excessive renal sodium excretion resulting from a centrally mediated process (through the secretion of brain natriuretic factor) and can be distinguished from SIADH as it is associated with dehydration instead of the hypervolemia seen in SIADH [21, 22]. However the two conditions may be difficult to distinguish, as normovolemia may be present in SIADH after the initial phase, leading to hyponatremia.

SIADH has the following clinical features: retention of water with plasma hypo-osmolality, normal or slightly increased blood volume, and inappropriate urine osmolality with respect to plasma osmolality. Laboratory tests usually show hyponatremia <130 mEq/l and Posm <270 mosm/kg. Other findings include urine sodium concentration >20 mEq/l (inappropriate natriuresis). Sodium excretion usually exceeds sodium intake at the start of the syndrome. Later on, urine sodium concentration may be normal, reflecting dietary intake. Criteria were developed in 1967 and have remained essentially unchanged since then [23].

Plasma renin activity is invariably low, but aldosterone is usually unsuppressed. Plasma AVP concentrations are usually in the normal range and abnormal only in relation to plasma osmolality. The diagnostic procedure usually includes routine evaluation of plasma and urine electrolytes.

References

1 Robertson GL, Aycinena P, Zerbe RL: Neurogenic disorders of osmoregulation. Am J Med 1982;72: 339–353.

2 Robertson GL: Thirst and vasopressin function in normal and disordered states of water balance. J Lab Clin Med 1983:101:351–371.

3 Thompson CJ, Bland J, Burd J, Baylis PH: The osmotic thresholds for thirst and vasopressin release are similar in healthy man. Clin Sci (Lond). 1986;71: 651–656.

4 Kanno K, Sasaki S, Kirata Y, Ishikawa S, Fushimi K, Nakanishi S, Bichet DG, Marumo F: Urinary excretion of aquaporin-2 in patients with diabetes insipidus. N Engl J Med 1995;332:1540–1545.

5 Czernichow P, Pomarede R, Basmaciogullari A, Rappaport R: Diabetes insipidus in children. I. Arginine-vasopressin determination in plasma during short dehydration test. Acta Paediat Scand 1979; 277(suppl):64–68.

6 Edelman CJ, Barnett HL Jr, Stark H, Boikis H, Soriano A Jr: Standardized test of renal concentrating capacity in children. Am J Dis Child 1967;114: 639–644.

7 Frazier SD, Kutnik LA, Achmidt RT, Smith FG Jr: A water deprivation test for the diagnosis of diabetes insipidus in children. Am J Dis Child l967;114:157–160.

8 Czernichow P, Pomarede R, Brauner R, Rappaport R: Neurogenic diabetes insipidus in children; in Czernichow P, Robinson AG (eds): Diabetes Insipidus in Man. Basel, Karger, 1984, pp 190–209.

9 Pomarede R, Moriette G, Czernichow P, Relier JP: Etude de la vasopressine plasmatique chez les enfants prématurés soumis à la ventilation artificielle. Arch Fr Pédiatr 1978;35(suppl):75–83.

10 Zerbe RL, Robertson GL: A comparison of plasma vasopressin measurements with a standard indirect test in the differential diagnosis of polyuria. N Engl J Med 1981;305:1539–1546.

11 Aaronson AS, Svenningsen NW: DDAVP test for estimation of renal concentrating capacity in infants and children. Arch Dis Child 1974;49:654–650.

12 Harrington AR, Vatin H: Impaired urinary concentration after vasopressin: its gradual correction in hypothalamic diabetes insipidus. J Clin Invest 1968; 47:502–512.

13 Fujisawa I, Nishimura K, Asato R, Togashi K, Itoh K, Noma S, Kawamura Y, Sago T, Nimani S, Nakano Y: Posterior lobe of the pituitary in diabetes insipidus: MR findings. J Comput Assist Tomogr 1987;11: 221–229.

14 Donadieu J, Rolon MA, Pion I, Thomas C, Doz F, Barkaoui M, Robert A, Deville A, Mazingue F, David M, Brauner R, Cabrol S, Garel C, Polak M, French LCH Study Group: Incidence of growth hormone deficiency in pediatric-onset Langerhans cell histiocytosis: efficacy and safety of growth hormone treatment. J Clin Endocrinol Metab 2004;89:604–609.

15 Léger J, Velasquez A, Garel C, Hassan M, Czernichow P: Thickened pituitary stalk on magnetic resonance imaging in children with central diabetes insipidus. J Clin Endocrinol Metab 1999;84:1954–1960.

16 Donadieu J, Rolon MA, Thomas C, Brugieres L, Plantaz D, Emile JF, Frappaz D, David M, Brauner R, Genereau T, Debray D, Cabrol S, Barthez MA, Hoang-Xuan K, Polak M, French LCH Study Group: Endocrine involvement in pediatric-onset Langerhans' cell histiocytosis: a population-based study. J Pediatr 2004;144:344–350.

17 Maghnie M, Cosi G, Genovese E, Manca-Bitti ML, Cohen A, Zecca S, Tinelli C, Gallucci M, Bernasconi S, Boscherini B, Severi F, Arico M: Central diabetes insipidus in children and young adults. N Engl J Med 2000;343:998–1007.

18 Czernichow P: Central diabetes insipidus; in Rappaport R, Amselem S (eds): Hypothalamic-Pituitary Development: Genetic and Clinical Aspects. Endocrine Development. Basel, Karger, 2001, vol 4, pp 162–174.

19 Paxon CL, Stoener JW, Denson SE, Adcock EW, Morris F: Syndrome of inappropriate antidiuretic hormone secretion in neonates with pneumothorax or atelectasis. J Pediatr 1977;91:459–463.

20 Feldman BJ, Rosenthal SM, Vargas GA, Fenwick RG, Huang EA, Matsuda-Abedini M, Lustig R, Mathias RS, Portale AA, Miller W, Gitelman SE: Nephrogenic syndrome of inappropriate antidiuresis. N Engl J Med 2005;352:1884–1890.

21 Peters JP, Welt LG, Sims EA, Orloff J, Needham J: 'A salt-wasting syndrome associated with cerebral disease'. Trans Assoc Am Physicians 1950;63:57–64.

22 Harrigan MR: Cerebral salt wasting syndrome: a review. Neurosurgery 1996;38:152–60.

23 Bartter FC, Schwartz WB: The syndrome of inappropriate secretion of antidiuretic hormone. Am J Med 1967;42:790–806.

Michel Polak
Pediatric Endocrinology, Hôpital Necker Enfants Malades
AP-HP, Université Paris Descartes, 149, rue de Sèvres
FR–75015 Paris (France)
Tel. +33 1 44 49 48 03, Fax +33 1 44 38 16 48, E-Mail michel.polak@nck.aphp.fr

Ranke MB, Mullis P-E (eds): Diagnostics of Endocrine Function in Children and Adolescents, ed 4.
Basel, Karger, 2011, pp 210–234

Diagnostic Investigations in Inherited Endocrine Disorders of Sodium Regulation

Paolo Ferrari[a] · Mario G. Bianchetti[b]

[a]Department of Nephrology, Fremantle Hospital and School of Medicine and Pharmacology, University of Western Australia, Perth, W.A., Australia; [b]Department of Paediatrics, Ospedale San Giovanni, Bellinzona, Switzerland

In this chapter we will focus primarily on endocrine disorders that are the consequence of abnormal biosynthesis, metabolism or target organ response of hormones that regulate renal sodium (Na^+) handling and are ultimately characterized by a decrease or increase in total body Na^+. The most important organ system for Na^+ regulation is the kidney. The adrenal steroid hormone aldosterone plays a central role in regulating renal Na^+ reabsorption in the cortical collecting duct of the kidney, which is the major site of regulated Na^+ handling along the nephron. In addition to angiotensin II, other stimulators of aldosterone are ACTH, which stimulates transiently aldosterone secretion, high potassium and vasopressin, while natriuretic peptides inhibit aldosterone synthesis [1]. Other adrenal steroids such as 11-deoxycorticosterone (DOC), but also cortisol, have approximately the same in vitro affinity for the mineralocorticoid receptor, although physiologically in vivo these hormones do not show mineralocorticoid action. Defects or disturbances in steroid hormone biosynthesis or target organ response to steroid hormones lead to either Na^+ loss, which is life threatening in the neonatal period, or Na^+ retention causing hypertension. Rapid and accurate diagnosis of these conditions is required to avoid severe complications. During the last few years advances in molecular genetics have identified many basic genetic defects for a number of clinical syndromes. This knowledge has considerably increased our understanding of the basic pathways involved in Na^+ and water homoeostasis and of the pathophysiology of these syndromes, particularly hypertension. Early diagnosis and identification will help prevent severe complications, but it has to be emphasized that the complicated cascade of aldosterone action is still relatively poorly understood. Further syndromes may exist which once identified will help to better understand the basic physiology of aldosterone action.

Deceptively, and perhaps paradoxically, endocrine disorders of Na^+ regulation are not characterized by marked abnormalities in plasma Na^+ concentration and therefore clinical suspicion of these disorders is not raised by the presence of striking hyper- or hyponatremia. Hypernatremia reflects a deficit of total body water (TBW) relative to total body Na^+ content and usually implies either limited access to water or impaired thirst mechanism. Common causes are net pure water losses (hypodipsia, diabetes insipidus), net hypotonic fluid losses either of renal (loop diuretics, osmotic diuresis, some intrinsic renal diseases), gastrointestinal (vomiting, enterocutaneous fistula, diarrhea) or cutaneous (burns, excessive sweating) origin, or net hypertonic Na^+ gains (hypertonic saline infusions or enemas). On the other hand, hyponatremia reflects an excess of TBW relative to total body Na^+ content, usually because of impaired renal water excretion, due most often to an inability to suppress ADH release. Common causes include diuretic use, diarrhea, heart and liver failure, and nephrotic syndromes. These conditions will not be discussed in detail in this chapter.

Regulation of Body Sodium

In terrestrial animals including humans the monovalent cation Na^+ accounts for over 90% of the osmotically active solute and it is the main determinant of the extracellular fluid (ECF) and hence the water content of the body. Salt and water homoeostasis in the body is tightly regulated by a variety of control mechanisms, including endocrine, paracrine and neural factors that maintain extracellular fluid osmolality within the extremely narrow range (280–290 mosm/kg), which is vitally essential for proper cell function.

The kidney plays a central role in the regulating of salt and water balance [2]; in mammals, 99% of the filtered Na^+ is reabsorbed by the nephron and the amount of Na^+ excreted equals the amount of Na^+ ingested. Na^+ is freely filtered by the glomerulum and despite the quantitative importance of Na^+ reabsorption in the proximal tubule and loop of Henle (~97%) there is surprisingly little known about the regulation of Na^+ handling in these nephron segments. The cortical collecting tubule handles roughly 2% of filtered Na^+, but has the ability to modulate Na^+ concentration. In this nephron segment Na^+ transport is controlled by aldosterone. Normal regulation of salt and water homeostasis in mammals is controlled in a negative-feedback loop by the renin-angiotensin-aldosterone system [3]. The key players of this system are renin, released by the juxtaglomerular cells of the afferent arterioles and macula densa cells of the kidney and aldosterone produced by the adrenal glands. Aldosterone exerts its physiological action by binding to receptors that belong to a transcription factor superfamily, which also includes proteins necessary for the regulation of steroid synthesis. Aldosterone regulates Na^+ homeostasis by stimulating Na^+ reabsorption via the amiloride-sensitive Na^+ channel in the apical membrane and

Na$^+$/K$^+$-ATPase in the basolateral membrane. These receptors, channels and pumps are linked together and form a complex system which is regulated and controlled at various levels. The genetic basis is known for a number of components; mutations causing defects or overactivity of these systems are the basis for a variety of inherited diseases with the clinical picture of either salt retention or salt loss [4]. Since Na$^+$ reabsorption in the distal nephron is coupled with enhanced tubular secretion of potassium and protons, hypokalemia and metabolic alkalosis are also common metabolic features of hormonal disorders causing Na$^+$ retention, while hyperkalemia and metabolic acidosis are common metabolic features of hormonal disorders causing Na$^+$ loss.

Adrenal Steroid Biosynthesis

The major adrenal steroid hormones are synthesized in different areas of the adrenal cortex: glucocorticoids in the zona fasciculata, androgens and estrogens in the zona reticularis and aldosterone in the zona glomerulosa (fig. 1). Knowledge of these pathways is critical in the understanding of the different forms of defects in the function of the enzymes involved in adrenal steroid hormone synthesis such as congenital adrenal hyperplasia and familial hypoaldosteronism and familial hyperaldosteronism.

Cholesterol is the substrate for the synthesis of all steroid hormones. In humans, cholesterol for adrenal steroidogenesis is taken up from circulating HDL by the receptor system for SR-B1 (scavenger receptor, class B, type 1). SR-B1 expression is stimulated by transcription factors such as SF-1, and Sp1 and is inhibited by the DAX-1 transcription factor. Four distinct cytochrome P450 enzymes are involved in adrenal glucocorticoid biosynthesis: (1) conversion of pregnenolone to progesterone (3β-hydroxysteroid dehydrogenase); (2) conversion of progesterone to 17α-hydroxyprogesterone or pregnenolone to 17α-hydroxypregnelone (17α-hydroxylase); (3) conversion of 17α-hydroxyprogesterone to 11-deoxycortisol (21-hydroxylase), and (4) conversion of 11-deoxycortisol to cortisol (11β-hydroxylase) (fig. 1).

Fig. 1. Biosynthesis of steroid hormones. The first committed step in steroid hormone biosynthesis is the conversion of cholesterol to pregnenolone. The conversion of cholesterol to pregnenolone entails 3 steps, all mediated by P450 side-chain cleavage enzyme, which is under pituitary hormone control (ACTH or LH depending on the tissue). From pregnenolone, steroid biosynthesis can proceed either through the so-called 'delta-5' pathway (17α-hydroxypregnenolone, DHEA, testosterone), or through the 'delta-4' pathway (progesterone onwards). Progesterone is the starting point for mineralocorticoid synthesis, whereas glucocorticoids are derived from its metabolite, 17α-hydroxyprogesterone. Estrogens are formed from androgens (androstenedione and/or testosterone). Most reactions are irreversible. D = Desmolase; HSD = hydroxysteroid dehydrogenase; OH = hydroxylase.

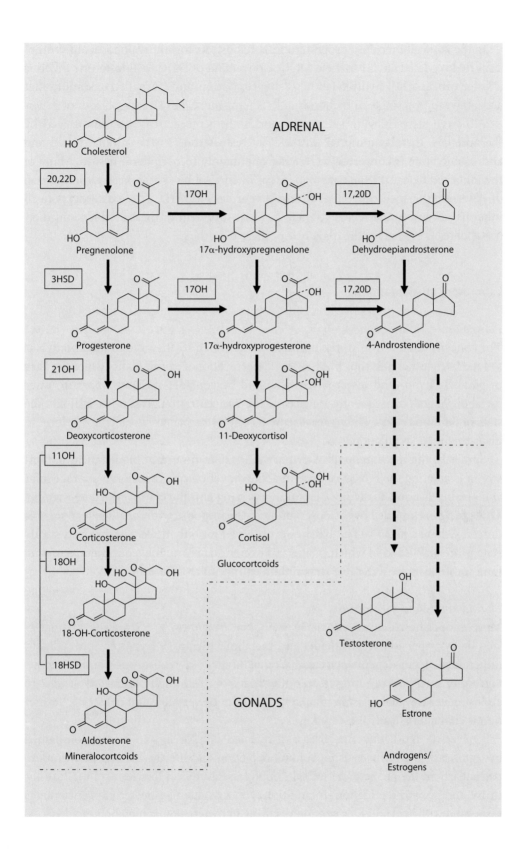

In the zona glomerulosa progesterone, the substrate for mineralocorticoid synthesis is hydroxylated at C21 to yield DOC. Conversion of DOC to aldosterone involves a 3-step process (11β-hydroxylation, 18-hydroxylation, and 18-methyl oxidation) that are catalyzed by a single mitochondrial P450 enzyme, CYP11B2 (fig. 1).

Although steroids with 19C atoms and androgenic activity are synthesized by the adrenals, there is minimal synthesis of testosterone in the adrenal gland and androstenedione is converted to testosterone mainly in peripheral tissues. Many of the inherited defects in the enzymatic steps of cortisol biosynthesis result in a group of syndromes termed congenital adrenal hyperplasia (CAH). These disorders are all inherited as autosomal-recessive traits [5]. Measurement of these steroids and their metabolites is crucial for the diagnosis of these disorders.

Laboratory Investigations

Plasma and Urinary Sodium

The concentration of Na^+ in the plasma is determined by the ratio of total body Na^+ to total body water and thus plasma Na^+ concentration and osmolality generally vary in parallel. Hypo- and hypernatremia should be considered disturbances of water metabolism and, consequently, the plasma Na^+ concentration gives no insight into the state of total body Na^+. Thus, measurements of plasma Na^+ are usually not helpful in disorders of Na^+ regulation.

Similarly, the measurement of urinary Na^+ is an important biochemical parameter in evaluating the renal response to acute depletion or expansion of extracellular volume, but is also usually not helpful in assessing chronic Na^+ overload or wasting. This can be exemplified by the observation of the response to diuretics in normal volunteers, where a negative Na^+ balance is observed for only three days before a steady state is re-established in which intake and excretion are roughly equivalent, allowing for a commensurate water loss to maintain extracellular fluid osmolality.

Plasma and Urinary Potassium

Most endocrine diseases associated with Na^+ retention are clinically characterized by hypertension, hypokalemia and metabolic alkalosis. Hypertension is due to mineralocorticoid-dependent excessive renal tubular Na^+ reabsorption and concomitant water retention resulting in volume expansion. Although plasma Na^+ levels are almost never elevated, plasma potassium (K^+) can be very low and urinary K^+ excretion is characteristically increased.

Conversely, most endocrine diseases associated with Na^+ loss are often accompanied by significant water loss causing volume depletion and life-threatening dehydration, particularly in the neonatal period, although less severe salt loss results in failure-to-thrive and growth retardation. In addition, Na^+ loss due to aldosterone deficiency is associated with acid and K^+ retention resulting in hyperkalemic metabolic acidosis.

Clearly, in these conditions hypo- and hyperkalemia are the result of either excessive or deficient aldosterone activity. The degree of aldosterone activity can be estimated by measuring the tubular fluid K^+ concentration at the end of the cortical collecting tubule, the site responsible for most of K^+ secretion. This measurement can be estimated clinically from calculation of the transtubular potassium gradient (TTKG) using osmolality and K^+ in plasma and urine [6], and is an index of the gradient of K^+ achieved at K^+ secretory sites, independent of urine flow rate:

TTKG = [Urine K^+ : (urine osmolality/plasma osmolality)] : plasma K^+

Use of the TTKG assumes that negligible amounts of K^+ are secreted or reabsorbed distal to these sites and that the final urinary K^+ concentration then depends on water reabsorption in the medullary collecting ducts.

This formula is accurate as long as the urine osmolality exceeds that of the plasma (so that the K^+ concentration of the cortical collecting tubule can be estimated) and the urine Na^+ concentration is >25 mmol/l (so that Na^+ delivery is not limiting).

An inadequately high renal K^+ loss is present when TTKG >2 for plasma K^+ <3.5 mmol/l or TTKG >6 for plasma K^+ 3.5–4.0 mmol/l. TTKG values <6 indicate an inappropriate renal response to hyperkalemia.

Determination of Plasma Renin Activity and Immunoreactive Renin
Circulating renin levels are traditionally measured using the plasma renin activity (PRA) assay in a blood sample collected in prechilled EDTA-coated vials immediately centrifuged at 4°C. The plasma has to be kept frozen until assayed to prevent cryo-activation of prorenin. For the assay an aliquot of thawed plasma is mixed with the angiotensinase inhibitor PMSF, neomycin (to prevent degradation by bacteria) and maleic acid (to optimize pH at 6.0). The sample is incubated for 3 and 18 h in a water bath at 37°C, respectively. The reaction is stopped by chilling the sample in an ice bath. The angiotensin I produced during incubation is quantitated by radioimmunoassay using ^{125}I-angiotensin I and polyclonal antibodies. For each sample endogenous angiotensin I of a corresponding unincubated plasma aliquot is subtracted [7].

The advent of commercially available simple assay kits measuring plasma immunoreactive renin (irR) concentration, rather than the more complex PRA, has made plasma renin measurements more attractive and practical. Unlike PRA the irR does not take into account the actual plasma concentration of angiotensinogen, the substrate of renin. The assay uses a two-site immunoradiometric assay for the measurement of active renin protein. Two different types of antibodies to human active renin are used to 'sandwich' directly the active renin molecule. The first polyclonal antibody, fixed to a polystyrol tube, recognize both active and inactive renin. The second monoclonal ^{125}I-labelled antibody specifically binds only to the active form of renin. After incubation the excess tracer is removed and the radioactivity which is proportional to the plasma concentration of active renin is measured [7]. The irR assays have the advantage that results can be readily compared between different laboratories, because the results are expressed in units of the internationally accepted renin

Table 1. Normal values of plasma aldosterone by age

	Supine, nmol/l (ng/dl)	Upright, nmol/l (ng/dl)
Adults	54–540 (1.5–15)	110–900 (3–25)
Pubertal children (11–15 years)	70–720 (2–20)	140–1,620 (4–45)
Prepubertal children (2–10 years)	100–1,260 (3–35)	180–2,890 (5–80)
Children (1–2 years)	180–1,800 (5–50)	
Infants (1–12 months)	180–3,250 (5–90)	
Newborn	35–6,500 (1–180)	

standard. Results of PRA assays cannot be expressed in this way, because the angiotensin I generation is determined not only by the plasma concentration of renin, but also by incubation conditions, which differ in different laboratories [7]. Normal PRA values range from 0.5 to 4 ng/ml/h, whereas normal values for irR range from 15 to 100 mU/l using the Nichols Advantage® immunochemiluminometric assay (Nichols Institute Diagnostics) and 5–20 ng/l using the BioRad Renin III immunoradiometric assay (Bio-Rad Laboratories Ltd., Hertfordshire, UK). Plasma renin varies with age, sodium intake and posture. In newborns, PRA can be as high as 10 ng/ml/h and these values slowly decline but high values can be seen up until the age of 5 years.

Determination of Plasma Aldosterone
Aldosterone measurement in plasma is usually done by solid-phase radioimmunoassay technique using specific antibodies. Normal values in the plasma range from 54 to 540 pmol/l (1.5–15 ng/dl) in the supine position and 110–900 pmol/I (3–25 ng/dl) in the upright position in normal adults on a regular salt diet (table 1) [7]. Aldosterone levels vary during the day, are highest in the morning and lowest in the evening; they follow cortisol but are not under direct ACTH control [1]. Aldosterone levels increase with upright posture, a test which is useful to evaluate aldosterone levels in various hypertensive states, but not useful in disorders with Na^+ loss.

Determination of Urinary Aldosterone and Its Metabolites
In the urine, aldosterone is excreted mainly as its tetrahydrometabolite (THAldo) and aldosterone-18-glucuronide, only a minor percentage is excreted as free aldosterone. Measured by standard radioimmunoassay, normal values for urinary aldosterone secretion are usually reported to range from 5 to 70 μg per 24 h. These values not only reflect free aldosterone, but also other metabolites with cross-reactivity with the antibody used in the assay. Moreover, results depend on the correct collection of a 24-hour urine and are influenced by the amount of dietary salt; the greater the amount of dietary salt, the lower the level of aldosterone. Results are also inappropriate if kidney

Ferrari · Bianchetti

Table 2. A selection of urinary steroid metabolites of particular significance in the diagnosis of steroid disorders and normal range by gender

	Male	Female	Abnormal
21-Hydroxylase deficiency			
17HP/(THE+THF+5αTHF)	0.01–0.10	0.01–0.13	>0.25
PT/(THE+THF+5αTHF)	0.04–0.29	0.01–0.13	>0.25
100*PT'ONE/(THE+THF+5αTHF)	0.06–0.79	0.03–2.03	>10
17α-Hydroxylase deficiency			
(THA+THB+5αTHB)/(THE+THF+5αTHF)	0.05–0.17	0.05–0.23	>10
(THA+THB+5αTHB)/(AN+ET)	0.06–0.34	0.06–0.28	>10
100*THDOC/(THE+THF+5αTHF)	0.05–0.74	0.03–5.21	>10
3ß-Hydroxysteroid dehydrogenase deficiency			
DHEA/(THE+THF+5αTHF)	0.00–0.30	0.01–0.25	>1
5PT/(THE+THF+5αTHF)	0.00–0.11	0.02–0.10	>1
11ß-Hydroxylase deficiency			
100*THS/(THE+THF+5αTHF)	0.29–1.75	0.60–2.91	>10
100*THDOC/(THE+THF+5αTHF)	0.05–0.74	0.03–5.21	>10
Pseudohypoaldosteronism			
THALDO (µg/24 h)	10–58	6–63	>90
100*THALDO/(THE+THF+5αTHF)	0.2–1.0	0.2–1.6	>5
Hypoaldosteronism			
THALDO (µg/24 h)	10–58	6–63	<2
18-OH-THA/THALDO	1.97–7.90	1.63–5.67	>20
(THA+THB+5αTHB)/(THE+THF+5αTHF)	0.05–0.17	0.05–0.23	>1
Glucocorticoid-remediable aldosteronism			
18-OH-F (µg/24 h)	6–410	6–153	
18-OH-F/total F metabolites	<0.075	<0.075	>0.075
11ß-Hydroxysteroid dehydrogenase deficiency			
Free F/E	0.28–0.85	0.33–0.67	>1
(THF+5αTHF)/THE	0.66–1.44	0.55–1.27	>3
(F+E)/(THE+THF+5αTHF)	0.01–0.08	0.03–0.14	>0.1

AN = Androsterone; ET = etiocholanolone; DHEA = dehydroepiandrosterone; TH = tetrahydro; A = 11-dehydro-corticosterone; B = corticosterone; E = cortisone; F = cortisol; S = 11-deoxycortisol; ALDO = aldosterone; DOC = deoxycorticosterone; PT = pregnanetriol; PT'ONE = 11-oxo- pregnanetriol; 5PT = 5-pregnan3β,17α,20α-triol; 17HP = 17-hydroxypregnanolone; 18-OH-F = 18-hydroxycortisol; 18-OH-THA = 18-hydroxytetrahydrocompound A.

function is reduced. Again, THAldo can be measured by radioimmunoassay; there are specific antibodies available, but more accurately using GC-MS or HPLC-MS [8].

Determination of the Urinary Steroid Profile
Urinary steroid profiling provides the most accurate quantitative information on the steroid biosynthetic and catabolic pathways and is the most sensitive and specific method to demonstrate a defect in adrenal steroid biosynthesis [8]. It is essential for identification of inborn errors of steroid metabolism, and useful in other disorders with altered steroid secretion [8]. Steroids, mostly in the form of glucuronide and sulphate conjugates, are extracted using solid-phase cartridges, followed by enzymatic hydrolysis, re-extraction of free steroids, formation of methoxime-trimethylsilyl derivatives and analysis by GC and GC-MS [8]. The measurement of steroid precursor/product ratios is a particularly robust method independent of 24-hour excretion or values relative to creatinine to assess disturbance of adrenal steroid biosynthesis [8] (table 2). These ratios represent the ratio of the urinary metabolite of an adrenal precursor (e.g. 17-OHP) to the urinary metabolites of the product (cortisol). Reference values are listed in table 2. Generally, commercial laboratories do not offer the determination of most of these steroids, so one has to rely on laboratories with a special research interest.

Endocrine Disorders Resulting in Sodium Retention (table 3; fig. 2)

The majority of the known inherited endocrine diseases resulting in Na^+ retention affect the mineralocorticoid axis either because of activation of the mineralocorticoid receptor (MR) by products of abnormal adrenal steroid biosynthesis, abnormal metabolism of cortisol in mineralocorticoid target cells, mutations of the MR or because of mutations of the MR-inducible ion channels (fig. 1) [9]. These disorders are clinically characterized by hypertension due to concomitant water retention resulting in volume expansion. Plasma Na^+ levels are never elevated, although in most cases plasma K^+ is very low [9, 10], except in cases of pseudohypoaldosteronism type 2 [11]. The latter is a consequence of mutations in a modulator of the distal tubular NaCl cotransporter, resulting in overactivation of ion transporter, which in turn leads to Na^+ and fluid retention and hypertension; with suppression hyporeninemia and relative hypoaldosteronism as a secondary consequence of volume expansion.

Mutations of the 11β-Hydroxylase or 17α-Hydroxylase Genes (Congenital Adrenal Hyperplasia)

The two forms of CAH associated with hypertension due to mineralocorticoid excess are the 11β-hydroxylase deficiency, wherein DOC is present in excess along with

Table 3. Inherited endocrine disorders resulting in sodium retention and hypertension

Cause	Genetic abnormality activity	Abnormal steroid with mineralocorticoid	Plasma		
			renin	aldosterone	potassium
Congenital adrenal hyperplasia		deoxycorticosterone	⇓	⇓	⇓
11β-Hydroxylase deficiency	CYP11B1				
17α-Hydroxylase deficiency	CYP17				
Glucocorticoid-remediable aldosteronism		18OH-cortisol	⇓	=/⇑	⇓
Glucocorticoid-remediable	chimeric CYP11B1/ CYP11B2				
Apparent mineralocorticoid excess		cortisol	⇓	⇓	⇓
11β-Hydroxysteroid dehydrogenase type 2 deficiency	HSD11B2				
Geller syndrome		progesterone	⇓	⇓	⇓
Activating mutation of the mineralocorticoid receptor	MLR				
Liddle syndrome		–	⇓	⇓	⇓
ENaC β-subunit mutation	SCNN1B				
ENaC γ-subunit mutation	SCNN1G				
Familial pseudohypo-aldosteronism type 2		–	⇓	⇓	⇑
Mutations in lysine-deficient kinase 1 and 4	WNK1/WNK4				

CYP11B1 = Cytochrome P450, subfamily XIB, polypetide 1 (11ß-hydroxylase); CYP11B2 = Cytochrome P450, subfamily XIB, polypetide 2 (aldosterone synthase); CYP17 = Cytochrome P450, subfamily XVII (17α-hydroxylase); HSD11B2 = 11ß-hydroxysteroid dehydrogenase type 2; MLR = mineralocorticoid receptor; SCNN1B/G = sodium channel, nonvoltage gated 1, ß/γ subunit; WNK = With No Lysine (K) kinase; AR = autosomal-recessive; AD = autosomal-dominant.

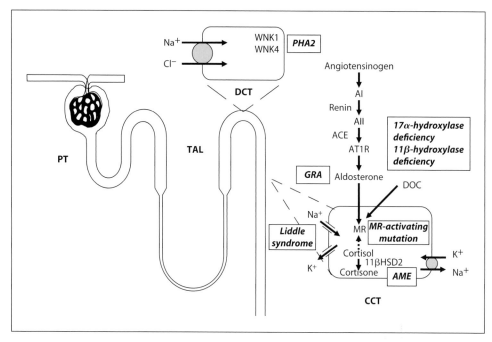

Fig. 2. Inherited endocrine disorders resulting in sodium retention. The diagram shows a nephron, the filtering unit of the kidney, with the relevant molecular pathways mediating NaCl reabsorption in individual renal cells, along with the pathway of the renin-angiotensin system, the major regulator of renal salt reabsorption. Inherited diseases affecting these pathways causing NaCl retention are indicated. PT = Proximal tubule; TAL = thick ascending limb of the loop of Henle; DCT = distal convoluted tubule; CCT = cortical collecting tubule; PHA2 = pseudohypoaldosteronism type 2; GRA = glucocorticoid-remediable aldosteronism; AME = apparent mineralocorticoid excess; AI = angiotensin I; ACE = angiotensin-converting enzyme; AII = angiotensin II; MR = mineralocorticoid receptor; 11βHSD2 = 11β-hydroxysteroid dehydrogenase type 2; DOC = deoxycorticosterone.

adrenal androgens and the 17α-hydroxylase deficiency, which also has an excess of DOC, but a deficiency of androgen production (table 3; fig. 2) [9]. Although these are rare causes of hypertension, partial enzymatic deficiencies have been observed in hirsute women [12], so some hypertensive adolescents may have unrecognized, subtle forms of CAH. These disorders are described in more detail by Flueck [this vol.]. A deficiency of the enzyme 11β-hydroxylase (CYP11B1) is usually diagnosed in infancy, because the defect sets off production of excessive androgens, which causes virilization [13]. The enzyme deficiency prevents the hydroxylation of 11-deoxycortisol to cortisol, resulting in cortisol deficiency and also prevents the conversion of DOC to corticosterone and aldosterone [13]. Because of DOC's mineralocorticoid activity, patients exhibit salt retention and hypertension with hypokalemic alkalosis and low plasma renin. The syndrome is diagnosed by finding high levels of 11-deoxycortisol and DOC in the urine and plasma, the characteristic steroid profile is elevation of urinary 17-hydroxycorticosteroids and DOC [14]. The enzymatic defect has been

Ferrari · Bianchetti

attributed to several mutations in the CYP11B1 gene [15]. The treatment is cortisol replacement; mineralocorticoid replacement may also be necessary. A deficiency of the enzyme 17α-hydroxylase (CYP17) is associated with an absence of sex hormones, leading to incomplete masculinization in males and primary amenorrhea in females. 17α-Hydroxylase is necessary for both cortisol and estrogen synthesis. Lack of these hormones results in increases in ACTH and FSH. Production of excessive corticosterone and DOC results in hypertension and hypokalemic alkalosis (table 3; fig. 2). The ensuing volume expansion inhibits renin release and therefore the synthesis of aldosterone. Oshiro et al. [16] also described a mutation in the CYP17 gene in an adult female referred because of hypertension and amenorrhea. Thus, adolescents with hypertension and hypokalemia or abnormal sexual development should be considered suspect.

Diagnosis

11β-Hydroxylase Deficiency. Clinical: Virilization, hypertension. Biochemical: Low plasma K^+, high urinary K^+, low plasma renin and aldosterone, low plasma cortisol, high plasma 11-deoxycortisol and DOC. Increased urinary 100*THS/ (THE+THF+5αTHF) and 100*THDOC/(THE+THF+5αTHF) ratios.

17α-Hydroxylase Deficiency. Clinical: Incomplete masculinization, hypertension. Biochemical: Low plasma K^+, high urinary K^+, low plasma renin and aldosterone, high plasma progesterone and DOC, low plasma 17α-hydroxyprogesterone, 11-deoxycortisol and cortisol. Increased urine 100*THDOC/(THE+THF+5αTHF) and (THA+THB+5αTHB)/(THE+THF+5αTHF) ratios

Chimeric 11β-Hydroxlase – Aldosterone Synthase Gene (Glucocorticoid Remediable Aldosteronism)

Glucocorticoid-remediable aldosteronism (GRA) is an autosomal-dominant form of hypertension with normal growth and sexual development characterized by low plasma renin activity, but variably increased aldosterone secretion (table 3; fig. 2) [17]. The hypertension, variable hyperaldosteronism, and abnormal steroid production are all under the control of ACTH and suppressible by glucocorticoids such as dexamethasone. In GRA there are high levels of the abnormal adrenal steroids 18-oxocortisol and 18-hydroxycortisol (18-OH-F) whereas plasma aldosterone levels may be variable [18, 19]. GRA is the result of aldosterone synthase (CYP11B2) activity under the control of ACTH (which normally regulates CYP11B1) and results from an unequal crossing-over involving the CYP11B1 and CYP11B2 genes (table 3). Aldosterone synthase, like steroid 11β-hydroxylase, is expressed in both adrenal fasciculata and glomerulosa; the two genes are 95% identical and lie on chromosome 8q immediately adjacent in a head-to-tail orientation with the CYP11B2 gene 5′ to the CYP11B1 gene [9]. Chimeric gene duplication between the CYP11B1 and CYP11B2 genes is the cause of GRA [19]. This chimeric gene encodes for the aldosterone synthase (functional elements of CYP11B2) but is under control of ACTH (regulatory elements of CYP11B1).

The number of reported cases with 'classic GRA' is very small; however, this condition might be underestimated. A report on 21 affected members on approximately 1,000 descendants of an English convict in Australia [18] revealed an extreme phenotypic heterogeneity in GRA, associated with hybrid genes showing somewhat different crossover points linking the CYP11B1 and CYP11B2 portions. Some of the affected members had only mild hypertension and normal biochemistry, including normokalemia and were clinically indistinguishable from patients with essential hypertension; and some remained normotensive until late in life [18]. Thus, in hypertensive patients of young age and family history with an absent postural increase in plasma aldosterone, treatment with glucocorticoid should be given for 4–6 weeks. An abnormal activity of the CYP11B2 may be characterized phenotypically by elevated urinary excretion THAldo and aldosterone or the decline of plasma aldosterone in response to dexamethasone. Preferably, GC/MS analysis of the urine with 18-OH-F assay should be performed whenever available.

Diagnosis
Clinical: Hypertension, correction by dexamethasone. Biochemical: Low plasma K^+, high urinary K^+, low plasma renin, high plasma 18-oxocortisol and 18-OH-F, variable aldosterone. Increased urinary 18-OH-F/total cortisol metabolites ratio.

Mutations of the 11β-Hydroxysteroid Dehydrogenase Type 2 Gene (Apparent Mineralocorticoid Excess)

Mutations in the gene encoding for the enzyme 11β-hydroxysteroid dehydrogenase type 2 (11βHSD2) cause a rare monogenic juvenile hypertensive syndrome called apparent mineralocorticoid excess (AME), which was first described by Ulick et al. [20] in 1979. Cortisol and aldosterone have the same in vitro affinity for the mineralocorticoid receptor (MR), although in vivo only aldosterone acts as a physiologic agonist of the MR, despite circulating levels of cortisol in humans and corticosterone in rodents being three orders of magnitude higher than aldosterone levels. In mineralocorticoid target organs the enzyme 11βHSD2 metabolizes 11-hydroxy steroids, to their inactive keto forms, thus protecting the nonselective MR from activation by glucocorticoids (table 3; fig. 2). The enzyme is highly expressed in all Na^+-transporting epithelia, particularly in the kidney and colon, but also in human placenta and vascular wall.

In AME, mutations in the HSD11B2 gene result in an enzyme with abolished or markedly decreased activity, which causes renal Na^+ retention, urinary K^+ wasting and low renin, low aldosterone salt-dependent hypertension [9, 21]; the symptoms of the disease respond to spironolactone or amiloride administration or a low salt diet. The condition is diagnosed by demonstrating an increase ratio of active to inactive cortisol metabolites in the urine, usually expressed as the urinary (THF+5αTHF)/THE ratio.

Although patients with homozygous mutations from different families show varying degrees of severity in terms of biochemical features [9, 21], most patients with classic AME syndrome have characteristic signs of severe 11βHSD2 deficiency. In those instances, birth weights are significantly lower than that of their unaffected sibs, and the patients are short, underweight and hypertensive for their age. It has become evident that depending on the degree of loss of enzyme activity, HSD11B2 mutations can cause a spectrum of hypertension ranging from a severe, life-threatening disease in early childhood to a milder form diagnosed only in adults. Heterozygous carriers of HSD11B2 mutations have been reported to have slightly raised urinary (THF+5αTHF)/THE ratios, suffer from hypertension or develop isolated hypertension of later onset, but have no other characteristic signs of AME. Cases of homozygous mutations in HSD11B2 producing mild deficiency in 11βHSD2 activity have been reported to present with low-renin hypertension, but without the phenotypic features of AME [9, 21]. Along with other findings these data suggest that an impaired 11βHSD2 activity may play a role in the pathogenesis of essential hypertension in some patients and that this may be genetically determined. The prevalence of mutations in the coding region of the HSD11B2 gene in the general population is estimated to be <1/250,000 in Caucasians [9].

Diagnosis
Clinical: Hypertension, failure to thrive, nephrocalcinosis, correction by spironolactone. Biochemical: Low plasma K^+, high urinary K^+, low plasma renin and aldosterone. Increased urinary (THF+5αTHF)/THE and free cortisol/cortisone ratios. No other abnormality in steroid profile.

Mutations of the Mineralocorticoid Receptor Gene (Geller Syndrome)

In a screening for mutation of all coding regions of the MR among 75 independent patients with severe hypertension, suppressed plasma renin activity, low aldosterone, and no other underlying cause of hypertension a 15-year-old boy was found to be heterozygous for a missense mutation, resulting in substitution of a leucine for serine at codon 810 (S810L) [22] (table 3; fig. 2). The S810L mutation lies in the MR hormone-binding domain, altering an amino acid that is conserved in all MRs from Xenopus to human but not found in other nuclear receptors. This mutation results in constitutive MR activity and alters receptor specificity, with progesterone and other steroids lacking 21-hydroxyl groups, normally MR antagonists, becoming potent agonists. Spironolactone was also a potent agonist of MR-L810, suggesting that this medication is contraindicated in MR-L810 carriers [22]. Among the 23 relatives of the index patient analyzed, 11 had been diagnosed with severe hypertension before age 20, a rare trait in the general population, whereas the remaining 12 had unremarkable blood pressures. Carriers of the mutant allele revealed a marked increase in blood pressure, suppression of aldosterone secretion and a trend toward lower plasma K^+ levels [22]. Two females later found to be MR-L810 carriers had previously undergone 5 pregnancies. Since progesterone levels normally increase 100-fold in pregnancy it was not surprising to notice that all pregnancies had been complicated by marked exacerbation of hypertension. To date no further cases of activating mutations of the MR have been reported.

Diagnosis
Clinical: Hypertension, exacerbation in pregnancy. Biochemical: Low plasma K^+, high urinary K^+, low plasma renin and aldosterone. Decreased urinary THALDO (<2 µg/24 h), no other abnormality in steroid profile.

Mutations of the Epithelial Sodium Channel Genes (Liddle Syndrome)

In the early 1960s Liddle et al. [23] described a young female with hypertension associated with hypokalemic alkalosis not due to hyperaldosteronism but rather to a renal tubular defect. Renal failure eventually developed in this patient, who received a cadaveric renal transplant in 1989, following which her disorder resolved with normalization of the aldosterone and renin responses to salt restriction. This condition, later called Liddle syndrome or pseudoaldosteronism, is characterized by hypoaldosteronism, hypokalemia, and decreased renin and angiotensin (table 3; fig. 2). Further studies demonstrated that amiloride and triamterene, but not spironolactone, were effective treatments for hypertension and hypokalemia in patients with this syndrome as long as dietary salt intake was restricted [24]. This form of mineralocorticoid hypertension is inherited as an autosomal-dominant trait.

The cloning of epithelial Na^+ channel (ENaC) led to the discovery that this hereditary monogenic form of hypertension was caused by mutations deleting the PY motif present in the C-terminus of the β- or γ-ENaC subunits [25]. The ENaC, expressed on the apical side of the cells from the distal tubule and cortical collecting duct, is the key modulator of Na^+ transport in the kidney [25] (fig. 2, 3). Expression and function of this transporter are under control of aldosterone [26]. In Liddle syndrome, the channel is hyperactive, due to two factors: an increased number of channels present at the cell surface and an increased intrinsic activity of ENaC. Increased expression and activity of ENaC causes Na^+ and water retention, which in turn leads to an increase in blood volume, hypertension, suppression of plasma renin and low aldosterone in plasma and urine. Thus, the associated endocrine disorder of hyporeninemia and hypoaldosteronism is a secondary consequence of volume expansion.

Ferrari · Bianchetti

Diagnosis

Clinical: Hypertension, correction by amiloride. Biochemical: Low plasma K$^+$, high urinary K$^+$, low plasma renin and aldosterone. Decreased urinary THALDO (<2 µg/24 h): No other abnormality in steroid profile.

Mutations of the Lysine Deficient Kinase 1 and 4 Genes (Pseudohypoaldosteronism Type 2 or Gordon Syndrome)

Pseudohypoaldosteronism type 2 or Gordon syndrome is a familial form of hypertension with an autosomal-dominant mode of inheritance [11]. Patients have suppressed plasma renin activity and present with symptoms of severe hypertension as a result of increase renal Na$^+$ reabsorption, and hyperkalemia and metabolic acidosis as a result of reduced renal K$^+$ and H$^+$ excretion [11]. The disorder is particularly responsive to thiazide diuretics. Investigations show normal renal and adrenal function. Although aldosterone concentrations are seemingly in the normal range, they are inappropriately low for the level of hyperkalemia, hence the designation of the condition as 'pseudohypoaldosteronism'. The clinical phenotype of pseudohypoaldosteronism type 2 is opposite to Gitelman syndrome, a disease caused by dysfunction of the thiazide-sensitive NaCl cotransporter (SLC12A3) in the distal tubule (table 3; fig. 2). Pseudohypoaldosteronism type 2 is the consequence of mutations in the WNK1 and WNK4 genes. The encoded proteins of these genes are members of a family of serine/threonine kinases known as WNK (*With No K*, lysine) because of the atypical positioning of a conserved lysine residue within the catalytic domain [27]. Mutations in both the WNK1 and WNK4 genes result in the overactivation of the NaCl cotransporter, which causes Na$^+$ and fluid retention and thus hypertension. The associated endocrine disorder (hyporeninemia and relative hypoaldosteronism) is a secondary consequence of volume expansion. In vitro studies indicate that WNK4 suppresses SLC12A3 activity [28]. On the other hand, WNK1 does not affect SLC12A3 activity directly, but it completely prevents WNK4 inhibition of SLC12A3. Some WNK4 mutations that cause pseudohypoaldosteronism type 2 demonstrate diminished activity, suggesting that WNK4 mutations lead to loss of SLC12A3 inhibition. Gain-of-function WNK1 mutations would be expected to inhibit WNK4 activity, thereby activating SLC12A3, contributing to the phenotype of pseudohypoaldosteronism type 2 [28]. Thus, WNK4 and WNK1 interact to regulate the thiazide-sensitive NaCl transporter activity, indicating that WNKs form a Na$^+$ regulatory pathway of the distal nephron.

Diagnosis

Clinical: Hypertension, correction by thiazide. Biochemical: High plasma K$^+$, low urinary K$^+$, low plasma renin and aldosterone. Decreased urinary THALDO (<2 µg/24 h), no other abnormality in steroid profile.

Endocrine Disorders Resulting in Sodium Loss (table 4; fig. 3)

Endocrine diseases associated with Na^+ loss are always accompanied by significant water loss causing volume depletion and life-threatening dehydration, particularly in the neonatal period.

Aldosterone and cortisol are the major steroids synthesized in the adrenals. Adrenal steroidogenesis can be defective at various levels and salt loss results from aldosterone deficiency and probably to a certain extent from the hypersecretion of steroids with aldosterone antagonistic activity [29]. The clinical picture depends upon the degree of the enzymatic deficiency but also upon the involvement of the cortisol pathway. Plasma Na^+ levels are seldom extremely low, but the associated acid and K^+ retention can result in life-threatening metabolic acidosis and hyperkalemia.

The most frequent causes of congenital adrenal insufficiency are associated with so-called CAH [30]. The most common form of CAH is a defect in the 21-hydroxylase enzyme system associated with androgen excess causing virilization of newborn female infants [30]. Other enzymatic defects of adrenal steroidogenesis causing CAH include the 3β-hydroxysteroid dehydrogenase deficiency and mutations in the StAR protein. Mutations in two other genes important for the development of the adrenals, the steroidogenic factor 1, encoded by the FTZ-F1 gene and the DAX-1 gene result in generalized adrenal insufficiency including low aldosterone and cortisol levels causing Na^+ wasting and cause congenital adrenal hypoplasia [31]. These disorders almost invariably affect gonadal steroid synthesis causing defects of genital differentiation and are discussed in more detail by Flueck [this vol.].

Mutations of the 3β-Hydroxylase or 21-Hydroxylase Genes (Congenital Adrenal Hyperplasia)

The two forms of CAH associated with significant water loss causing volume depletion due to mineralocorticoid deficiency are 21-hydroxylase deficiency, which also has an excess of 17-hydroxyprogesterone (17-OHP) and excessive androgen production, and 3β-hydroxysteroid dehydrogenase deficiency, wherein high ratios of δ-5-pregnenolone to progesterone in serum or pregnanetriol to pregnanediol in urine are present [30] (table 4; fig. 3).

A deficiency of the enzyme 21-hydroxylase (CYP21A2) accounts for approximately 95% of cases of CAH and it is also one of the most common inherited disorders. In the zona fasciculata of the adrenal cortex, the enzyme 21-hydroxylase converts 17-OHP to 11-deoxycortisol [30, 32]. Mutations in the CYP21A2 gene result in impaired generation of 11-deoxycortisol and thus defective cortisol synthesis. In turn, ACTH levels increase, resulting in overproduction of cortisol precursors proximal to the block, particularly 17-OHP. This causes excessive production of androgens, resulting in virilization. Biochemical abnormalities include high serum concentrations of

Ferrari · Bianchetti

Table 4. Inherited endocrine disorders resulting in sodium loss and volume depletion

Cause	Inheritance	Genetic abnormality	Abnormal steroid	Plasma		
				renin	aldosterone	potassium
Congenital adrenal hyperplasia				⇑	⇓	⇑
21-Hydroxylase deficiency	AR	CYP21A2	17OHP, testosterone			
3β-Hydroxysteroid dehydrogenase deficiency	AR	HSD3B2	δ5-pregnenolone, DHEA			
Congenital hypoaldosteronism				⇑	⇓	⇑
18-Hydroxylase deficiency	AR	CYP11B2	low 18-OHB/aldo			
18-Oxidase deficiency	AR	CYP11B2	high 18-OHB/aldo			
Pseudohypoaldosteronism type 1				⇑	⇑	⇑
ENaC α/β/γ subunit mutations	AR	SCNN1A, 1B, 1G	–			
Mineralocorticoid receptor mutations	AD	MLR	–			
Antenatal Bartter syndrome				⇑	⇑	⇑
Na-K-Cl cotransporter mutation furosemide-sensitive	AR	SLC12A1	–			
Potassium channel mutations	AR	KCNJ1	–			
Barttin mutations (subunit of Na-K-Cl cotransporter and potassium channel)	AR	BSND	–			
Classic Bartter syndrome				⇑	⇑	⇑
Chloride channel mutations	AR	CLCNKB	–			
Gitleman syndrome				⇑	⇑	⇑
Na-Cl cotransporter mutations, thiazide-sensitive	AR	SLC12A3	–			

CYP21A2 = Cytochrome P450, subfamily XXIA, polypetide 2 (21-hydroxylase); HSD3B2 = 3β-hydroxysteroid dehydrogenase type 2; SCNN1A/B/G = sodium channel, nonvoltage gated 1, a/β/γ subunit; MLR = mineralocorticoid receptor; SLC12A1 = solute carrier family 12, member 1; KCNJ1 = potassium channel, subfamily J, member 1; CLCNKB = chloride channel kidney B; SLC12A3 = solute carrier family 12, member 3; AR = autosomal recessive; AD = autosomal dominant.

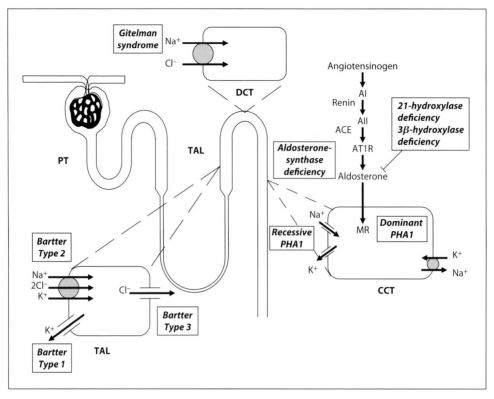

Fig. 3. Inherited endocrine disorders resulting in sodium loss. The diagram shows a nephron, the filtering unit of the kidney, with the relevant molecular pathways mediating NaCl reabsorption in individual renal cells, along with the pathway of the renin-angiotensin system, the major regulator of renal salt reabsorption. Inherited diseases affecting these pathways causing NaCl loss are indicated. PT = Proximal tubule; TAL = thick ascending limb of the loop of Henle; DCT = distal convoluted tubule; CCT = cortical collecting tubule; PHA1 = pseudohypoaldosteronism type 1; AI = angiotensin I; ACE = angiotensin-converting enzyme; AII = angiotensin II; MR = mineralocorticoid receptor.

androstenedione and testosterone, and increased urinary excretion of metabolites of cortisol precursors, particularly pregnanetriol, pregnanetriol glucuronide, and 17-ketosteroids. Classic 21-hydroxylase deficiency results in one of two clinical syndromes: a salt-losing form or a non-salt-losing, simple virilizing form. The salt-losing form of 21-hydroxylase deficiency presents in boys and girls with a salt-losing adrenal crisis in the neonatal period (hyponatremia, hyperkalemia, and failure to thrive), with girls also showing signs of ambiguous genitalia. The non-salt-losing form of 21-hydroxylase deficiency presents in girls at an early age because of ambiguous genitalia and in boys as toddlers with signs of puberty. The characteristic biochemical abnormality in patients with classic 21-hydroxylase deficiency is an elevated serum concentration of 17-OHP and most affected neonates have concentrations >3.5 µg/dl (>105 nmol/l). In 21-hydroxylase-deficient CAH, salt loss is present in 60% of affected

Ferrari · Bianchetti

patients and can be confirmed when plasma K^+ reaches levels above 6 mmol/l and plasma Na^+ falls below 130 mmol/l. Measurement of urine Na^+ in a spot urine can be useful, in particular if one can show Na^+ excretion in the face of low plasma Na^+. Plasma renin is high and plasma and urine aldosterone values as well as DOC levels are significantly decreased or not measurable, but serum 17-OHP values are not dissimilar to those found in the non-salt-losing form.

Deficiency of 3β-hydroxysteroid dehydrogenase (HSD3B2) results in decreased synthesis of cortisol, aldosterone, androgens and estrogens. Cortisol deficiency leads to increased ACTH secretion and therefore accumulation of excessive amounts of steroid precursors such as δ5-pregnenolone, 17α-hydroxypregnenolone, and dehydroepiandrosterone (DHEA) and DHEA sulphate. Most patients present in early infancy with clinical manifestations of both cortisol and aldosterone deficiency, with vomiting, volume depletion, hyponatremia, and hyperkalemia. Females may have mild virilization of their external genitalia, presumably due to excess DHEA and males have varying degrees of failure of normal genital development, ranging from hypospadia to male pseudohermaphroditism.

Diagnosis
21-Hydroxylase Deficiency. Clinical: Virilization. Biochemical: Low plasma renin and aldosterone, low plasma 11-deoxycortisol and cortisol, high plasma androstenedione and testosterone. Increased urinary 17HP/(THE+THF+5αTHF) and 17HP/(THE+THF+5αTHF) ratios. Salt-losing form: High plasma renin, low plasma aldosterone and DOC, low plasma Na^+, high plasma K^+.

3β-Hydroxysteroid Dehydrogenase. Clinical: Mild virilization, feeding difficulties, vomiting, volume depletion. Biochemical: Low plasma Na^+, high plasma K^+, high plasma renin, low plasma aldosterone and cortisol, high plasma ratio of δ5-pregnenolone to progesterone. Increased urinary DHA/(THE+THF+5αTHF) and 5PT/(THE+THF+5αTHF) ratios.

Mutations of the Aldosterone Synthase Gene (Corticosterone Methyloxidase Deficiency)

The aldosterone synthase (CYP11B2) gene encodes a steroid 11/18β-hydroxylase expressed in the zona glomerulosa of the adrenal to synthesize the mineralocorticoid aldosterone. The enzyme catalyzes 3 reactions: the 11β-hydroxylation of DOC to corticosterone (B); the 18-hydroxylation of corticosterone to 18-hydroxycorticosterone (18-OHB); and the 18-oxidation of 18-hydroxycorticosterone to aldosterone. Congenital isolated hypoaldosteronism is a rare inherited disorder caused by mutations in CYP11B2 that is transmitted as an autosomal-recessive trait [33, 34] (table 4; fig. 3). The clinical presentation is typical of aldosterone deficiency; affected infants have recurrent dehydration, salt wasting, and failure to thrive. Aldosterone synthase type I deficiency is caused by a defect in the penultimate biochemical step of aldosterone biosynthesis, the 18-hydroxylation of corticosterone (B) to 18-hydroxycorticosterone (18-OHB). This enzymatic defect results in decreased aldosterone and salt-wasting. This disorder is characterized by low plasma concentrations of products derived from corticosterone (18-OHB and aldosterone) and low urinary excretion of their metabolites [34]. Aldosterone synthase type II deficiency is caused by a defect in the final biochemical step of aldosterone biosynthesis, the 18-oxydation of 18-OHB to aldosterone. This enzymatic defect results in decreased aldosterone and salt-wasting associated with an increased serum ratio of 18-OHB to aldosterone. In aldosterone synthase type II deficiency the secretion of 18-OHB is typically increased. These patients have a low ratio of corticosterone to 18-OHB and increased urinary excretion of the major metabolite of 18-OHB, tetrahydro-18-hydroxy, 11-dehydrocorticosterone (18-OH-THA) [34]. Plasma renin is elevated in both disorders, and aldosterone is often very low. The ratio of plasma 18-OHB/aldosterone can be used to differentiate between the two disorders. There is no difference between the degree of salt loss in both types. Although the severity of salt-losing symptoms decreases with age, the abnormal steroid pattern persists throughout life.

Diagnosis

Aldosterone Synthase Deficiency. Clinical: Hypotension, failure to thrive. Biochemical: Low plasma Na^+, high plasma K^+, high plasma renin, low plasma aldosterone, high plasma corticosterone. Differentiation: Type 1 – plasma 18-OHB/aldosterone <10; type 2 – plasma 18-OHB/aldosterone >100.

Mutations of the Epithelial Sodium Channel or Mineralocorticoid Receptor (Pseudohypoaldosteronism Type 1)

Type 1 pseudohypoaldosteronism is a hereditary disease characterized by salt wasting resulting from target organ unresponsiveness to mineralocorticoids. Pseudohypoaldosteronism type 1 is present in two forms: as an autosomal-recessive trait or as an autosomal-dominant or sporadic form. Both forms are responsive to supplementary Na^+, but not to mineralocorticoids (table 4; fig. 3). The autosomal-recessive pseudohypoaldosteronism type 1 is caused by mutation in the α-subunit (SCNN1A), the β-subunit (SCNN1B), or the γ-subunit (SCNN1G) of the ENaC. This disorder presents in infancy with failure to thrive due to salt wasting, but also with cystic fibrosis-like symptoms such as recurring lower respiratory tract infections and persistently elevated sweat and saliva. Marked aldosterone excess is present in all reported cases and renin levels are increased in most. Salt-losing symptoms do not improve with age and severe salt loss including crisis, shock and death can occur at any age. In contrast, the autosomal-dominant form of pseudohypoaldosteronism type 1 is caused by loss-of-function mutations in the mineralocorticoid receptor gene and is life-threatening only during the neonatal period [35]. In childhood, salt loss recovers and relatively mild disorder persists which does not require any therapy [35]. On a biochemical basis the two forms cannot be differentiated, with both forms showing hyperkalemic acidosis and significant urinary Na$^+$ loss despite often marked hyponatremia. Renin and aldosterone levels are extremely elevated and treatment with mineralocorticoids is unable to influence the Na$^+$ excretion. A therapeutic trial with 0.1–0.2 mg fludrocortisone for 2–3 days with no response of the Na$^+$ excretion is considered diagnostic. Therapy consists of daily oral sodium supplementation and in the severe form sodium bicarbonate may be necessary to correct the metabolic acidosis.

Diagnosis
Autosomal-Recessive Pseudohypoaldosteronism Type I. Clinical: Vomiting, failure to thrive, short stature, also recurring lower respiratory tract infections and persistently elevated sweat and saliva electrolyte values. Biochemical: Low plasma Na$^+$, high plasma K$^+$, high plasma renin, high plasma aldosterone.

Autosomal-Dominant Pseudohypoaldosteronism Type I. Clinical: Vomiting, failure to thrive, short stature. Biochemical: Low plasma Na$^+$, high plasma K$^+$, high plasma renin, high plasma aldosterone.

Mutations Resulting in Impaired Sodium Chloride Reabsorption in the Loop of Henle (Bartter Syndromes) or Distal Tubule (Gitelman Syndrome)

Bartter syndromes and Gitelman syndrome, which result from an impairment in one of the transporters involved in NaCl reabsorption in the loop of Henle and distal tubule, respectively, present with a characteristic set of metabolic abnormalities including hypokalemia, metabolic alkalosis, hyperplasia of the juxtaglomerular apparatus (the source of renin in the kidney), hyperreninemia and hyperaldosteronism (table 4; fig. 3).

Mutations in the Thick Ascending Loop of Henle (Bartter Syndromes)

Bartter syndrome refers to a group of disorders that are unified by autosomal-recessive transmission and impaired salt reabsorption in the thick ascending loop (TAL) of Henle. Clinical disease results from defective renal reabsorption of NaCl in the TAL where 30% of filtered salt is normally reabsorbed [36, 37]. Pronounced salt wasting is accompanied by hypokalemic metabolic alkalosis, and high urinary excretion of K$^+$ and hypercalciuria. Plasma renin and aldosterone are elevated despite a normal or low blood pressure, secondary to salt and fluid loss, which causes volume depletion (table 4, fig. 3).

Antenatal Bartter syndrome type 1 is caused by mutation in the sodium-potassium-chloride cotransporter-2 gene (SLC12A1). Antenatal Bartter syndrome type 2, which is clinically and biochemically indistinguishable from type 1, is caused by mutation in the potassium channel ROMK1 gene (KCNJ1). The very recently described Bartter syndrome type 4, which is also clinically and biochemically indistinguishable from type 1 and 2, is caused by a mutation in Barttin, a subunit required for proper function of the sodium-potassium-chloride cotransporter-2 and the potassium channel ROMK1. In addition to fluid loss, patients with Bartter syndrome type IV present with sensorineural hearing loss.

Classic Bartter syndrome, also called Bartter syndrome type 3, is caused by mutation in the kidney chloride channel B gene (CLCNKB).

Mutations of the Thiazide-Sensitive NaCl Cotransporter Gene (Gitelman Syndrome)

Gitelman syndrome is widely described as a benign or milder variant of Bartter syndrome. Gitelman syndrome patients typically present at older ages without overt hypovolemia, but with hypokalemia and hypomagnesemia associated with renal K^+ and magnesium wasting, as well as hypocalciuria [38, 39]. There is usually a marked increase in plasma renin and aldosterone, responsible for hypokalemia and metabolic alkalosis. The Gitelman variant of Bartter syndrome is caused by mutation in the thiazide-sensitive NaCl cotransporter (SLC12A3).

Diagnosis
Patients with antenatal Bartter syndrome (types 1, 2 and 4) are born prematurely after a pregnancy complicated by polyhydramnios and present with nephrocalcinosis. Hypokalemia and metabolic alkalosis are often absent at presentation in this peculiar form of this syndrome.

The clinical presentation of classic (type 3) Bartter syndrome is heterogeneous: most patients present in infancy with failure to thrive, salt wasting, and polyuria; however, some patients present later in childhood with symptoms that resemble Gitelman syndrome.

Gitelman disease is sometimes not diagnosed until late childhood or even adulthood. Cramps are observed in almost all patients. Affected patients may also present with tetany, particularly in association with vomiting and diarrhea. Fatigue may also be observed, and polyuria and nocturia are found in a minority of these patients.

References

1 White PC: Disorders of aldosterone biosynthesis and action. N Engl J Med 1994;331:250–258.

2 Frassetto L, Morris RC Jr, Sellmeyer DE, Todd K, Sebastian A: Diet, evolution and aging–the pathophysiologic effects of the post-agricultural inversion of the potassium-to-sodium and base-to-chloride ratios in the human diet. Eur J Nutr 2001; 40:200–213.

3 Corvol P, Michel JB, Evin G, Gardes J, Bensala-Alaoui A, Menard J: The role of the renin-angiotensin system in blood pressure regulation in normotensive animals and man. J Hypertens Suppl 1984;2:S25–S30.

4 Lifton RP: Molecular genetics of human blood pressure variation. Science 1996;272:676–680.

5 White PC: Genetic diseases of steroid metabolism. Vitam Horm 1994;49:131–195.

6 Ethier JH, Kamel KS, Magner PO, Lemann J Jr, Halperin ML: The transtubular potassium concentration in patients with hypokalemia and hyperkalemia. Am J Kidney Dis 1990;15:309–315.

7 Ferrari P, Shaw SG, Nicod J, Saner E, Nussberger J: Active renin versus plasma renin activity to define aldosterone-to-renin ratio for primary aldosteronism. J Hypertens 2004;22:377–381.

8 Shackleton CH: Profiling steroid hormones and urinary steroids. J Chromatogr 1986;379:91–156.

9 Ferrari P, Bonny O: Forms of mineralocorticoid hypertension. Vitam Horm 2003;66:113–156.

10 Lifton RP, Gharavi AG, Geller DS: Molecular mechanisms of human hypertension. Cell 2001;104:545–556.

11 Gordon RD: Syndrome of hypertension and hyperkalemia with normal glomerular filtration rate. Hypertension 1986;8:93–102.

12 Lucky AW, Rosenfield RL, McGuire J, Rudy S, Helke J: Adrenal androgen hyperresponsiveness to adrenocorticotropin in women with acne and/or hirsutism: adrenal enzyme defects and exaggerated adrenarche. J Clin Endocrinol Metab 1986;62:840–848.

13 Rosler A, Leiberman E, Sack J, Landau H, Benderly A, Moses SW, Cohen T: Clinical variability of congenital adrenal hyperplasia due to 11ß-hydroxylase deficiency. Horm Res 1982;16:133–141.

14 Levine LS, Rauh W, Gottesdiener K, Chow D, Gunczler P, Rapaport R, Pang S, Schneider B, New MI: New studies of the 11ß-hydroxylase and 18-hydroxylase enzymes in the hypertensive form of congenital adrenal hyperplasia. J Clin Endocrinol Metab 1980;50:258–263.

15 Geley S, Kapelari K, Johrer K, Peter M, Glatzl J, Vierhapper H, Schwarz S, Helmberg A, Sippell WG, White PC, Kofler R: CYP11B1 mutations causing congenital adrenal hyperplasia due to 11ß-hydroxylase deficiency. J Clin Endocrinol Metab 1996;81: 2896–2901.

16 Oshiro C, Takasu N, Wakugami T, Komiya I, Yamada T, Eguchi Y, Takei H: Seventeen alpha-hydroxylase deficiency with one base pair deletion of the cytochrome P450c17 (CYP17) gene. J Clin Endocrinol Metab 1995;80:2526–2529.

17 Sutherland DJ, Ruse JL, Laidlaw JC: Hypertension, increased aldosterone secretion and low plasma renin activity relieved by dexamethasone. Can Med Assoc J 1966;95:1109–1119.

18 Gordon RD: Heterogeneous hypertension. Nat Genet 1995;11:6–9.

19 Lifton RP, Dluhy RG, Powers M, et al: Hereditary hypertension caused by chimaeric gene duplications and ectopic expression of aldosterone synthase. Nat Genet 1992;2:66–74.

20 Ulick S, Levine LS, Gunczler P, Zanconato G, Ramirez LC, Rauh W, Rosler A, Bradlow HL, New MI: A syndrome of apparent mineralocorticoid excess associated with defects in the peripheral metabolism of cortisol. J Clin Endocrinol Metab 1979;49:757–764.

21 Morineau G, Sulmont V, Salomon R, Fiquet-Kempf B, Jeunemaitre X, Nicod J, Ferrari P: Apparent mineralocorticoid excess: report of six new cases and extensive personal experience. J Am Soc Nephrol 2006;17:3176–3184.

22 Geller DS, Farhi A, Pinkerton N, Fradley M, Moritz M, Spitzer A, Meinke G, Tsai FT, Sigler PB, Lifton RP: Activating mineralocorticoid receptor mutation in hypertension exacerbated by pregnancy. Science 2000;289:119–123.

23 Liddle GW, Bledsoe T, Coppage WSJ: A familial renal disorder simulating primary aldosteronism but with negligible aldosterone secretion. Trans Am Assoc Physicians 1963;76:199–213.

24 Wang C, Chan TK, Yeung RT, Coghlan JP, Scoggins BA, Stockigt JR: The effect of triamterene and sodium intake on renin, aldosterone, and erythrocyte sodium transport in Liddle's syndrome. J Clin Endocrinol Metab 1981;52:1027–1032.

25 Shimkets RA, Warnock DG, Bositis CM, Nelson-Williams C, Hansson JH, Schambelan M, Gill JR Jr, Ulick S, Milora RV, Findling JW, Canessa CM, Rossier BC, Lifton RP: Liddle's syndrome: heritable human hypertension caused by mutations in the beta subunit of the epithelial sodium channel. Cell 1994;79:407–414.

26 Horisberger JD, Rossier BC: Aldosterone regulation of gene transcription leading to control of ion transport. Hypertension 1992;19:221–227.

27 Wilson FH, Disse-Nicodeme S, Choate KA, Ishikawa K, Nelson-Williams C, Desitter I, Gunel M, Milford DV, Lipkin GW, Achard JM, Feely MP, Dussol B, Berland Y, Unwin RJ, Mayan H, Simon DB, Farfel Z, Jeunemaitre X, Lifton RP: Human hypertension caused by mutations in WNK kinases. Science 2001;293:1107–1112.

28 Yang CL, Angell J, Mitchell R, Ellison DH: WNK kinases regulate thiazide-sensitive NaCl cotransport. J Clin Invest 2003;111:1039–1045.

29 Kuhnle U, Hinkel GK, Hubl W, Reichelt T: Pseudohypoaldosteronism: family studies to identify asymptomatic carriers by stimulation of the renin-aldosterone system. Horm Res 1996;46:124–129.

30 Gruneiro-Papendieck L, Prieto L, Chiesa A, Bengolea S, Bossi G, Bergada C: Neonatal screening program for congenital adrenal hyperplasia: adjustments to the recall protocol. Horm Res 2001;55:271–277.

31 Ferraz-de-Souza B, Achermann JC: Disorders of adrenal development. Endocr Dev 2008;13:19–32.

32 Krone N, Arlt W: Genetics of congenital adrenal hyperplasia. Best Pract Res Clin Endocrinol Metab 2009;23:181–192.

33 Ulick S, Wang JZ, Morton DH: The biochemical phenotypes of two inborn errors in the biosynthesis of aldosterone. J Clin Endocrinol Metab 1992;74:1415–1420.

34 White PC: Aldosterone synthase deficiency and related disorders. Mol Cell Endocrinol 2004;217:81–87.

35 Geller DS, Zhang J, Zennaro MC, Vallo-Boado A, Rodriguez-Soriano J, Furu L, Haws R, Metzger D, Botelho B, Karaviti L, Haqq AM, Corey H, Janssens S, Corvol P, Lifton RP: Autosomal dominant pseudohypoaldosteronism type 1:mechanisms, evidence for neonatal lethality, and phenotypic expression in adults. J Am Soc Nephrol 2006;17:1429–1436.

36 Seyberth HW: An improved terminology and classification of Bartter-like syndromes. Nat Clin Pract Nephrol 2008;4:560–567.

37 Simon DB, Karet FE, Rodriguez-Soriano J, Hamdan JH, DiPietro A, Trachtman H, Sanjad SA, Lifton RP: Genetic heterogeneity of Bartter's syndrome revealed by mutations in the K+ channel, ROMK. Nat Genet 1996;14:152–156.

38 Bettinelli A, Bianchetti MG, Girardin E, et al: Use of calcium excretion values to distinguish two forms of primary renal tubular hypokalemic alkalosis: Bartter and Gitelman syndromes. J Pediatr 1992;120:38–43.

39 Simon DB, Nelson-Williams C, Bia MJ, Ellison D, Karet FE, Molina AM, Vaara I, Iwata F, Cushner HM, Koolen M, Gainza FJ, Gitleman HJ, Lifton RP: Gitelman's variant of Bartter's syndrome, inherited hypokalaemic alkalosis, is caused by mutations in the thiazide-sensitive NaCl cotransporter. Nat Genet 1996;12:24–30.

Paolo Ferrari, MBBS, MD, FRACP, FASN
Department of Nephrology
Fremantle Hospital, University of Western Australia
Alma Street, Perth, Western Australia 6160 (Australia)
Tel. +61 8 9431 3600, Fax +61 8 9431 3619, E-Mail paolo.ferrari@health.wa.gov.au

Ranke MB, Mullis P-E (eds): Diagnostics of Endocrine Function in Children and Adolescents, ed 4.
Basel, Karger, 2011, pp 235–259

Investigation of Calcium Disorders in Children

Les Perry[a] · Jeremy Allgrove[b]

[a]Department of Clinical Biochemistry, Pathology and Pharmacy Block, Barts and the London NHS Trust, and
[b]Royal London Hospital, London, UK

Disorders of calcium, phosphate and magnesium metabolism, although relatively rare in childhood, are important firstly because they can often cause considerable morbidity and secondly because the vast majority of them are treatable. However, in order to be able to offer suitable treatment, a definitive diagnosis must be reached. A thorough understanding of the mechanisms that give rise to these disorders together with appropriate laboratory investigation will usually allow such a diagnosis to be made.

There are four principal factors, vitamin D and its metabolites, parathyroid hormone (PTH), parathyroid hormone-related peptide (PTHrP) and calcitonin (CT) that are involved in calcium metabolism and one, fibroblast growth factor 23 (FGF23), that influences phosphate. Each of these is measurable in plasma and will be discussed in detail in this chapter. Normal values for these factors are shown in table 1. In addition there are several other factors, including alkaline phosphatase (ALP) and cyclic adenosine monophosphate (cAMP) that also play an important part in the investigation of calcium disorders and will also be discussed. Investigation of genetic mutations, which are responsible for many of the disorders seen in children, will not be discussed in detail and the methods of assessing bone turnover will not be covered. Changes in plasma and urine calcium, phosphate, magnesium, alkaline phosphatase and each of these humoral factors, together with the principal clinical features and genetic abnormalities that occur in different pathological states are shown in table 2.

General Considerations

The first step in identifying a problem related to calcium metabolism is to undertake baseline investigations. These include routine measurement of plasma calcium, phosphate, albumin, alkaline phosphatase, creatinine and magnesium. If an abnormality

Table 1. Normal levels of biochemical parameters and calciotropic agents in blood and urine.

Serum (fasting)		
Calcium[1] (total)	2.2–2.6 mmol/l	8.4–10.6 mg/dl
Ionised calcium (Ca^{2+})	1.1–1.3 mmol/l	
Phosphate		
Infants	1.6–2.6 mmol/l	5–8 mg/dl
Children[2]	1.3–1.9 mmol/l	4.6 mg/dl
Adults	0.6–1.5 mmol/l	2–4.6 mg/dl
Alkaline phosphatase		
Children[3]	200–600 IU/l	
Adults	60–170 IU/l	
Parathyroid hormone (PTH1–84)[4]	1.1–5.8 pmol/l	10–55 pg/ml
Parathyroid-related peptide (PTHrP)[4]	<2.5 pmol/l	
Calcitonin		
Infants <6 months[4]	<40 ng/ml	
Children 6 months <3 years[4]	<15 ng/ml	
>3 years[4]	<5 ng/ml	
Fibroblast growth factor 23 (FGF23)		
Intact[4]	<55 pg/ml	
C-terminal[4]	<150 RU/ml	
25-Hydroxyvitamin D (25OHD)[5]	50–150 nmol/l	20–60 ng/ml
1,25-Dihydroxyvitamin D (1,25(OH)$_2$D)		
Infants	70–360 pmol/l	30–150 pg/ml
Children	70–220 pmol/l	30–90 pg/ml
Adults	50–120 pmol/l	20–50 pg/ml
Urine (second morning fasting)		
Calcium excretion	0.1 mmol/kg/d	4 mg/kg/d
Calcium/creatinine (Ca/Cr)	0.7 mmol/mmol	0.25 mg/mg
Magnesium (Mg/Cr)	1.0 mmol/mmol	0.2 mg/mg
Tubular reabsorption of phosphate (TRP)		
Children	85–97%	
Adults	80–95%	
Tubular maximum for phosphate in relation to glomerular filtrate (TmP/GFR)		
0–14 years	1.3–2.6 mmol/l	4–8 mg/dl
Adults	0.8–1.5 mmol/l	2.5–4.7 mg/dl

[1]Corrected for albumin according to the formula: $Ca_{Corr} = Ca_{Total} + (0.02*(40-Alb))$, where Ca_{Total} is measured in mmol/l and albumin in g/l. [2]Levels are briefly somewhat higher during the adolescent growth spurt and are maximal about 4 months before the peak of the adolescent growth spurt. [3]Levels are higher during adolescence and reflect the increased growth rate, being highest at the peak of the growth spurt. [4]Details of normal values for all of these parameters are somewhat limited in children. The normal ranges are age-dependent and may vary according to the precise assay being used. [5]These values are thought to be adequate for normal bone health. There is now increasing evidence to suggest that levels >70-80 nmol/l are ideal for maximising the health of the cardiovascular and immune systems and for reducing the risk of some forms of cancer and diabetes. In the absence of dietary supplementation, there is an annual variation in 25OHD values that reflect sunlight exposure.

in calcium metabolism is identified, plasma 25OHD and PTH should always be measured as well. In addition, a measurement of urinary calcium, phosphate and creatinine may point to a diagnosis. Blood samples should always be taken for later measurement of 1,25-dihydroxyvitamin D ($1,25(OH)_2D$) if this is deemed necessary later and it is helpful to take a further sample for DNA analysis if, as is often the case, a genetic mutation is suspected.

Radiological assessment is also frequently helpful. This includes plain X-rays of the wrist and knee where rickets is suspected, the remainder of the skeleton if a skeletal dysplasia is thought to be present or if evidence of fracture or vertebral collapse is considered possible. Dual energy X-ray absorptiometry (DXA) scan may also be indicated and scintigraphy such as skeletal bone scan or SestaMIBI scan of the parathyroids may also be indicated. Ultrasound may be helpful, particularly in identifying the presence of nephrocalcinosis, and CT scan readily identifies soft tissue calcification that may not be seen on conventional X-ray. This chapter concentrates on the laboratory investigations only.

Calcium

Approximately 40% of plasma calcium is bound to albumin. Of the remainder, most (about 50% of the total) is free ionised and it is this that determines neuromuscular function and is controlled by the calciotropic factors. The remaining 10% is complexed to other anions such as citrate. In order to allow for variations in serum albumin, it is usual practice to make an adjustment for this to obtain a 'corrected' calcium level. The most commonly used formula is:

$$Ca_{Corr} = Ca_{Total} + 0.02*(40\text{-Alb}),$$

where Ca_{Corr} is the 'corrected' calcium, Ca_{Total} is the observed calcium and Alb is the observed albumin level and the calcium is expressed in mmol/l and the albumin in g/l although the validity of this formula has been questioned and several other formulae have been suggested [1]. The normal range is 2.20–2.60 mmol/l (some laboratories give a slightly wider range) and, after the neonatal period, varies little throughout life. As an alternative to estimating the 'corrected' calcium, it is possible relatively easily to measure ionised calcium (Ca^{2+}) directly. Most modern blood gas machines are capable of doing this. The normal range for Ca^{2+} is 1.1–1.3 mmol/l.

Phosphate and Creatinine

Both phosphate and creatinine are measured routinely in serum, no corrections being required. The importance of measuring serum phosphate is that it may give a guide to diagnosis. Phosphate levels change with age, being highest in the early years with a secondary rise during adolescence, peaking about four months before the peak of

Table 2. Details of principal biochemical findings, radiological and clinical features and, where relevant, genetic abnormalities in the most common forms of rickets, hypocalcaemia and hypercalcaemia

Disorder	Calcium	Phosphate	ALP	PTH	25OHD
Hypocalcaemia					
Rickets					
A. Nutritional					
1. Congenital	↓	↓	↑	↑↑	↓↓
2. Dilated cardiomyopathy	↓↓	↑	↑	↑	↓↓
3. Classical rickets	↓	↓	↑↑	↑↑	↓↓
4. Hypocalcaemia	↓↓	↑↑	↑ or N	↑	↓↓
5. Generalised aches and pains	N	N	N	N	↓
B. Vitamin D-dependent type I (VDRR1)	↓	↓	↑↑	↑	N
C. Vitamin D-dependent type II (VDDR2)	↓	↓	↑↑	↑	N
D. Hypophosphataemic					
1. X-linked dominant (XLHR)	N	↓↓	↑	N	N
2. Autosomal dominant (ADHR)	N	↓↓	↑	N	N
3. Autosomal recessive (ARHR)	N	↓↓	↑	N	N
4. Hereditary hypophosphataemia with hypercalciuria (HHRH)	N	↓↓	↑	N	N
5. Tumour-induced osteomalacia (TIO)	N	↓↓	↑	N	N
6. McCune-Albright syndrome (MAS)	N	↓↓	↑	N	N
7. Epidermal naevus syndrome	N	↓↓	↑	N	N
Hypoparathyroidism					
A. Primary hypoparathyroidism					
1. Isolated primary hypoparathyroidism	↓	↑	N or ↓	↓ or U/D	N

$1,25(OH)_2D$	UCa/ Creat	X-ray appearances	Clinical features	Mutation
↓	↓	generalised rickets	respiratory impairment, clinical rickets	–
↓	↓	usually rickets	cardiac failure, hypocalcaemic seizures	–
↓, N or ↑	↓	generalised rickets	clinical rickets, bowed legs, swollen wrists, 'rickety rosary'	–
↓	↓	may be normal	hypocalcaemic seizures	–
?	?N	normal	normal	–
↓	↓	generalised rickets	clinical rickets	1a-hydroxylase gene
↑↑↑	↓	generalised rickets	clinical rickets, may have alopecia	vitamin D receptor
N or ↓	N	rickets	clinical rickets	PHEX
N or ↓	N	rickets	clinical rickets	FGF23
N or ↓	N	rickets	clinical rickets	DMP1
N or ↓	↑	rickets	clinical rickets	Na-Pi co-transporter
N or ↓	N	rickets	clinical rickets	–
N or ↓	N	rickets	clinical rickets	GNAS
N or ↓	N	rickets	clinical rickets. widespread epidermal naevi	–
N or ↓	↓	normal, may be undermineralised	hypocalcaemic seizures, tingling, carpopedal spasms	preproPTH, PTH, GCMB, ?SOX3

Table 2. Continued

Disorder	Calcium	Phosphate	ALP	PTH	25OHD
2. Hypoparathyroid sensorineural deafness renal anomalies (HDR)	↓	↑	N or ↓	↓ or U/D	N
3. Hypoparathyroid mental and growth retardation dysmorphic features (Kenny-Caffey and Sanjad-Sakati syndromes)	↓	↑	N or ↓	↓ or U/D	N
4. DiGeorge/Velocardiofacial	↓	↑	N or ↓	↓ or U/D	N
5. Autosomal-dominant hypocalcaemia	↓	↑	N or ↓	↓ or U/D	N
B. Pseudohypoparathyroidism type 1a	↓	↑	N or ↓	↓ or U/D	N
B. Pseudohypoparathyroidism type 1b	↓	↑	N or ↓	↓ or U/D	N
Hypercalcaemia					
Primary hyperparathyroidism					
Familial isolated primary hyperparathyroidism (FIPHPT)	↑	N or ↓	N or ↑	↑	N
Multiple endocrine neoplasia type I	↑	N or ↓	N or ↑	↑	N
Multiple endocrine neoplasia type IIA	↑	N or ↓	N or ↑	↑	N
Multiple endocrine neoplasia type IIB	↑	N or ↓	N or ↑	↑	N
Multiple endocrine neoplasia type IIC	N	N	N	N	N
Multiple endocrine neoplasia type IV	↑	N or ↓	N or ↑	↑	N
Hyperparathyroid jaw-tumour syndrome	↑	N or ↓	N or ↑	↑	N

1,25(OH)$_2$D	UCa/ Creat	X-ray appearances	Clinical features	Mutation
N or ↓	↓	normal, may be undermineralised	hypocalcaemic seizures, deafness, renal anomalies	GATA3
N or ↓	↓	normal, may be undermineralised	hypocalcaemic seizures, mental retardation, etc.	TBCE
N or ↓	↓	normal, may be undermineralised	hypocalcaemic seizures etc, developmental problems, swallowing and speech abnormalities, cardiac defects	TBX1 as part of microdeletion of 22q
N or ↓	↑	normal, may be undermineralised	hypocalcaemic seizures, nephrocalcinosis	CaSR
N or ↓	↓	normal, may be undermineralised	hypocalcaemic seizures, etc., developmental problems, mild hypothyroidism. aho	GNAS
N or ↓	↓	normal, may be undermineralised	hypocalcaemic seizures, etc., mild hypothyroidism. normal intelligence	GNAS associated methylation defects
N or ↑	N or ↑	periosteal microcysts, rickets-like changes, +ve sestamibi scan	constipation, lethargy, muscle weakness, thirst, polyuria, psychiatric disturbance	MEN1, HRPT2, HRPT3
N or ↑	N or ↑	as for FIPHPT		MEN1
N or ↑	N or ↑	as for FIPHPT		Ret proto-oncogene
N or ↑	N or ↑	as for FIPHPT		Ret proto-oncogene
N	N	normal		Ret proto-oncogene
N or ↑	N or ↑	as for FIPHPT		CDKN1B
N or ↑	N or ↑	as for FIPHPT	hyperparathyroidism, jaw tumours, renal abnormalities, parathyroid carcinoma	HRPT2

Table 2. Continued

Disorder	Calcium	Phosphate	ALP	PTH	25OHD
Familial isolated hyperparathyroidism	↑	N or ↓	N or ↑	↑	N
Familial benign (hypocalciuric) hypercalcaemia	↑	N or ↓	N	N	N
Neonatal severe hyperparathyroidism	↑	N or ↓	N or ↑	↑	N
Parathyroid adenomas	↑	N or ↓	N or ↑	↑	N
Parathyroid carcinoma	↑	N or ↓	N or ↑	↑	N

the adolescent growth spurt [2]. Creatinine rises with age. In hypoparathyroid states, calcium is low whereas phosphate is elevated, whilst in secondary hyperparathyroid states (e.g. vitamin D deficiency rickets), calcium may be somewhat low but phosphate is also low as a result of inhibition of renal tubular reabsorption by PTH. In addition, in hypophosphatemic rickets, where serum calcium is usually normal, phosphate is usually low as a result of impaired renal tubular handling of phosphate (see below).

Urinary Calcium, Phosphate and Creatinine

The value of taking a urine sample for estimation of calcium, phosphate, creatinine and, if necessary, magnesium cannot be underestimated. In measuring urinary calcium, it is easiest to measure the calcium/creatinine ratio in the second morning urine sample [3, 4]. Some authors recommend measuring the clearance ratio (i.e. fractional excretion) of calcium and creatinine as this also takes into account the plasma calcium and creatinine concentrations. In hypoparathyroid states, renal tubular reabsorption of calcium is low but the low filtered load of calcium results in a low urinary calcium excretion. The one exception to this is where the hypoparathyroidism is caused by an activating mutation in the calcium sensing receptor (CaSR), in which case hypocalcaemia is accompanied by inappropriately high urinary calcium excretion.

In contrast, hypercalcaemia caused either by primary hyperparathyroidism or vitamin D intoxication is usually accompanied by hypercalciuria. When hypercalcaemia is caused by an inactivating mutation of the CaSR, urinary calcium excretion is inappropriately low.

Perry · Allgrove

1,25(OH)$_2$D	UCa/ Creat	X-ray appearances	Clinical features	Mutation
N or ↑	N or ↑	as for FIPHPT		HRPT3
N	↓	no abnormalities	usually asymptomatic	CaSR
N or ↑	N or ↑	severe 'rachitic' changes with 'moth-eaten' appearances of growth plates	respiratory difficulties, abnormal chest shape, dehydration, cachexia	CaSR
N or ↑	N or ↑	as for FIPHPT		PRAD1/PTH
N or ↑	N or ↑	as for FIPHPT	depends on extent, if any, of metastases	HRPT2

Urinary phosphate measurement is particularly useful when assessing renal tubular handling of phosphate. This is particularly so when hypophosphataemic rickets is suspected. The first step in making this diagnosis is to measure the fractional excretion of phosphate (FE$_{PO4}$) which can easily be done from a simultaneous measurement of urine and plasma phosphate and creatinine. It can be done on a 'spot' urine and serum, although some authors argue that it is best done on a three hour timed urine sample taken fasting in order to control for changes in phosphate intake [5].

The formula for calculating FE$_{PO4}$ is:

$$FE_{PO4} = [U_{PO4}]/[P_{PO4}] \times [P_{Creat}]/[U_{Creat}],$$

where U$_{PO4}$ and P$_{PO4}$ are the urine and plasma concentrations of phosphate and P$_{Creat}$ and U$_{Creat}$ are the plasma and urine concentrations of creatinine. Note that this has no units but the measurements of phosphate and of creatinine must be in the same units. In this respect it is important to note that plasma creatinine is usually reported as μmol/l whilst urine creatinine is often in mmol/l. Once the FE$_{PO4}$ has been calculated, the Tubular Reabsorption of phosphate (TRP) can be deduced as:

$$TRP = 100*(1-FE_{PO4}),$$

and is expressed as a percentage. The normal range for TRP varies during life and is higher in children (table 1).

This calculation is dependent on two assumptions:
1 Since the TRP is effectively comparing the clearance of phosphate with the clearance of creatinine, it assumes that clearance of creatinine approximates to glomerular filtration rate (GFR). Whilst this is generally true, it may not be so in conditions such as chronic renal failure, where plasma creatinine is significantly elevated. In

practice, this is of no great consequence since plasma creatinine rises as GFR falls and, once it is less that 30 ml/min/1.73 m^2, elevated plasma phosphate becomes of clinical significance. TRP is more concerned with hypophosphataemic states.

2 The plasma phosphate is high enough to saturate the tubular reabsorptive process. Because TRP is dependent on the plasma phosphate, in the presence of a very low plasma phosphate, and hence low filtered load, the TRP may be normal even if renal tubular handling is impaired. To overcome this problem, it is necessary to measure the theoretical tubular maximal phosphate reabsorption (TmPO$_4$/GFR). Although it can be calculated, the easiest way to do this is to refer to the nomogram of Walton and Bijvoet [6]. This removes the effect of plasma phosphate and provides a figure that is measured in mmol/l (or mg/dl). As with TRP, the value varies with age (table 1).

Under pathological circumstances, hyperparathyroid states and hypophosphataemic rickets lower TRP and TmPO$_4$/GFR whilst the reverse is true in hypoparathyroidism.

Magnesium

Measurement of plasma magnesium should not be forgotten as part of the initial investigations. Hypomagnesaemia, although rare, is an important cause of hypoparathyroidism and may give a clue to the diagnosis [7]. In addition to acquired hypomagnesaemia, in which urinary magnesium excretion is generally reduced, there are several genetic conditions that lead to hypomagnesaemia. Some of these are associated with hypermagnesuria and some with hypomagnesuria and measurement of urinary magnesium may be helpful in the differential diagnosis [8].

Alkaline Phosphatase

This enzyme hydrolyses phosphate in a number of tissues. Circulating alkaline phosphatase (ALP) is derived mainly from bone and liver but also from intestine and placenta. The different forms of ALP have slightly different properties, mainly related to their heat lability and, in the event that there is uncertainty about the origins of circulating ALP, it is possible to use this property to distinguish between the various forms. Bone-specific ALP (B$_s$ALP) is mainly derived from osteoblasts and is the most heat labile. Measurement of B$_s$ALP is not a routine procedure but may occasionally be helpful, especially if there is a need to distinguish between liver and bone-derived ALP.

Raised ALP reflects increased osteoblast activity and is seen whenever bone turnover is increased. Normal values vary during life and, in children, reflect the growth rate, being highest during infancy and adolescence. During the latter, maximum ALP is seen at the height of the growth spurt and then declines rapidly towards normal adult values thereafter [2]. Very raised values are particularly seen in rickets and ALP measurements, which may occasionally reach as high as 8,000 IU/l, form part of the monitoring process. Following the start of treatment of rickets, there may be an initial rise in ALP before it begins to fall. Some rise in ALP is also seen following fractures as the bone heals. Hyperparathyroidism is also associated with raised ALP, and a slightly increased ALP, particularly if this is bone derived, may help to distinguish osteogenesis imperfecta (OI) from idiopathic juvenile osteoporosis (IJO). In contrast, hypophosphatasia is characterised by low levels of ALP in which case the diagnosis can be confirmed by also measuring phosphoethanolamine, which is raised as this is also a natural substrate for ALP [9].

Vitamin D Metabolism

Vitamin D_3 (cholecalciferol) is a secosteroid that is principally derived from the action of ultraviolet light (UVB) at a wavelength of 270–290 nm on the cholesterol precursor, dehydrocholesterol. A second precursor, ergosterol, is present in plants, particularly fungi, and undergoes a similar conversion to a secosteroid, ergocalciferol (vitamin D_2). Cholecalciferol results from cleavage of the steroid B ring (hence the term seco-, or cut, steroid) with an additional eight carbon side chain present at the 17-position of the steroid molecule. Thus, it is a 25-carbon molecule. It is already hydroxylated at the 3-position and is otherwise known as calciol. Ergocalciferol is identical in structure to cholecalciferol apart from the presence of a double bond between positions 20 and 21 in the side chain. Both are metabolised in a similar fashion and are thought to be equipotent. The presence of cholecalciferol in plasma results from a combination not only principally of its synthesis in the skin, but also from dietary sources, whilst ergocalciferol is derived entirely from the latter, mainly as a result of food fortification. When plasma levels are satisfactory and dietary fortification has not been employed, 80% of vitamin D is derived from natural synthesis and consists mainly of cholecalciferol. This has implications for laboratory investigation of vitamin D metabolism. The term vitamin D (calciferol) is used where neither chole- nor ergocalciferol is specified. Inadequate supplies of vitamin D, either as a result of insufficient sunlight exposure or failure to give adequate nutritional supplements, result in nutritional vitamin D deficiency.

Vitamin D and its metabolites circulate in plasma bound to a specific vitamin D binding protein (DBP). This is an α_2-globulin synthesised by the liver with a molecular weight of 56–58 kD. DBP circulates in micromolar concentrations (about 6 µM or 350 µg/ml), far exceeding the requirement for vitamin D transport. The protein has a higher affinity for 25OHD than for vitamin D or $1,25(OH)_2D$. There are no clinical indications for measurement of DBP.

Following synthesis, vitamin D undergoes two hydroxylation steps in order to become fully active. The first, which takes place in the liver, occurs at position 25 and results in 25OHD, also known as calcidiol. This is the principal circulating metabolite and is what is measured when a vitamin D level is requested. Its concentration gives a good idea of how replete the subject is with vitamin D. Levels of 25OHD are not closely controlled and are largely dependent on the quantity of vitamin D synthesised and how much dietary supplementation has been provided. Excessive sunlight exposure does not result in vitamin D toxicity since, under this circumstance, cholecalciferol is diverted into inactive metabolites. Failure of 25-hydroxylation is very uncommon and only occurs in a few conditions.

The final hydroxylation takes place at the 1-position and results in the highly active metabolite, $1,25(OH)_2D$, also known as calcitriol. This hydroxylation step is stimulated by the enzyme 25-hydroxyvitamin D 1α-hydroxylase and takes place mainly in the kidney but also, during pregnancy, in the placenta and, in pathological circumstances, in macrophages and some granulomas. Its synthesis is normally tightly controlled and is principally stimulated by PTH (and therefore indirectly by low plasma calcium) and hypophosphataemia. Fibroblast growth factor 23 (FGF23) and 24,25-dihydroxyvitamin D $(24,25(OH)_2D)$ inhibit its formation. Mutations in the 1α-hydroxylase gene result in inappropriately low synthesis of $1,25(OH)_2D$ which causes vitamin D-dependent rickets type 1 (VDDR1), and impaired $1,25(OH)_2D$ synthesis also occurs in chronic renal insufficiency. Inappropriately raised levels are found in a number of granulomatous conditions, of which subcutaneous fat necrosis is the most important in children.

$24,25(OH)_2D$, an inactive vitamin D metabolite resulting from hydroxylation at the 24- rather than the 1-position, is synthesised as an alternative to $1,25(OH)_2D$ when plasma calcium is within the normal range and PTH levels are low. Its function is not known for certain but it is thought to act to prevent levels of $1,25(OH)_2D$ becoming too high. 25OHD has limited vitamin D activity and circulates in nanomolar concentrations whilst $1,25(OH)_2D$ is highly active and circulates in picomolar concentrations (table 2). Measurement of $1,25(OH)_2D$ plays no part in the diagnosis of vitamin D deficiency as it may be low, normal or high depending on whether or not there has been some vitamin D exposure. For a more detailed description of the metabolism of vitamin D and the enzymes involved, see Allgrove [8].

$1,25(OH)_2D$ acts on a specific vitamin D receptor that is present in many tissues. It is a member of the steroid/thyroid receptor superfamily and has a surface receptor that combines with the ligand and is transported to the nucleus where it stimulates DNA formation. If the vitamin D receptor is defective, $1,25(OH)_2D$ levels may be very elevated, even as high as nanomolar, especially if additional calcitriol or 1α-hydroxycolecalciferol (alfacalcidol) have been administered. This situation is seen particularly in vitamin D dependent rickets type 2 (VDDR2), which is more appropriately called vitamin D receptor defect.

Measurement of Vitamin D Metabolites in Plasma

25OHD constitutes the major circulating form of vitamin D in humans. Physiological concentrations of other metabolites include $24,25(OH)_2D$ and $1,25(OH)_2D$ which circulate at approximately 10 and 0.1% those of 25OHD. Since these metabolites circulate at lower concentrations their 'interference' will have minimal impact on the total vitamin D result. Only determinations of the concentrations of 25-hydroxyvitamin D and $1,25(OH)_2D$ have been shown to have clinical importance. The body naturally can produce D_3 but patients can be supplemented with either D_3 or D_2. Methods for vitamin D analysis must therefore be able to measure both D_2 and D_3 forms equally.

Vitamin D is very lipophilic and, historically, assays of vitamin D comprised 3 steps:

1 Separation of the vitamin D components from lipids that interfere with analysis.
2 Chromatographic separation of vitamin D metabolites using either Sephadex LH-20 or, more frequently, high pressure liquid chromatography (HPLC).
3 Quantification of the vitamin D metabolites using competitive protein binding or immunoassay.

The purification steps 1 and 2 are very laborious and time consuming compared with step 3. Liquid extraction to remove lipid components that affect the assay is achieved using various solvents, predominantly acetonitrile or absolute ethanol.

Like PTH assays, 25OHD assays are dominated by the automated immunoassay platforms of which globally there are ~5 major ones.

Assays are classified into:
– Radioimmunoassay (~17% methods).
– HPLC (~3% methods).
– Liquid chromatography and tandem mass spectrometry (LCMSMS) (~10% methods).
– Immunometric assays where the 'isotopic signal' has been replaced with a non-isotopic signal, e.g. (electro-)chemiluminescence or enzyme (~70%).

Radioimmunoassay using ^{125}I-labelled commercial kits has long been the method of choice for assessing 25OHD status. However, as the figures above show, there has more recently been a big move away from isotopic to non-isotopic methods partly due to a decrease in the use of isotopes generally, but also due to the introduction of automation to cope with the significant increase in workload. The reader is advised to look at the automated platform kit insert for the exact details of the test principle.

Our own laboratory has recently introduced a semi-automated method linked with LCMSMS to measure simultaneously $25OHD_2$ and $25OHD_3$. In this process 0.15 ml is mixed with deuterated $25OHD_2$ and $25OHD_3$ internal standard in a deep-well microtitre plate using the Tecan robotic system. The Tecan then dispenses a protein disruption solution (zinc sulphate) followed by methanol to denature the lipid complexes. The microtitre plate is centrifuged to precipitate the debris and returned to the Tecan instrument. After initial priming of a solid-phase elution plate, vitamin D is extracted from the supernatant into a standard microtitre plate. This is placed in the LCMSMS instrument where sample is injected into it and, following ultra-performance liquid chromatography (UPLC), the vitamin D_2 and D_3 products are quantified using mass spectrometry.

The emergence of LCMSMS, a new 'physico-chemical' method which some have suggested might be a candidate reference technique, has highlighted several concerns about 25OHD analysis:

1 Firstly, there is no agreed International Standard. Recent vitamin D external quality assessment schemes (DEQAS) data have demonstrated that the variation in the source and the matrix of calibrator material has a significant impact on method bias. In January 2008, DEQAS distributed a human based commercial standard (ChromSystems, GmbH) to all users of the HPLC and LCMSMS methods and asked laboratories to analyse this sample and then to recalculate their results against this 'common standard' to see if this would decrease the between laboratory variation (%CV). HPLC results were relatively unaffected but LCMSMS methods showed much closer agreement when the same standard was used. This was particularly noticeable for $25OHD_3$ [10].

2 Secondly, there is variation in some manufacturers' methods in their reported and actual cross reactivity with vitamin D_2. One manufacturer (Roche) states that their method is marketed only as a vitamin D_3 kit.

3 Thirdly, the differences in bias may affect classification as to whether a patient is vitamin D deficient, insufficient or sufficient.

Manual immunoassays generally use 0.5 ml to produce a result in duplicate while the automated platforms use significantly less (0.2–0.25 ml) and report $25OHD_3$ results down to ~20 nmol/l (8 ng/ml). HPLC and LCMSMS methods use 0.15 ml and can report down to ~5 nmol/l (2 ng/ml).

Manual assays have between assay CV of about 8% at 25 nmol/l (10 ng/ml) while the automated immunoassay platforms, HPLC and LCMSMS have CV ~8% at 10 nmol/l (4 ng/ml). The lower limit of reporting and lower limit of quantitation varies with each analytical method.

The interpretation of 25OHD results is controversial but there seems to be some agreement that results less than 25 nmol/l indicate vitamin D deficiency while results between 25 and 50 nmol/l suggests vitamin D insufficiency. However, full sufficiency is probably not achieved unless levels are above 75 nmol/l and a target range of 75–150 (median 100) nmol/l suggests vitamin D adequacy. A Vitamin D concentration greater than 200 nmol/l is suggestive of toxicity although this not always accompanied by symptoms which may not occur until much higher levels are achieved.

Measurement of 1,25-Dihydroxyvitamin D in Plasma

Plasma concentrations of $1,25(OH)_2D$ are not affected by sunlight but, since 25OHD circulates at concentrations approximately one-thousand times greater than $1,25(OH)_2D$, cross reactivity with the former becomes significant. The methods used for $1,25(OH)_2D$ are dominated by radioimmunoassay. One RIA manufacturer also produces an enzymoimmunoassay (EIA). Recently, there is increased use of tandem mass spectrometry.

An original method developed by Reinhardt et al. [11] involved serum extraction with acetonitrile and crude purification on a C18 Sep-Pak cartridge. Final purification on a silica Sep-Pak cartridge used 5% isopropanol in hexane. Quantification of $1,25(OH)_2D$ used a radioreceptor assay with the receptor being extracted from calf thymus.

Immunoassay techniques have managed to obviate the organic solvent extraction techniques. Patient samples are delipidated with magnesium chloride and $1,25(OH)_2D$ is extracted from potential cross-reactants by incubation for 90 min with a highly specific solid phase monoclonal anti-$1,25(OH)_2D$ antibody (known as immunoextraction). The immunoextraction gel is then washed and the purified $1,25(OH)_2D$ is eluted directly into glass tubes. The eluate is then used in a standard (radio-/enzyme-)immunoassay. Tandem mass spectrometry also involves some sample preparation but the use of UPLC and chromatography is able to reach the performance levels of the immunoassays. Tandem mass spectrometry is able simultaneously to determine the $1,25(OH)_2D_2$ and $1,25(OH)_2D_3$ levels. Whether this will prove to be of clinical value has yet to be determined, so meanwhile the results are still reported as totals.

Manual immunoassays generally use 1.0 ml serum to produce a result in duplicate though they can use 0.5 ml for paediatric samples. All the assays seem to be able to measure down to ~5 pmol/l (~2 pg/ml).

The between assay CV's of about 20% at 20 nmol/l (8.3 pg/ml) and ~10% at 160 pmol/l (67 pg/ml) is a fair reflection of the complexity of these manual assays. The differences in $1,25(OH)_2D$ concentrations between methods is difficult to interpret as there is no agreed International Reference material.

Total $1,25(OH)_2D$ reference ranges for adults for the RIA and the EIA methods are similar (40–190 pmol/l) with lower levels reported in patients with end-stage renal failure (<40 pmol/l). Values for normal infants (72–360 pmol/l or 30–150 pg/ml) and older children (70–220 pmol/l or 30–90 pg/ml) have been reported using the now discontinued Nichols Institute Diagnostics radioimmunoassay kit.

The reader should be aware that, at present, the major manufacturer of the RIA and EIA kits has reported that the RIA method may overestimate the amount of $1,25(OH)_2D$ while the EIA tends to underestimate concentrations in circulation of patients on Vitamin D_2 therapy.

Indications for Measurement of Vitamin D Metabolites

With the increasing recognition that vitamin D deficiency occurs commonly, particularly as 'normal' values of 25OHD have been revised upwards, measurement of 25OHD is becoming more routine. In our own hospital, which is situated within an area containing a population with a high ethnic minority, particularly from South Asia, approximately 25,000–30,000 assays are performed annually and assays are run daily. In addition, the average cost of a single assay has declined and is now approximately GBP 8 (~EUR 9, USD 12.5). This makes it more feasible to measure 25OHD in a large number of patients and results can be obtained within 24 h.

Measurement of 25OHD is indicated at presentation in any child with:

- Hypocalcaemia, particularly if accompanied by seizures, cardiac failure, etc.
- Rickets.
- Generalised limb aches and pains.
- With chronic renal failure [12].
- Hypercalcaemia if vitamin D intoxication is suspected.
- As a screening procedure if other family members have been identified as having vitamin D deficiency.
- Vitamin D deficiency to assess adequacy of replacement therapy.

Measurement of $1,25(OH)_2D$ is much less frequently indicated and is confined to:

- Those instances where hypercalcaemia and low PTH suggests the possibility of vitamin D intoxication (e.g. subcutaneous fat necrosis).
- Rickets in the absence of hypophosphataemia or vitamin D deficiency as a cause suggests the possibility of 1a-hydroxylase deficiency or vitamin D receptor abnormality.
- Chronic renal failure if PTH is elevated (although it is important to exclude vitamin D deficiency as a cause of the raised PTH) [12].

It is not indicated as a diagnostic test in vitamin D deficiency.

Parathyroid Hormone

PTH is an 84 amino acid polypeptide hormone that is synthesised and secreted by the parathyroid glands. Only the first 34 amino acids are required for full hormone activity and the function of the remainder of the molecule is not properly understood. Its secretion is determined principally by the plasma ionised calcium (Ca^{2+}) concentration and is controlled by a calcium-sensing receptor (CaSR) located on the surface of the parathyroid glands and also in renal tubules. PTH secretion is mediated via a magnesium-dependent G-protein coupled second messenger. Magnesium deficiency can interfere with this process and may lead to hypoparathyroidism which can only be reversed by correcting the magnesium deficiency. Secretion of PTH occurs in a sigmoid fashion in response to Ca^{2+} which is normally maintained within very narrow limits of 1.1–1.3 mmol/l. For further details of the function of the CaSR and its relationship with PTH, see Allgrove [8].

Very little PTH is stored within the glands. PTH is secreted after cleavage from a pre,pro-precursor which contains a further 31 amino acids on the N-terminal end of the molecule. For a detailed description of the synthesis of PTH, see Habener and

Potts [13, 14]. Following secretion, the half-life of PTH in the circulation is very short – about 2 min – after which it is cleaved into several inactive fragments. These circulate in plasma and are excreted via the kidney.

PTH acts on a specific receptor, the PTHrP/PTH1 receptor. A second receptor, the PTH2 receptor is present in brain but PTHrP is not a ligand for this. The PTH1 receptor is linked to its intracellular actions by a G-protein coupled second messenger that is common to a number of polypeptide hormones including thyroid-stimulating hormone (TSH), the gonadotrophins, and growth hormone-releasing hormone (GHRH). The receptors are mainly present in renal tubules, where renal tubular reabsorption of phosphate is inhibited, and bone, principally on osteoblasts. Under normal physiological conditions, when PTH is secreted in low quantities in a tonic fashion, it acts as an anabolic agent for bone but, when circumstances arise in which extra calcium is required in the circulation, it acts as a catabolic agent to promote bone resorption in order to restore calcium to normal. The excess phosphate that is resorbed at the same time is eliminated by the phosphaturic actions of PTH on renal tubules. The resorptive effect is mediated by osteoclasts which increase their action under the influence of osteoblasts via changes in the levels of Rank Ligand (RANKL) and its inhibitory ligand, osteoprotegerin, which are both products of osteoblasts, and which determine the activity of osteoclasts.

Measurement of PTH (in Plasma)

Measurement of PTH is complicated by the heterogeneity of the circulating forms [15] but the concentration of intact PTH is relatively independent of glomerular filtration and reflects the biologically active portion of the hormone. The lack of an agreed International Reference material for intact PTH complicates between method comparisons.

PTH assays are dominated by the (semi-)automated immunoassay platforms of which globally there are <10 major manufacturers. Assays are classified into:
- Radioimmunoassay.
- Immunometric assays where the 'isotopic signal' has been replaced with a non-isotopic signal, e.g. (electro-)chemiluminescence, or an enzyme.

There has been a significant switch from radioimmunoassays, which were initially introduced to measure the C-terminal fraction of the PTH molecule [16]. The introduction of the immunometric assay, which uses two antibodies targeted at different areas of the PTH molecule, has increased the analytical sensitivity of the assay (i.e. how low can the assay measure reproducibly), but has also increased the analytical specificity of the assay (i.e. the ability to measure the intact PTH molecule and not its other molecular forms).

The intact PTH (iPTH) immunometric assays use two, usually monoclonal, antibodies. One is the 'capture' antibody and is targeted at one end of the molecule (e.g.

Siemens Immulite®; PTH 44–84) while the other is the signal antibody and is targeted to the other end of the molecule (Siemens Immulite PTH 1–34). The iPTH thus becomes the 'jam in the sandwich' which is why these types of assays are called sandwich assays.

For immunoradiometric assays, the signal is ^{125}I-labelled antigen. However, to obviate the use of isotopic material and its well known disadvantages such as instability due to radiolytic damage of the labelled protein, short tracer half-life and contact with radioactive material, the signal became non-isotopic. The advent of non-isotopic signals and the coupling of one of the monoclonal antibodies to a 'solid-phase' to expedite antibody-bound and free antigen separation, has facilitated the introduction of automated immunoassay platforms. Automation has significantly replaced manual immunoassays.

Most automated platforms separate the antibody-bound PTH using either magnetised solid-phase (Roche Elecsys®; Beckman Access®; Abbott Architect®) or the antibodies have been coupled to a bead (Siemens Immulite; DiaSorin Liaison®).

A simplified analytical process is that calibrator, internal quality control (IQC) or patient plasma sample is mixed with paramagnetic particles coated with a capture antibody. The sample is 'washed' to remove excess PTH not bound to the antibody. A second antibody coupled to a 'signal' is then added. This will bind to any PTH present in the reaction mixture to form a complex. Excess material not bound is then washed away and the trigger for the signal is added to the complex to complete the reaction. The amount of signal present is proportional to the intensity of the signal generated. The reader is advised to look at the automated platform kit insert for the exact details of the test principle.

These automated platforms can use either serum or plasma, although those assays that use alkaline phosphatase as the enzyme to generate the chemiluminescent signal can give lower results if the EDTA tube is under filled as the excess EDTA in the assay sequesters Ca^{2+} ions used by the enzyme.

Manual immunoassays generally use 0.4 ml to produce a result in duplicate while the automated platforms use significantly less (0.05–0.1 ml). In addition, the precision of the automated assays is superior to that of the manual assays. Consequently, analytical sensitivity is improved. The manual assays have between assay CV of about 8% at 1 pmol/l (~10 pg/ml) while the automated immunoassay platforms have CV < 5%. The detection limit of PTH assays is about 0.1 pmol/l (~1 pg/ml).

The normal range for PTH in healthy children and adults is approx 1–6 pmol/l (~10–60 ng/l) with no detectable age or sex dependent variation. Some laboratories will quote a slightly different range depending on their methodology. Crucial to this is the patient's need to be vitamin D replete.

Recent audit and United Kingdom External Quality Assessment Scheme (UKNEQAS) data have shown that some methods can give results up to three times different from the lowest to highest. Despite these significant between-method differences in bias, the reference range quoted is approximately the same for all the methods [17].

Perry · Allgrove

The absence of an International Standard precludes assessment of absolute accuracy of method calibration. However, comparative recovery data using the National Institute for Biological Standards and Control (NIBSC) reference reagent (RR 95/646) suggests that assay bias would be reduced if assays were calibrated accurately. The RR 95/646 is a preparation of recombinant human PTH (1–84) and has been proposed as a candidate material for an International Standard for PTH. Its universal adoption might cause a significant change in observed patient concentrations but would also minimise the between method differences currently experienced. Because of their nature, these assays do not detect PTH 1–34 in the circulation and cannot be used to assay PTH levels following treatment with PTH 1–34.

Indications for PTH Measurement

PTH should be measured in any child who presents with:
- Hypocalcaemia (vitamin D deficiency is not an indication not to measure it).
- Hypercalcaemia, especially where primary hyperparathyroidism is suspected and as part of the monitoring process in:
- hypophosphataemic rickets,
- chronic renal disease,
- some rare causes of hyperphosphataemic familial tumoral calcinosis.

Assessment of PTH Responsiveness

PTH acts via a second messenger, the stimulatory G-protein, which, when PTH-responsive cells, particularly renal tubules, are activated, normally gives rise to an increase in cAMP production. This can be measured in both plasma and urine under controlled circumstances. The so-called Ellsworth-Howard test was developed to enable responsiveness to be demonstrated, particularly in order to distinguish between hypoparathyroidism and pseudohypoparathyroidism (PHP). In practice, this test is rarely, if ever, undertaken nowadays both because synthetic PTH, either 1–34 or 1–84, has not, until recently, been available commercially and still is not available in quantities that are useful for this test without considerable wastage, and because the diagnosis of PHP has been overtaken by genetic methods that are able more precisely to identify the underlying mutation. Details of the test are therefore not given here but the reader is referred to the previous edition of this book should they be needed [18]. Measurement of cAMP is not a routine test but commercial kits are available if needed for research purposes.

In essence, stimulation by PTH results in a brisk response of cAMP of both plasma and urine in both normal subjects and those with hypoparathyroidism, whilst in PHP these responses are blunted or absent. Resistance of the cAMP response to

PTH can also be demonstrated in some patients with vitamin D deficiency, probably as a result of down regulation of the PTH receptors when PTH levels are moderately elevated. This may give confusion with some types of PHP and it is essential to ensure that vitamin D deficiency is corrected if necessary prior to undertaking this test.

Parathyroid Hormone-Related Peptide

PTHrP is a peptide whose presence was first suspected in studies of PTH bioactivity in neonatal cord blood in which significant PTH-like bioactivity was demonstrated despite the absence of immunoreactivity [19]. It was subsequently shown that this is responsible for maintaining the positive gradient of calcium across the placenta during foetal life although it is not normally present in measurable amounts during post natal life. It was also shown that some cases of hypercalcaemia associated with malignancy are caused by inappropriate secretion of PTHrP [20]. Whilst PTHrP probably acts as a classical hormone in utero and produces PTH-like hypercalcaemic effects in some cases of hypercalcaemia of malignancy, it also has important paracrine effects on chondrocyte proliferation and maturation.

Alternate splicing of PTHrP mRNA results in three different proteins of 139, 141 and 173 amino acids. They are identical in their C-terminal region as far as amino acid 139 and show close homology with PTH in the first 13 amino acids. PTHrP acts equipotently with PTH on the PTH1 receptors but does not stimulate PTH2 receptors. Assays for PTHrP are principally used in the diagnosis of hypercalcaemia of malignancy.

Measurement of PTHrP in Plasma

The variety of molecular forms of PTHrP means that immunoassay remains difficult. The absence of an agreed International standard also compounds comparison between methods. Assays for PTHrP include a two-site 1–72 IRMA and an N-terminal RIA. In normal and pathological samples the two methods showed a good correlation in PTHrP results and good discrimination between normal, primary hyperparathyroid and malignant humoral hypercalcaemia subjects. However, the IRMA was reported to be more sensitive and more practical than the RIA [21].

Blood samples should preferably be collected in the presence of protease inhibitors. The optimal collection technique is to use a lithium heparin tube with the protease inhibitor, aprotinin (Trasylol), at 500 kU/l. An EDTA tube is an acceptable alternative. Blood samples should be separated by centrifugation within two hours of collection and the plasma should be immediately assayed or stored frozen. Plasma samples stored frozen should be assayed within 30 days.

The kits have good precision performance with between run precision of <10% over the concentration range 30–900 ng/l. The analytical sensitivity is claimed to be 3 ng/l but in reality results are not reported if <20 ng/l.

The PTHrP antiserum has no cross-reactivity with other PTH and PTH fragments.

Normal ranges have been difficult to establish in children and are likely to show some degree of variability with age and to be assay-dependent. Most authors have suggested that levels below 2.5–3 pg/ml are within normal.

Indications for Measuring PTHrP

Measurement of PTHrP is rarely indicated in children. The only situation where it is needed is where hypercalcaemia is accompanied by undetectable PTH with no evidence of raised $1,25(OH)_2D$. In practice, this usually means that the hypercalcaemia is being caused by PTHrP secretion by a tumour and the origin of this should then be actively sought.

Calcitonin

Calcitonin (CT) is a 31 amino acid peptide that is secreted by the C-cells of the thyroid gland. It is secreted in response to hypercalcaemia and has an effect that is largely opposite to that of PTH [22]. However, it has little physiological effect in postnatal life although it probably plays an important role in promoting bone mineralisation during fetal life. Assays of CT are principally used for screening for medullary carcinoma of the thyroid which mainly occurs in multiple endocrine neoplasia type 2.

Measurement of Calcitonin

Measurement of calcitonin is complicated by the heterogeneity of the circulating forms especially in pathological cases. The lack of an agreed International Standard with a defined mass content means assessment of absolute accuracy between methods in not possible.

Calcitonin assays are classified into:
– Immunoradiometric (IRMA).
– Non-isotopic immunometric assays where the 'isotopic signal' has been replaced with a non-isotopic signal, e.g. chemiluminescence, or an enzyme.

The reader is advised to look at the automated platform kit insert for the exact details of the test principle.

Manual immunoassays generally use 0.2 ml serum to produce a result in duplicate while the semi-automated platforms use less serum (0.05–0.1 ml). The manual assays have between assay CV of about 8% at 10 ng/l while the semi-automated immunoassay platforms have marginally improved precision with a CV <5% at the same concentration. The detection limit of calcitonin assays is about 1 ng/l.

There are very few data on normal ranges for children using the immunometric assays. Values for normal infants (<40 ng/l for children under 6 months of age) and older children (<15 ng/l for children 6 months to 3 years age) and for children over three years of age values were indistinguishable from adults. However, the adult reference range was reported as <5 ng/l for females and <12 ng/l for males. All these values have been reported using the now discontinued Nichols Institute Diagnostics Advantage automated chemiluminescence immunoassay analyser. We use the DiaSorin Liaison automated immunometric analyser and its adult reference range is similar to the Nichols method, namely, adult females <5 ng/l and adult males <19 ng/l. However, the normal range in serum for healthy adults is approx <13 ng/l for females and <30 ng/l for males using a manual ELISA kit illustrating the differences between methods which is probably calibration related.

In summary, the reader is advised to look at the automated platform kit insert for the exact details of the test principle and the reference ranges.

Fibroblast Growth Factor 23

Fibroblast growth factor 23 (FGF23) was first described in 2000 [23] and is now thought to act as a classical hormone in that it is secreted by one gland, in this case mainly osteocytes of bone, circulates in plasma and has an action that is manifest at a distant location, namely renal tubules. It is secreted in response to a number of stimuli, particularly hyperphosphataemia, and is thought to be the 'phosphotonin' whose presence had been suspected for some years before being finally discovered. It is influenced by a number of factors including the phosphate-regulating gene with homologies to endopeptidases on the X chromosome (PHEX), dentin matrix protein 1 (DMP1) and a number of other similar SIBLING proteins. FGF23 is inactivated by cleavage, between the arginine and serine residues at positions 179 and 180, into two inactive fragments. X-linked hypophosphataemic rickets (XLHR) is caused by mutations in the PHEX gene that probably interferes with the natural cleavage by influencing the subtilisin/furin activity that causes this cleavage. Autosomal-dominant hypophosphataemic rickets (ADHR) results from mutations in the FGF23 gene itself that inhibit cleavage which results in raised levels of intact circulating FGF23, whilst autosomal-recessive hypophophataemic rickets is the product of mutations in the DMP1 gene that also raise FGF23 levels. FGF23 levels are also raised in other forms of acquired hypophosphataemia such as the McCune-Albright and Epidermal Naevus syndromes. Thus, in all these syndromes, FGF23 levels are inappropriately raised. Tumours that cause oncogenic (OO), or tumour-induced osteomalacia (TIO) have been shown to over express FGF-23 mRNA making it likely that elevated concentrations of FGF-23 in the blood are the cause of renal phosphate wasting in this group of patients [24]. This probably occurs as a result of derepression of one or other of the genes controlling the SIBLING proteins mentioned above.

In contrast, in hereditary hypophosphataemic rickets with hypercalciuria (HHRH), FGF23 levels are low or absent since the hypophosphataemia which results from mutations in the sodium/phosphate co-transporter in renal tubules that causes the phosphate leak suppresses FGF23 synthesis.

There are also several syndromes associated with hyperphosphataemia and soft tissue calcification that are related to abnormalities in FGF23 metabolism. These are known as the hyperphosphataemic familial tumoral calcinoses, of which three kinds are described [5]. Levels of FGF23 found in these conditions vary according to the assay method used, depending on whether C-terminal or intact assays are employed.

Measurement of FGF23

There are two commercial ELISA kits available for FGF-23 analysis. Sample collection is critical in both methods as intact FGF-23 appears to be highly unstable resulting in decreased plasma concentrations with time. Specimen collection must be performed in an expeditious manner. The sample should be collected in the morning following an overnight fast into an EDTA collection tube. The sample should then be sent to the laboratory immediately and centrifuged to separate the plasma. The separated plasma is frozen immediately and stored frozen (–20°C) until analysis.

Assay sensitivity is reported as 1 ng/l and between assay imprecision is <7% at ~15 and 150 ng/l concentrations. There are few data reporting normal FGF23 levels in children and the results depend on whether a C-terminal or Intact molecule assay is being employed [25].

Indications for Measurement of FGF23

There are currently few indications for measurement of FGF23 and it remains a largely research-based procedure. However, it may be useful in monitoring treatment of the various forms of hypophosphataemic rickets [26] and, as newer treatments for these conditions, particularly the use of FGF23 antibodies, become available it is likely to acquire increasing importance. It can also be of value in determining the cause of some of the other conditions associated with abnormal phosphate metabolism such as TIO or hyperphosphataemic familial tumoral calcinoses.

Approach to the Laboratory Investigations of Calcium Disorders

Any child who presents with either hypocalcaemia, hypercalcaemia or rickets requires a systematic approach to diagnosis. In all cases it is essential to start with routine measurements of calcium (either total or ionised), phosphate, albumin, magnesium, creatinine, PTH and 25OHD. Urine should also be taken for measurement of calcium, phosphate, creatinine and, if necessary, magnesium. It is also helpful to take samples for measurement of $1,25(OH)_2D$ to be assayed later. At some stage, either at presentation or later, blood should also be taken for appropriate DNA analysis if it seems that there is a genetic cause of the pathology. However, the results of these investigations must be interpreted with caution. Thus, for instance, it is not possible to make a definitive diagnosis of either rickets or hypocalcaemia until vitamin D deficiency has been excluded or, if necessary, effectively treated.

Radiological examination to detect the presence of rickets or soft tissue calcification, ultrasound of the kidneys for nephrocalcinosis and CT scan of the head to assess the presence of intracranial calcification and nuclear medicine investigations such as SestaMIBI scan for parathyroid tumours may then be required to confirm a diagnosis of parathyroid tumour. Finally, close liaison with geneticists is required in order to be able to confirm a genetically determined condition.

Normal ranges for the main factors involved in mineral metabolism are shown in table 1 and details of the abnormalities of the measurable parameters in disorders of the principal causes of hypocalcaemia, hypercalcaemia and rickets are shown in table 2. By using these and taking a systematic approach to laboratory investigations, it should be possible to make a correct diagnosis. This should then lead to appropriate treatment which is possible in most cases.

References

1 Clase CM, Norman GL, Beecroft ML, Churchill DN: Albumin-corrected calcium and ionized calcium in stable haemodialysis patients. Nephrol Dial Transplant 2000;15:1841–1846.

2 Round JM, Butcher S, Steele R: Changes in plasma inorganic phosphorus and alkaline phosphatase activity during the adolescent growth spurt. Ann Hum Biol 1979;6:129.

3 Kruse K, Kracht U, Kruse U: Reference values for urinary calcium excretion and screening for hypercalciuria in children and adolescents. Eur J Pediatr 1984;143:25–31.

4 Shaw NJ, Wheeldon J, Brocklebank JT: The tubular maximum for calcium reabsorption: a normal range in children. Clin Endocrinol (Oxf) 1992;36:193–195.

5 Bergwitz C, Juppner H: Disorders of phosphate homeostasis and tissue mineralisation. Endocr Dev 2009;16:133–156.

6 Walton RJ, Bijvoet OL: Nomogram for derivation of renal threshold phosphate concentration. Lancet 1975;ii:309–310.

7 Allgrove J, Adami S, Fraher L, Reuben A, O'Riordan JL: Hypomagnesaemia: studies of parathyroid hormone secretion and function. Clin Endocrinol (Oxf) 1984;21:435–449.

8 Allgrove J: Physiology of calcium, phosphate and magnesium. Endocr Dev 2009;16:8–31.

9 Whyte MP: Enzyme defects and the skeleton; in Rosen CJ (ed): Primer on the Metabolic Bone Diseases and Disorders of Mineral Metabolism, ed 7. Washington, American Society for Bone and Mineral Research, 2008, pp 454–458.

10 ZRT Laboratories for DEQAS Optimal Clinical Relevance for LC-MS/MS Testing of Vitamin D: http://www.zrtlab.com/download-document/49-optimal-clinical-relevance-for-lc-ms/ms-testing-of-vitamin-d.html

11 Reinhardt TA, Horst RL, Orf JW, Hollis BW: A microassay for 1,25-dihydroxyvitamin D not requiring high performance liquid chromatography: application to clinical studies. J Clin Endocrinol Metab 1984;58:91–98.

12 National Kidney Foundation: K/DOQI clinical practice guidelines for bone metabolism and disease in chronic kidney disease. Am J Kidney Dis 2003; 42(suppl 3):S1–S201.

13 Habener JF, Potts JT Jr: Biosynthesis of parathyroid hormone. Part 1. N Engl J Med 1978;299:580–585.

14 Habener JF, Potts JT Jr: Biosynthesis of parathyroid hormone. Part 2. N Engl J Med 1978;299:635–644.

15 Berson SA, Yalow RS: Immunochemical heterogeneity of parathyroid hormone in plasma. J Clin Endocrinol Metab 1968;28:1037–1047.

16 Berson SA, Yalow RS, Aurbach GD, Potts JT: Immunoassay of bovine and human parathyroid hormone. Proc Natl Acad Sci USA 1963;49:613–617.

17 Cole DE, Webb S, Chan PC: Update on parathyroid hormone: new tests and new challenges for external quality assessment. Clin Biochem 2007;40:585–590.

18 Kruse K: Vitamin D and parathyroid; in Ranke MB (ed): Diagnostics of Endocrine Function in Children and Adolescents. Basel, Karger, 2003, pp 240–258.

19 Allgrove J, Adami S, Manning RM, O'Riordan JL: Cytochemical bioassay of parathyroid hormone in maternal and cord blood. Arch Dis Child 1985;60:110–115.

20 Mundy GR, Edwards JR: PTH-related peptide (PTHrP) in hypercalcemia. J Am Soc Nephrol 2008; 19:672–675.

21 Minebois-Villegas A, Audran M, Lortholary A, Legrand E, Boux DC-R, Jallet P: Performances of two kits for parathyroid hormone-related peptide (PTHrP) assay in the additional study of malignant hypercalcemias. Pathol Biol (Paris) 1995;43:799–805.

22 Copp DH: Calcitonin – a new hormone from the parathyroid which lowers blood calcium. Oral Surg Oral Med Oral Pathol 1963;16:872–877.

23 Yamashita T, Yoshioka M, Itoh N: Identification of a novel fibroblast growth factor, FGF-23, preferentially expressed in the ventrolateral thalamic nucleus of the brain. Biochem Biophys Res Commun 2000; 277:494–498.

24 Shimada T, Mizutani S, Muto T, et al: Cloning and characterization of FGF23 as a causative factor of tumor-induced osteomalacia. Proc Natl Acad Sci USA 2001;98:6500–6505.

25 Brown WW, Juppner H, Langman CB, Price H, Farrow EG, White KE et al.: Hypophosphatemia with elevations in serum fibroblast growth factor 23 in a child with Jansen's metaphyseal chondrodysplasia. J Clin Endocrinol Metab 2009;94:17–20.

26 Endo I, Fukumoto S, Ozono K, et al: Clinical usefulness of measurement of fibroblast growth factor 23 (FGF23) in hypophosphatemic patients: proposal of diagnostic criteria using FGF23 measurement. Bone 2008;42:1235–1239.

Dr. Jeremy Allgrove
Royal London Hospital, Whitechapel
London E1 1BB (UK)
Tel. +44 0 20 7377 7468, Fax +44 0 20 7377 7372
E-Mail Jeremy.allgrove@bartsandthelondon.nhs.uk

Ranke MB, Mullis P-E (eds): Diagnostics of Endocrine Function in Children and Adolescents, ed 4.
Basel, Karger, 2011, pp 260–272

Hyperinsulinism, Neonatal Hypoglycemia, New Mechanisms

Vassili Valayannopoulos[a] · Pascale de Lonlay[a] · Michel Polak[b]

[a]Metabolic Department and Reference Centre for Metabolic Diseases, and [b]Pediatric Endocrinology, AP-HP,
Reference Center for Rare Endocrine Disorders of Growth, INSERM U845, Necker-Enfants Malades Hospital,
Université Paris Descartes, Paris, France

Hypoglycemia, defined by a glucose plasma level below 3 mmol/l (55 mg/dl) in children and below 2 (1st 24 h of life) to 2.5 mmol/l (35–45 mg/dl) in neonates, can be a life-threatening situation that needs to be assessed rigorously in order to treat efficiently and avoid relapse that can be responsible for cerebral damage [1]. Hypoglycemia results from an impairment of glucose homeostasis and the diagnosis of its causes requires a good knowledge of the complex mechanisms which maintain blood glucose concentration between the narrow range of 2.5 and 6.6 mmol/l in the fasting or fed state [2]. The clinical history and presentation, when available, may allow diagnosing the cause of hypoglycemias in more than 90% of patients. Those diagnostic aspects will be developed in another chapter of this book and will therefore only be briefly exposed [pp. 273–293].

The main clinical criteria for diagnosis are the timing of hypoglycemia with respect to the last meal and the presence or absence of an enlarged liver (table 1). Associated symptoms, like responsiveness to glucagon administration, vomiting, bleeding or a multiorgan failure may also be essential to orientate diagnosis. Simple biochemical data such as blood lactate and blood and urine ketone bodies, easily measured in urine using a ketone-detecting dipstick, are also important diagnostic clues, especially in fasting hypoglycemias.

During feeding, the liver builds up energy stores in the form of glycogen and triglycerides, the latter being exported to adipose tissue. On the opposite, during fasting, it releases glucose and ketone bodies. The maintenance of a normal blood glucose level depends upon: (1) hepatic glycogenolytic and gluconeogenic enzymes; (2) an adequate supply of endogenous gluconeogenic substrates (amino acids, glycerol and lactate); (3) an adequate energy supply provided by β-oxidation of fatty acids needed to synthesize glucose and ketone bodies, the latter being exported to peripheral tissues

Table 1. Diagnostic clues, confirmation and molecular tests as well as specific treatment for the most frequent genetic causes of hypoglycemia.

Disease	Clues to diagnosis	Diagnostic tests	Specific treatment
Hyperinsulinism	pre- and post-prandial hypoglycemia, positive glucagon response, inappropriately high insulin levels for plasma glucose <2.7 mmol/l (50 mg/dl)	molecular screening SUR1/Kir 6.1/other genes [^{18}F]fluoro-DOPA PET scan	diazoxide, somatostatin, calcium channel blockers, pancreatic surgery
Fatty acid oxidation disorders	fasting hypoketotic (free fatty acids/ketone bodies >2 mmol/l) hypoglycemia, multi-organ failure, abnormal organic acids, acylcarnitins	overall FAO and specific enzymatic assays and molecular diagnosis enzymatic and molecular studies	prevent fasting and lipolysis by dietary treatment, MCT in long chain FAO disorders, L-carnitine
Glycogen storage disorders	short fasting hypoglycemia, permanent hepatomegaly, negative glucagon response, high lactate (when gluconeogensis also impaired), high triglycerides and uric acid	enzymatic and molecular studies	dietary treatment: raw cornstarch between meals, continuous night feeding
Neoglucogenesis disorders	fasting hypoglycemia, hepatomegaly during hypoglycemia, high lactate and alanine	enzymatic and molecular studies	prevent prolonged fasting and catabolic states
Ketone bodies synthesis	fasting hypoketotic hypoglycemia	enzymatic and molecular studies	prevent prolonged fasting and catabolic states
Ketolysis defects and organic acidurias	fasting hypoglycemia, severe ketoacidosis, coma	enzymatic and molecular studies	prevent prolonged fasting and catabolic states
Hormonal deficiencies	no specific timing for adrenal insufficiency, microphallus, growth failure, fasting hypoglycemia for GHD	function tests, molecular studies	hormonal treatment

and preferentially used as an alternative fuel to glucose; (4) a normal endocrine system for integrating and modulating these processes. At all these steps genetic causes can be described. The major signals, which control the transition between the fed (postprandial) and the fasting states, are glucose, insulin and glucagon blood levels

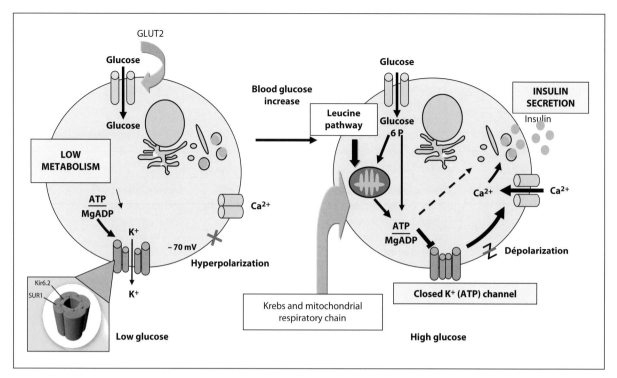

Fig. 1. Schematic representation of the regulation of insulin secretion by the pancreatic β-cell. GLUT2 catalyses glucose uptake by β-cells. Glucokinase, the enzyme that initiates β-cell glucose metabolism, has a high Km for glucose and, thus, the circulating concentrations of glucose directly determine the rate of glucose oxidation and subsequent release of insulin. Glucose and leucine, a potent positive allosteric effector of glutamate dehydrogenase (GDH) interacts with the Krebs cycle activity resulting in ATP synthesis in the mitochondria. This results in an increase of the intracellular ratio of ATP/ADP ratio that activates a plasma membrane protein, the sulfonylurea receptor (SUR1), to cause the closure of the potassium channel (K_{ATP}), leading to depolarization of the cell membrane, influx of extracellular calcium and release of insulin from storage granules. An increased GDH activity resulting by mutations of the GDH gene (dominant positive effect) is responsible for increased α-ketoglutarate levels and consecutively increased Krebs cycle activity and β-cell ATP/ADP ratio, and subsequently an exaggerated insulin release. These regulation mechanisms account for the efficacy of medical treatments such as diazoxide, somatostatin and in protein (leucine)-restricted diet on insulin secretion. GLUT2 = Glucose transporter; Krebs = Krebs cycle; Kir6.2 = inward-rectifying potassium channel; SUR1 = regulatory subunit of the potassium channel.

[3,4]. A diagnostic algorithm including the genetic studies is presented in table 1. Based on the origin of the glucose in blood, it is possible to divide glucose homeostasis time course into 5 phases. The timing of hypoglycemia with respect to the last meal is a valuable diagnostic element. The diagnostic algorithm is presented in figure 1. The glucagon test is a useful diagnostic test for short-fasting hypoglycemia (<8 h of fasting). It is considered as 'positive' when blood glucose levels double within the first 15 min following the injection of 1 mg of glucagon parenterally. Hereditary

intolerance of galactose and fructose are two rare causes of postprandial hypoglycemia that are not displayed in the table 1 and are always associated to specific digestive signs (vomiting) and liver dysfunction.

Recently new causes of hypoglycemia such as glucose transporter disorders, respiratory chain disorders and congenital disorders of glycosylation have been identified. In addition, new genes and syndromes have been reported in hyperinsulinism (HI), which can be considered as the mirror of diabetes. In this article, we will focus in new genetic causes of hypoglycemia that give insight in the complex regulatory mechanism of blood glucose but also cite the more classic endocrine ones.

Congenital Hyperinsulinism

General Concept

Hyperinsulinism is a heterogeneous disorder of primary origin or in rare cases secondary to other defects. In the latter, hypoglycemia is not isolated. The diagnostic criteria for congenital hyperinsulinism (HI) are given in table 1. In the neonatal period diagnosis is often easy, mostly based on the severity of hypoglycemia occurring within 72 h after birth and the glucagon responsiveness. The majority of newborns display macrosomy at birth. Hypoglycemia is always severe, revealed by seizures in many cases, with risk of brain damage [1, 5, 6]. The rates of administered glucose required to prevent hypoglycemia are elevated to values close to 17 mg/kg/mn in our series. Most often, no other symptoms are associated with hypoglycemia. Facial dysmorphism with high forehead, large and bulbous nose with short columella, smooth philtrum and thin upper lip is frequently observed in all types of hyperinsulinism [6].

Hyperinsulinemic hypoglycemia is due to an inappropriate insulin secretion by the β cells of Langerhans islets. Insulin is the only hormone to lower glucose concentration in plasma. It does it by both inhibiting glucose release from hepatic glycogen and by increasing glucose uptake in muscle cells. This explains the two main characteristic clinical findings of neonatal HI: the high glucose requirement to correct hypoglycemia and the responsiveness of hypoglycemia to exogenous glucagon. Several pathways are involved in the regulation of insulin secretion by the pancreatic β-cell, and this helps to explain the effectiveness of the different medical treatments, such as oral diazoxide (5–15 mg/kg/day), somatostatin injections (10–50 μg/day in 3 injections or continuous infusion), calcium channel inhibitors (nifedipine 0.5–2 mg/kg/day) and protein (leucine) restricted diet [7– 9] (fig. 1).

Patients who are resistant to medical treatment and require surgical treatment have to be classified according to histological criteria [10]. A focal form is defined as a focal adenomatous hyperplasia. In the diffuse HI, histological abnormalities involve the whole pancreas [11]. In the absence of any distinctive clinical feature, a pancreatic venous catheterization and sampling of glucose, insulin and C-peptide [11] and pancreatic arteriography were until recently the only preoperative procedures available for locating the site of insulin secretion. Recently, an 18-fluoro-DOPA PET scan has shown efficacy in distinguishing focal from diffuse forms. Pancreatic β-cells are neuroendocrine cells and can take up [18F]fluoro-L-dopa converted into dopamine by DOPA decarboxylase. A good correlation between the localization of DOPA decarboxylase and proinsulin in normal pancreas and in both diffuse and focal HI tissues has been demonstrated by immunochemistry studies on pancreatic surgical samples [12].

Dysfunction of ATP-Sensitive Potassium Channel

The most common mechanism underlying HI is dysfunction of the pancreatic ATP-sensitive potassium channel (K^+_{ATP}). The two subunits of the K^+_{ATP} channel are encoded by the sulfonylurea receptor gene *(SUR1 subunit by ABCC8)* and the inward-rectifying potassium channel gene *(KIR6.2 subunit by KCNJ11)*, both located in the 11p15.1 region. HI 'channelopathies' are due to inhibiting SUR1 or KIR6.2 mutations. These mutations can lead to type 1 channelopathy without channel activity, or to type 2 channelopathy with a decreased channel activity due either to defective function, or to decreased number of channels. Heterogeneous outcome is observed for the same mutation as some cells manifest a type 1 channelopathy, others a type 2 channelopathy, and other mutated cells have a normal activity of the potassium channel [13, 14]. This observation could be explained by interactions with modulator genes, exogenous factors, or variable degree of penetrance of the mutation.

Mutations of *SUR1* gene are responsible for 50–60% of HI, whether focal or diffuse HI, especially in neonates. More than 100 distinct mutations, distributed throughout the *SUR1* gene, have already been described. Mutations of *KIR6.2* gene are less frequent and are responsible for 10–15% of HI [15, 16].

The histopathological lesions associated with neonatal HI may be described as diffuse or focal. Focal adenomatous islet cell hyperplasia is sporadic and has been demonstrated to arise in individuals who have a germline mutation in the paternal allele of the sulfonylurea-receptor *SUR1* gene or the inward-rectifying potassium-channel *Kir6.2* in addition to a somatic loss of the maternally derived chromosome region 11p15 in adenomatous pancreatic β-cells. Diffuse HI may be familial and arises from the autosomal recessive inheritance of mutations in both *SUR1* and *Kir6.2* genes. The therapeutic outcome for the patients is heavily dependent upon distinguishing between the two histopathological lesions. Diffuse HI, which are unresponsive to medical treatment, require extensive pancreatectomy with a high risk of diabetes. Conversely, focal HI can be cured by limited pancreatectomy. Genetic counseling is dramatically different as focal HI is considered a sporadic molecular event with a very low recurrence risk, while diffuse HI is inherited in a recessive pattern for neonatal onset forms and dominant or sporadic transmission for late onset HI [17].

Hyperinsulinism may be also due to metabolic causes where increase of the ATP/ADP ratio in pancreatic β-cells is responsible for inappropriate insulin secretion (fig. 1). In these cases, the K^+_{ATP} channels are functional explaining the fact that hypoglycemia responds to treatment by diazoxide.

Valayannopoulos · de Lonlay · Polak

Hyperinsulinism-Hyperammonemia Syndrome

The second most common form of congenital hyperinsulinism, the hyperinsulinism/hyperammonemia syndrome (HIHA), is associated with dominantly expressed missense mutations of the mitochondrial enzyme, glutamate dehydrogenase (GDH). GDH catalyzes the oxidative deamination of glutamate to α-ketoglutarate plus ammonia. HIHA mutations impair GDH sensitivity to its allosteric inhibitor, GTP, resulting in a gain of enzyme function and increased sensitivity to its allosteric activator, leucine. The phenotype is dominated by hypoglycemia, usually postprandial, following high-protein meals, as well as fasting hypoglycemia. Plasma ammonia levels are increased 3–5 times normal due to expression of mutant GDH in liver, probably reflecting increased ammonia release from glutamate as well as impaired synthesis of N-acetyl glutamate, due to reduction of hepatic glutamate pools. Ammonia levels are unaffected by feeding or fasting [18]. However, some patients present epilepsy and mental retardation that may be related to effects of GDH mutations in the brain, perhaps in combination with effects of recurrent hypoglycemia and chronic hyperammonemia [19].

Dominantly Expressed Glucokinase Mutations

Glucokinase (GK) mutations are a rare cause of HI [20]. They result in a gain of function by increased affinity of GK for glucose leading to inappropriate insulin secretion. These mutations are remote from the glucose-binding site and suggest an allosteric regulation defect.

Short Chain 3-Hydroxyacyl-CoA Dehydrogenase Deficiency

A few hyperinsulinemic patients have been reported to have a mutation in the gene encoding short-chain 3-hydroxyacyl-CoA dehydrogenase (SCHAD), an enzyme participating in mitochondrial fatty acid oxidation. The patients present with neonatal severe hyperinsulinism, enhanced levels of 3-hydroxybutyryl-carnitine in their blood plasma and greatly reduced SCHAD activity in fibroblasts. Urine metabolite analysis showed that SCHAD deficiency resulted in specific excretion of 3-hydroxyglutaric acid [21]. Recent reports suggest that mitochondrial fatty acid oxidation influences insulin secretion through a K^+_{ATP} channel-independent mechanism [22].

Exercise-Induced Hyperinsulinism

Exercise-induced hyperinsulinism is a novel, autosomal-dominant form of HI, which has been identified in two families. The patients suffer from hypoglycemic symptoms only when performing strenuous physical exercise [23]. The underlying mechanism of hypoglycemia is unclear, but probably linked to anaerobic glycolysis as pyruvate administration leads to increased insulin secretion and hypoglycemia and seems to be a reliable diagnostic test of this condition.

Many other genes could also be involved in HI, particularly those playing a role in insulin secretion, as recently described with *HNF4A* mutations in maturity-onset diabetes (MODY) and HI [24] and mutations of the insulin receptor (*INSR*) gene that was recently implicated in a dominant form of hyperinsulinemic hypoglycemia [25]. Patients presented with postprandial as well as fasting hyperinsulinemic hypoglycemia associated with resistance to insulin. Mutations in the gene encoding prohormone convertase-1 leading to abnormal or absent proinsulin processing are also responsible for hyperinsulinemic-like hypoglycemia, associated with diarrhea and obesity [26].

Genetic Syndromes Associated with Hyperinsulinism and Hypoglycemia

Finally, hyperinsulinemic hypoglycemia can be 'syndromic' as observed in the following overlapping syndromes:

Overgrowth Syndromes with Diazoxide-Senitive Hypoglycemia
Beckwith-Wiedemann Syndrome (BWS). BWS has to be searched when exomphalos, macroglossia, or gigantism including length are noted, since the patients have a increased risk of developing specific tumors [27]. BWS results from several identified genetic and epigenetic molecular events including paternal isodisomy, abnormal methylation of *IGF2/H19*, chromosomal aberrations involving the 11p15 region, and *CDKN1C* mutation. Hypoglycemia in BWS patients has been associated with paternal uniparental disomy of 11p15 rather than other genetic abnormalities, but the pathophysiological mechanism leading to hyperinsulinic hypoglycemia is still unclear as no evidence for duplication of *INS*, *HRAS1* and *IGF2* or overexpression of the *INS* and *IGF2* genes was found [28, 29]. Simpson-Golabi-Behmel syndrome (SGBS) is an X-linked condition that shows phenotypic similarities to Beckwith-Wiedemann syndrome Shared clinical features of BWS and SGBS include macrosomia, macroglossia, cleft palate, visceromegaly, earlobe creases, hernias, neonatal hypoglycemia, and a risk of embryonal tumors [30].

Perlman Syndrome and Sotos Syndrome. Two overgrowth syndromes that have been associated with congenital hyperinsulinism [31, 32]. The mechanisms of hypoglycemia in syndromic HI with gigantism remain unclear. Hyperplasia of β-cells, due to the overexpression of IGF2 and/or an imbalance between IGF2 and tumor suppressor genes (H19, P57) has been suggested. In Sotos syndrome a majority of patients displayed mutations on the NSD1 gene, that could be involved in imprinting of the 11p15 region [31].

Usher Syndrome Type 1C
Usher syndrome type 1 describes the association of profound, congenital sensorineural deafness, vestibular hypofunction and childhood onset retinitis pigmentosa. It is an autosomal recessive condition and is subdivided on the basis of linkage analysis into types 1A through 1E. Usher type 1C maps to the region containing the genes

ABCC8 and KCNJ11 (encoding components of ATP-sensitive K$^+$ (KATP) channels), which may be deleted in patients who present with hyperinsulinism [33].

Kabuki Syndrome
Kabuki syndrome (KS) is a rare multiple congenital syndrome with an estimated frequency of 1/32,000 in Japan. Five major criteria delineate KS namely postnatal short stature, skeletal anomalies, moderate mental retardation, dermatoglyphic anomalies, and a characteristic facial dysmorphism. Some rare and atypical features have been reported including chronic and/or severe diarrhea, diaphragmatic defects, pseudarthrosis of the clavicles, vitiligo and persistent hypoglycemia. Hypoglycemia in KS, which can be underestimated, may be to due to HI or to growth hormone deficiency. The molecular basis of KS remains unknown.

Congenital Disorders of Glycosylation
Congenital disorders of glycosylation (CDG) are genetic defects in the assembly of the carbohydrate moiety of glycoconjugates. This results in abnormal structure and function of proteins in many organs. The clinical spectrum of the disease in children is heterogeneous. Phosphomannose-mutase deficiency (CDG type Ia) is a multisystemic disease with dysmorphic features (abnormal fat distribution and inverted nipples), significant neurologic involvement (hypotonia, hyporeflexia, ataxia, convulsions, and psychomotor retardation), and failure to thrive. Other features are cerebellar hypoplasia, hypothyroidism, thyroxin-binding globulin (TBG) deficiency, strabismus, retinitis pigmentosa, vomiting, feeding difficulties, hepatomegaly, liver fibrosis, elevated transaminase concentration, coagulopathy, and hypoalbuminemia. Children may have cardiomyopathy, pericardial effusion, protein-losing enteropathy, or lymphedema. In phosphomannose-isomerase deficiency (CDG type Ib) neurologic symptoms are usually absent. Clinical presentations are hypoglycemia, hypothyroidism, TBG deficiency, vomiting, feeding difficulties, diarrhea, failure to thrive, protein-losing enteropathy, hepatomegaly, elevated transaminase concentration, congenital hepatic liver fibrosis, and coagulopathy. Children with CDG type Ia and those with type Ib may have hyperinsulinemia and hypoglycemia, occurring most frequently during episodes of gastroenteritis [8]. Children with CDG type Ib should be treated with mannose. Patients with CDG type I can be identified by isoelectric focusing of serum transferrin, enzyme analysis, and/or DNA analysis.

Endocrine Causes

Growth Hormone Signaling Deficiency and Growth Hormone Resistance
Whereas insulin dominates periprandially, growth hormone (GH) may be viewed as the primary anabolic hormone during stress and fasting [34]. GH exerts anabolic effects directly and through stimulation of IGF-1, insulin, and free fatty acids (FFA).

When subjects are well nourished, the GH-induced stimulation of IGF-1 and insulin is important for anabolic storage and growth of lean body mass (LBM), adipose tissue, and glycogen reserves. During fasting and other catabolic states, GH predominantly stimulates the release and oxidation of FFA, which leads to decreased glucose and protein oxidation and preservation of LBM and glycogen stores. The most prominent metabolic effect of GH is a marked increase in lipolysis and FFA levels. GH is a counter-regulatory hormone that antagonizes the hepatic and peripheral effects of insulin on glucose metabolism via mechanisms involving the concomitant increase in FFA flux and uptake. This ability of GH to induce insulin resistance is significant for the defense against hypoglycemia. Children with profound GH deficiency and resistance are prone therefore to hypoglycemia, especially the youngest ones [35–38, see 39 for a comprehensive review].

Primary Adrenal Deficiency and Corticotroph Deficiency
Fasting hypoglycemia is well described in adrenal insufficiency, due to the well described role of cortisol on glucose metabolism. In the fasted state, cortisol stimulates several processes that collectively serve to increase and maintain normal concentrations of glucose in blood. These effects include: (1) Stimulation of gluconeogenesis, particularly in the liver: this pathway results in the synthesis of glucose from non-hexose substrates such as amino acids and lipids. Enhancing the expression of enzymes involved in gluconeogenesis is probably the best known metabolic function of glucocorticoids. (2) Mobilization of amino acids from extrahepatic tissues: these serve as substrates for gluconeogenesis. (3) Inhibition of glucose uptake in muscle and adipose tissue: a mechanism to conserve glucose. (4) Stimulation of fat breakdown in adipose tissue: the fatty acids released by lipolysis are used for production of energy in tissues like muscle, and the released glycerol provide another substrate for gluconeogenesis [40]. Hypoglycemia is more common in secondary adrenal insufficiency possibly due to concomitant growth hormone insufficiency and in isolated ACTH deficiency [41].

Metabolic Causes of Hypoglycemia not Associated to Hyperinsulinism
Glucose Transporter Deficiencies
Fanconi-Bickel Syndrome (GLUT2 Deficiency). Here is the place to recall the fascinating story of the Fanconi Bickel syndrome (FBS), the pathophysiology of which was recently identified [42, 43]. FBS is a rare well-defined clinical entity, inherited in an autosomal recessive mode. It is characterized by hepatorenal glycogen accumulation. Fasting hypoglycemia, as well as postprandial hyperglycemia and hypergalactosemia, indicate an impaired utilization of these two monosaccharides, and a proximal renal tubular dysfunction. In contrast to other types of glycogen storage diseases caused by enzymatic defects of glycogenolysis, FBS has recently been shown to result from a defective monosaccharide transporter, GLUT2, in cell membranes of different tissues. It thus represents the first disease with hypoglycemia caused by a defect of a member

of the facilitative glucose transporter family. The diagnosis of this disorder, easily suspected on the very suggestive clinical pattern, relies upon the molecular investigation of the GLUT2 gene [43]. Defects in GLUT1 activity, another glucose transporter, is responsible for infantile seizures, acquired microcephaly, and developmental delay [44] but not hypoglycemia. This deficiency results in reduced cerebrospinal fluid glucose concentrations (hypoglycorrhachia) and reduced erythrocyte glucose transporter activities in the patients. The appropriate diagnosis is important as a ketogenic diet can improve symptoms.

Respiratory Chain Deficiency. We recently described 2 patients affected with respiratory chain deficiency (complex III and complex IV deficiency) who presented with isolated recurrent attacks of fasting hypoglycemia [45]. During a fasting test, the first patient showed evidence for impaired gluconeogenesis (progressive increase of plasma lactate and no decrease of alanine levels), whereas the second patient appeared to have impaired fatty acid oxidation (hypoketotic hypoglycemia with increased levels of non esterified fatty acids). In both cases lack of ATP has been suggested to be responsible for secondary deficiency of ATP-dependant enzymes of gluconeogenesis.

Citrin Deficiency. A deficiency of citrin, which is encoded by the SLC25A13 gene, causes both adult-onset type II citrullinemia (CTLN2) and neonatal intrahepatic cholestasis (NICCD). The clinical features of the disease in neonates and infants include mainly severe intrahepatic cholestasis with fatty liver and variable accompanying clinical features, namely: failure to thrive, hemolytic anemia, bleeding tendencies and ketotic hypoglycemia. Laboratory data show elevated serum bile acid levels, hypoproteinemia, low levels of vitamin K-dependent coagulation factors, and hypergalactosemia. Hypercitrullinemia is detected in most patients. Most of the reported patients were given a lactose-free and/or medium chain triglycerides-enriched formula and lipid-soluble vitamins. Symptoms resolved in most patients by 12 months of age. However a few patients suffered from progressive liver failure and underwent liver transplantation before their first birthday. Another patient developed citrullinemia type II (CTLN2) at age of 16 years [46, 47].

Conclusions and Research Directions

In our experience, most of the genetic causes of hypoglycemia are rather easy to elucidate. The diagnosis relies upon a limited number of parameters, mostly clinical and some simple biological tests. New genetic syndromes have been discovered most of them associated to hyperinsulinic hypoglycemia and new genes will probably be discovered implicated in hypoglycemia, namely all the genes playing a role in glucose regulation.

References

1 Hawdon JM: Hypoglycaemia and the neonatal brain. Eur J Pediatr 1999;158(suppl 1):S9–S12.

2 Cornblath M, Schwartz R, Aynsley-Green A, Lloyd JK: Hypoglycemia in infancy: the need for a rational definition. a Ciba Foundation discussion meeting. Pediatrics 1990;85:834–837.

3 Pagliara AS, Karl IE, Haymond M, Kipnis DM: Hypoglycemia in infancy and childhood. I. J Pediatr 1973;82:365–379.

4 Van den Berghe G: The role of the liver in metabolic homeostasis: implications for inborn errors of metabolism. J Inherit Metab Dis 1991;14:407–420.

5 de Lonlay-Debeney P, Poggi-Travert F, Fournet JC, Sempoux C, Vici CD, Brunelle F, Touati G, Rahier J, Junien C, Nihoul-Fekete C, Robert JJ, Saudubray JM: Clinical features of 52 neonates with hyperinsulinism. N Engl J Med 1999;340:1169–1175.

6 de Lonlay P, Cormier-Daire V, Amiel J, Touati G, Goldenberg A, Fournet JC, Brunelle F, Nihoul-Fekete C, Rahier J, Junien C, Robert JJ, Saudubray JM: Facial appearance in persistent hyperinsulinemic hypoglycaemia. Am J Med Genet 2002;111:130–133.

7 de Lonlay P, Cuer M, Vuillaumier-Barrot S, Beaune G, Castelnau P, Kretz M, Durand G, Saudubray JM, Seta N: Hyperinsulinemic hypoglycemia as a presenting sign in phosphomannose isomerase deficiency: a new manifestation of carbohydrate-deficient glycoprotein syndrome treatable with mannose. J Pediatr 1999;135:379–383.

8 Kane C, Shepherd RM, Squires PE, Johnson PR, James RF, Milla PJ, Aynsley-Green A, Lindley KJ, Dunne MJ: Loss of functional KATP channels in pancreatic beta-cells causes persistent hyperinsulinemic hypoglycemia of infancy. Nat Med 1996;2:1344–1347.

9 Lindley KJ, Dunne MJ, Kane C, Shepherd RM, Squires PE, James RF, Johnson PR, Eckhardt S, Wakeling E, Dattani M, Milla PJ, Aynsley-Green A: Ionic control of beta cell function in nesidioblastosis: a possible therapeutic role for calcium channel blockade. Arch Dis Child 1996;74:373–378.

10 Rahier J, Sempoux C, Fournet JC, Poggi F, Brunelle F, Nihoul-Fekete C, Saudubray JM, Jaubert F: Partial or near-total pancreatectomy for persistent neonatal hyperinsulinaemic hypoglycaemia: the pathologist's role. Histopathology 1998;32:15–19.

11 Dubois J, Brunelle F, Touati G, Sebag G, Nuttin C, Thach T, Nikoul-Fekete C, Rahier J, Saudubray JM: Hyperinsulinism in children: diagnostic value of pancreatic venous sampling correlated with clinical, pathological and surgical outcome in 25 cases. Pediatr Radiol 1995;25:512–516.

12 de Lonlay P, Simon-Carre A, Ribeiro MJ, Boddaert N, Giurgea I, Laborde K, Bellanne-Chantelot C, Verkarre V, Polak M, Rahier J, Syrota A, Seidenwurm D, Nihoul-Fekete C, Robert JJ, Brunelle F, Jaubert F: Congenital hyperinsulinism: pancreatic [^{18}F]fluoro-L-dihydroxyphenylalanine (DOPA) positron emission tomography and immunohistochemistry study of DOPA decarboxylase and insulin secretion. J Clin Endocrinol Metab 2006;91:933–940.

13 Cosgrove KE, Antoine MH, Lee AT, Barnes PD, de Tullio P, Clayton P, McCloy R, De Lonlay P, Nihoul-Fekete C, Robert JJ, Saudubray JM, Rahier J, Lindley KJ, Hussain K, Aynsley-Green A, Pirotte B, Lebrun P, Dunne MJ: BPDZ 154 activates adenosine 5′-triphosphate-sensitive potassium channels: in vitro studies using rodent insulin-secreting cells and islets isolated from patients with hyperinsulinism. J Clin Endocrinol Metab 2002;87:4860–4868.

14 Glaser B, Kesavan P, Heyman M, Davis E, Cuesta A, Buchs A, Stanley CA, Thornton PS, Permutt MA, Matschinsky FM, Herold KC: Familial hyperinsulinism caused by an activating glucokinase mutation. N Engl J Med 1998;338:226–230.

15 Dunne MJ, Cosgrove KE, Shepherd RM, Aynsley-Green A, Lindley KJ: Hyperinsulinism in infancy: from basic science to clinical disease. Physiol Rev 2004;84:239–275.

16 Fernandez-Marmiesse A, Salas A, Vega A, Fernandez-Lorenzo JR, Barreiro J, Carracedo A: Mutation spectra of ABCC8 gene in Spanish patients with Hyperinsulinism of Infancy (HI). Hum Mutat 2006;27:214.

17 Valayannopoulos V, Vaxillaire M, Aigrain Y, Jaubert F, Bellanne-Chantelot C, Ribeiro MJ, Brunelle F, Froguel P, Robert JJ, Polak M, Nihoul-Fekete C, de Lonlay P: Coexistence in the same family of both focal and diffuse forms of hyperinsulinism. Diabetes Care, 2007.

18 Straub SG, Cosgrove KE, Ammala C, Shepherd RM, O'Brien RE, Barnes PD, Kuchinski N, Chapman JC, Schaeppi M, Glaser B, Lindley KJ, Sharp GW, Aynsley-Green A, Dunne MJ: Hyperinsulinism of infancy: the regulated release of insulin by KATP channel-independent pathways. Diabetes 2001;50:329–339.

19 Stanley CA: Hyperinsulinism/hyperammonemia syndrome: insights into the regulatory role of glutamate dehydrogenase in ammonia metabolism. Mol Genet Metab 2004;81(suppl 1):S45–S51.

20 Raizen DM, Brooks-Kayal A, Steinkrauss L, Tennekoon GI, Stanley CA, Kelly A: Central nervous system hyperexcitability associated with glutamate dehydrogenase gain of function mutations. J Pediatr 2005;146:388–394.

21 Molven A, Matre GE, Duran M, Wanders RJ, Rishaug U, Njolstad PR, Jellum E, Sovik O: Familial hyperinsulinemic hypoglycemia caused by a defect in the SCHAD enzyme of mitochondrial fatty acid oxidation. Diabetes 2004;53:221–227.

22 Hardy OT, Hohmeier HE, Becker TC, Manduchi E, Doliba NM, Gupta RK, White P, Stoeckert CJ, Jr., Matschinsky FM, Newgard CB, Kaestner KH: Functional genomics of the beta-cell: short-chain 3-hydroxyacyl-coenzyme A dehydrogenase regulates insulin secretion independent of K+ currents. Mol Endocrinol 2007;21:765–773.

23 Otonkoski T, Kaminen N, Ustinov J, Lapatto R, Meissner T, Mayatepek E, Kere J, Sipila I: Physical exercise-induced hyperinsulinemic hypoglycemia is an autosomal-dominant trait characterized by abnormal pyruvate-induced insulin release. Diabetes 2003;52:199–204.

24 Pearson ER, Boj SF, Steele AM, Barrett T, Stals K, Shield JP, Ellard S, Ferrer J, Hattersley AT: Macrosomia and hyperinsulinaemic hypoglycaemia in patients with heterozygous mutations in the HNF4A gene. PLoS Med 2007;4:e118.

25 Hojlund K, Hansen T, Lajer M, Henriksen JE, Levin K, Lindholm J, Pedersen O, Beck-Nielsen H: A novel syndrome of autosomal-dominant hyperinsulinemic hypoglycemia linked to a mutation in the human insulin receptor gene. Diabetes 2004;53: 1592–1598.

26 Jackson RS, Creemers JW, Farooqi IS, Raffin-Sanson ML, Varro A, Dockray GJ, Holst JJ, Brubaker PL, Corvol P, Polonsky KS, Ostrega D, Becker KL, Bertagna X, Hutton JC, White A, Dattani MT, Hussain K, Middleton SJ, Nicole TM, Milla PJ, Lindley KJ, O'Rahilly S: Small-intestinal dysfunction accompanies the complex endocrinopathy of human proprotein convertase 1 deficiency. J Clin Invest 2003;112:1550–1560.

27 Cohen MM Jr: Beckwith-Wiedemann syndrome: historical, clinicopathological, and etiopathogenetic perspectives. Pediatr Dev Pathol 2005;8:287–304.

28 Henry I, Jeanpierre M, Barichard F, Serre JL, Mallet J, Turleau C, de Grouchy J, Junien C: Duplication of HRAS1, INS, and IGF2 is not a common event in Beckwith-Wiedemann syndrome. Ann Genet 1988; 31:216–220.

29 Spritz RA, Mager D, Pauli RM, Laxova R: Normal dosage of the insulin and insulin-like growth factor II genes in patients with the Beckwith-Wiedemann syndrome. Am J Hum Genet 1986;39:265–273.

30 Hughes-Benzie R, Allanson J, Hunter A, Cole T: The importance of differentiating Simpson-Golabi-Behmel and Beckwith-Wiedemann syndromes. J Med Genet 1992;29:928.

31 Baujat G, Rio M, Rossignol S, Sanlaville D, Lyonnet S, Le Merrer M, Munnich A, Gicquel C, Cormier-Daire V, Colleaux L: Paradoxical NSD1 mutations in Beckwith-Wiedemann syndrome and 11p15 anomalies in Sotos syndrome. Am J Hum Genet 2004;74:715–720.

32 Henneveld HT, van Lingen RA, Hamel BC, Stolte-Dijkstra I, van Essen AJ. Perlman syndrome: four additional cases and review. Am J Med Genet 1999;86:439–446.

33 Bitner-Glindzicz M, Lindley KJ, Rutland P, Blaydon D, Smith VV, Milla PJ, Hussain K, Furth-Lavi J, Cosgrove KE, Shepherd RM, Barnes PD, O'Brien RE, Farndon PA, Sowden J, Liu XZ, Scanlan MJ, Malcolm S, Dunne MJ, Aynsley-Green A, Glaser B: A recessive contiguous gene deletion causing infantile hyperinsulinism, enteropathy and deafness identifies the Usher type 1C gene. Nat Genet 2000; 26:56–60.

34 Møller N, Lunde Jørgensen JO: Effects of growth hormone on glucose, lipid, and protein metabolism in human subjects. Endocr Rev 2009;30:152–177.

35 Brasel JA, Wright JC, Wilkins L: An evaluation of 75 patients with hypopituitarism beginning in childhood. Am J Med 1965;38:494–498.

36 Jaquet D, Touati G, Rigal O, Czernichow P: Exploration of glucose homeostasis during fasting in growth hormone-deficient children. Acta Paediatr 1998;87:505–510.

37 Chernausek SD, Backeljauw PF, Frane J, Kuntze J, Underwood LE, GH: Insensitivity Syndrome Collaborative Group: Long-term treatment with recombinant insulin-like growth factor (IGF)-I in children with severe IGF-1 deficiency due to growth hormone insensitivity. J Clin Endocrinol Metab 2007;92:902–910.

38 Rosenfeld RG, Hwa V: The growth hormone cascade and its role in mammalian growth. Horm Res 2009;71(suppl 2):36–40.

39 Aynsley-Green A, McGann A, Deshpande S: Control of intermediary metabolism in childhood with special reference to hypoglycaemia and growth hormone. Acta Paeditr Scand Suppl 1991;377:43–52.

40 Bornstein SR: Predisposing factors for adrenal insufficiency. N Engl J Med 2009;360:2328–2339.

41 Lamolet B, Pulichino AM, Lamonerie T, Gauthier Y, Brue T, Enjalbert A, Drouin J: A pituitary cell-restricted T box factor, Tpit, activates POMC transcription in cooperation with Pitx homeoproteins. Cell 2001;104:849–859.

42 Santer R, Schneppenheim R, Dombrowski A, Gotze H, Steinmann B, Schaub J: Mutations in GLUT2, the gene for the liver-type glucose transporter, in patients with Fanconi-Bickel syndrome. Nat Genet 1997;17:324–326.

43 Santer R, Schneppenheim R, Suter D, Schaub J, Steinmann B: Fanconi-Bickel syndrome–the original patient and his natural history, historical steps leading to the primary defect, and a review of the literature. Eur J Pediatr 1998;157:783–797.

44 Seidner G, Alvarez MG, Yeh JI, O'Driscoll KR, Klepper J, Stump TS, Wang D, Spinner NB, Birnbaum MJ, De Vivo DC: GLUT-1 deficiency syndrome caused by haploinsufficiency of the blood-brain barrier hexose carrier. Nat Genet 1998; 18:188–191.

45 Mochel F, Slama A, Touati G, Desguerre I, Giurgea I, Rabier D, Brivet M, Rustin P, Saudubray JM, DeLonlay P: Respiratory chain defects may present only with hypoglycemia. J Clin Endocrinol Metab 2005;90:3780–3785.

46 Hachisu M, Oda Y, Goto M, Kobayashi K, Saheki T, Ohura T, Noma S, Kitanaka S: Citrin deficiency presenting with ketotic hypoglycaemia and hepatomegaly in childhood. Eur J Pediatr 2005;164: 109–110.

47 Ohura T, Kobayashi K, Tazawa Y, Abukawa D, Sakamoto O, Tsuchiya S, Saheki T: Clinical pictures of 75 patients with neonatal intrahepatic cholestasis caused by citrin deficiency (NICCD). J Inherit Metab Dis 2007;30:139–144.

Michel Polak, MD, PhD
Pediatric Endocrinology, Hôpital Necker Enfants Malades
149, rue de Sèvres
FR–75015 Paris (France)
Tel. +33 1 44 49 48 03/02, Fax +33 1 44 38 16 48, E-Mail michel.polak@nck.aphp.fr

Ranke MB, Mullis P-E (eds): Diagnostics of Endocrine Function in Children and Adolescents, ed 4.
Basel, Karger, 2011, pp 273–293

Hypoglycaemia in Infants and Children

Khalid Hussain

Clinical and Molecular Genetics Unit, Developmental Endocrinology Research Group, Institute of Child Health,
University College London and Great Ormond Street Hospital for Children NHS Trust, London, UK

Hypoglycaemia is a common biochemical problem observed in the neonatal, infancy and childhood periods. However, despite the commonality there is confusion about the definition and the appropriate management. Hypoglycaemia can be due to many different causes. For example the most severe forms of hypoglycaemia occur due to hyperinsulinism (hyperinsulinaemic hypoglycaemia; HH) whereas 'ketotic' hypoglycaemia presents typically during an intercurrent illness. An understanding of normal glucose physiology and biochemistry will not only help the clinician to understand the biochemical basis of hypoglycaemia but also to organise appropriate investigations and institute the correct management. The early recognition and prompt management of hypoglycaemia is the cornerstone in preventing brain injury. The aim of this chapter is to provide a brief background to normal glucose physiology, review the mechanisms that help maintain normoglycaemia and then, from a clinical perspective, focus on the clinical approach to a patient with hypoglycaemia and finally to review the different causes of hypoglycaemia in the childhood period.

Definition

The definition of hypoglycaemia remains one of the most contentious and confusing areas (especially in the newborn) in glucose physiology [1]. This confusion stems from the fact that there is poor correlation between plasma glucose concentrations, the onset of clinical symptoms, and the long-term neurological sequelae. It is difficult to define a blood glucose level that will require intervention since there is uncertainty over the level and duration of hypoglycaemia that can cause neurological damage.

Several different approaches have been used to define hypoglycaemia (based on clinical manifestations, epidemiology, acute changes in metabolic, endocrine responses and on neurologic function, and on long-term neurologic outcome) but none of these approaches is satisfactory [2]. The approach based on neurophysiological responses to falling blood glucose concentrations has led to the proposal that hypoglycaemia should be defined as a concentration less than 2.6 mmol/l as measured with a laboratory research method [3]. However, around 20% of entirely normal full-term infants have blood glucose concentrations less than this in the first 48 h after delivery. These infants demonstrate concurrent hyperketonaemia and the assumption (which still needs to be proved) is that the babies will not demonstrate neural dysfunction at this time because of the protective effect of the availability of alternative fuels.

Recently, it has been recommended that operational thresholds are used when assessing an interventional response in a patient with hypoglycaemia [1]. An operational threshold is defined as the concentration of plasma or whole blood glucose at which clinicians should consider intervention, based on the evidence currently available in the literature. Significant hypoglycaemia is not and can never be defined by a single number that can be applied universally to every individual patient. Rather, it is characterized by a value(s) that is unique to each individual and varies with both their state of physiologic maturity and the influence of pathology. It can be defined as the concentration of glucose in the blood or plasma at which the individual demonstrates a unique response to the abnormal milieu caused by the inadequate delivery of glucose to a target organ (for example, the brain). It is therefore clear that hypoglycaemia is a continuum and the blood glucose concentration should be interpreted in the context of the clinical presentation, counter-regulatory hormonal responses and in relation to the intermediate metabolites.

Metabolic and Endocrine Changes at the Time of Birth

At birth the healthy term newborn must adapt to an independent existence. The transplacental supply of nutrients including glucose is interrupted and the newborn must now initiate metabolic and endocrine responses to maintain adequate circulating blood glucose concentrations. For extrauterine adaptation there must be adequate glycogen stores, intact and functional glycogenolytic, gluconeogenic and lipogenic mechanisms and appropriate counter-regulatory hormonal responses.

A normal infant at term shows an immediate postnatal fall in blood glucose concentrations during the first 2–4 h from values close to maternal levels to around 2.5 mmol/l [4]. The trigger for the metabolic and endocrine adaptation with reference to glucose control is unclear but surges in catecholamines and glucagon secretion are thought to be important. The raised plasma insulin to glucagon ratio is reversed at birth allowing glucagon to activate adenylate cyclase and increase the activity of cAMP-dependent protein kinase A. This in turn activates phosphorylase kinase which facilitates glucose release. The catecholamine surge activates lipolysis and lipid oxidation resulting in increases in the levels of glycerol and free fatty acids. Free fatty acids are then used to generate ketone bodies which are used as an alternative source of fuel. Healthy term breastfed babies have significantly lower blood glucose concentrations than those who were bottle-fed, but their ketone body concentrations are elevated in response to breast feeding.

Major changes occur in the function of several physiological systems after birth which enables the neonate to adapt to postnatal nutrition [5]. Successful enteral feeding in healthy term newborns triggers the secretion of gut peptides and plays a key role in triggering a cascade of developmental changes in gut structure and function, and in the relation of pancreatic endocrine secretion to intermediary metabolism [5]. Hence full-term infants are functionally and metabolically programmed to make the transition from their intrauterine-dependent environment to their extrauterine existence without the need for metabolic monitoring or interference with the natural breastfeeding process. This complex metabolic and endocrine adaptation process is incomplete and compromised when the infant is born prematurely or following intrauterine growth retardation.

Endocrine and Metabolic Changes during Feeding and Fasting

A normal (fasting blood glucose levels 3.5–5.5 mmol/l) circulating blood glucose concentration is vital for brain function. Any defect that leads to hypoglycaemia will cause hypoglycaemic brain injury. Glucose homeostasis is regulated systemically by hormones such as insulin and glucagon, and at the cellular level by energy status [6]. A complex network of transcription factors, coactivators and corepressors coordinate changes in blood glucose levels. Despite periods of feeding and fasting, in normal individuals plasma glucose remains in a narrow range.

This tight control of glucose concentration is determined by a balance between glucose absorption from the intestine, production by the liver, and uptake in muscle and fat. The liver can produce glucose by breaking down glycogen (glycogenolysis) and by de novo synthesis of glucose from non-carbohydrate precursors such as lactate, pyruvate, glycerol and alanine (gluconeogenesis). Glycogenolysis occurs more rapidly, beginning within 2–3 h after a meal in humans, but gluconeogenesis assumes a much greater importance with prolonged fasting. In liver, glycogen is mainly stored as a glucose reservoir for other tissues. As a consequence, the level of hepatic glycogen changes considerably (between 1 and 100 mg) with the feeding condition.

Hepatic gluconeogenesis plays a key role in the maintenance of glucose homeostasis. Key hormones such as insulin, glucagon and glucocorticoids regulate the rate of hepatic gluconeogenesis [7]. The rate of gluconeogenesis is controlled principally by the activities of certain unidirectional enzymes, such as phosphoenolpyruvate carboxykinase (PEPCK), fructose-1,6-bisphosphatase and glucose-6-phosphatase (G6Pase). The genes encoding these proteins are powerfully controlled at the transcriptional level by key hormones, particularly insulin, glucagon and glucocorticoids. In the fasted state, insulin levels drop while glucagon secretion goes up resulting in increased glycogenolysis and gluconeogenesis. In the fed state, insulin suppresses gly-cogenolysis and hepatic glucose production.

Prolonged fasting is characterized by low insulin concentrations and high gluca-gon, glucocorticoids, and adrenaline (noradrenaline) concentrations in plasma. This hormonal profile promotes the hydrolysis of triacylglycerols in adipose tissue, thereby increasing the concentration of free fatty acids in plasma. The fatty acids are taken up by the liver, where they are either re-esterified to triacylglycerol and secreted as very-low-density lipoprotein (VLDL) or oxidized in the mitochondria via beta-oxidation. During late stages of fasting, free fatty acids become the predominant substrate for energy production. The majority of fatty acids are only partially oxidized to acetyl-coenzyme A (acetyl-CoA), which then condenses with itself to form ketone bodies, an important fuel for the brain. Figure 1 outlines the process of glycolysis, fatty acid oxi-dation and the citric acid cycle. The energy released in the process of beta-oxidation is used by the liver to carry out gluconeogenesis from substrates such as glycerol, lactate, and amino acids. Thus, efficient hepatic fatty acid oxidation is obligatory to the metabolic response to fasting. Figure 2 shows the relationship between serum non-esterified fatty acids and serum ketone bodies.

Counter-Regulatory Hormonal Responses

During the post-absorptive phase (4- to 6-hour interval following the ingestion of a meal) plasma glucose concentrations are maintained by interactions between insulin and the various counter-regulatory hormones including glucagon, cortisol, growth hormone (GH), adrenaline and noradrenaline [8]. Glucagon allows the controlled release of stored glycogen from the liver and insulin restrains the effects of glucagon by preventing accelerated lipolysis and proteolysis. GH and cortisol play an essential role in the regulation of a normal blood glucose concentration by setting the sensitivity of the peripheral tissues to glucagon and insulin. Both of these hormones counter-act the actions of insulin on glucose metabolism. Both hormones reduce the peripheral utilization of glucose as well as increasing the rates of gluconeogenesis. Cortisol as with GH decreases insulin induced peripheral utilization of glucose, increases hepatic glucose production and stimulates protein breakdown. This has the effect of provid-ing amino acids for gluconeogenesis.

Diagnostic Approach to a Patient with Hypoglycaemia

The careful clinical history, description of symptoms, physical examination and a sys-tematic step by step approach are the cornerstones of diagnosis (fig. 3). Given the complexity of the metabolic and endocrine adaptations that occur at birth, hypogly-caemia occurs more commonly during the first days after birth than at any other time

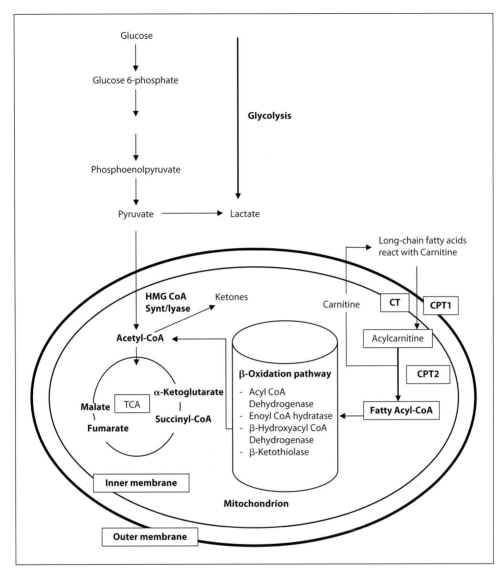

Fig. 1. Outline of glycolysis, carnitine and fatty acid metabolism. Long-chain fatty acids require carnitine for transportation into the mitochondria. Once inside the mitochondria the fatty-acyl CoA undergoes β-oxidation yielding acetyl-CoA. This can then either be converted to ketone bodies or enter the citric acid cycle. CT = Carnitine translocase; CPT = carnitine palmitoyl transferase; TCA = tricyclic acid cycle.

of life. Furthermore, it is a transient phenomenon in the majority of the cases. The symptoms of hypoglycaemia may be very non-specific (table 1) hence any symptomatic child must have a blood glucose level measured and documented.

In the neonatal period the clinical history should include details of pregnancy and delivery, birth weight, gestational age of the infant, noting in particular any

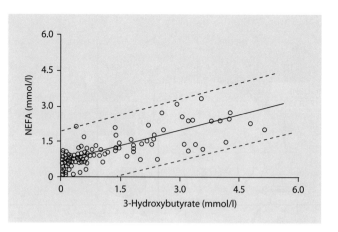

Fig. 2. Relationship between the NEFA and ketone body ratio in children undergoing diagnostic fasting studies (mean and 95th centiles). HH causes suppression of lipolysis and ketone body generation thus leading to low NEFA and ketone body ration. Children with a fatty acid oxidation disorder will have high fatty acids and low ketone bodies.

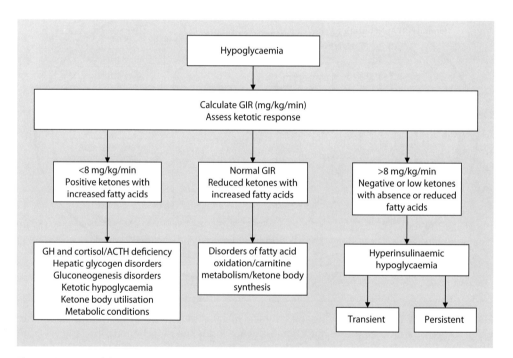

Fig. 3. Suggested diagnostic approach to a patient presenting with hypoglycaemia. An assessment of the glucose infusion rate (GIR) required to maintain normoglycaemia with the ketone body response will help classify patients into the three main subgroups.

evidence for foetal distress, birth asphyxia and smallness for dates. The relationship of a hypoglycaemic episode to the most recent meal can be important diagnostically. Hypoglycaemia occurring after a short fast (2–3 h) may be suggestive of glycogen storage disease. Hypoglycaemia occurring after a long fast (12–14 h) may suggest a

Table 1. Symptoms of hypoglycaemia may be very non-specific

Symptoms of hypoglycaemia
The blood glucose concentration must be measured in any patient with any symptom
Any non-specific symptom may indicate hypoglycaemia
Feeding poorly
Irritability
Lethargy
Stupor
Apnoea, cyanotic spells
Hypothermia
Hypotonia, limpness
Tremor
Confusion
Loss of memory
Inattention
Seizures
Coma

disorder of gluconeogenesis. Postprandial hypoglycaemia may indicate galactosaemia, hereditary fructose intolerance, insulin receptor mutations or the dumping syndrome. A family history of sudden infant deaths may be a clue to an unrecognized, inherited metabolic disorder. Any provocation factors such as an upper respiratory tract infection or an episode of gastro-enteritis leading to hypoglycaemia should be documented.

From the history and physical examination, certain at risk groups of infants (table 2) can be identified on the basis of obvious conditions that are usually associated with transient hypoglycaemia and need monitoring.

The recognition and diagnosis of hypoglycaemia in the neonatal period depends on routine monitoring of blood glucose levels at frequent intervals after birth in asymptomatic infants at risk, and in any infant who demonstrates any symptom which might be suggestive of hypoglycaemia. Again in this group it is important to monitor blood glucose in relation to the time of feeds. Thus, a blood glucose concentration that increases after a feed is probably less worrying than one which is persistently low. If low concentrations are obtained during routine bedside monitoring in asymptomatic high risk infants or at the time of symptoms in symptomatic infants it is necessary to confirm the result in the laboratory, but intervention does not need to wait for the result in infants who are severely symptomatic and in whom reagent strip test results suggest hypoglycaemia. Resolution of symptoms after glucose confirms that they were due to hypoglycaemia.

Other important points from the history and examination include the presence or absence of maternal diabetes or rhesus incompatibility. Increased birth weight and

Table 2. Risk factors for hypoglycaemia

Risk factors which may be associated with hypoglycaemia
Prematurity
Intra-uterine growth retardation
Maternal diabetes mellitus (insulin dependent and gestational)
Perinatal asphyxia
Erythroblastosis fetalis
Beckwith-Wiedemann syndrome
Macrosomia
Any 'sick' infant
Polycythaemia
Hypothermia
Congenital heart disease
Midline defects (cleft lip or palate)
Micropenis
Ambiguous genitalia
Infections such as malaria

macrosomia should raise the possibility of neonatal hyperinsulinism. Distinctive physical signs such as transverse ear lobe creases, exomphalos and macroglossia should raise the possibility of the Beckwith-Wiedemann syndrome (BWS), whilst the presence of micropenis and undescended testes might indicate the presence of hypopituitarism. Mid-line defects, including cleft palate, could also indicate congenital hypopituitarism whilst the existence of ambiguous genitalia could indicate congenital adrenal hyperplasia.

Hepatomegaly should always be looked for and is associated with abnormal glycogen metabolism, defects in gluconeogenesis and galactosaemia. Moderate hepatomegaly due to glycogen accumulation may, however, also develop in infants with hyperinsulinism who are receiving very high infusion rates of glucose to maintain normoglycaemia. In the childhood period, particular attention should be paid to the rate of growth, micropenis, undescended testes, skin pigmentation, blood pressure and weight loss.

After the clinical history has been taken and the examination completed a diagnostic cascade of appropriate tests is necessary.

Blood Sample at Time of Hypoglycaemia

By far the most important investigation is the obtaining of a blood sample at the time of hypoglycaemia. The blood glucose must be considered in the context of the whole fuel economy and in the light of concurrent hormone concentrations. Essential diagnostic information can be obtained by measuring the basic metabolites and hormones

Table 3. Recommended routine baseline investigations in patients with suspected hypoglycaemia

---

Blood (normal range and response to hypoglycaemia)
Glucose (3.5–5.6 mmol/l)
Insulin (should be undetectable when hypoglycaemic)
Cortisol (450–500 nmol/l at time of hypoglycaemia but response can be variable)
Lactate (1–2 mmol/l)
Growth hormone (variable response and poor specificity)
Non-esterified fatty acids (level depends on the degree of fasting)
3β-Hydroxybutyrate (level depends on the degree of fasting)
Carnitine (free and total)
Blood spot acyl-carnitine
Ammonia (<40 μmol/l)

Urine
Ketones
Organic acids
Reducing substances

---

listed in table 3, in the blood sample drawn at the time of hypoglycaemia. The next urine sample, which is passed, should also be deep frozen for subsequent assay for abnormal constituents. Once the basic investigations are complete further investigations can be planned accordingly if required (as guided by the results of the preliminary investigations (table 4).

Reagent strips in combination with a reflectance meter are the most common method of measuring bedside blood glucose levels. However, it is important to remember that these should be used as a guide (can be inaccurate) and the blood glucose concentration should always be checked in the laboratory. Whole blood glucose is approximately 15% lower than serum glucose levels because of the lower glucose content and intracellular water content of the red cells. Glucose concentrations in venous blood are 10% lower than arterial blood. The blood sample for glucose measurement should be collected in a fluoride container to inhibit glycolysis. It should also be analysed immediately because, even in the presence of fluoride, the blood glucose concentration will decrease over time.

Diagnostic Fast

In many conditions hypoglycaemia occurs only in relation to periods of low caloric intake or starvation. Starvation tests are potentially very dangerous and they must be conducted only under strictly controlled conditions by staff experienced in their administration, with a secure intravenous infusion available for immediate correction

Table 4. Suggested investigations depending on the underlying mechanism leading to the hypoglycaemia

---

Fatty acid oxidation disorder/disorders of carnitine metabolism
- Fatty acid flux studies (skin biopsy for fibroblast culture)
- Serum carnitine levels
- Genetic analysis

Suspected glycogen storage disease
- Cholesterol, triglycerides
- Urate, Liver function tests
- Genetic analysis

Gluconeogenesis
- Leucocyte fructose 1,6-bisphosphatase activity
- Liver phosphorylase
- Genetic analysis

Hepatic glycogen synthase disease (GSD 0)
- Pre and postprandial blood glucose and lactate profiles
- Genetic analysis

Ketone body synthesis/utilisation disorder
- HMG CoA/succinyl-CoA: 3-oxoacid CoA-transferase (SCOT) mutational analysis
- Liver biopsy

Suspected metabolic disease
- Red cell galactose-1-phophateuridyltransferase activity (galactosaemia)
- Plasma amino acids (maple syrup urine disease)
- Urinary succinylacetone (tyrosinaemia)
- Transferrin isoelectric focussing (congenital disorder of glycosylation CDG)
- Pyruvate
- Acetoacetate
- Mitochondrial respiratory chain complex activity

Insulinoma
- MRI or CT scan
- Intra-operative ultrasound
- Genetic testing for MEN1

Hyperinsulinaemic hypoglycaemia (non-insulinoma)
- Protein (leucine) loading studies (HI/HA syndrome)
- Exercise provocation tests (exercise induced hyperinsulinism)
- If unresponsive to medical therapy then ^{18}F-DOPA-PET/CT scan to differentiate diffuse from focal disease
- Mutational analysis of known genes

Unexplained
- 'Ketotic' hypoglycaemia (diagnosis of exclusion)
- Urine toxicology (specifically request for the possible offending agent)

---

of hypoglycaemia [9]. The hazards are greatest in defects in fatty acid oxidation, since the induced hyper-fatty acidaemia carries a risk of inducing a cardiac arrhythmia. Sequential measurements of intermediary metabolites and glucose are taken throughout the fast, with the crucial blood sample being drawn when hypoglycaemia occurs. The urine sample passed then or after restoration of normoglycaemia should be deep frozen for measurement of organic acids and other abnormal metabolites.

Other measurements from this specimen obtained at the time of hypoglycaemia can also help in diagnosis. Thus, cortisol deficiency will be revealed by showing a low cortisol concentration. Further tests to define the integrity of the hypothalamo-pituitary adrenal axis are mandatory if a low cortisol level is found at the time of hypoglycaemia since cortisol deficiency may be lethal if not corrected by appropriate replacement therapy. Low growth hormone levels at the time of fasting hypoglycaemia do not rule out or indicate deficiency [10]. If this deficiency is suspected from abnormal growth then a validated test such a glucagon provocation test should be performed.

The documentation of abnormal urinary organic acids is particularly helpful when hypoglycaemia is due to methylmalonic acidaemia, maple syrup urine disease (MSUD) or mitochondrial beta-oxidation defects. In the latter, clues to the deficient enzymes are provided by the chain length of the dicarboxylic acids in the urine and the presence of hydroxyl groups or unsaturated bonds. The presence of urinary glycine conjugates may also be diagnostic of fatty acid oxidation defects.

Emergency Management of Hypoglycaemia

1 Hypostop (apply gel onto the inside of the cheek) or sugary drink if the patient is conscious.
2 Intravenous glucose (give 1–2 ml/kg of 10% dextrose as a bolus).
3 Glucagon (in emergency give 1 mg stat intramuscularly). Glucagon can cause rebound hypoglycaemia so the patient should be admitted to hospital. Glucagon is most effective in patients with hyperinsulinaemic hypoglycaemia and least effective in patients with glycogen storage diseases.

Overview of the Different Causes of Hypoglycaemia in Childhood

Hypoglycaemia in childhood can be due to many causes. These can be broadly summarized into those due to hormonal abnormalities such as hyperinsulinism, cortisol or growth hormone deficiency, defects of hepatic glycogen release/storage, defects in gluconeogenesis, defects in carnitine metabolism, defects in fatty acid oxidation, postprandial, metabolic and unknown causes such as idiopathic ketotic hypoglycaemia. Table 5 summarises the different causes of hypoglycaemia.

Table 5. Differential diagnosis of hypoglycaemia

Hyperinsulinaemic hypoglycaemia (including post-prandial)
Transient: infant of diabetic mother/perinatal asphyxia/rhesus disease/intra-uterine growth retardation/Beckwith-Wiedemann syndrome
Congenital: *ABCC8/KCNJ11/ GCK/ GDH/HADH/HNF4A/ SLC16A1*
Insulinoma
Dumping syndrome
Insulin receptor mutations and antibodies
Non-insulinoma pancreatogenous hypoglycaemia (adults)
Gastric bypass surgery for morbid obesity

Hormonal deficiency/ Resistance
Adrenocorticotrophic/cortisol /growth hormone/glucagon/adrenaline (no human case reported with adrenaline deficiency yet)
Laron syndrome (resistance to growth hormone)

Defects in hepatic glycogen release/storage
Glycogen storage diseases: glucose-6-phosphatase, amylo-1,6-glucosidase deficiency, liver phosphorylase deficiency
Glycogen storage disease type 0

Defects in gluconeogenesis
Fructose-1,6-bisphosphatase deficiency
PEPCK deficiency
Pyruvate carboxylase deficiency

Carnitine metabolism
Carnitine deficiency (primary and secondary)
Carnitine palmitoyl transferase deficiency (CPT1 and CPT2)
Carnitine transporter defects

Fatty acid oxidation
Medium chain acyl-CoA dehydrogenase (MCAD) deficiency
Very-long-chain acyl-CoA dehydrogenase (VLCAD) deficiency
Short-chain acyl-CoA dehydrogenase (SCAD) deficiency
Long/short chain- L-3-hydroxy-acyl CoA (L/SCHAD) deficiency

Defects in ketone body synthesis/utilisation
HMG CoA synthase deficiency/HMG CoA lyase deficiency
Succinyl-CoA: 3-oxoacid CoA-transferase (SCOT) deficiency

Metabolic conditions (common ones)
Organic acidaemias (propionic/methylmalonic)
Maple syrup urine disease, galactosaemia, fructosaemia, tyrosinaemia
Hereditary fructose intolerance
Glutaric aciduria type 2
Mitochondrial respiratory chain complex deficiencies
Congenital disorders of glycosylation (CGD)

Drug induced
Sulphonylurea/insulin/beta-blocker/salicylates/alcohol

Table 5. Continued

Miscellaneous causes (mechanism(s) not clear)
Idiopathic ketotic hypoglycaemia (diagnosis of exclusion)
Infections (sepsis, malaria), congenital heart disease
Glucose transporter (GLUT2)

Hypoglycaemia due to Hormonal Abnormalities

Hyperinsulinaemic Hypoglycaemia

Hyperinsulinaemic hypoglycaemia (HH) is the commonest cause of recurrent and severe hypoglycaemia in the neonatal and infancy period. It is characterized by the excessive and inappropriate secretion of insulin in relation to the prevailing blood glucose concentration [11]. HH can be either persistent or transient. In adolescents or older children presenting with HH, insulinoma must be considered as a possibility. An insulinoma may be a part of multiple endocrine neoplasia (MEN1) and hence a family history may provide a diagnostic clue in the familial cases. HH presents primarily in the newborn period and during the first 2–6 months after birth in term and preterm neonates. The characteristic metabolic and endocrine profile in a blood sample drawn at the time of hypoglycaemia is one of hyperinsulinaemic, hypoketotic, hypo fatty acidaemic hypoglycaemia with inappropriately raised insulin and accompanied by high concentrations of C-peptide levels. High intravenous infusion rates of glucose may be required to maintain a blood glucose concentration above 3.5 mmol/l. The level of insulin in the blood may not necessarily be particularly high [12]. The diagnostic criteria for HH are listed in table 6.

Management

The immediate imperative is to give sufficient glucose to maintain blood glucose concentrations above 3.5 mmol/l. Infusion rates in excess of 4–6 mg/kg/min may be necessary, rarely; infusion rates >20 mg/kg/min may be needed. Having stabilised the blood glucose concentration, it is then imperative to determine whether or not the patient will respond to the conventional medical therapy of a combination of diazoxide (5–20 mg/kg/day given orally) together with a diuretic [12]. The administration of glucagon by continuous infusion (starting dose 1.0–10 μg/kg/h) concurrently with a continuous infusion of the somatostatin analogue octreotide (initial dose 5–35 μg/kg/day) may confer substantial benefit. Those patients that show no response to medical therapy will require surgery [12]. It is now imperative to differentiate focal from diffuse disease prior to surgery. This is now done using ^{18}F-DOPA-PET/CT scan [13]. Figure 4 outlines the management of patients with HH.

Table 6. Diagnostic criteria for HH

Glucose infusion rate >8 mg/kg/min	

Calculated as $\dfrac{\%\ of\ dextrose\ infused \times Mls/h}{Weight \times 6}$

Laboratory blood glucose <3 mmol/l with
- Detectable serum insulin/C-peptide (insulin levels need not be very high)
- Suppressed/inappropriately low serum ketone bodies
- Suppressed/ inappropriately low serum fatty acids
- Serum ammonia level may be raised (HI/HA syndrome)
- Raised plasma hydroxybutyrylcarnitine and urinary 3-hydroxyglutarate (HADH deficiency)

Other supportive evidence (when diagnosis is in doubt or further investigations required)
- Positive glycaemic (>1.5 mmol/l) response to intramuscular/intravenous glucagon
- Positive glycaemic response to a subcutaneous/intravenous dose of octreotide
- Low levels of serum IGFBP-1 (as insulin negatively regulates IGFBP-1)

Hydroxyacyl-coenzyme A dehydrogenase (HADH), hyperinsulinism and hyperammonaemia syndrome (HI/HA); insulin-like growth factor-binding protein 1 (IGFBP-1)

Postprandial Hyperinsulinaemic Hypoglycaemia

Postprandial hyperinsulinaemic hypoglycaemia (PPHH) refers to the development of hypoglycaemia within a few hours of meal ingestion. It is associated with inappropriate insulin secretion in response to the meal. The most common cause is due to the 'dumping' syndrome in infants who have undergone gastro-oesophageal surgery [14]. PPHH occurs in the insulin autoimmune syndrome (which is characterized by the presence of insulin-binding autoantibodies in subjects that have not been previously exposed to exogenous insulin) and in patients with insulin receptor mutations. Most other causes of PPHH have been reported in adults.

Hypoglycaemia due to Hormone Deficiency

Deficiency of glucagon, adrenaline, GH and cortisol can cause hypoglycaemia. Glucagon and adrenaline deficiency is extremely rare and so far no true human genetically proven defect in glucagon and adrenaline deficiency have been described. Serum GH and cortisol respond differently to spontaneous hypoglycaemia and that induced by the insulin tolerance test. This is not related to the pulsatile nature of GH secretion but may be related to the rate of fall of the blood glucose concentration. Hence a low serum growth hormone value at the time of spontaneous hypoglycaemia may not necessarily indicate growth hormone deficiency [10].

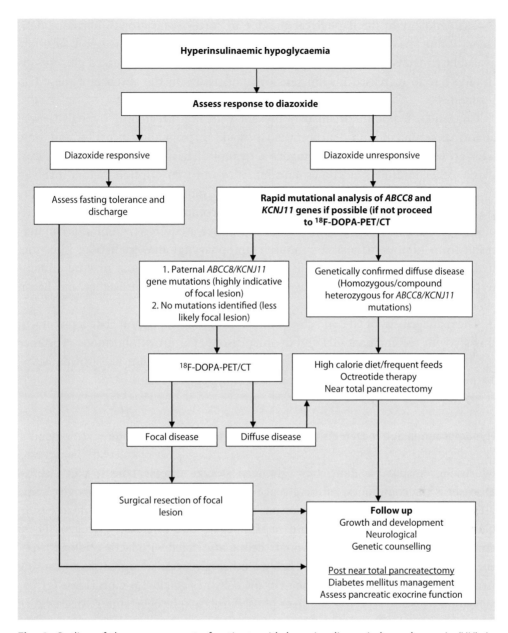

Fig. 4. Outline of the management of patients with hyperinsulinaemic hypoglycaemia (HH). In those patients that show no response to diazoxide therapy it is imperative to distinguish between focal and diffuse HH as the management of the two subgroups is radically different. Patients with focal HH only require a limited pancreatectomy whereas patients with diffuse HH will require a near (95–98%) pancreatectomy. Not all patients with medically unresponsive HH require a PET scan. This should only be performed in patients with a paternally inherited mutation in either *ABCC8* or *KCNJ11* genes.

The aetiology of the hypoglycaemia due to cortisol and growth hormone deficiency is due to a combination of factors including reduced gluconeogenic substrate availability (decreased mobilization of fats and proteins) and increased glucose utilization due to increased insulin sensitivity of tissues in the absence of these two hormones.

Congenital hypopituitarism may present with life-threatening hypoglycaemia, abnormal serum sodium concentrations, shock, microphallus in males, and, only later, growth failure. Causes of congenital hypopituitarism include septo-optic dysplasia, other midline syndromes, and mutations of transcription factors involved in pituitary gland development. Children with acquired hypopituitarism typically present with growth failure and may have other complaints depending on the aetiology and the extent of missing pituitary hormones. Acquired hypopituitarism may result from tumours (most commonly craniopharyngioma), radiation, infection, hydrocephalus, vascular anomalies, and trauma. Hypoglycaemia may be a manifestation of hormone resistance syndromes (such as ACTH resistance and Laron syndrome).

The management of GH and cortisol deficiency involves appropriate replacement therapy with recombinant GH and hydrocortisone. For growth hormone resistance syndrome (such as Laron syndrome) recombinant IGF-1 (insulin-like growth factor-1) therapy can be used but this also can lead to hypoglycaemia

Hypoglycaemia due to Defects in Hepatic Glycogen Release/Storage

Glucose-6-phosphatase deficiency (glycogen storage disease type I, Von Gierkes Disease) is the commonest of the glycogen storage diseases causing hypoglycaemia [15]. The deficiency of this enzyme results in the inability to release free glucose from glucose-6-phosphate, with resultant hepatomegaly due to stored glycogen. These children present with recurrent hypoglycaemia associated with lactic acidosis, hyperuricaemia and hyperlipidaemia. The two other glycogen storage diseases causing hypoglycaemia are due to deficiencies of the enzymes amylo-1,6-glucosidase (glycogen storage disease type III) and liver phosphorylase (glycogen storage disease VI). The clinical and biochemical features of GSDIII subjects are quite heterogeneous.

The clinical manifestations of GSDIII are represented by hepatomegaly, hypoglycaemia, hyperlipidaemia, short stature and, in a number of subjects, cardiomyopathy and myopathy. Glycogen-storage disease type VI (GSDVI) represents a heterogeneous group of hepatic glycogenoses with mild clinical manifestations and benign course. Patients typically exhibit prominent hepatomegaly, growth retardation, and variable but mild episodes of fasting hypoglycaemia and hyperketosis during childhood. Hyperlacticacidaemia and hyperuricaemia characteristically are absent. In addition, patients may demonstrate elevated serum transaminases, hyperlipidaemia, hypotonia, and muscle weakness.

Hepatic glycogen synthase deficiency is a rare cause of hypoglycaemia in childhood [16]. The characteristic features include fasting hypoglycaemia, with hyperketonaemia but with normal lactate. After a meal the plasma lactate will increase as glucose is channelled along the glycolytic pathway with hyperglycaemia. Mutations in the liver glycogen synthase gene (GYS2) localized on chromosome 12p12.2 have been described in some patients. The management of hepatic glycogen storage diseases involves the avoidance of prolonged fasting. This is achieved by giving continuous overnight feeding and/or uncooked cornstarch.

Hypoglycaemia due to Defects in Gluconeogenesis

Gluconeogenesis, or the formation of glucose from mainly lactate/pyruvate, glycerol, glutamine and alanine, plays an essential role in the maintenance of normoglycaemia during fasting. Inborn deficiencies are known in each of the four enzymes of the glycolytic-gluconeogenic pathway that ensure a unidirectional flux from pyruvate to glucose: pyruvate carboxylase, phosphoenolpyruvate carboxykinase (PEPCK), fructose-1,6-bisphosphatase, and glucose-6-phosphatase [17]. Gluconeogenesis can essentially be viewed as a reversal of glycolysis but with few important differences. Patients with defects in gluconeogenesis present with fasting hypoglycaemia and lactic acidosis [17]. Pyruvate carboxylase deficiency may lead to a more widespread clinical presentation with lactic acidosis, severe mental and developmental retardation, and proximal renal tubular acidosis. The management of patients with defects in gluconeogenesis also involves the avoidance of prolonged fasting by giving continuous overnight feeding and or cornstarch.

Hypoglycaemia due to Disorders of Carnitine Metabolism and Defects of Fatty Acid Oxidation

Serious clinical consequences may occur if fatty-acid oxidation (FAO) is impaired, including hypoglycaemic seizures, muscle damage, cardiomyopathy, metabolic acidosis, and liver dysfunction [18]. Fatty acids are taken up by hepatocytes and muscle, where they are subsequently activated to their coenzyme A (CoA) esters. FAO disorders are individually rare, but they are collectively common because of the number of different enzymes affected. They are typically inherited in an autosomal-recessive pattern. When defects occur in fatty-acid degradation, excess acylcarnitine intermediates accumulate in the tissues, including heart, liver, and skeletal muscle, which can lead to organ dysfunction [19]. The diversion of acyl-CoA intermediates into beta-oxidation results in accumulation of toxic dicarboxylic acids. Acylcarnitines that spill into the blood provide a marker for diagnosis, including early detection on newborn screening. The diagnosis of some FAO disorders may require more invasive specimens to be tested because substrate profiles alone can be normal or only mildly abnormal. Cultured skin fibroblasts are useful for testing enzyme activity or metabolism of labelled fatty-acid substrates.

Primary carnitine deficiency is an autosomal-recessive disorder of fatty acid oxidation that can present at different ages with hypoketotic hypoglycaemia and cardiomyopathy and/or skeletal myopathy [20]. This disease is suspected based on reduced levels of carnitine in plasma and confirmed by measurement of carnitine transport in the patient's fibroblasts. Carnitine transport is markedly reduced (usually <5% of normal) in fibroblasts from patients with primary carnitine deficiency. The 'hepatic' carnitine palmitoyl transferase 1 (CPT1) isoform is expressed in liver, kidney and fibroblasts and at low levels in the heart, while the other isoform (muscle) occurs in skeletal muscle and is the predominant form in heart. Patients with hepatic isoform of CPT1 deficiency present with hypoketotic hypoglycaemia, hepatomegaly with raised transaminases, renal tubular acidosis, transient hyperlipidaemia and, paradoxically, myopathy with elevated creatinine kinase or cardiac involvement and seizures and coma in the neonatal period [20]. The typical biochemical finding in the urine is dicarboxylic acids of chain lengths C6-C10.

CPT2 deficiency has several clinical presentations [21]. The infantile-type CPT2 deficiency presents as severe attacks of hypoketotic hypoglycaemia, occasionally associated with cardiac damage commonly responsible for sudden death before 1 year of age. In addition to these symptoms, features of brain and kidney dysorganogenesis are frequently seen in the neonatal-onset CPT2 deficiency, almost always lethal during the first month of life [21]. Treatment is based upon avoidance of fasting and/or exercise, a low-fat diet enriched with medium chain triglycerides and carnitine.

The commonest disorder of fatty acid beta-oxidation is medium-chain acyl-CoA dehydrogenase (MCAD). This is an autosomal-recessive condition characterized by intolerance to prolonged fasting, recurrent episodes of hypoglycaemic coma with medium-chain dicarboxylicaciduria, impaired ketogenesis, and low plasma and tissue carnitine levels [22]. MCAD deficiency usually presents between infancy and 2 years of age, although onset of symptoms can occur as early as the first days of life to as late as 6 years. Children are typically asymptomatic except during times of fasting and metabolic stress, usually associated with a viral illness. They present with fasting non-ketotic hypoglycaemia associated with vomiting, lethargy, apnoea, coma, encephalopathy, and sudden death. If undiagnosed, 20–25% of affected patients will die during the first episode. Routine laboratory studies during an acute illness may show hypoketotic hypoglycaemia, metabolic acidosis, lactic acidosis, hyperammonaemia, increased blood urea nitrogen and transaminases, and elevated uric acid. Serum and urine free carnitine levels may be normal or low. Elevated suberylglycine and hexanoylglycine (dicarboxylic acid esters of glycine) are typically found in urine.

Enzyme deficiency can be shown in fibroblasts. Screening of the *ACADM* gene often identifies a common A985G mutation that accounts for 85% of mutations [23]. Some of the children detected with newborn screening have a genotype that may not be associated with clinical manifestations. The disorder may be severe, and even fatal, in young patients. Other defects of beta-oxidation (long-chain acyl-CoA dehydrogenase) may present with hypoketotic hypoglycaemia associated with neurological (hypotonia) and cardiovascular complications (cardiomyopathy). The pattern of dicarboxylicaciduria accumulation is characteristic for each enzymatic defect of the beta-oxidation spiral.

As is true for the defects in carbohydrate metabolism leading to hypoglycaemia, treatment of the fatty acid oxidation defects involves avoidance of fasting and provision of adequate glucose. Restriction of dietary fat intake and supplemental L-carnitine therapy are recommended.

Hypoglycaemia due to Defects in Ketone Body Synthesis/Utilization

Ketone bodies are an alternative form of fuel to glucose especially for the brain. Each ketone body is synthesized from the combination of acetyl-CoA and acetoacetyl-CoA to from hydroxymethylglutaryl-CoA (HMG-CoA), which is then split by HMG-CoA lyase to yield acetoacetate. Acetoacetate is then converted to β-hydroxybutyrate. Defects in either the synthesis or the utilization of ketone bodies may lead to hypoglycaemia. Hereditary deficiency of mitochondrial HMG-CoA synthase can cause episodes of severe hypoketotic hypoglycaemia [24]. Typical biochemical findings include hypoketosis, elevated free fatty acids, normal acylcarnitines, and specific urinary organic acids during acute episodes. A rare cause of hypoglycaemia due to the inability to utilize ketone bodies is deficiency of succinyl-CoA:3-oxoacid CoA-transferase (SCOT) [25]. This is characterized by intermittent ketoacidotic crises and persistent ketosis. The management of patients with defects in ketone body synthesis and utilisation also involves the avoidance of prolonged fasting.

Idiopathic Ketotic Hypoglycaemia

Idiopathic ketotic hypoglycaemia usually presents between the ages of 18 months and 5 years and remits spontaneously by the ages of 9–10 years. The typical history is of a child who may miss a meal and develops hypoglycaemia usually following an upper respiratory tract infection. The hypoglycaemic episodes seem to be unpredictable, only developing sometimes. Biochemically the hypoglycaemia is associated with raised ketone bodies and free fatty acids with suppressed insulin levels. Ketotic hypoglycaemia is characterised by low levels of plasma alanine [26] but the precise mechanism responsible for the hypoglycaemia is not understood.

Idiopathic ketotic hypoglycaemia is a poorly defined term and may include groups of conditions in which there is no clear cause of the hypoglycaemia. Conditions such as hepatic glycogen synthase deficiency and acetoacetyl CoA thiolase deficiency have been reported as presenting with ketotic hypoglycaemia. Ketotic hypoglycaemia is a diagnosis of exclusion and may be due to a mismatch between glucose demand and glucose production [27, 28].

Miscellaneous Causes of Hypoglycaemia

Metabolic
Hypoglycaemia can also occur due to a number of metabolic conditions including galactosaemia, fructosaemia, tyrosinaemia, organic acidaemias, maple syrup urine disease, glutaric aciduria type II, and in mitochondrial respiratory chain defects [29]. Hereditary fructose intolerance, caused by catalytic deficiency of aldolase B (fructose 1,6-phosphate aldolase) is a recessively inherited condition in which affected homozygotes develop hypoglycaemic and severe abdominal symptoms after taking foods containing fructose and cognate sugars. Continued ingestion of noxious sugars leads to hepatic and renal injury and growth retardation.

Factitious
Hypoglycaemia can also be induced pharmacologically, either intentionally as a diagnostic tool, accidentally as a complication of the treatment of diabetes mellitus, or as a consequence of poisoning either with insulin itself or with drugs such as sulphonylureas, which stimulate insulin release [30]. Whenever severe hypoglycaemia occurs with documented hyperinsulinism, the possibility of Munchausen syndrome by proxy should be considered. The possibility of malicious administration of insulin or an oral sulphonylurea should always be suspected in cases of sudden onset of hypoglycaemia in a previously healthy child. In the case of insulin administration the clue in the biochemistry will be a raised insulin level with normal C-peptide.

References

1 Cornblath M, Hawdon JM, Williams AF, Aynsley-Green A, Ward-Platt MP, Schwartz R, Kalhan SC: Controversies regarding definition of neonatal hypoglycemia: suggested operational thresholds. Pediatrics 2000;105:1141–1145.
2 Williams AF: Hypoglycaemia of the newborn: a review. Bull World Health Org 1997;75:261–290.
3 Koh THHG, Aynsley-Green A, Tarbit M, Eyre JA: Neural dysfunction during hypoglycaemia. Arch Dis Child 1988;63:1353–1358.
4 Hawdon JM, Ward Platt MP, Aynsley-Green A: Patterns of metabolic adaptation for preterm and term infants in the first neonatal week. Arch Dis Child 1992;67(spec No):357–365.

5 Aynsley-Green A, Lucas A, Bloom SR: The control of the adaptation of the human neonate to postnatal nutrition. Acta Chir Scand Suppl 1981;507:269–281.
6 Gerich JE, Cryer P, Rizza R: Hormonal mechanisms in acute glucose counter-regulation: the relative roles of glucagon, epinephrine, norepinephrine, growth hormone and cortisol. Metabolism 1980;29:1164–1175.
7 Kahn CR, Granner DK, Newgard CB, Spiegelman BM: Control of hepatic gluconeogenesis through the transcriptional coactivator PGC-1. Nature 2001;413:131–138.

8   Smith U, Attvall S, Eriksson J, Fowelin J, Lönnroth P, Wesslau C: The insulin-antagonistic effect of the counterregulatory hormones – clinical and mechanistic aspects. Adv Exp Med Biol 1993;334:169–180.

9   Morris AA, Thekekara A, Wilks Z, Clayton PT, Leonard JV, Aynsley-Green A: Evaluation of fasts for investigating hypoglycaemia or suspected metabolic disease. Arch Dis Child 1996;75:115–119.

10 Hussain K, Hindmarsh P, Aynsley-Green A: Spontaneous hypoglycaemia in childhood is accompanied by paradoxical serum cortisol and growth hormone counter-regulatory hormonal responses. J Clin Endocrinol Metab 2003;88:3715–3723.

11 Kapoor RR, Flanagan SE, James C, Shield J, Ellard S, Hussain K: Hyperinsulinaemic hypoglycaemia. Arch Dis Child 2009;94:450–457.

12 Aynsley-Green A, Hussain K, Hall J, Saudubray JM, Nihoul-Fékété C, Debeney P, Brunelle F, Otonkoski T, Thornton P, Lindley JK: The practical management of hyperinsulinism in infancy. Arch Dis in Child Fetal Neonatal Ed 2000;82:F98–F107.

13 Otonkoski T, Nanto-Salonen K, Seppanen M, Veijola R, Huopio H, Hussain K, Tapanainen P, Eskola O, Parkkola R, Ekstrom K, Guiot Y, Rahier J, Laakso M, Rintala R, Nuutila P, Minn H: Noninvasive diagnosis of focal hyperinsulinism of infancy with [¹⁸F]-DOPA positron emission tomography. Diabetes 2006;55:13–18.

14 Tack J, Arts J, Caenepeel P, De Wulf D, Bisschops R: Pathophysiology, diagnosis and management of postoperative dumping syndrome. Nat Rev Gastroenterol Hepatol 2009;6:583–590.

15 Ozen H: Glycogen storage diseases: new perspectives. World J Gastroenterol 2007;13:2541–2553.

16 Gitzelmann R, Spycher MA, Feil G, Müller J, Seilnacht B, Stahl M, Bosshard NU: Liver glycogen synthase deficiency: a rarely diagnosed entity. Eur J Pediatr 1996;155:561–567.

17 van den Berghe G: Disorders of gluconeogenesis. J Inherit Metab Dis 1996;19:470–477.

18 Stanley CA: New genetic defects in mitochondrial fatty acid oxidation and carnitine deficiency. Adv Pediatr 1987;34:59–88.

19 Sim KG, Hammond J, Wilcken B: Strategies for the diagnosis of mitochondrial fatty acid beta-oxidation disorders. Clin Chim Acta 2002;323:37–58.

20 Longo N, Amat di San Filippo C, Pasquali M: Disorders of carnitine transport and the carnitine cycle. Am J Med Genet C Semin Med Genet 2006; 142C:77–85.

21 Bonnefont JP, Demaugre F, Prip-Buus C, Saudubray JM, Brivet M, Abadi N, Thuillier L: Carnitine palmitoyltransferase deficiencies. Mol Genet Metab 1999; 68:424–440.

22 Schatz UA, Ensenauer R: The clinical manifestation of MCAD deficiency: challenges towards adulthood in the screened population. J Inherit Metab Dis 2010;33:513–520.

23 Carroll JC, Gibbons CA, Blaine SM, Cremin C, Dorman H, Honeywell C, Meschino WS, Permaul J, Allanson J: Genetics: newborn screening for MCAD deficiency. Can Fam Physician 2009;55:487.

24 Hegardt FG: Mitochondrial 3-hydroxy-3- methylglutaryl-CoA synthase: a control enzyme in ketogenesis. Biochem J 1999;338:569–582.

25 Berry GT, Fukao T, Mitchell GA, Mazur A, Ciafre M, Gibson J, Kondo N, Palmieri MJ: Neonatal hypoglycaemia in severe succinyl-CoA: 3-oxoacid CoA-transferase deficiency. J Inherit Metab Dis 2001;24: 587–595.

26 Pagliara AS, Kari IE, De Vivo DC, Feigin RD, Kipnis DM: Hypoalaninemia: a concomitant of ketotic hypoglycemia. J Clin Invest 1972;51:1440–1149.

27 Bodamer OA, Hussein K, Morris AA, Langhans CD, Rating D, Mayatepek E, Leonard JV: Glucose and leucine kinetics in idiopathic ketotic hypoglycaemia. Arch Dis Child 2006;91:483–486.

28 Huidekoper HH, Duran M, Turkenburg M, Ackermans MT, Sauerwein HP, Wijburg FA: Fasting adaptation in idiopathic ketotic hypoglycemia: a mismatch between glucose production and demand. Eur J Pediatr 2008;167:859–865.

29 Mochel F, Slama A, Touati G, Desguerre I, Giurgea I, Rabier D, Brivet M, Rustin P, Saudubray JM, DeLonlay P: Respiratory chain defects may present only with hypoglycemia. J Clin Endocrinol Metab 2005;90:3780–3785.

30 Glatstein M, Garcia-Bournissen F, Scolnik D, Koren G, Finkelstein Y: Hypoglycemia in a healthy toddler. Ther Drug Monit 2009;31:173–177.

Dr. K. Hussain
Developmental Endocrinology Research Group, Clinical and Molecular Genetics Unit
Institute of Child Health, University College London
30 Guilford Street, London WC1N 1EH (UK)
Tel. +44 20 7 905 2128, Fax +44 20 7 404 6191, E-Mail K.Hussain@ich.ucl.ac.uk

Ranke MB, Mullis P-E (eds): Diagnostics of Endocrine Function in Children and Adolescents, ed 4.
Basel, Karger, 2011, pp 294–309

Insulin Resistance in Childhood and Adolescence

Stefan Ehehalt · Andreas Neu

University Children's Hospital, Pediatric Endocrinology and Diabetes, Tuebingen, Germany

Diagnosing Diabetes and Insulin Resistance

Diagnosing diabetes used to be a simple task. Clinical symptoms such as polydipsia and polyuria, weight loss and fatigue gave reasons for blood glucose measurement. Elevated measurements of blood glucose and classical symptoms were sufficient criteria for diagnosing diabetes in childhood, which was as a rule considered to be type 1 diabetes.

With the emerging number of reports on an increasing prevalence of obese children and children at risk for type 2 diabetes, the diagnostic situation in pediatric diabetology has changed. Insulin resistance (IR) was recognized to be a condition of its own leading to hyperinsulinemia and eventually to type 2 diabetes. In contrast to the diagnostic assessment of diabetes, the path of diagnosing IR is less clear and depends on the given situation in an individual.

In adulthood, IR is known to be important in the pathogenesis of the metabolic syndrome and cardiovascular disease [Reaven, 1988; Facchini et al., 2001]. The more recent literature even describes an association between hyperinsulinemia and both cancer development and neurodegeneration [Becker et al., 2009; Frasca et al., 2008; de la Monte, 2009]. In childhood, there is less evidence about what IR really means. Despite this fact, IR is of importance because it is associated with childhood obesity which has reached epidemic proportions globally [WHO, 2009]. Furthermore, IR in childhood is also associated with cardiovascular and metabolic risk factors including nonalcoholic fatty liver disease [Denzer et al., 2009; Ten and Maclaren, 2004].

Definition

Multiple definitions of IR exist, but none of them is generally accepted [Arslanian, 2005].

Based on glucose metabolism, IR is 'a less effective response of tissues to insulin in terms of glucose uptake and inhibition of gluconeogenesis' [Becker et al., 2009].

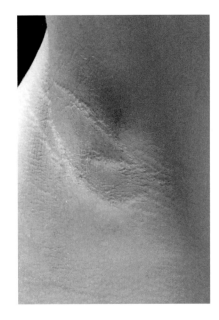

Fig. 1. Acanthosis nigricans of the left axilla.

The skeletal muscle is of importance as the majority of glucose uptake occurs there [DeFronzo, 1992].

Based on insulin action, IR can be defined as 'an impaired ability of plasma insulin at usual concentrations to adequately promote peripheral glucose disposal, suppress hepatic glucose, and inhibit very-low-density lipoprotein (VLDL) output' [Ten and Maclaren, 2004].

Based on the clinical picture, IR can be defined by the 'phenotype of IR' which can include, among others: visceral obesity, acanthosis nigricans (fig. 1), hirsutism, hypertension, hepatic steatosis, and hyperandrogenism [Ten and Maclaren, 2004].

Risk Factors of Childhood Insulin Resistance

Obesity
A major factor in the development of IR is obesity with a negative correlation between insulin sensitivity and BMI/body fat [Arslanian and Suprasongsin, 1996; Bacha et al., 2006]. However, not every obese person is always insulin resistant and IR can also occur in normal-weight individuals [Springer et al., 2010]. It is well known that body fat distribution and fat deposition in muscle and liver (ectopic fat) are important determinants of insulin sensitivity in adulthood [Ferrannini et al., 1997; Machann et al., 2005; Springer et al., 2010; Stefan et al., 2005]. In childhood and adolescence, the contribution of visceral adipose tissue to IR is well-established, while there are only

few reports indicating that ectopic fat deposition is associated with decreased insulin sensitivity [Springer et al., 2010; Weiss et al., 2003].

Waist circumference alone is a strong predictor of in vivo insulin sensitivity [Lee et al., 2006]. Therefore, waist circumference measurements should be included in the clinical evaluation of childhood obesity [Lee et al., 2006].

Prematurity, Low Birth Weight and Rapid Catch-Up Growth
Lower insulin sensitivity and higher blood pressure are more common in young adults born preterm than in controls. Furthermore, restricted prenatal growth and rapid catch-up seem to be important for the early pathogenesis of IR and other diseases like hypertension [Rotteveel et al., 2008]. These findings provide evidence for a 'Metabolic Programming' (Barker Hypothesis) early in life [Barker and Osmond, 1986; Barker and Clark, 1997].

Sleeping Disorders
Sleep-disordered breathing occurs in 2–5% of adults in western countries [Young et al., 2002] and in 1–6% of children [Rosen et al., 2003]. Obesity and sleep apnea seem to be mutual risk factors. Typical symptoms are loud snoring, sleep fragmentation, and sleep-associated intermittent hypoxemia [Redline et al., 2007]. Sleep-disordered breathing has been associated with IR, obesity, cardiovascular disease, and hypertension [Philips et al., 2005]. Mechanisms for these effects are not yet fully understood, but intermittent hypoxia may contribute to the morbidity of metabolic syndrome by inducing inflammation and oxidative stress and by an increased sympathetic vascular reactivity [Tsaoussoglou et al., 2009; O'Brien and Gozal, 2005].

Pubertal Status
Impaired insulin sensitivity during development is not always a permanent phenomenon. For example, insulin sensitivity decreases significantly during puberty, but increases to near prepubertal levels when pubertal development is complete [Moran et al., 1999; Cutfield et al., 1990].

Ethnicity
Relating to ethnicity, Hispanic, African-American, Pima Indian, and Asian children are more insulin resistant compared with matched Caucasian children [Goran et al., 2002; Arslanian et al., 2002; Whincup et al., 2002]. These studies indicate that there might be a genetic basis for the ethnicity-related differences in insulin sensitivity.

Consequences of Childhood Insulin Resistance

IR itself is not considered a disease. Therefore, according to the statement of an Expert Committee, there is no need to screen for IR in children, and there is no use of medication to treat children with IR in the absence of specific diagnoses like type 2 diabetes or polycystic ovary syndrome [International Expert Committee, 2009; Lévy-Marchal et al., 2010]. This recommendation is based on the following observations: (1) For insulin levels, there is no clear cut-off value separating 'normal' from 'abnormal' [Arslanian, 2005]. (2) It is not clear if metformin does improve insulin sensitivity in obese adolescents without type 2 diabetes or polycystic ovarian syndrome and if it could prevent progression towards type 2 diabetes [International Expert Committee, 2009; Lévy-Marchal et al., 2010; Clarson et al., 2009]. Therefore, not insulin levels but obesity should be treated, since the latter is the major trigger for childhood IR [International Expert Committee, 2009; Lévy-Marchal et al., 2010; Henry et al., 1986; Miyatake et al., 2002].

Type 2 Diabetes, Metabolic Syndrome, and Cardiovascular Disease

It is not clear if IR predicts the development of type 2 diabetes. However, IR itself is associated with the metabolic syndrome [Lee et al., 2008]: The 'Muscatine Study' showed that risk factors of cardiovascular disease begin in childhood and that BMI is the strongest childhood predictor of adult metabolic syndrome [Burns et al., 2009]. In agreement with this study, longitudinal observations of children, adolescents, and young adults enrolled in the 'Bogalusa Heart Study' showed that childhood obesity is linked to IR, dyslipidemia, and hypertension leading to an increased cardiovascular risk later in life [Berenson, 2005].

Nonalcoholic Fatty Liver Disease

Nonalcoholic fatty liver disease (NAFLD) was first described in adults at the end of the 1970s [Adler and Schaffner, 1979; Ludwig et al., 1980]. The frequency of NAFLD varies with ethnicity (Asian: 10.2%; black: 1.5%; Hispanic: 11.8%; white: 8.6% [Schwimmer et al., 2005]), with gender (German children: 41.1% in boys vs. 17.2 % in girls [Denzer et al., 2009]) and pubertal status (German children: highest frequency in boys with Tanner stage 5 (51.2%) and lowest in girls with Tanner stage 5 (12.2%) [Denzer et al., 2009]). Different forms of NAFLD exist ranging from simple steatosis to steatohepatitis to advanced fibrosis and cirrhosis [Angulo, 2002]. It is controversial in whom and when a liver biopsy is indicated [Björnsson, 2008].

NAFLD is associated with visceral obesity and IR [Denzer et al., 2009]. Children with histologically proven NAFLD have higher rates of abnormal glucose tolerance during an OGTT. Because of the strong correlation between NAFLD and IR, increased visceral fat, and hypoadiponectinemia, NAFLD has been described as 'core feature of the metabolic syndrome' [Burgert et al., 2006]. Currently, there are no evidenced-based guidelines for how to medically treat NAFLD in children [Alisi et al., 2009]. It has been shown that weight-loss can normalize levels of alanine aminotransferase (ALT) and reduce fatty liver infiltration, while the degree of fibrosis remained unchanged [Huang et al., 2005].

Polycystic Ovary Syndrome

Polycystic ovary syndrome (PCOS) is the leading cause of infertility in women [Azziz et al., 2009; Diamanti-Kandarakis, 2010]. There are several definitions of PCOS given in the literature. According to the 'Androgen Excess and PCOS Society Task Force', PCOS should be defined by the presence of hyperandrogenism (clinical and/ or biochemical), ovarian dysfunction (oligo-anovulation and/or polycystic ovaries), and the exclusion of related disorders. There is substantial controversy regarding the methods for assessing IR in PCOS. Nevertheless, it is assumed that between 50 and 70% of women with PCOS have demonstrable IR [Azziz et al., 2009]. Moreover, β-cell dysfunction appears to be prevalent in PCOS. However, the severity of the abnormality is also positively related to a family history of type 2 diabetes [Ehrmann et al., 2005].

Measurement

Measurement of insulin sensitivity includes both the assessment of the sensitivity of body tissue to insulin and the determination of insulin secretion of the β-cell in response to rising glucose levels. The 'golden standard' techniques for measuring insulin sensitivity are clamp studies. These studies are time-consuming and difficult to perform [Arslanian, 2005], particularly during childhood (see below). Thus, several mathematical models have been proposed to simplify the assessment of IR. However, the clinical use of these models is under controversial debate [Arslanian, 2005]. One of the essential aspects causing this controversy is the lack of a globally standardized insulin assay. Thus, according to the 'Insulin Standardization Workgroup', 'measurements of insulin sensitivity and secretion are currently done only for research purposes and are only comparable within individual studies' [Staten et al., 2010]. This position is contrary to the finding that measures of insulin sensitivity can help to identify children at risk for obesity-associated comorbidities like NAFLD [Denzer et al., 2009].

Fasting Levels of Insulin

In adulthood, obesity is associated with higher levels of fasting insulin than those observed in normal weight individuals [Kim et al., 2004].

Test Procedure. Testing is performed after an overnight fasting period of 10–12 h. Baseline venous blood sample is drawn for the determination of serum insulin.

Stability of Insulin. At room temperature: in whole blood only 15 min, in serum/ plasma 1 day; refrigerated to 4–8°C (serum/plasma): 6 days; at –20°C (serum/plasma): 6 months. Hemolyzed samples must not be used [Guder and Nolte, 2009; Thomas, 2005].

In adults, fasting levels of insulin greater than 15 μU/ml, or insulin peak (post-OGTT) levels of more than 150 μU/ml and/or more than 75 μU/ml at 120 min of OGTT are considered to be hyperinsulinemic [Reaven et al., 1993]. In children, there is neither a clear cutoff between normal and abnormal nor a standardized methodology how to measure fasting insulin [International Expert Committee, 2009; Lévy-Marchal et al., 2010]. Testing the circulating level of insulin against insulin sensitivity measured by using the euglycemic insulin clamp, the correlation was reported to be r = –0.51 for children with a BMI ≥ 85th percentile [Schwartz et al., 2008]. Comparing fasting insulin to parameters of IR of the Minimal Model, a correlation of r = –0.58 (p < 0.0001) was shown [Cutfield and Hofman, 2005].

It seems reasonable to measure not only fasting insulin but also fasting glucose levels and/or to do an oral glucose tolerance test in patients who are at risk for the metabolic syndrome.

Clamp Studies

Clamp studies are complex and not suitable for routine clinical praxis or in large epidemiological studies [Schwartz et al., 2008]. The method at its present form has been developed by DeFronzo et al. [1979]. In pediatrics, only few investigators are experienced in this technique. For children and adolescents, the test procedure has been described in detail by Arslanian [2005]. In the following, we refer to this protocol.

Prior to the test, a weight-maintaining diet rich in carbohydrates is recommended. Testing is performed after an overnight fasting period of 12 h.

Hyperinsulinemic-Euglycemic Clamp

The hyperinsulinemic-euglycemic clamp technique provides insights into the insulin sensitivity of hepatic and peripheral tissues of an individual [Arlsanian, 2005]. Under steady state plasma glucose conditions, the hepatic glucose production is suppressed. In this case, the amount of glucose infused is equal to the amount of glucose metabolized by the total body. If endogenous glucose production is not suppressed, total-body glucose uptake equals to the amount of endogenous glucose production plus exogenous glucose infusion rate. Hepatic glucose production can be quantified by means of isotopes [Arslanian et al., 1997]. Protein and fat metabolism can be determined if the administration of multiple isotopes is combined with indirect calorimetry [Arslanian, 2005], (fig. 2).

Test Preparation. An antecubital catheter for infusions; a heated superficial hand vein catheter for frequent sampling of arterialized blood [Abumrad et al., 1981; Ferrannini and Mari, 1998]; accurate, regularly calibrated pumps; glucose (20% dextrose); short-acting human insulin; a frequently calibrated bedside glucose analyzer.

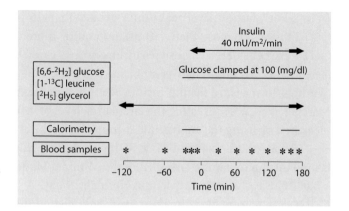

Fig. 2. Study protocol to assess glucose, protein (leucine) and lipid (glycerol) metabolism, and the effect of insulin during a hyperinsulinemic-euglycemic clamp combined with multiple stable isotope infusions. From Arslanian [2005].

Test Procedure. After baseline measurements, insulin infusion is started (5–120 mU/m²/min, usually 40 mU/m²/min, dependent on the desired steady state plasma insulin concentration). 2–10 min later, glucose infusion is started (about 1–2 mg/kg/min). In case of hyperglycemia (diabetic patients), blood glucose is lowered to normal values before glucose infusion gets started. In the following, blood glucose measurements are done every 2.5–5 min. Glucose infusion rate is adjusted appropriately to maintain plasma glucose concentration at the basal level and to prevent hypoglycemia.

Test duration: 2–4 h.

Test measurements (among others): insulin sensitivity = insulin-stimulated glucose disposal rate/steady-state insulin levels during the last 30 min of the clamp [Arslanian et al., 2002; Lee et al., 2007].

For example (mean ± SD): African-American children and adolescents (mean age 12.3 ± 0.2 years): insulin sensitivity = 6.5 ± 0.5 mg × kg^{-1} × min^{-1}/µU/ml versus American white children and adolescents (mean age 12.9 ± 0.2 years): insulin sensitivity = 7.2 ± 0.6 mg × kg^{-1} × min^{-1}/µU/ml [Lee et al., 2007].

The metabolic clearance rate of insulin = insulin infusion rate/increase in plasma insulin concentration above basal [DeFronzo et al., 1979; Sherwin et al., 1974].

For example (mean ± SD): African-American children (aged 10.0–14.3 years): 17.9 ± 0.8 µmol × kg FFM^{-1} × min^{-1} versus American white children (aged 9.9–14.3 years): 20.7 ± 1.1 µmol × kg FFM^{-1} × min^{-1} [Hannon et al., 2008].

Normal glucose-tolerant black and white children (mean age 8.7 ± 1.4 years): 0.106 ± 0.033 mg × kg^{-1} × min^{-1}/µU/ml [Uwaifo, 2002].

Glucose disposition index = insulin sensitivity × first-phase insulin [Arslanian et al., 2002]. In order to maintain glucose homeostasis, insulin secretion has to increase if insulin sensitivity decreases [Arslanian 2005] (fig. 3).

For example (mean ± SD): African-American adolescents (aged 10.0–14.3 years): 10.3 ± 1.0 versus American white adolescents (aged 9.9–14.3 years): 6.3 ± 0.7 µmol × kg FFM^{-1} × min^{-1}, p = 0.002 [Hannon et al., 2008].

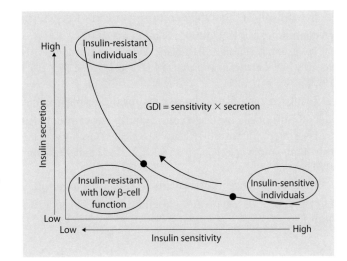

Fig. 3. Hyperbolic relationship between insulin sensitivity and secretion. GDI = Glucose disposition index. Source: Arslanian [2005], Bergman et al. [2002], Weyer et al. [1999].

Hyperglycemic Clamp

During a controlled hyperglycemic condition, the response of the β-cell to glucose and the amount of glucose metabolized can be assessed [DeFronzo et al., 1979; Arslanian et al., 1997, 2001; Hovorka and Jones, 1994]. During hyperglycemia, the hepatic gluconeogenesis is completely suppressed in healthy individuals. If not (e.g. in diabetic patients), hepatic glucose production can be determined by isotopes [Arslanian, 2005].

Test preparation: see above (without insulin).

Test procedure: baseline measurements before the clamp. Priming dose of glucose (dextrose 25–50%) over 2 min to raise blood glucose concentration quickly (usually to 225 mg/dl ± 10%), followed by a maintenance dose of glucose (dextrose 20%) over a period of 2 h [DeFronzo et al., 1979].

0.5 min after the bolus to 15 min (every 2.5 min): measurements of plasma glucose, insulin, and C-peptide. 15–120 min: blood is drawn every 5 min for glucose measurement, and every 15 min for insulin and C-peptide determination.

The glucose priming bolus (mg) can be calculated as follows [Arslanian, 2005]: 225 mg/dl minus the mean of three baseline fasting plasma glucose levels [mg/dl] × individual's weight [kg] × glucose distribution factor [dl/kg] [1.5 for children of normal weight and 1.1 for overweight and obese children].

Test measurements (among others): first-phase insulin secretion = mean of 5 determinations within the first 15 min.

For example (mean ± SD): black Americans (mean age 10.0 ± 0.2 years): 76.9 ± 6.8 μU/ml versus white Americans (mean age 10.7 ± 0.3 years): 52.1 ± 6.4 μU/ml (p = 0.016) [Arslanian and Suprasongsin, 1997].

Second-phase insulin secretion = mean of 8 determinations from 15 to 120 min [Arslanian et al., 1997, 2001; Saad et al., 2002].

For example (mean ± SD): black Americans (mean age 10.0 ± 0.2 years): 89.7 ± 11.1 μU/ml versus white Americans (mean age 10.7 ± 0.3 years): 78.1 ± 8.5 μU/ml (p = 0.2 [Arslanian et al., 1997].

Insulin sensitivity = glucose disposal rate/plasma insulin concentration during the last 60 min of the hyperglycemic clamp experiment [Austin et al., 1994].

For example (mean ± SD): black Americans (mean age 10.0 ± 0.2 years): 17.4 ± 2.7 versus white Americans (mean age 10.7 ± 0.3 years): 21.6 ± 2.8 mg/kg × min per μU/ml [n.s., Arslanian et al., 1997].

Rate of glucose metabolism = rate of exogenous glucose infusion minus urinary glucose loss, typically calculated from 60 to 120 min [mg/kg/min] [Arslanian, 2005].

The 'Minimal Model'

Previously, intravenous glucose tolerance test (ivGTT) and tolbutamide test were widely used to assess β-cell function. Today, both tests are part of the procedures for the 'Minimal Model'.

The Minimal Model Analysis of the 'Frequently Sampled Intravenous Glucose Tolerance Test' (FSIVGTT) was developed to measure insulin sensitivity and β-cell glucose sensitivity from the response to intravenous glucose by means of computer modeling [Bergman et al., 1981]. The correlation between the minimal model analysis and the glucose clamp is significant [Saad et al., 1994].

The Modified Minimal Model (MMM) [Cutfield et al., 1990]: the MMM is the adoption of the Minimal Model to children. It is considered to be safe, accurate, and valid [Cutfield et al., 1990].

Test Preparation. A catheter for infusions; a catheter for frequent sampling of blood; glucose (25% dextrose); tolbutamide diluted in sterile water; a bedside glucose analyzer.

Test Procedure. Prior to the test, a weight-maintaining diet rich in carbohydrates is recommended. Testing is performed after an overnight fasting period of 10–12 h. Baseline samples are drawn at –30, –15, and 0 min. At time point zero, 0.3 g/kg 25% dextrose is injected over 1 min. Twenty minutes later, tolbutamide (5 mg/kg) is injected over 30 s.

Duration of the Test. MMM: 180 min, abbreviated MMM: 90 min.

Blood samples are taken for glucose and insulin measurements (abbreviated MMM time points may vary) at 1, 2, 3, 4, 5, 6, 8, 10, 12, 14, 19, 22, 23, 24, 25, 27, 30, 35, 40, 50, 60, 70, 80, and 90 min, and (MMM) 100, 120, 140, 160, and 180 min [Vuguin et al., 2001].

Test Measurements (Among Others). The insulin sensitivity index (S_I) and the acute insulin response (AIR) can be calculated using the Minimod computer program as reported by Cutfield et al. [1990].

For example, a study conducted by Cutfield and associates, showed the following Insulin sensitivity index S_I in American children (90-min abbreviated test [Cutfield et al., 1990]).

Prepubertal children (8.7 ± 2.0 (mean ± SEM) years old, n = 29): S_I = 6.57 ± 0.45.
Pubertal children (13.4 ± 1.8 years old, n = 16): S_I = 2.92 ± 0.45.
Postpubertal group (18.2 ± 0.9 years old, n = 12): S_I = 4.63 ± 0.86.

The acute insulin response (AIR) is an index of insulin-secreting capacity, calculated from the insulin output in the first 19 min.

For example, median AIR was 366 (interquartile range, 216–459) mU/l in normal-weight prepubertal children of New Zealand (mean age 8.2 ± 0.4 years old, n = 15) [Hunter et al., 2004].

Surrogate Measures of Insulin Resistance

Surrogate measures of IR could be a useful tool for both daily clinical practice and research (e.g., for large cohort studies) [Schwartz et al., 2008]. Unfortunately, in childhood and adolescence, the literature is conflicting and well accepted normal values with any of the described methods are still missing [Ten and Maclaren, 2004]. The following methods are presented in detail because they have been widely used in adult, and subsequent, in pediatric studies [Bonora et al., 2000; Katz et al., 2000; Schwartz et al., 2008].

Homeostasis Model Assessment (HOMA)
HOMA estimates steady state beta cell function (%B) and insulin sensitivity (%S), as percentages of a normal reference population. It reflects the balance between hepatic glucose output and insulin secretion [Turner et al., 1979; Wallace et al., 2004].

Test Procedure. Testing is performed after an overnight fasting period of 10–12 h. Baseline samples are drawn at 0 min: plasma glucose, insulin.

The formulas for HOMA and for % β-cell function are as follows [Matthews et al., 1985]:

HOMA = [fasting glucose (mmol/l) × fasting insulin (mU/l)]/22.5, or NPG (mmol/l) × NPI (pmol/l) × 135^{-1}
% β-cell function = 20 × plasma insulin (mU/l)/(plasma glucose (mmol/l) – 3.5).

In childhood and adolescence, the correlation between HOMA and fasting insulin is high (r = 0.99) [Schwartz et al., 2008]. Conwell et al. [2004] reported in obese children and adolescents that HOMA correlates strongly with insulin sensitivity assessed by the MMM. This high correlation, however, could not be found in another study conducted in children by Rössner et al. [2008]. Comparing HOMA and clamp-derived IR unadjusted for fatness (M), the correlation was r = –0.53. After removal of fatness from the estimate of glucose disposal (M_{LBM}), the correlation became lower. In the heavier children, the reported correlations are higher (BMI ≥85th percentile): HOMA versus M: r = –0.60 and HOMA versus M_{LBM}: r = –0.40 [Schwartz et al.,

Table 1. Gender- and age group-specific HOMA-IR

	Age, years	Mean (95% CI)	5th (95% CI)	25th (95% CI)	50th (95% CI)	75th (95% CI)	95th (95% CI)
Boys	9 (n = 342)	0.95 (0.87–1.03)	0.33 (0.29–0.36)	0.55 (0.52–0.61)	0.83 (0.76–0.86)	1.15 (1.05–1.22)	1.88 (1.71–2.49)
	13 (n = 370)	1.66 (1.50–1.82)	0.58 (0.48–0.65)	0.91 (0.87–0.99)	1.40 (1.28–1.52)	2.04 (1.83–2.16)	3.28 (2.95–3.80)
	16 (n = 375)	1.55 (1.43–1.67)	0.61 (0.56–0.70)	0.94 (0.90–0.99)	1.28 (1.21–1.36)	1.69 (1.57–1.85)	3.31 (2.96–4.01)
Girls	9 (n = 369)	1.13 (0.94–1.32)	0.34 (0.28–0.39)	0.63 (0.56–0.68)	0.90 (0.84–0.96)	1.29 (1.18–1.36)	2.07 (1.87–2.39)
	13 (n = 352)	1.90 (1.73–2.06)	0.79 (0.68–0.83)	1.25 (1.14–1.31)	1.62 (1.52–1.75)	2.27 (2.10–2.41)	3.86 (3.34–4.42)
	16 (n = 436)	1.60 (1.52–1.68)	0.68 (0.62–0.75)	1.03 (0.98–1.12)	1.42 (1.35–1.53)	2.01 (1.82–2.14)	3.10 (2.80–3.38)

Representative sample of Quebec youth (n = 2,244 individuals; 9, 13, and 16 years of age) [Allard et al., 2003]. CI = Confidence interval.

2008]. It should be noted that the correlation between HOMA and clamp studies is higher in adulthood (e.g. r = 0.88) [Matthews, 1985].

There are several studies providing data of HOMA in childhood and adolescence. But again, well-accepted normal values are still missing. For example, the gender- and age group-specific distribution of HOMA-IR values corresponding to a representative sample of Quebec youth is given in table 1 [Allard et al., 2003].

The above-mentioned formula for HOMA overestimates insulin sensitivity and underestimates β-cell function. Therefore, the computer-generated model of HOMA (HOMA2 or 'updated HOMA model') was developed [Wallace et al., 2004; Cutfield et al., 2003]. The computer program is available at http://www.dtu.ox.ac.uk/index.php?maindoc = /homa/index.php. The model helps to determine insulin sensitivity and ß-cell function from fasting plasma glucose and RIA insulin, specific insulin, or C-peptide concentrations. The formula can only be used in a steady state situation [Wallace et al., 2004].

Quantitative Insulin Sensitivity Check Index (QUICKI)
For adults, Katz et al. [2000] and associates have developed an alternative IR index based on fasting insulin and fasting glucose values. Plasma glucose and insulin are determined after an overnight fasting period of 10–12 h:

QUICKI = 1/(log [fasting insulin in mU/l] + log [fasting glucose in mg/dl])

Ehehalt · Neu

For American children and adolescents, Schwartz et al. [2008] have reported the following values (323 children and adolescents, mean age 13 years) (mean ± SD): for the whole cohort: 0.15 ± 0.02; for adolescents with a BMI <85th percentile: 0.16 ± 0.02; for adolescents with a BMI ≥85th percentile: 0.14 ± 0.02. In this study, QUICKI was significantly correlated with clamp-derived measures of insulin sensitivity in children with a BMI ≥85th percentile (r = 0.53–0.62). However, other authors reported significantly lower correlations [Cutfield et al., 2003].

Oral Glucose Tolerance Test/Whole-Body Insulin Sensitivity Index (WBISI)
The Index of whole-body insulin sensitivity (WBISI) has been developed by Matsuda and DeFronzo [1999] and validated in adults. It provides an approximation of whole-body insulin sensitivity from the oGTT. According to Yeckel et al. [2004], WBISI represents a good estimate (r = 0.78) for clamp-derived insulin sensitivity (glucose disposed, M-value).

Test Procedure. Prior to the test, a weight-maintaining diet rich in carbohydrates is recommended. Testing is performed after an overnight fasting period of 10–12 h. Baseline samples are drawn at 0 min (plasma glucose, insulin). At time point zero, a glucose solution is given to drink (1.75 g/kg body weight, maximum 75 g). Blood samples are taken for plasma glucose and insulin measurements at 30, 60, 90 and 120 (150 and 180 min).

The Whole-Body Insulin Sensitivity Index is calculated as follows:

WBISI = (10,000/square root of [fasting glucose (mg/dl) × fasting insulin (µU/ml)] × [mean glucose (mg/dl) × mean insulin (µU/ml) during OGTT]).

For example (mean ± SD): for American children and adolescents (n = 56, aged 8–18 years, mean BMI 36.7 ± 0.8) with impaired glucose tolerance, WBISI (Tertile 0) was calculated to be 1.02 ± 0.09. For American children and adolescents (n = 107, aged 8–18 years, mean BMI 34.6 ± 0.7) with normal glucose tolerance, WBISI (Tertile 3) was calculated to be 3.38 ± 0.11 [Yeckel et al., 2004].

Conclusions

Most of the tests mentioned require research like settings as they are time consuming and expensive. Thus, they are not useful for clinical purposes. From our point of view, oral glucose tolerance testing including measurements of fasting insulin rather seem to be adequate and sufficient tools in most cases.

The clinician should be aware of the clinical picture (visceral obesity, acanthosis nigricans) and of the consequences of IR. However, IR itself is not a disease. Therefore, insulin levels should not be treated but obesity (especially visceral fat, and fat deposition in muscle and liver) which is one of the major risk factors for IR.

References

Abumrad NN, Rabin D, Diamond MP, Lacy WW: Use of a heated superficial hand vein as an alternative site for the measurement of amino acid concentrations and for the study of glucose and alanine kinetics in man. Metabolism 1981;30:936–940.

Adler M, Schaffner F: Fatty liver hepatitis and cirrhosis in obese patients. Am J Med 1979;67:811–816.

Alisi A, Manco M, Vania A, Nobili V: Pediatric nonalcoholic fatty liver disease in 2009. J Pediatr 2009;155: 469–474.

Allard P, Delvin EE, Paradis G, Hanley JA, O'Loughlin J, Lavallée C, Levy E, Lambert M: Distribution of fasting plasma insulin, free fatty acids, and glucose concentrations and of homeostasis model assessment of insulin resistance in a representative sample of Quebec children and adolescents. Clin Chem 2003; 49:644–649.

Angulo P: Nonalcoholic fatty liver disease. N Engl J Med 2002;346:1221–1231.

Arslanian SA: Clamp techniques in paediatrics: what have we learned? Horm Res 2005;64:16–24.

Arslanian SA, Lewy VD, Danadian K: Glucose intolerance in obese adolescents with polycystic ovary syndrome: roles of insulin resistance and β-cell dysfunction and risk of cardiovascular disease. J Clin Endocrinol Metab 2001;86:66–71.

Arslanian SA, Saad R, Lewy V, Danadian K, Janosky J: Hyperinsulinemia in african-american children: decreased insulin clearance and increased insulin secretion and its relationship to insulin sensitivity. Diabetes 2002;51:3014–3019.

Arslanian S, Suprasongsin C: Insulin sensitivity, lipids, and body composition in childhood: is 'syndrome X' present? J Clin Endocrinol Metab 1996;81:1058–1062.

Arslanian S, Suprasongsin C, Janosky JE: Insulin secretion and sensitivity in black versus white prepubertal healthy children. J Clin Endocrinol Metab 1997; 82:1923–1927.

Austin A, Kalhan SC, Orenstein D, Nixon P, Arslanian S: Roles of insulin resistance and beta-cell dysfunction in the pathogenesis of glucose intolerance in cystic fibrosis. J Clin Endocrinol Metab 1994;79:80–85.

Azziz R, Carmina E, Dewailly D, Diamanti-Kandarakis E, Escobar-Morreale HF, Futterweit W, Janssen OE, Legro RS, Norman RJ, Taylor AE, Witchel SF: The Androgen Excess and PCOS Society criteria for the polycystic ovary syndrome: the complete task force report, Fertil Steril 2009;91:456–488.

Bacha F, Saad R, Gungor N, Arslanian SA: Are obesity-related metabolic risk factors modulated by the degree of insulin resistance in adolescents? Diabetes Care 2006;29:1599–1604.

Barker DJ, Clark PM: Fetal undernutrition and disease in later life. Rev Reprod 1997;2:105–112.

Barker DJ, Osmond C: Infant mortality, childhood nutrition, and ischaemic heart disease in England and Wales. Lancet 1986;i:1077–1081.

Becker S, Dossus L, Kaaks R: Obesity related hyperinsulinaemia and hyperglycaemia and cancer development. Arch Physiol Biochem 2009;115:86–96.

Berenson GS: Obesity–a critical issue in preventive cardiology: the Bogalusa Heart Study. Prev Cardiol 2005;8:234–241.

Bergman RN, Ader M, Huecking K, VanCitters G: Accurate assessment of β-cell function: the hyperbolic correction. Diabetes 2002;51:S212–S220.

Bergman RN, Phillips LS, Cobelli C: Physiologic evaluation of factors controlling glucose tolerance in man: measurement of insulin sensitivity and beta-cell glucose sensitivity from the response to intravenous glucose. J Clin Invest 1981;68:1456–1467.

Björnsson E: The clinical aspects of non-alcoholic fatty liver disease. Minerva Gastroenterol Dietol 2008;54: 7–18.

Bonora E, Targher G, Alberiche M, Bonadonna RC, Saggiani F, Zenere MB, Monauni T, Muggeo M: Homeostasis model assessment closely mirrors the glucose clamp technique in the assessment of insulin sensitivity. Diabetes Care 2000;23:57–63.

Burgert TS, Taksali SE, Dziura J, Goodman TR, Yeckel CW, Papademetris X, Constable RT, Weiss R, Tamborlane WV, Savoye M, Seyal AA, Caprio S: Alanine aminotransferase levels and fatty liver in childhood obesity: associations with insulin resistance, adiponectin, and visceral fat. J Clin Endocrinol Metab 2006;91:4287–4294.

Burns TL, Letuchy EM, Paulos R, Witt J: Childhood predictors of the metabolic syndrome in middle-aged adults: the Muscatine study. J Pediatr 2009;155:S5. e17– S5.e26.

Clarson CL, Mahmud FH, Baker JE, Clark HE, McKay WM, Schauteet VD, Hill DJ: Metformin in combination with structured lifestyle intervention improved body mass index in obese adolescents, but did not improve insulin resistance. Endocrine 2009;36:141–146.

Conwell LS, Trost SG, Brown WJ, Batch JA: Indexes of insulin resistance and secretion in obese children and adolescents: a validation study. Diabetes Care 2004;27:314–319.

Cutfield WS, Bergman RN, Menon RK, Sperling MA: The modified minimal model: application to measurement of insulin sensitivity in children. J Clin Endocrinol Metab 1990;70:1644–1650.

Cutfield WS, Hofman PL: Simple fasting methods to assess insulin sensitivity in childhood. Horm Res 2005;64:25–31.

Cutfield WS, Jefferies CA, Jackson W, Robinson EM, Hofman PL: Evaluation of HOMA and QUICKI as measures of insulin sensitivity in prepubertal children. Pediatr Diabetes 2003;4:119–125.

DeFronzo RA: Pathogenesis of type 2 (non-insulin dependent) diabetes mellitus: a balanced overview. Diabetologia 1992;35:389–397.

DeFronzo RA, Tobin JD, Andres R: Glucose clamp technique: a method for quantifying insulin secretion and resistance. Am J Physiol 1979;237:E214–E223.

de la Monte SM: Insulin resistance and Alzheimer's disease. BMB Rep 2009;31;42:475–481.

Denzer C, Thiere D, Muche R, Koenig W, Mayer H, Kratzer W, Wabitsch M: Gender-specific prevalences of fatty liver in obese children and adolescents: roles of body fat distribution, sex steroids, and insulin resistance. J Clin Endocrinol Metab 2009;94:3872–3881.

Diamanti-Kandarakis E: PCOS in adolescents. Best Pract Res Clin Obstet Gynaecol 2010;24:173–183.

Ehrmann DA, Kasza K, Azziz R, Legro RS, Ghazzi MN: Effects of race and family history of type 2 diabetes on metabolic status of women with polycystic ovary syndrome. J Clin Endocrinol Metab 2005;90:66–71.

Facchini FS, Hua N, Abbasi F, Reaven GM: Insulin resistance as a predictor of age-related diseases. J Clin Endocrinol Metab 2001;86:3574–3578.

Ferrannini E, Mari A: How to measure insulin sensitivity. J Hypertens 1998;16:895–906.

Ferrannini E, Natali A, Bell P, Cavallo-Perin P, Lalic N, Mingrone G: Insulin resistance and hypersecretion in obesity. European Group for the Study of Insulin Resistance (EGIR). J Clin Invest 1997;100:1166–1173.

Frasca F, Pandini G, Sciacca L, Pezzino V, Squatrito S, Belfiore A, Vigneri R: The role of insulin receptors and IGF-I receptors in cancer and other diseases. Arch Physiol Biochem 2008;114:23–37.

Guder WG, Nolte J (eds): Das Laborbuch. Munich, Elsevier, 2009.

Goran MI, Bergman RN, Cruz ML, Watanabe R: Insulin resistance and associated compensatory responses in African-American and Hispanic children. Diabetes Care 2002;25:2184–2190.

Hannon TS, Bacha F, Lin Y, Arslanian SA: Hyperinsulinemia in African-American adolescents compared with their American white peers despite similar insulin sensitivity: a reflection of upregulated beta-cell function? Diabetes Care 2008;31:1445–1447.

Henry RR, Weist-Kent TA, Scheafer L, Kolterman OG, Olefsky JM: Metabolic consequences of very low caloric diet therapy in obese non-insulindependent diabetic and nondiabetic subjects. Diabetes 1986;35:155–161.

Hovorka R, Jones RH: How to measure insulin secretion. Diabetes Metab Rev 1994;10:91–117.

Huang MA, Greenson JK, Chao C, Anderson L, Peterman D, Jacobson J, Emick D, Lok AS, Conjeevaram HS: One-year intense nutritional counseling results in histologic improvement in patients with non-alcoholic steatohepatitis: a pilot study. Am J Gastroenterol 2005;100:1072–1078.

Hunter WA, Cundy T, Rabone D, Hofman PL, Harris M, Regan F, Robinson E, Cutfield WS: Insulin sensitivity in the offspring of women with type 1 and type 2 diabetes. Diabetes Care 2004;27:1148–1152.

International Committee Advises: Don't Measure Fasting Insulin in Children. New York, 2009, http://www.diabetesincontrol.com/index.php?option = com_content&view = article&id = 8408&catid = 53& Itemid = 8

Katz A, Nambi S, Mather K, Baron AD, Follmann DA, Sullivan G, Quon MJ: Quantitative insulin sensitivity check index: a simple accurate method for assessing insulin sensitivity in humans. J Endocrinol Metab 2000;85:2402–2410.

Kim SH, Abbasi F, Reaven GM: Impact of degree of obesity on surrogate estimates of insulin resistance. Diabetes Care 2004;27:1998–2002.

Lavine JE, Schwimmer JB: Nonalcoholic fatty liver disease in the pediatric population. Clin Liver Dis 2004;8:549–558, viii–ix.

Lee S, Bacha F, Arslanian SA: Waist circumference, blood pressure, and lipid components of the metabolic syndrome. J Pediatr 2006;149:809–816.

Lee S, Bacha F, Gungor N, Arslanian S: Waist circumference is an independent predictor of insulin resistance in black and white youths. J Pediatr 2006;148:188–194.

Lee S, Bacha F, Gungor N, Arslanian S: Comparison of different definitions of pediatric metabolic syndrome: relation to abdominal adiposity, insulin resistance, adiponectin, and inflammatory biomarkers. J Pediatr 2008;152:177–184.

Lee S, Gungor N, Bacha F, Arslanian S: Insulin resistance: link to the components of the metabolic syndrome and biomarkers of endothelial dysfunction in youth. Diabetes Care 2007;30:2091–2097.

Lévy-Marchal C, Arslanian S, Cutfield W, Sinaiko A, Druet C, Marcovecchio ML, Chiarelli F, ESPE-LWPES-ISPAD-APPES-APEG-SLEP-JSPE, Insulin Resistance in Children Consensus Conference Group: Insulin Resistance in Children: consensus, perspective, and future directions. J Clin Endocrinol Metab 2010, Sep 8 [Epub ahead of print].

Ludwig J, Viggiano TR, McGill DB, Oh BJ: Nonalcoholic steatohepatitis: Mayo Clinic experiences with a hitherto unnamed disease. Mayo Clin Proc 1980;55: 434–438.

Machann J, Thamer C, Schnoedt B, Stefan N, Stumvoll M, Haring HU, Claussen CD, Fritsche A, Schick F: Age and gender related effects on adipose tissue compartments of subjects with increased risk for type 2 diabetes: a whole body MRI/MRS study. Magn Reson Mater Phy 2005;18:128–137.

Matsuda M, DeFronzo RA: Insulin sensitivity indices obtained from oral glucose tolerance testing: comparison with the euglycemic insulin clamp. Diabetes Care 1999;22:1462–1470.

Matthews DR, Hosker JP, Rudenski AS, Naylor BA, Treacher DF, Turner RC: Homeostasis model assessment: insulin resistance and beta-cell function from fasting plasma glucose and insulin concentrations in man. Diabetologia 1985;28:412–419.

Miyatake N, Nishikawa H, Morishita A, Kunitomi M, Wada J, Suzuki H, Takahashi K, Makino H, Kira S, Fujii M: Daily walking reduces visceral adipose tissue areas and improves insulin resistance in Japanese obese subjects. Diabetes Res Clin Pract 2002;58:101–107.

Moran A, Jacobs DR Jr, Steinberger J, Hong CP, Prineas R, Luepker R, Sinaiko AR: Insulin resistance during puberty: results from clamp studies in 357 children. Diabetes 1999;48:2039–2044.

O'Brien LM, Gozal D: Autonomic dysfunction in children with sleep-disordered breathing. Sleep 2005;28:747–752.

Phillips B: Sleep-disordered breathing and cardiovascular disease. Sleep Medicine Reviews 2005;9:131–140.

Reaven GM: Banting lecture 1988: role of insulin resistance in human disease. Diabetes 1988;37:1595–1607.

Reaven GM, Chen YD, Hollenbeck CB, Sheu WH, Ostrega D, Polonsky KS: Plasma insulin, C-peptide, and proinsulin concentrations in obese and non-obese individuals with varying degrees of glucose tolerance. J Clin Endocrinol Metab 1993;76:44–48.

Redline S, Storfer-Isser A, Rosen CL, Johnson NL, Kirchner HL, Emancipator J, Kibler AM: Association between metabolic syndrome and sleep-disordered breathing in adolescents. Am J Respir Crit Care Med 2007;176:401–408.

Rössner SM, Neovius M, Montgomery SM, Marcus C, Norgren S: Alternative methods of insulin sensitivity assessment in obese children and adolescents. Diabetes Care 2008;31:802–804.

Rosen CL, Larkin EK, Kirchner HL, Emancipator JL, Bivins SF, Surovec SA, Martin RJ, Redline S: Prevalence and risk factors for sleepdisordered breathing in 8- to 11-year-old children: association with race and prematurity. J Pediatr 2003;142:383–389.

Rotteveel J, van Weissenbruch MM, Twisk JW, Delemarre-Van de Waal HA: Infant and childhood growth patterns, insulin sensitivity, and blood pressure in prematurely born young adults. Pediatrics 2008;122:313–321.

Saad MF, Anderson RL, Laws A, Watanabe RM, Kades WW, Chen YD, Sands RE, Pei D, Savage PJ, Bergman RN: A comparison between the minimal model and the glucose clamp in the assessment of insulin sensitivity across the spectrum of glucose tolerance: Insulin Resistance Atherosclerosis Study. Diabetes 1994;43:1114–1121.

Saad RJ, Danadian K, Lewy V, Arslanian SA: Insulin resistance of puberty in African-American children: lack of a compensatory increase in insulin secretion. Pediatr Diabetes 2002;3:4–9.

Schwartz B, Jacobs DR Jr, Moran A, Steinberger J, Hong CP, Sinaiko AR: Measurement of insulin sensitivity in children: comparison between the euglycemic-hyperinsulinemic clamp and surrogate measures. Diabetes Care 2008;31:783–788.

Schwimmer JB, Behling C, Newbury R, Deutsch R, Nievergelt C, Schork NJ, Lavine JE: Histopathology of pediatric nonalcoholic fatty liver disease. Hepatology 2005;42:641–649.

Sherwin RS, Kramer KJ, Tobin JD, Insel PA, Liljenquist JE, Berman M, Andres R: A model of the kinetics of insulin in man. J Clin Invest 1974;53:1481–1492.

Springer F, Nguyen HP, Machann J, Schweizer R, Ranke MB, Binder G, Schick F, Ehehalt S: Normal-weight 14-year-old girl with acanthosis nigricans and markedly increased hepatic steatosis: evidence for the important role of ectopic fat deposition in the pathogenesis of insulin resistance in childhood and adolescence. Horm Res Paediatric 2010 Sep 15. [Epub ahead of print]

Staten MA, Stern MP, Miller WG, Steffes MW, Campbell SE: Insulin Standardization Workgroup: Insulin assay standardization: leading to measures of insulin sensitivity and secretion for practical clinical care. Diabetes Care 2010;33:205–256.

Stefan N, Machann J, Schick F, Claussen CD, Thamer C, Fritsche A, Häring HU: New imaging techniques of fat, muscle and liver within the context of determining insulin sensitivity. Horm Res 2005;64(suppl 3):38–44.

Ten S, Maclaren N: Insulin resistance syndrome in children. J Clin Endocrinol Metab 2004;89:2526–2539.

Thomas L: Labor und Diagnose, ed 6. Marburg, Die Medizinische Verlagsgesellschaft mbH, 2005.

Tsaoussoglou M, Bixler EO, Calhoun S, Chrousos GP, Sauder K, Vgontzas AN: Sleep-disordered breathing in obese children is associated with prevalent excessive daytime sleepiness, inflammation, and metabolic abnormalities. J Clin Endocrinol Metab 2009; 95:143–150.

Turner RC, Holman RR, Matthews D, Hockaday TD, Peto J: Insulin deficiency and insulin resistance interaction in diabetes: estimation of their relative contribution by feedback analysis from basal plasma insulin and glucose concentrations. Metabolism 1979;28:1086–1096.

Uwaifo GI, Fallon EM, Chin J, Elberg J, Parikh SJ, Yanovski JA: Indices of insulin action, disposal, and secretion derived from fasting samples and clamps in normal glucose-tolerant black and white children. Diabetes Care 2002;25:2081–2087.

Vuguin P, Saenger P, Dimartino-Nardi J: Fasting insulin ratio: a useful measure of insulin resistance in girls with premature adrenarche. JCEM 2001;86:4618–4621.

Wallace TM, Levy JC, Matthews DR: Use and abuse of HOMA modeling. Diabetes Care 2004;27:1487–1495.

Weiss R, Dufour S, Taksali SE, Tamborlane WV, Petersen KF, Bonadonna RC, Boselli L, Barbetta G, Allen K, Rife F, Savoye M, Dziura J, Sherwin R, Shulman GI, Caprio S: Prediabetes in obese youth: a syndrome of impaired glucose tolerance, severe insulin resistance, and altered myocellular and abdominal fat partitioning. Lancet 2003;362:951–957.

Weyer C, Bogardus C, Mott DM, Pratley RE: The natural history of insulin secretory dysfunction and insulin resistance in the pathogenesis of type 2 diabetes mellitus. J Clin Invest 1999;104:787–794.

Whincup PH, Gilg JA, Papacosta O, Seymour C, Miller GJ, Alberti KG, Cook DG: Early evidence of ethnic differences in cardiovascular risk: cross sectional comparison of British South Asian and white children. BMJ 2002;324:635.

World Health Organization: Obesity and Overweight. http://www.who.int/dietphysicalactivity/publications/facts/obesity/en/

Yeckel CW, Weiss R, Dziura J, Taksali SE, Dufour S, Burgert TS, Tamborlane WV, Caprio S: Validation of insulin sensitivity indices from oral glucose tolerance test parameters in obese children and adolescents. J Clin Endocrinol Metab 2004;89:1096–1101.

Young T, Peppard PE, Gottlieb DJ: Epidemiology of obstructive sleep apnea: a population health perspective. Am J Respir Crit Care Med 2002:1217–1239.

Prof. Dr. Andreas Neu
University Children's Hospital Tuebingen, Pediatric Endocrinology and Diabetes
Hoppe-Seyler Strasse 1
DE–72076 Tübingen (Germany)
Tel. +49 7071 2983781, Fax +7071 295475, E-Mail andreas.neu@med.uni-tuebingen.de

Ranke MB, Mullis P-E (eds): Diagnostics of Endocrine Function in Children and Adolescents, ed 4.
Basel, Karger, 2011, pp 310–330

Endocrine Function of the Testis

Paul-Martin Holterhus[a] · John W. Honour[b] · Martin O. Savage[b]

[a]Department of Pediatrics, Division of Pediatric Endocrinology and Diabetes, Christian-Albrechts-University Kiel/
University Hospital of Schleswig-Holstein, Campus Kiel, Kiel, Germany; [b]Department of Chemical Pathology, UCL
Hospitals, London, UK

Testicular function is important during fetal life, in early infancy and throughout puberty when it is responsible for the transition from childhood to adult life. Expression of the SRY (sex-determining region Y) gene and further downstream genes such as SOX9 (sex-determining region Y-box 9), DMRT1 (doublesex and mab-3-related transcription factor 1) and MAMLD1 (mastermind-like domain containing 1; previously known as CXorf6 – chromosome X open reading frame 6) determine differentiation of the bipotent gonadal anlagen into the testes. Between the 6th and 12th weeks of gestation, testosterone secreted by the Leydig cells leads to virilization of the external genitalia while anti-müllerian hormone from the Sertoli cells inhibits development of the müllerian duct derivates. During childhood, from 6 months to the onset of puberty at 9–14 years, testicular function is in a quiescent phase. At puberty, there is an increase in gonadotrophin-stimulated Leydig cell activity, together with secretion of inhibin from the seminiferous tubules [Sinclair et al., 1990; Manasco et al., 1995; Raymond et al., 1999; Fukami et al., 2006].

Assessment of testicular endocrine function is relevant to a wide range of disorders that affect male genital differentiation during embryogenesis leading to 46,XY DSD (disorders of sex development) and during male secondary sexual development in puberty (table 1). 46,XY DSD can also become apparent for the first time during puberty due to virilization and masculinization of a child raised as female.

Many of such disorders are monogenic diseases, e.g. defects of androgen biosynthesis [Richter-Unruh et al., 2004; Boehmer et al., 1999], androgen insensitivity syndrome (AIS) [Ahmed et al., 2000a; Holterhus et al., 2000], hypogonadotrophic hypogonadism, e.g. Kallmann's syndrome [Maya-Nunez et al., 1998; Dodé et al., 2009] and other molecular defects of the hypothalamo-pituitary control of testicular function [de Roux, 2006]. Some defects of testicular androgen biosynthesis can also comprise adrenal biosynthesis, e.g. in 3β-hydroxysteroid dehydrogenase type II deficiency [Welzel et al., 2008] leading to additional glucocorticoid and mineralocorticoid

Table 1. Assessment of testicular endocrine function

Clinical assessment
1. History and family history
2. General physical examination
3. Examination of the external genitalia including measurement of testicular volume

Laboratory investigations
1. Basal plasma concentrations of
   a. Testosterone
   b. Dihydrotestosterone
   c. Androstenedione
      specifically determined by RIA following extraction and chromatography or by LC-MS/MS (liquid chromatography tandem mass spectrometry)
2. Human chorionic gonadotrophin stimulation test
3. Plasma concentrations of luteinizing-hormone and follicle-stimulating hormone
4. Inhibin B, anti-müllerian hormone, sex hormone-binding globulin

Specific and optional investigations depending on the individual clinical condition
1. Karyotype analysis (alternative investigations: fluorescent in situ hybridization with X and Y specific probes on buccal mucosa cells, SRY-specific PCR on blood leukocyte DNA)
2. Urinary steroid profile by GC-MS (gas chromatography mass spectrometry)
3. Plasma steroid profile including adrenal steroids by LC-MS/MS (liquid chromatography tandem mass spectrometry)
4. Imaging: ultrasound, MRI
5. Laparoscopy
6. Gonadal biopsy (especially in combination with laparoscopy)
7. Gene-specific molecular analyses (genomic DNA sequencing)
8. Array CGH (comparative genomic hybridization)
9. Functional analyses on cultured genital skin fibroblasts (5α-reductase activity, androgen binding analysis, expression analyses) in rare cases

deficiency. In contrast, genes originally associated with both, adrenal and testicular development and function, e.g. SF-1 [Achermann et al., 1999] can be associated with only gonadal insufficiency [Köhler et al., 2008]. Hypogonadotrophic hypogonadism can be part of an overriding genetic defect of pituitary development (PROP1) leading to panhypopituitarism [Wu et al., 1998] with further hormonal deficiencies of clinical relevance. AIS may be present even in the absence of an androgen receptor gene mutation presumably caused by deficiency of androgen receptor co-regulators [Adachi et al., 2000] or defective androgen receptor transcription due to unknown causes [Holterhus et al., 2005] which makes diagnosis difficult in some cases.

In poorly masculinized males there can be abnormalities of both fetal and pubertal testicular function. A different situation is the 'vanishing testis syndrome' in which the testicular defect originates in the fetus only after normal virilization of the external genitalia thus compromising puberty. In other situations the defect is of postnatal origin, e.g. acquired hypopituitarism or hypogonadism due to treatment of leukemia by chemotherapy or irradiation. Therefore, timing of the testicular defect is an important determinant for the pattern of clinical manifestations. In either case, the clinical and endocrine evaluation of testicular function is relevant to the diagnosis, the clinical management and the future welfare of the patient.

Physiology of Testicular Endocrine Function

Testosterone synthesis and production in the male embryo begins at about 8 weeks of gestation and is maximal at 12–13 weeks. During this critical period of genital development, Leydig cell secretion is mainly stimulated by placental human chorionic gonadotrophin (HCG). Peripheral conversion of testosterone by 5α-reductase is the main source of the circulating dihydrotestosterone which plays the key role in development of the prostate, phallus and scrotum. At the same time, anti-müllerian hormone (AMH) (müllerian-inhibiting substance; MIS), a glycoprotein, is secreted by the Sertoli cells. AMH actively suppresses development of the müllerian duct derivates.

A surge of testosterone secretion during the first 6 months of infancy was first demonstrated by Forest et al. [1973]. The physiological significance of this phenomenon is still not understood. During most of childhood, plasma testosterone levels are then usually below 1 nmol/l. The testosterone concentrations increase progressively from the start of puberty although early activity is confined to the night time. Therefore, blood sampling in boys in early puberty should occur in the morning. Testosterone is responsible for male secondary sexual development.

Clinical Assessment of Testicular Function

The history and family history should be documented carefully. Since many monogenic disorders of testosterone biosynthesis follow an autosomal-recessive mode of inheritance, possible consanguinity of the parents and whether or not other family members are affected should be enquired about. Moreover, the ethnic origin of the patient and the parents is of high potential importance since mutations of androgen biosynthesis genes, e.g. HSD17B3 (17β-hydroxysteroid dehydrogenase type III) are often 'endemic' in certain regions of the world [Boehmer et al., 1999]. The ethno-socio-cultural background is certainly an important piece of diagnostic information for later interdisciplinary clinical management in cases with DSD. In AIS there is usually an X-chromosomal recessive mode of inheritance with the mothers being carriers. However, up to 1/3 of the mutations of the androgen receptor gene in AIS typically occur de novo and in 1/3 of the latter, a somatic mosaic of mutated and wild-type

Holterhus · Honour · Savage

androgen receptor is present which may significantly alter the expected family tree and the expected clinical findings [Holterhus et al., 1997, 1999; Hiort et al., 1998].

Careful examination of the external genitalia is mandatory. Palpation of the gonads is performed to determine their location and their size. Unilateral undescended testis is a frequent congenital abnormality. Both unilateral and bilateral undescended testis can be observed in association with DSD, e.g. testosterone biosynthesis defects, AIS as well as defects in the production or action of anti-müllerian hormone [Josso et al., 1997]. In rare cases, nonpalpable testes can be a symptom of completely virilized 46,XX females due to 21-hydroxylase deficiency. Undescended testis can also be a first clinical clue of a later pubertal manifestation of hypogonadotrophic hypogonadism as in Prader-Willi syndrome or in Kallmann's syndrome. Testicular enlargement, which should be measured using a Prader orchidometer, is usually the first sign of puberty. A testicular volume of 4 ml (gonadarche) or greater indicates the onset of puberty induced by the action of LH. A testis volume of 15–25 ml is characteristic for the adult male genitalia. Furthermore, the scrotum and the phallus are examined.

In the newborn with DSD, the degree of external genital virilization has to be documented. Different scoring systems have been suggested for the undervirilized genetic male [Sinnecker et al., 1996; Ahmed et al., 2000b]. The size of the phallus can vary from a normal 'clitoris' to a normal penis. Penile size can be compared with age-dependent percentiles [Winter and Faiman, 1972]. The position of the urethral meatus should be noted. The degree of virilization and therefore the degree of embryonic testicular endocrine function is not least reflected by the degree of distal-to-proximal fusion of the genital midline forming the scrotum. In cases with DSD, the appearance of the external genitalia at birth can range from normal male to different degrees of genital ambiguity to completely female external genitalia. In cases with 46,XY DSD due to a defect of androgen biosynthesis or androgen action, there is a short and blind ending vagina. However, in cases with gonadal dysgenesis there is also decreased AMH production by the testes during embryogenesis giving rise to the clinically variable persistence of the portio uteri and the corpus uteri.

The general physical examination has always to be part of a comprehensive clinical workup in presumed disorders of testicular endocrine function with or without DSD. This includes the body proportions and auxologic parameters which become more and more important at the time of expected puberty (e.g. upper/lower length ratio, presence of gynecomastia (e.g. Klinefelter's syndrome), male versus female shaped abdomen and hips (e.g. in partial AIS), musculature (weak in partial AIS due to missing effects of all androgens but high production of estrogens by aromatization; normal in 5α-reductase type II deficiency due to normal anabolic testosterone actions on musculature during puberty), distribution of body hair and voice. In particular in cases with DSD, additional malformations should be documented, for example microcephaly, hypertelorism, epicanthic folds, anteverted nostrils in gonadal dysgenesis due to DMRT1 deletion.

In some interdisciplinary teams joint clinical examination of patients by the pediatric endocrinologist and the human geneticist has been implemented and helps to plan imaging or complex molecular diagnostics. In some cases mental retardation (e.g. in DMRT1 deletions, Prader-Willi syndrome) is part of the symptoms. Knowledge of the normal progression of pubertal development which is generally scored according to Marshall and Tanner [1970] stages is essential for the diagnosis of testicular defects during adolescence. The degree and rate of virilization can be used as an in vivo 'bioassay' of Leydig cell function. Impaired testicular function will be shown by impaired pubertal progress. Due to the secular trend of pubertal onset to a younger age, the absence of any signs of puberty at the age of 14 years in the boy may currently be considered to be an abnormal delay of puberty [Styne and Grumbach, 2008].

Laboratory Assessment of Testicular Function

It is important to interpret hormone results against reference ranges that are appropriate for age and stage of development. There are marked differences in results with different methodologies particularly for androgens [Kulle et al., 2010] and proteins such as sex hormone-binding globulin [Bukowski et al., 2000].

Basal Plasma Androgen Determinations
In the last 40 years or so radioimmunoassays (RIA) were widely used. When investigating the neonate, it is important to remember that there are high blood concentrations of steroid sulphates (dehydroepiandrosterone, 17-hydroxypregnenolone) from the fetal adrenal cortex that can interfere in the immunoassay methods which are still frequently in use. Some of these methods, however, use extraction of the steroids into an organic solvent and chromatography (e.g. HPLC) prior to RIA. These combined techniques provide sufficient sensitivity and specificity for many clinical conditions in pediatric endocrinology, especially in neonates, compared with RIA based on neat sera alone [von Schnakenburg et al., 1980; Dörr et al., 1988]. However, this method is cumbersome, time-consuming and therefore expensive and restricted to only few remaining specialized pediatric laboratories. Furthermore, differences in the techniques used in the different laboratories and changing specificities of RIA antibodies hamper comparability and thus implementation of widely usable and comparable normal ranges and cut-offs for diseases associated with testicular endocrine function. Problems have inevitably been encountered with automated methods in the laboratory. In immunoassays, results for testosterone in newborns have been reported to be grossly elevated [Fuqua et al., 1995] due to interferences from fetal and placental steroids.

GC-MS has also been found to be a very reliable quantitative method for plasma androgens [Wudy et al., 1992, 1995] because of the high specificity through separation of steroids in the sample extract. Comparisons of GC-MS results with clinical samples assayed by direct and extracted RIA methods show close agreement with the

Table 2. Male androgen levels – median (range) – by age [Kulle et al., 2010]

Age	n	Androstenedione		Testosterone		Dihydrotestosterone	
		ng/dl	nmol/l	ng/dl	nmol/l	ng/dl	nmol/l
<1 week	8	18 (<3–34)	0.62 (<0.1–1.2)	20 (6–78)	0.70 (0.2–2.7)	3 (<3–20)	0.10 (<0.1–0.7)
2 weeks–2 months	19	40 (11–94)	1.40 (0.4–3.3)	164 (14–363)	5.70 (0.5–12.6)	3 (<3–75)	0.10 (<0.1–2.6)
3–5 months	12	17 (3–54)	0.60 (0.1–1.9)	35 (3–89)	1.20 (0.1–3.1)	3 (<3–23)	0.10 (<0.1–0.8)
6–11 months	4	5 (3–9)	0.16 (0.1–0.3)	3 (3–12)	0.10 (0.1–0.4)	3 (<3–12)	0.10 (<0.1–0.4)
1–3 years	9	3 (3–23)	0.10 (0.1–0.8)	12 (3–20)	0.40 (0.1–0.7)	3 (<3–38)	0.10 (<0.1–1.3)
4–6 years	10	15 (3–43)	0.52 (0.1–1.5)	12 (3–26)	0.40 (0.1–0.9)	3 (3–23)	0.10 (0.1–0.8)
7–9 years	10	11 (3–51)	0.40 (0.1–1.8)	7 (3–23)	0.24 (0.1–0.8)	4 (3–17)	0.15 (0.1–0.6)
10–12 years	18	26 (3–72)	0.90 (0.1–2.5)	21 (3–161)	0.75 (0.1–5.6)	7 (3–55)	0.25 (0.1–1.9)
13–15 years	26	50 (3–192)	1.75 (0.1–6.7)	226 (3–507)	7.84 (0.1–17.6)	28 (3–93)	0.96 (0.1–3.2)
16–18 years	20	59 (23–163)	2.08 (0.8–5.7)	350 (115–691)	12.14 (4–24)	39 (3–55)	1.35 (0.1–1.9)

extracted RIAs. In the meantime, different techniques based on liquid chromatography tandem mass spectrometry (LC MS/MS) have been developed to detect A, T and DHT [Albrecht and Styne, 2007; Gallagher et al., 2007; Wang et al., 2008; Mitamura et al., 2005; Cawood et al., 2005, Shiraishi et al., 2008; Turpeinen et al., 2008]. In contrast to immunoassays, these methods are largely independent of matrix effects or cross reactivity. In our own laboratory, we have recently established a robust LC-MS/MS method allowing for sensitive, specific and high-throughput (180 samples per 24 h) determination of A, T and DHT simultaneously from 100 μl of plasma or serum as well as the accompanying reference values covering the whole pediatric age range (tables 2–4) [Kulle et al., 2010].

Directly after birth, normal plasma testosterone concentrations can be up to 15 nmol/l when measured with RIA in an extraction assay. The testosterone concentrations

Table 3. Male androgen levels – median (range) by Tanner stage [Kulle et al., 2010]

Tanner stage	n	Androstenedione		Testosterone		Dihydrotestosterone	
		ng/dl	nmol/l	ng/dl	nmol/l	ng/dl	nmol/l
P1 <6 months	41	26 (3–29)	0.90 (0.1–1.0)	72 (3–92)	2.50 (0.1–3.2)	3 (3–87)	0.10 (0.1–3.0)
P1 6 months–9 years	35	10 (3–51)	0.35 (0.1–1.8)	8 (3–69)	0.28 (0.1–2.4)	3 (3–38)	0.10 (0.1–1.3)
P1 >9 years	13	23 (3–46)	0.80 (0.1–1.6)	10 (3–29)	0.34 (0.1–1)	9 (3–29)	0.30 (0.1–1)
P2	11	26 (3–71)	0.90 (0.1–2.5)	89 (9–383)	3.10 (0.3–13.3)	12 (3–52)	0.40 (0.1–1.8)
P3	11	43 (17–95)	1.50 (0.6–3.3)	194 (35–409)	6.75 (1.2–14.2)	17 (3–55)	0.60 (0.1–1.9)
P4	10	57 (3–117)	2.00 (0.1–4.1)	288 (29–455)	10.00 (1–15.8)	28 (3–52)	0.95 (0.1–1.8)
P5	18	77 (23–192)	2.66 (0.8–6.7)	326 (144–691)	11.32 (5–24.0)	38 (6–93)	1.30 (0.2–3.2)

fall over the first weeks of life as HCG is cleared from the circulation. From 2 weeks of age to 2 months after birth the concentrations of the androgens testosterone and dihydrotestosterone increase to approach the lower limits of normal adult male concentrations and then decline over the next 3–4 months [von Schnakenburg et al., 1980; Kulle et al., 2010]. LH is the stimulus to T secretion during this period [Andersson et al., 1998]. In premature boys, the plasma testosterone concentrations for postconceptional age are similar to those of term babies. The rapid decline in plasma testosterone concentrations in the immediate postnatal period and subsequent rise is related to postnatal age and not to gestational age. The secondary rise lags somewhat behind in premature infants, and peak values are significantly higher and remain elevated for a longer period of time than in term infants [Forest et al., 1980].

During childhood, testosterone concentrations are below 1 nmol/l which may be near the detection limit of some RIA assays but which is still well within the detection limit of LC MS/MS methods (0.1 nmol/l) [Kulle et al., 2010] (tables 2–4). In prepuberty, testosterone is still below 1 nmol/l and at the age of 10 years rises continuously up to 24 nmol/l in the adult male. Androstenedione increases up to 3 nmol/l during 'minipuberty' as measured by LC MS/MS, decreases to below 1 nmol /l during early childhood and then begins to rise during late childhood before testosterone indicating adrenal origin due to adrenarche reaching highest values of up to 6 nmol/l at the

Table 4. Male androgen levels – range (median) – by testicular volume [Kulle et al., 2010]

Testicular volume	n	Androstenedione		Testosterone		Dihydrotestosterone	
		ng/dl	nmol/l	ng/dl	nmol/l	ng/dl	nmol/l
1–2 ml < 6 months	40	26 (3–92)	0.90 (0.1–3.2)	72 (3–432)	2.55 (0.1–15.0)	2.9 (<3–98)	0.10 (<0.1–3.4)
1–2 ml 6 months– 9 years	26	9 (3–63)	0.30 (0.1–2.2)	3 (3–43)	0.10 (0.1–1.5)	2.9 (<3–38)	0.10 (<0.1–1.3)
1–2 ml > 9 years	7	17 (3–37)	0.60 (0.1–1.3)	10 (3–29)	0.34 (0.11–1)	6 (3–20)	0.20 (0.1–0.7)
3–4 ml	7	23 (3–66)	0.80 (0.1–2.3)	23 (3–288)	0.80 (0.1–10)	9 (3–49)	0.30 (0.1–1.7)
5–10 ml	9	43 (3–94)	1.50 (0.1–3.3)	94 (34–432)	3.27 (1.2–15.0)	26 (3–49)	0.90 (0.1–1.7)
11–15 ml	15	60 (3–117)	2.10 (0.1–4.1)	273 (49–472)	9.50 (1.7–16.4)	38 (9–55)	1.31 (0.3–1.9)
> 15 ml	10	74 (14–192)	2.60 (0.5–6.7)	403 (144–691)	14.00 (5–24.0)	39 (9–93)	1.35 (0.3–3.2)

age of 13–15 years (table 2). DHT generally follows the excursions of testosterone at a lower concentration level and shows a peak plasma concentration of up to 3 nmol/l at Tanner genital stage P5 (table 3). Because of the above-discussed methodological aspects and because of increasing use of the LC-MS/MS method in steroid determination, we decided to present LC-MS/MS based normative data of A, T and DHT according to age, Tanner stage and testicular volume. It has to be noted that existing clinical experience is still mostly based on RIA methods which includes the HCG test.

Specific Considerations in Infants
Testosterone measurements coinciding with the spontaneous neonatal surge are helpful in two clinical situations. Firstly, in 46,XY DSD (table 5), a low testosterone level will indicate either impaired synthesis of this hormone or a dysgenetic gonad whereas a normal or even elevated level will indicate a defect of peripheral androgen action [Ng et al., 2000]. The postnatal T, LH and FSH surge does not, however, occur in complete androgen insensitivity syndrome [Bouvattier et al., 2002]. Secondly, in the infant with micropenis suspected of having Kallmann's syndrome, low testosterone

Table 5. Selected causes of 46,XY DSD [adapted from Hughes et al., 2006]

A   Disorders of gonadal development
1. Ovotesticular DSD
2. Complete or partial gonadal dysgenesis (SRY, SOX9, SF1, WT1, DHH, WNT4-duplication, DAX1-duplication, etc.)
3. Gonadal regression

B   Disorders of androgen biosynthesis and androgen action
1. Disorders of androgen biosynthesis
    – LH receptor defect
    – Smith-Lemli-Opitz syndrome
    – Steroidogenic acute regulatory protein (STAR) deficiency
    – P450 side chain cleavage (SCC) deficiency
    – 3β-Hydroxysteroid dehydrogenase type II deficiency
    – 17α-Hydroxylase/17,20-lyase deficiency
    – P450 oxidoreductase deficiency
    – 17β-Hydroxysteroid dehydrogenase type III deficiency
    – 5α reductase type II deficiency
2. Disorders of androgen action
    – Complete and partial androgen insensitivity syndrome (AIS)

C   Different causes
1. Syndromic forms
    – Cloacal exstrophy
    – Aarskog syndrome
    – Hand-foot-genital syndrome
2. Syndrome of persistent müllerian structures (AMH, AMH receptor)
3. Vanishing testis syndrome
4. Isolated hypospadias
5. Cryptorchidism

and gonadotrophin levels will support a diagnosis of gonadal failure. Testosterone should be measured during the first 3 days or during the 3 months after day 10 of life to avoid the naturally low levels between days 5 and 8.

46,XY DSD due to defects of androgen biosynthesis caused by inactivating mutations of genes coding for the steroid biosynthesis enzymes (fig. 1) are often characterized by typical steroid hormone constellations. In case of stimulated Leydig cells in 'minipuberty' or in puberty these may be characterized by an elevation of the precursor steroid and by a diminution of the final synthetic product. Typical examples are the elevation of androstenedione and an increased androstenedione to testosterone ratio in 17β-hydroxysteroid dehydrogenase type III deficiency, an increase of the Δ5 steroids 17OH-pregnenolone and DHEA in 3β-hydroxysteroid dehydrogenase type II deficiency and an elevation of the ratio of testosterone to dihydrotestosterone in 5α-reductase type II deficiency [Ahmed et al., 2000c].

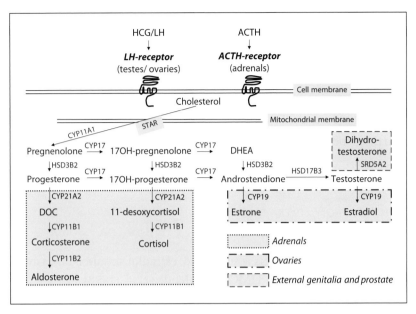

Fig. 1. Enzyme defects in testosterone biosynthesis. Androgen biosynthesis defects involving adrenal steroid biosynthesis: STAR = steroid acute regulatory protein; CYP11A1 = P450 side chain cleavage; HSD3B2 = 3β-hydroxysteroid dehydrogenase type II; CYP17 = 17α-hydroxylase/17, 20-lyase. Androgen biosynthesis defects involving only the testicular Leydig cells: HSD17B3 = 17β-hydroxysteroid dehydrogenase type III. Androgen biosynthesis defects involving peripheral activation of testosterone to dihydrotestosterone: SRD5A2 = 5α-reductase type II.

Specific Considerations during Puberty

As mentioned more above, in the early stages of puberty, testosterone production occurs during the night and only early morning blood samples will be useful. Later in puberty, testosterone is produced throughout the day and night, and timing of blood samples is not critical anymore. Plasma concentrations of testosterone are usually low until pubertal stage 2–3 but can vary considerably between individuals and reach quite high values in single cases [von Schnakenburg et al., 1980; Manasco et al., 1995, Kulle et al., 2010]. At the clinical level, any defect of androgen production will be accompanied by impaired pubertal virilization. The measurement of plasma androgens is, however, essential in the investigation of hypogonadism in late adolescence and adult life. The finding then of a subnormal adult value indicates the need for investigation and potential androgen replacement.

HCG Test

In the pediatric patient aged 6 months to 8 years, basal gonadal steroids are frequently undetectable in plasma, and gonadal function can only be assessed by Leydig cell stimulation using HCG. Measurement of testosterone in this test is particularly helpful in the child with bilateral cryptorchidism in order to have evidence for the presence or

Table 6. HCG test protocols

Test	Age	HCG regimen	Timing of androgen samples
1	all ages	5,000 IU /m^2, only 1 injection on day 0	day 0, day 3 (after 72 h)
2	infancy and childhood	1,000 IU i.m. daily × 3	days 0 and 3
3	infancy and childhood	1,000 IU i.m. twice weekly × 6	day 0 and 24 h after the last injection
4	adolescence	2,000 IU i.m. on days 0 and 3	days 0, 3 and 5

absence of testicular tissue. If an ovotestis is suspected, estradiol should be measured in a human menopausal gonadotrophin HMG test [Mendez et al., 1998].

HCG Test Protocols
The test is based on the principle that samples for steroids are taken before and after HCG injection. Many different protocols are used for HCG administration [Tapanainen et al., 1983; Dunkel et al., 1985; Forest et al., 1988; Ahmed et al., 1999]. Excellent Leydig cell stimulation has been demonstrated using a single injection of 5,000 IU/m^2 body surface area with plasma testosterone measured 24 or 72 h later. Repeated injections don't seem to have diagnostic benefits over a single injection [Dunkel et al., 1985].

Androgen Responses to HCG
The normal testosterone response to HCG depends on the age of the patient. Of note, the values given here have not been re-validated with recent LC-MS/MS technology but they are based on RIA methods. In infancy, a normal testosterone increment after HCG may vary from 2-fold to 10- or even 20-fold. During childhood, the increment is between 5-and 10-fold [Ahmed et al., 1999]. Increments in plasma testosterone are typically between 2.0 and 8.5 nmol/l with peak values between 2.3 and 8.7 nmol/l. During puberty, as the basal concentration is higher, the increment is less, i.e. 2- to 3-fold. If there is no response to a short HCG test, a prolonged test over 2 weeks (table 6) should be performed, and a 5- to 10-fold increment from the basal testosterone level will be a normal response. The ratios of androstenedione to testosterone, and of testosterone to dihydrotestosterone become exaggerated in the HCG test and are therefore more reliable with respect to diagnosis of 17β-hydroxysteroid dehydrogenase type III or 5α-reductase type II deficiency [Ng et al., 2000].

SHBG
Measurement of plasma sex hormone-binding globulin (SHBG) may indicate a disturbance of testicular function or androgen action. Normally, SHBG levels are around

100 nmol/l in prepubertal boys and fall progressively throughout puberty to around 60 nmol/l [Belgorosky et al., 1987]. Persistent elevation or a lack of decrease in SHBG following HCG stimulation may indicate a failure of testicular testosterone production, as in anorchia, or a defect of peripheral androgen action, as in AIS [Belgorosky et al., 1982; Ciaccio et al., 1989, Bertelloni et al., 1997]. In vivo androgen sensitivity can also be assessed elegantly by measuring the decrease of SHBG in response to oral administration of the synthetic anabolic steroid stanozolol [Sinnecker et al., 1997]. Stanozolol is a documented transcriptional activator of AR signaling [Holterhus et al., 2002; Werner et al., 2006]. A decrease of <63.4% compared with the basal value before medication is considered a normal androgen sensitivity. In AIS, there is decreasing downregulation with decreasing receptor function. In complete AIS, SHBG downregulation in response to stanozolol is usually abolished [Sinnecker et al., 1997]. Of note, patients with somatic mosaicism of an inactivating AR gene mutation may have discordant results [Holterhus et al., 1997; Holterhus et al., 1999].

Adrenal Steroid Measurement
Some rare defects of androgen biosynthesis can also affect adrenal steroid biosynthesis (fig. 1). In particular, they include: STAR (steroid acute regulatory protein) affecting cholesterol transport, CYP11A1 (P450 side chain cleavage) affecting the cholesterol to pregnenolone conversion, HSD3B2 (3β-hydroxysteroid dehydrogenase type II) affecting the conversion of the Δ5 to Δ4 steroids as well as CYP17 (17α-hydroxylase and 17,20-lyase activities, respectively), producing different adrenal phenotypes with and without ACTH-mediated excess production of mineralocorticoids (17α-hydroxylase deficiency) (fig. 1). Therefore, many of these defects may present with early adrenal crisis due to lack of sufficient basal and/or stress-induced cortisol and mineralocorticoid biosynthesis. In newborn DSD patients with presumed disorder of androgen biosynthesis, clinical examination, short-term follow-up as well as laboratory testing should consider this possibility in order to prevent adrenal crisis (e.g. general examination, clinical assessment of hydration, weight gain during the first weeks of life, pigmentation of the skin; baseline determination of glucose, electrolytes and cortisol, in some cases adrenal steroid profiling by LC-MS/MS or urinary steroid profiling). In the Smith-Lemli-Opitz syndrome, there is a defect in cholesterol synthesis [Tint et al., 1994] and adrenal insufficiency has also been described [Andersson et al., 1999]. Mutations in DAX-1 cause X-linked adrenal hypoplasia congenital (AHC) which is the leading clinical problem in the newborn due to early adrenal crisis. AHC is associated with hypogonadotrophic hypogonadism in puberty [Achermann et al., 1999; Reutens et al., 1999; Achermann and Jamesson, 2001].

Urinary Steroid Determinations
An informative analysis of the metabolites of androgens and other steroids in urine is possible by gas chromatography mass spectrometry (GS-MS). GC-MS displays the metabolites of cortisol and adrenal androgens as well as precursor hormones and is

particularly helpful in the diagnosis of defects of androgen biosynthesis with and without adrenal insufficiency [Honour and Brook, 1997].

An abnormally high ratio of 5β- to 5α-reduced metabolites of androgens is seen in urine of children with 5α-reductase type II deficiency although the excretion rates are extremely low until 4 years of age. From 3 months of age a diagnosis is supported from a high ratio of 5β- to 5α reduced metabolites of cortisol (THF to allo-THF). A urine profile that shows no androgen or cortisol metabolites but an excess of corticosterone metabolites supports the diagnosis of 17α-hydroxylase deficiency. Metabolites of DHEA and 17-hydroxypregnenolone are raised when the adrenal and gonadal 3β-hydroxysteroid dehydrogenase type II is impaired. Low excretion rates of all steroids are seen in lipoid adrenal hyperplasia due to defects in the STAR gene [Achermann et al., 2001] and when adrenal and gonadal insufficiency is due to mutations in the DAX-1 gene [Achermann, 1999]. In the Smith-Lemli-Opitz syndrome, Δ7 and Δ8 metabolites of 16-hydroxy-DHA, pregnenolone and 16-hydroxypregnenolone are seen in the urine steroid profile [Shackleton et al., 1999].

Determinations of Luteinizing Hormone and Follicle-Stimulating Hormone and the Luteinizing Hormone-Releasing Hormone Test
Determinations of plasma gonadotrophins are unlikely to give diagnostic information in newborn infants with ambiguous genitalia. In the pubertal child with primary testicular failure, basal LH and follicle-stimulating hormone (FSH) levels may be elevated. In testicular dysgenesis, FSH is a more sensitive index of seminiferous tubular damage. When plasma basal gonadotrophins are elevated, the response to luteinizing hormone-releasing hormone (LHRH, 60 μg/m² (max. 100 μg), 0 and 30 min) is unlikely to provide any further diagnostic information. In AIS, testosterone and gonadotrophins are usually within or above the normal range.

In pubertal patients with hypogonadotrophic hypogonadism, testicular function may be low because of lack of stimulation from gonadotrophin-releasing hormone (GnRH). An LHRH test can localize the primary defect to the hypothalamus. In some patients, the distinction between hypogonadotrophic hypogonadism and constitutional delay of puberty may be difficult. In these cases, a GnRH agonist test (e.g. Nafarelin, 1 μg/kg (max. 100 μg) s.c.) is useful [Ehrmann et al., 1989; Ghai et al., 1995; Kletter et al., 1996]. Different criteria of normal and pathological test results have been published. A maximum LH peak after 4 h <6.2 U/l [Ghai et al., 1995] and/or a testosterone increase after 24 h of <1 nmol/l [Kletter et al., 1996] support hypogonadotrophic hypogonadism.

Miscellaneous Investigations
Inhibin B
Inhibin B which is secreted by the Sertoli cells has low plasma concentrations in boys with testicular damage (delayed diagnosis of cryptorchidism; after testicular torsion) and in patients with testicular dysgenesis [Kubini et al., 2000]. It is well correlated with the testosterone response to HCG.

Anti-Müllerian Hormone

AMH is produced by the Sertoli cells and is responsible for regression of the müllerian ducts. In testicular dysgenesis leading to ambiguous or completely female external genitalia due to reduced or abolished testicular androgen production, the additional absence of AMH results in the persistence of müllerian duct derivates which is always an important ultrasound finding in the differential diagnosis of DSD. Defects in AMH action may be the result of mutations in the gene encoding the protein or the AMH receptor. In DSD patients with defects of androgen synthesis or action AMH can be secreted normally and therefore, ultrasound will confirm absence of mullerian structures in these cases. AMH is secreted at high levels until puberty, concentrations are 500–1,000 pmol/l 2 weeks after birth and decline by 10 years of age be to less than 500 pmol/l. In patients with persistent müllerian duct syndrome due to AMH gene mutations and anorchia serum AMH is undetectable and low in hypogonadotrophic hypogonadism [Rey et al., 1999].

Imaging

Ultrasound is an important noninvasive method to investigate and locate the testes. Ultrasound of the abdomen should include the kidney, the adrenals and the search for müllerian remnants, e.g. in testicular dysgenesis. Magnetic resonance imaging is additionally valuable when searching the gonads, especially in older children due to the larger size of the gonads. In newborns or very young children who need sedation for MRI anyway, laparoscopic search for the gonads by an experienced pediatric surgeon or pediatric urologist should be considered.

Testicular Biopsy

Testicular biopsy should not be performed routinely, for example in patients with cryptorchidism, as damage to the testicular tissue may result. Biopsy should be restricted to children with DSD due to gonadal dysgenesis and to unclear cases where histology of the testicular tissue can help to establish a diagnosis if clinical and hormonal data are inconclusive. Experience in histological examination of testicular specimens is required to detect pre-malignant [Savage and Lowe, 1990] and disease-specific changes. Testicular biopsy with the aim of detecting carcinoma in situ may be indicated in cases of suspected gonadal neoplasm.

In vitro Functional Studies on Cultured Genital Skin Fibroblasts

Cultured genital skin fibroblasts can be used for different bioassays investigating the last steps of the androgen pathway in patients with DSD. However, since most of the diagnoses investigated by these assays can be established by genomic DNA sequencing of the underlying genes as today's gold standard (table 7), these methods are only rarely indicated. The standard location of the biopsy is labial, labioscrotal or scrotal skin, but not foreskin which has a different embryological origin [Holterhus et al., 2007]. If a patient with DSD but not yet established diagnosis undergoes a

Table 7. Selected genes involved in endocrine function of the testes

Gene name	Chromosomal locus	Pathophysiology
SRY	Yp11.3	testicular dysgenesis
SOX9	17q24.3-q25.1	testicular dysgenesis
WT1	11p3	tesicular dysgenesis
SF1	9q33	testicular dysgenesis
MAMLD1 (CXorf6)	Xq28	testicular dysgenesis
DMRT1	9p24.3	testicular dysgenesis
DAX1	Xp21.3	testicular dysgenesis in case of duplication; adrenal hypoplasia congenita (AHC) plus hypogonadotrophic hypogonadism in case of mutations
WNT4	1p35	testicular dysgenesis
STAR	8p11.2	combined gonadal and adrenal defect of steroid biosynthesis due to impaired mitochondrial cholesterol transport
CYP11A1	15q23-24	combined gonadal and adrenal defect of steroid biosynthesis due to impaired conversion of cholesterol to pregnenolone
CYP17	10q24.3	combined gonadal and adrenal defect of steroid biosynthesis due to impaired 17α-hydroxylase and 17/20 lyase activity
HSD3B2	1p13.1	combined gonadal and adrenal defect of steroid biosynthesis due to impaired conversion of Δ5 to Δ4 steroids
POR (P450 oxidoreductase)	7q11.2	apparently combined 21-hydroxylase and 17α-hydroxylase and 17/20 lyase deficiency
HSD17B3	9q22	defect of testicular androgen biosynthesis due to impaired androstenedione to testosterone conversion
SRD5A2	2p23	defect of peripheral conversion of testosterone to dihydrotestosterone in androgen target tissues
AR	Xq11-12	androgen insensitivity syndrome
AMH	19p13.3-13.2	persistent müllerian duct syndrome
AMHR	12q13	persistent müllerian duct syndrome
LHRHR	4q21.2	hypogonadotrophic hypogonadism
GPR54	9p13.3	hypogonadotrophic hypogonadism

Table 7. Continued

Gene name	Chromosomal locus	Pathophysiology
KAL1	Xp22.3	hypogonadotrophic hypogonadism (Kallmann's syndrome)
FGFR1	8p12	hypogonadotrophic hypogonadism (Kallmann's syndrome)
PROKR2	20p13	hypogonadotrophic hypogonadism (Kallmann's syndrome)
PROK2	3q21.2	hypogonadotrophic hypogonadism (Kallmann's syndrome)
PROP1	5q	hypogonadotrophic hypogonadism due to multiple pituitary hormone deficiency
LHX3	9q34.3	hypogonadotrophic hypogonadism due to multiple pituitary hormone deficiency
HESX1	3p21.2-21.1	hypogonadotrophic hypogonadism due to multiple pituitary hormone deficiency
LHRH	2p21	leydig cell hypoplasia, hypergonadotrophic hypogonadism
GNAS1	20q13.2	McCune-Albright syndrome

surgical operation of the external genitalia, a genital skin culture should always be established.

In the ligand-binding assay, the specific binding of androgen (e.g. methyltrienolone) to the ligand-binding domain of the androgen receptor is tested. Absent or reduced androgen binding and/or an increased dissociation constant indicate AIS [Kaufman et al., 1976]. However, defects outside the ligand-binding domain of the androgen receptor are at most indirectly detected (e.g. reduced maximum binding due to reduced androgen receptor transcription and translation). Determination of 5α-reductase activity is also possible in cultured genital skin fibroblasts and is severely reduced in patients with 5α-reductase type II deficiency [Pinsky et al., 1978]. In some cases with AIS, no underlying mutation of the androgen receptor gene can be established. In these cases, reduced transcription and translation due to unknown causes [Holterhus et al., 2005] or an absent androgen receptor co-regulator [Adachi et al., 2000] have been shown in cultured genital skin fibroblasts. The latter investigations need high experience and should be performed in collaboration with a specialized centre. More recently, a bio-assay on genital skin fibroblasts has been established that measures the potency of the androgen receptor as a ligand-activated transcriptional activator. In patients with CAIS and PAIS, there is a severe reduction of DHT-mediated up-regulation of apolipoprotein D (APOD) transcription while in normal scrotal skin fibroblasts or in labia majora fibroblasts from 46,XY female patients with 17β-hydroxysteroid dehydrogenase type III deficiency, there is high induction of APOD [Appari et al., 2009]. As suggested above for transcription analysis and co-regulator analysis in fibroblasts this is a very specific test at the transition from basic endocrine science to clinical use and can currently be performed only by specialized labs.

Molecular Analysis of Genes Involved in Endocrine Function of the Testes

During the last 2 decades many genes involved in testicular development, androgen biosynthesis and androgen action have been identified. Table 7 summarizes genes of interest. Even gene sequencing is becoming easier and molecular testing will be more widely used.

References

Achermann JC, Ito M, Ito M, Hindmarsh PC, Jameson JL: A mutation in the gene encoding steroidogenic factor-1 causes XY sex reversal and adrenal failure in humans. Nat Genet 1999;22:125–126.

Achermann JC, Jameson JL: Advances in the molecular genetics of hypogonadotropic hypogonadism. J Pediatr Endocrinol Metab 2001;14:3–15.

Achermann JC, Meeks JJ, Jeffs B, Das U, Clayton PE, Brook CG, Jameson JL: Molecular and structural analysis of two novel StAR mutations in patients with lipoid congenital adrenal hyperplasia. Mol Genet Metab 2001;73:354–357.

Achermann JC, Gu WX, Kotlar TJ, Meeks JJ, Sabacan LP, Seminara SB, Habiby RL, Hindmarsh PC, Bick DP, Sherins RJ, Crowley WF Jr, Layman LC, Jameson JL: Mutational analysis of DAX1 in patients with hypogonadotropic hypogonadism or pubertal delay. J Clin Endocrinol Metab 1999;84:4497–4500.

Adachi M, Takayanagi R, Tomura A, Imasaki K, Kato S, Goto K, Yanase T, Ikuyama S, Nawata H: Androgen-insensitivity syndrome as a possible coactivator disease. N Engl J Med 2000;343:856–862.

Ahmed SF, Cheng A, Dovey L, Hawkins JR, Martin H, Rowland J, Shimura N, Tait AD, Hughes IA: Phenotypic features, androgen receptor binding, and mutational analysis in 278 clinical cases reported as androgen insensitivity syndrome. J Clin Endocrinol Metab 2000a;85:658–665.

Ahmed SF, Cheng A, Hughes IA: Assessment of the gonadotrophin-gonadal axis in androgen insensitivity syndrome. Arch Dis Child 1999;80:324–329.

Ahmed SF, Iqbal A, Hughes IA: The testosterone :androstenedione ratio in male undermasculinization. Clin Endocrinol (Oxf) 2000c;53:697–702.

Ahmed SF, Khwaja O, Hughes IA: The role of a clinical score in the assessment of ambiguous genitalia. BJU Int 2000b;85:120–124.

Albrecht L, Styne D: Laboratory testing of gonadal steroids in children. Pediatr Endocrinol Rev;2007;5 (Suppl 1):599–607.

Andersson AM, Toppari J, Haavisto AM, Petersen JH, Simell T, Simell O, Skakkebaek NE: Longitudinal reproductive hormone profiles in infants: peak of inhibin B levels in infant boys exceeds levels in adult men. J Clin Endocrinol Metab 1998;83:675–681.

Andersson HC, Frentz J, Martínez JE, Tuck-Muller CM, Bellizaire J: Adrenal insufficiency in Smith-Lemli-Opitz syndrome. Am J Med Genet 1999;82:382–384.

Appari M, Werner R, Wünsch L, Cario G, Demeter J, Hiort O, Riepe F, Brooks JD, Holterhus PM: Apolipoprotein D (APOD) is a putative biomarker of androgen receptor function in androgen insensitivity syndrome. J Mol Med. 2009;87:623–632.

Belgorosky A, Rivarola MA: Changes in serum sex hormone-binding globulin and in serum non-sex hormone-binding globulin-bound testosterone during prepuberty in boys. J Steroid Biochem 1987;27:291–295.

Belgorosky A, Rivarola MA: Sex hormone-binding globulin response to human chorionic gonadotropin stimulation in children with cryptorchidism, anorchia, male pseudohermaphroditism, and micropenis. J Clin Endocrinol Metab 1982;54:698–704.

Bertelloni S, Federico G, Baroncelli GI, Cavallo L, Corsello G, Liotta A, Rigon F, Saggese G: Biochemical selection of prepubertal patients with androgen insensitivity syndrome by sex hormone-binding globulin response to the human chorionic gonadotropin test. Pediatr Res 1997;41:266–271.

Boehmer AL, Brinkmann AO, Sandkuijl LA, Halley DJ, Niermeijer MF, Andersson S, de Jong FH, Kayserili H, de Vroede MA, Otten BJ, Rouwé CW, Mendonça BB, Rodrigues C, Bode HH, de Ruiter PE, Delemarre-van de Waal HA, Drop SL: 17Beta-hydroxysteroid dehydrogenase-3 deficiency: diagnosis, phenotypic variability, population genetics, and worldwide distribution of ancient and de novo mutations. J Clin Endocrinol Metab 1999;84:4713–4721.

Bouvattier C, Carel JC, Lecointre C, David A, Sultan C, Bertrand AM, Morel Y, Chaussain JL: Postnatal changes of T, LH, and FSH in 46,XY infants with mutations in the AR gene. J Clin Endocrinol Metab 2002;87:29–32.

Bukowski C, Grigg MA, Longcope C: Sex hormone-binding globulin concentration: differences among commercially available methods. Clin Chem 2000;46:1415–1416.

Cawood ML, Field HP, Ford CG, Gillingwater S, Kicman A, Cowan D, Barth JH: Testosterone measurement by isotope-dilution liquid chromatography-tandem mass spectrometry: validation of a method for routine clinical practice. Clin Chem 2005;51:1472–1479.

Ciaccio M, Rivarola M, Belgorosky A: Decrease of serum sex hormone-binding globulin as a marker of androgen sensitivity: correlation with clinical response. Acta Endocrinol (Copenh) 1989;120:540–544.

Dodé C, Teixeira L, Levilliers J, Fouveaut C, Bouchard P, Kottler ML, Lespinasse J, Lienhardt-Roussie A, Mathieu M, Moerman A, Morgan G, Murat A, Toublanc JE, Wolczynski S, Delpech M, Petit C, Young J, Hardelin JP: Kallmann syndrome: mutations in the genes encoding prokineticin-2 and prokineticin receptor-2. PLoS Genet 2006;2:e175.

Doerr HG, Sippell WG, Versmold HT, Bidlingmaier F, Knorr D: Plasma mineralocorticoids, glucocorticoids, and progestins in premature infants: longitudinal study during the first week of life. Pediatr Res 1988;23:525–529.

Dunkel L, Perheentupa J, Apter D: Kinetics of the steroidogenic response to single versus repeated doses of human chorionic gonadotropin in boys in prepuberty and early puberty. Pediatr Res 1985;19:1–4.

Ehrmann DA, Rosenfield RL, Cuttler L, Burstein S, Cara JF, Levitsky LL: A new test of combined pituitary-testicular function using the gonadotropin-releasing hormone agonist nafarelin in the differentiation of gonadotropin deficiency from delayed puberty: pilot studies. J Clin Endocrinol Metab 1989;69:963–967.

Forest MG, Cathiard AM, Bertrand JA: Evidence of testicular activity in early infancy. J Clin Endocrinol Metab 1973;37:148–151.

Forest MG, David M, David L, Chatelain PG, François R, Bertrand J: Undescended testis: comparison of two protocols of treatment with human chorionic gonadotropin: effect on testicular descent and hormonal response. Horm Res 1988;30:198–205.

Forest MG, de Peretti E, Bertrand J: Testicular and adrenal androgens and their binding to plasma proteins in the perinatal period: developmental patterns of plasma testosterone, 4-androstenedione, dehydroepiandrosterone and its sulfate in premature and small for date infants as compared with that of full-term infants. J Steroid Biochem 1980;12:25–36.

Fukami M, Wada Y, Miyabayashi K, Nishino I, Hasegawa T, Nordenskjöld A, Camerino G, Kretz C, Buj-Bello A, Laporte J, Yamada G, Morohashi K, Ogata T: CXorf6 is a causative gene for hypospadias. Nat Genet 2006;38:1369–1371.

Fuqua JS, Sher ES, Migeon CJ, Berkovitz GD: assay of plasma testosterone during the first six months of life: importance of chromatographic purification of steroids. Clin Chem;41:1146–1149.

Gallagher LM, Owen LJ, Keevil BG: Simultaneous determination of androstenedione and testosterone in human serum by liquid chromatography-tandem mass spectrometry. Ann Clin Biochem 2007;44:48–56.

Ghai K, Cara JF, Rosenfield RL: Gonadotropin releasing hormone agonist (nafarelin) test to differentiate gonadotropin deficiency from constitutionally delayed puberty in teenage boys: a clinical research center study. J Clin Endocrinol Metab 1995;80:2980–2986.

Hiort O, Sinnecker GH, Holterhus PM, Nitsche EM, Kruse K: Inherited and de novo androgen receptor gene mutations: investigation of single-case families. J Pediatr 1998;132:939–943.

Holterhus PM, Brüggenwirth HT, Hiort O, Kleinkauf-Houcken A, Kruse K, Sinnecker GH, Brinkmann AO: Mosaicism due to a somatic mutation of the androgen receptor gene determines phenotype in androgen insensitivity syndrome. J Clin Endocrinol Metab 1997;82:3584–3589.

Holterhus PM, Deppe U, Werner R, Richter-Unruh A, Bebermeier JH, Wünsch L, Krege S, Schweikert HU, Demeter J, Riepe F, Hiort O, Brooks JD: Intrinsic androgen-dependent gene expression patterns revealed by comparison of genital fibroblasts from normal males and individuals with complete and partial androgen insensitivity syndrome. BMC Genomics 2007;8:376.

Holterhus PM, Piefke S, Hiort O: Anabolic steroids, testosterone-precursors and virilizing androgens induce distinct activation profiles of androgen responsive promoter constructs. J Steroid Biochem Mol Biol 2002;82:269–275.

Holterhus PM, Sinnecker GH, Hiort O: Phenotypic diversity and testosterone-induced normalization of mutant L712F androgen receptor function in a kindred with androgen insensitivity. J Clin Endocrinol Metab 2000;85:3245–3250.

Holterhus PM, Werner R, Hoppe U, Bassler J, Korsch E, Ranke MB, Dörr HG, Hiort O: Molecular features and clinical phenotypes in androgen insensitivity syndrome in the absence and presence of androgen receptor gene mutations. J Mol Med 2005;83:1005–1013.

Holterhus PM, Wiebel J, Sinnecker GH, Brüggenwirth HT, Sippell WG, Brinkmann AO, Kruse K, Hiort O: Clinical and molecular spectrum of somatic mosaicism in androgen insensitivity syndrome. Pediatr Res 1999;46:684–690.

Honour JW, Brook CG: Clinical indications for the use of urinary steroid profiles in neonates and children. Ann Clin Biochem 1997;34:45–54.

Hughes IA, Houk C, Ahmed SF, Lee PA; LWPES Consensus Group; ESPE Consensus Group: Consensus statement on management of intersex disorders. Arch Dis Child 2006;91:554–563.

Josso N, Picard JY, Imbeaud S, di Clemente N, Rey R: Clinical aspects and molecular genetics of the persistent müllerian duct syndrome. Clin Endocrinol (Oxf) 1997;47:137–144.

Kaufman M, Straisfeld C, Pinsky L: Male pseudo-hermaphroditism presumably due to target organ unresponsiveness to androgens. Deficient 5alpha-dihydrotestosterone binding in cultured skin fibroblasts. J Clin Invest 1976;58:345–350.

Kletter GB, Rolfes-Curl A, Goodpasture JC, Solish SB, Scott L, Henzl MR, Beitins IZ: Gonadotropin-releasing hormone agonist analog (nafarelin): a useful diagnostic agent for the distinction of constitutional growth delay from hypogonadotropic hypogonadism. J Pediatr Endocrinol Metab 1996;9:9–19.

Köhler B, Lin L, Ferraz-de-Souza B, Wieacker P, Heidemann P, Schröder V, Biebermann H, Schnabel D, Grüters A, Achermann JC: Five novel mutations in steroidogenic factor 1 (SF1, NR5A1) in 46,XY patients with severe underandrogenization but without adrenal insufficiency. Hum Mutat 2008;29:59–64.

Kubini K, Zachmann M, Albers N, Hiort O, Bettendorf M, Wölfle J, Bidlingmaier F, Klingmüller D: Basal inhibin B and the testosterone response to human chorionic gonadotropin correlate in prepubertal boys. J Clin Endocrinol Metab. 2000;85:134–138.

Kulle AE, Riepe FG, Melchior D, Hiort O, Holterhus PM: A novel UPLC MS/MS method for the simultaneous determination of androstenedione, testosterone and dihydrotestosterone in pediatric blood samples: age and sex specific reference data. J Clin Endocrinol Metab 2010;95:2399–2409.

Manasco PK, Umbach DM, Muly SM, Godwin DC, Negro-Vilar A, Culler MD, Underwood LE: Ontogeny of gonadotropin, testosterone, and inhibin secretion in normal boys through puberty based on overnight serial sampling. J Clin Endocrinol Metab 1995;80:2046–2052.

Marshall WA, Tanner JM: Variations in the pattern of pubertal changes in boys. Arch Dis Child 1970;45:13–23.

Maya-Nuñez G, Zenteno JC, Ulloa-Aguirre A, Kofman-Alfaro S, Mendez JP: A recurrent missense mutation in the KAL gene in patients with X-linked Kallmann's syndrome. J Clin Endocrinol Metab 1998;83:1650–1653.

Mendez JP, Schiavon R, Diaz-Cueto L, Ruiz AI, Canto P, Söderlund D, Diaz-Sanchez V, Ulloa-Aguirre A: A reliable endocrine test with human menopausal gonadotropins for diagnosis of true hermaphroditism in early infancy. J Clin Endocrinol Metab 1998;83:3523–3526.

Mitamura K, Ogasawara C, Shiozawa A, Terayama E, Shimada K: Determination method for steroid 5alpha-reductase activity using liquid chromatography/atmospheric pressure chemical ionization-mass spectrometry. Anal Sci 2005;21:1241–1244.

Ng KL, Ahmed SF, Hughes IA: Pituitary-gonadal axis in male undermasculinisation. Arch Dis Child 2000;82:54–58.

Pinsky L, Kaufman M, Straisfeld C, Zilahi B, Hall CS: 5alpha-reductase activity of genital and nongenital skin fibroblasts from patients with 5alpha-reductase deficiency, androgen insensitivity, or unknown forms of male pseudohermaphroditism. Am J Med Genet 1978;1:407–416.

Raymond CS, Parker ED, Kettlewell JR, Brown LG, Page DC, Kusz K, Jaruzelska J, Reinberg Y, Flejter WL, Bardwell VJ, Hirsch B, Zarkower D: A region of human chromosome 9p required for testis development contains two genes related to known sexual regulators. Hum Mol Genet 1999;8:989–996.

Reutens AT, Achermann JC, Ito M, Ito M, Gu WX, Habiby RL, Donohoue PA, Pang S, Hindmarsh PC, Jameson JL: Clinical and functional effects of mutations in the DAX-1 gene in patients with adrenal hypoplasia congenita. J Clin Endocrinol Metab. 1999;84:504–511.

Rey RA, Belville C, Nihoul-Fékété C, Michel-Calemard L, Forest MG, Lahlou N, Jaubert F, Mowszowicz I, David M, Saka N, Bouvattier C, Bertrand AM, Lecointre C, Soskin S, Cabrol S, Crosnier H, Léger J, Lortat-Jacob S, Nicolino M, Rabl W, Toledo SP, Baş F, Gompel A, Czernichow P, Chatelain P, Rappaport R, Morel Y, Josso N: Evaluation of gonadal function in 107 intersex patients by means of serum antimüllerian hormone measurement. J Clin Endocrinol Metab 1999;84:627–631.

Richter-Unruh A, Verhoef-Post M, Malak S, Homoki J, Hauffa BP, Themmen AP: Leydig cell hypoplasia: absent luteinizing hormone receptor cell surface expression caused by a novel homozygous mutation in the extracellular domain. J Clin Endocrinol Metab 2004;89:5161–5167.

de Roux N: GnRH receptor and GPR54 inactivation in isolated gonadotropic deficiency. Best Pract Res Clin Endocrinol Metab 2006;20:515–528.

Savage MO, Lowe DG: Gonadal neoplasia and abnormal sexual differentiation. Clin Endocrinol (Oxf) 1990;32:519–533.

von Schnakenburg K, Bidlingmaier F, Knorr D: 17-Hydroxyprogesterone, androstenedione, and testosterone in normal children and in prepubertal patients with congenital adrenal hyperplasia. Eur J Pediatr 1980;133:259–267.

Shackleton CH, Roitman E, Kelley R: Neonatal urinary steroids in Smith-Lemli-Opitz syndrome associated with 7-dehydrocholesterol reductase deficiency. Steroids. 1999;64:481–490.

Shiraishi S, Lee PW, Leung A, Goh VH, Swerdloff RS, Wang C: Simultaneous measurement of serum testosterone and dihydrotestosterone by liquid chromatography-tandem mass spectrometry. Clin Chem 2008;54:1855–1863.

Sinclair AH, Berta P, Palmer MS, Hawkins JR, Griffiths BL, Smith MJ, Foster JW, Frischauf AM, Lovell-Badge R, Goodfellow PN: A gene from the human sex-determining region encodes a protein with homology to a conserved DNA-binding motif. Nature 1990;346:240–241.

Sinnecker GH, Hiort O, Nitsche EM, Holterhus PM, Kruse K: Functional assessment and clinical classification of androgen sensitivity in patients with mutations of the androgen receptor gene. German Collaborative Intersex Study Group. Eur J Pediatr 1997;156:7–14.

Styne DM, Grumbach MM: Puberty: Onogeny, neuroendocrinology, physiology, and disorders; in Kronenberg MM, Melmed S, Polonsky KS, Larsen PR (eds): William Textbook of Endocrinology. Philadelphia, Saunders Elsevier, 2008, chap 24, pp 969–1166.

Tapanainen J, Martikainen H, Dunkel L, Perheentupa J, Vihko R: Steroidogenic response to a single injection of hCG in pre- and early pubertal cryptorchid boys. Clin Endocrinol (Oxf) 1983;18:355–562.

Tint GS, Irons M, Elias ER, Batta AK, Frieden R, Chen TS, Salen G: Defective cholesterol biosynthesis associated with the Smith-Lemli-Opitz syndrome. N Engl J Med 1994;330:107–113.

Turpeinen U, Linko S, Itkonen O, Hamalainen E: Determination of testosterone in serum by liquid chromatography-tandem mass spectrometry. Scand J Clin Lab Invest 2008;68:50–57.

Wang C, Shiraishi S, Leung A, Baravarian S, Hull L, Goh V, Lee PW, Swerdloff RS: Validation of a testosterone and dihydrotestosterone liquid chromatography tandem mass spectrometry assay: interference and comparison with established methods. Steroids 2008;73:1345–1352.

Welzel M, Wüstemann N, Simic-Schleicher G, Dörr HG, Schulze E, Shaikh G, Clayton P, Grötzinger J, Holterhus PM, Riepe FG: Carboxyl-terminal mutations in 3beta-hydroxysteroid dehydrogenase type II cause severe salt-wasting congenital adrenal hyperplasia. J Clin Endocrinol Metab 2008;93:1418–1425.

Werner R, Schütt J, Hannema S, Röpke A, Wieacker P, Hiort O, Holterhus PM: Androgen receptor gene mutations in androgen insensitivity syndrome cause distinct patterns of reduced activation of androgen-responsive promoter constructs. J Steroid Biochem Mol Biol 2006;101:1–10.

Winter JS, Faiman C: Pituitary-gonadal relations in male children and adolescents. Pediatr Res 1972;6:126–135.

Wu W, Cogan JD, Pfäffle RW, Dasen JS, Frisch H, O'Connell SM, Flynn SE, Brown MR, Mullis PE, Parks JS, Phillips JA 3rd, Rosenfeld MG: Mutations in PROP1 cause familial combined pituitary hormone deficiency. Nat Genet 1998;18:147–149.

Wudy SA, Wachter UA, Homoki J, Teller WM: 17alpha-Hydroxyprogesterone, 4-androstenedione, and testosterone profiled by routine stable isotope dilution/ gas chromatography-mass spectrometry in plasma of children. Pediatr Res 1995;38:76–80.

Wudy SA, Wachter UA, Homoki J, Teller WM, Schackleton CH: Androgen metabolism assessment by routine gas chromatography/mass spectrometry profiling of plasma steroids. 1. Unconjugated steroids. Steroids 1992;57:319–324.

Paul-Martin Holterhus
Department of Pediatrics, Division of Pediatric Endocrinology and Diabetes
Christian-Albrechts-University Kiel/University Hospital of Schleswig-Holstein, Campus Kiel
Schwanenweg 20, DE–24105 Kiel (Germany)
Tel. +49 431 597 1626, Fax +49 431 597 1675, E-Mail holterhus@pediatrics.uni-kiel.de

Ranke MB, Mullis P-E (eds): Diagnostics of Endocrine Function in Children and Adolescents, ed 4.
Basel, Karger, 2011, pp 331–349

Normal Ovarian Function and Assessment of Ovarian Reserve in Children and Young People

Robert J. Johnston[a] · W. Hamish B. Wallace[b]

[a]Royal Hospital for Sick Children, and [b]Section of Child Life and Health, Department of Reproductive Health and Developmental Sciences, University of Edinburgh, Edinburgh, UK

The ovary is a complex organ with an essential role in reproduction, normal growth and development and bone health. Over recent years with increasing understanding of chronic disorders of childhood and improved survival in conditions such as cancer and cystic fibrosis it is recognised that ovarian function is affected by therapies as well as underlying chronic illness. Additionally, there has been improved understanding and recognition of genetic conditions associated with loss of ovarian function. As a result healthcare professionals are increasingly faced with patients in whom assessment of ovarian function at an early stage may be important. In this chapter we will detail the normal development of the human ovary, summarise the conditions of childhood associated with loss of ovarian function, and detail our current understanding of the assessment of this complex organ during childhood and adolescence.

The Human Ovary

Normal Ovarian Development and Follicular Depletion
Our current understanding of human ovarian reserve presumes that the ovary establishes several million non-growing follicles (NGFs) during the second half of intrauterine life, which is followed by a decline to the menopause when approximately 1,000 remain at an average age of 50–51 years. Baker was the first to demonstrate germ cells multiply rapidly during the first half of gestation to reach 6×10^6, followed by a rapid decline to reduce to approximately 2×10^6 at term [1]. With approximately 450 ovulatory monthly cycles in the normal human reproductive

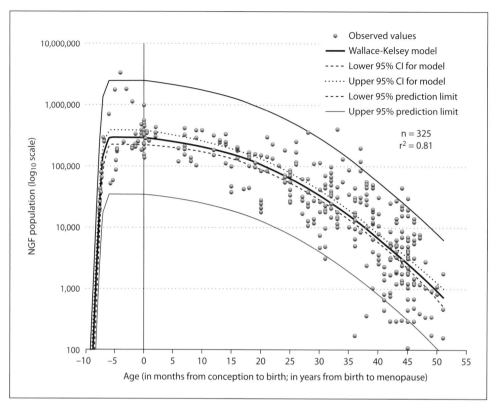

Fig. 1. The best model for the establishment of the NGF population after conception, and the subsequent decline until menopause is described by $\log_{10}(NGF) = (a/4)(1 + erf((x\text{-}b + c/2)/(d\sqrt{2})))(1 - erf((x\text{-}b - c/2)/(e\sqrt{2})))$, with parameters a = 5.56 (95% CI 5.38–5.74), b = 25.6 (95% CI 24.9–26.4), c = 52.7 (95% CI 51.1–54.2), d = 0.074 (95% CI 0.062–0.085), and e = 24.5 (95% CI 20.4–28.6). The model has a correlation coefficient $r^2 = 0.81$, fit standard error = 0.46 and F value = 364. This figure shows the dataset (n = 325), the model, the 95% prediction limits of the model, and the 95% CI for the model.

lifespan, this progressive decline in NGF numbers is attributed to follicle death by apoptosis. Wallace and Kelsey have described the first model of human ovarian reserve from conception to menopause that best fits the combined histological evidence [2]. This model allows us to estimate the number of NGFs present in the ovary at any given age, and suggests that 81% of the variance in NGF populations is due to age alone (fig. 1). Further analysis demonstrated that 95% of the NGF population variation is due to age alone for ages up to 25 years. The remaining 5% is due to factors other than age, e.g. smoking, BMI, parity and stress. We can speculate that as chronological age increases, factors other than age become more important in determining the rate at which NGFs are lost through apoptosis.

There is speculation that this widely held tenet of mammalian ovarian function may require revision. A report in 2004 suggested the presence of germ stem cells in the adult mouse ovary [3], and two subsequent reports by the same group suggested the ability of bone marrow-derived cells to give rise to new immature oocytes [4]. Bone marrow transplantation was shown to partially restore the fertility of busulphan-treated mice [5] although all offspring derived from the host germline. These murine studies provide a basis for re-evaluating the regenerative capacity of the mammalian ovary and new approaches for overcoming fertility loss. While the emerging evidence thus appears to provide evidence in support of the existence of germ stem cells within adult mouse ovary the Wallace-Kelsey model of ovarian follicle decline provides no supporting evidence of neo-oogenesis in normal human physiological ageing.

Premature ovarian failure (POF), also known as primary ovarian insufficiency is caused by premature depletion of NGFs and is characterised by the absence of menarche (primary amenorrhoea) with growth impairment or premature menopause before the age of 40 years (secondary amenorrhoea).

Summary of the Normal Hypothalamic-Pituitary-Gonadal Axis

In normal menstruating women, ovarian function depends on pituitary gonadotrophin production – follicle-stimulating hormone (FSH) stimulates the granulosa cells of the growing follicle to proliferate and produce oestradiol. Ovulation occurs in response to the mid-cycle surge of luteinising hormone (LH), following which the corpus luteum produces progesterone, which prepares the endometrium to receive the fertilized ovum (fig. 2).

At birth the hypothalamic-pituitary axis is active for only a transient period following which it remains quiescent until puberty. At the onset of puberty, the initiation of pulsatile gonadotrophin-releasing hormone (GnRH) from the hypothalamus leads to gonadotrophin (FSH/LH) release from the pituitary, which in turn supports maturation of oocytes within the ovary. The consequent release of hormones, principally oestrogen, from the granulosa cells, is responsible for the development of secondary sexual characteristics.

Follicle development and atresia is a continuous process occurring throughout the reproductive lifespan (fig. 3). A large number of NGFs leave the resting follicle pool each day and start to develop, however only one of which is destined to become a mature oocyte each cycle, the majority becoming atretic. This process of maturation takes approximately 90 days, but it is only in the later stages of oocyte maturation, once there is antral follicle development, that the follicle becomes gonadotrophin dependent. The number of NGFs present at any time will determine reproductive lifespan and ovarian reserve.

Anti-müllerian hormone (AMH) which is produced by the granulosa cells of growing follicles, shows a marked decline in levels with advancing age [6]. AMH levels may reflect total NGF numbers becoming undetectable following the menopause. Inhibin-B is produced by small growing follicles after cyclic recruitment and thus is at its highest in the early follicular phase of the menstrual

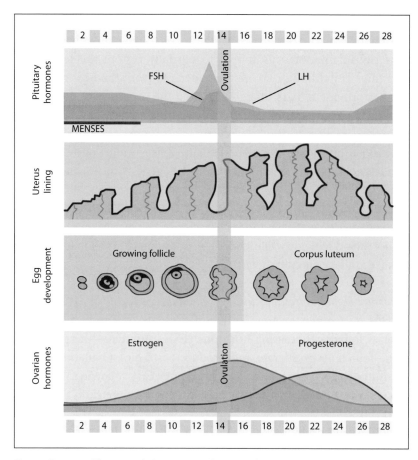

Fig. 2. Timing of hormonal changes in relation to follicle and endometrial development during the 28 days of the menstrual cycle.

cycle. Inhibin-B is involved in the feedback regulation of FSH secretion from the pituitary.

With advancing age, depletion of NGFs occurs associated with a fall in AMH levels. There is a decline in production of inhibin-B with subsequent reduced negative feedback on FSH production leading to elevated levels of FSH. This process is postulated to be responsible for the maintenance of oestradiol levels until late in the transition to menopause.

Aetiology of Premature Ovarian Failure

Premature ovarian failure (POF) is uncommon in children and adolescents, affecting 1 in 10,000 by age 20 years. The causes are heterogeneous and may be acquired,

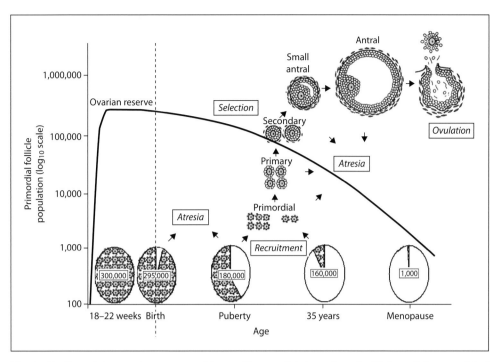

Fig. 3. Decline of the ovarian reserve with age. The graph is based on the Wallace-Kelsey model of ovarian reserve [2] and shows the establishment of follicles during gestation and subsequent decline throughout life. The pie charts along the bottom of the diagram represent the proportion of primordial follicles left in the ovaries at key times in reproductive life and the average population of primordial follicles are given. Finally, the main stages in the recruitment and development of the follicles are shown.

genetic or idiopathic in origin (table 1). The following is a summary of those conditions leading to POF illustrating current understanding of this diverse range of conditions.

Iatrogenic Causes

Treatment for Cancer and Autoimmune Conditions
Iatrogenic POF is caused by treatments for cancer or autoimmune conditions. In a Childhood Cancer Survivor Study (CCSS) 8% of all survivors of childhood cancer experienced a non-surgical premature menopause, compared with 0.8% of sibling controls [7]. Any radiation or chemotherapy-induced damage to the ovary may lead to POF. Animal studies have shown there to be a reduction of the ovarian follicle pool following chemotherapy and radiotherapy [8, 9]. It is understood that cancer therapy may affect the number of primordial follicles and directly reduce reproductive

Table 1. Aetiology of premature ovarian failure

Iatrogenic	surgery
	chemotherapy
	radiotherapy
Autoimmune	polyglandular autoimmune syndrome
	autoimmune polyendocrinopathy-candidiasis-ectodermal-dystrophy (APECED)
Chromosome-X defects	Turner syndrome
	Fragile-X syndrome (FMR1 premutation)
Syndromic defects	congenital disorders of glycosylation
	galactosaemia
	blepharophimosis-ptosis-epicanthus inversus syndrome (BPES)
	pseudohypoparathyroidism type 1a
Isolated defects	FSH-receptor mutation
	LH-receptor mutation
	FOXL2 mutation
	BMP15 mutation
Idiopathic	sporadic or familial

lifespan and accelerate menopause [10], the risk to the ovary being determined by the nature of the treatment used.

Pelvic, abdominal or whole body radiotherapy may lead to loss of primordial follicles resulting in impaired ovarian function [11, 12]. The effective sterilizing dose (ESD: dose of fractionated radiotherapy (Gy) at which premature ovarian failure occurs immediately after treatment in 97.5% of patients) decreases with increasing age at treatment. ESD at birth is 20.3 Gy; at 10 years 18.4 Gy, at 20 years 16.5 Gy, and at 30 years 14.3 Gy [13]. Chemotherapy with procarbazine and alkylating agents such as cyclophosphamide, melphalan and busulphan has the potential to cause premature ovarian failure. After chemotherapy-induced ovarian dysfunction there may be recovery some years later; however, these patients are at high risk of developing a premature menopause. If ovarian failure occurs before puberty induction of puberty may be required for the normal development of secondary sexual characteristics and to preserve bone health.

Autoimmune Causes
Autoimmune polyendocrinopathy-candidiasis-ectodermal-dystrophy (APECED) is an autosomal-recessive condition characterised by chronic superficial candidiasis, autoimmune destruction of endocrine glands and ectodermal dystrophy. It is caused by mutation of the autoimmune regulator gene (AIRE) mapped to 21q22.3.

Hypogonadism is present in 60% of females over 12 years of age, half of whom experienced pubertal failure [14].

Genetic Associations

Two normally functioning X-chromosomes are required for normal ovarian function. Genes for POF have been localised to Xq21.3-Xq27 (POF1) following studies of deletions in various pedigrees, Xq13.3-Xq21.1 (POF2) is implicated by the analysis of balanced X:autosomal translocations. Chromosomal aneuploidy has been associated with acceleration of germ cell apoptosis during foetal life the mechanism of which remains unclear [15].

Turner syndrome is the most widely known genetic cause of ovarian hypofunction, resulting in severe POF with failure of menarche and growth impairment. Turner syndrome affects approximately 1 in 2,500 female births; 50% have monosomy X (45, X), 5–10% carry the long arm of an X-chromosome with a normal X-chromosome 46x,i(Xq), and the remainder have mosaicism (45,X/46,XX). Only 10% of girls with monosomy X will achieve menarche, however in those with mosaicism 40% will menstruate before developing a premature menopause at a later stage.

Lesser degrees of ovarian failure have been associated with partial X-chromosome deletions, inversions and duplications. Balanced X-chromosome: autosome translocations are also common causes of POF such as DIAPH2 (Xq22) mutations of which leads to disruption of oogenesis and spermatogenesis [16]. Several different genetic mechanisms are known to be responsible for POF, although further understanding is hindered by a lack of candidate genes, small pedigrees and few fortuitous autosomal translocations.

The Fragile X Mental Retardation (FMR1) gene located at Xq27.3 is mutated in Fragile-X syndrome, a common cause of inherited mental retardation. Here expansions of the CGG trinucleotide repeat in the 5′ untranslated region (UTR) of FMR1. In carriers, the size of the repeat tract is between 60 and 200 repeats and is known as premutation. Alingham-Hawkins et al. [17] found a significant incidence of premature menopause in carriers of the premutation when compared to unaffected control (16% vs. 0.4%). Only premutation carriers are affected by POF. Full-mutation carriers and their non-carrier sisters, who appear to have the same risk as the general population [18]. Premenopausal premutation carriers have higher FSH levels [18].

Syndromic Effects

Galactosaemia
Galactosaemia is a rare autosomal-recessive metabolic condition due to impaired galactose 1-phosphate uridyltransferase (GALT) metabolism. Despite neonatal diagnosis

and optimal dietary management long-term complications can include cognitive, motor and speech delays. More than 80% experience POF [16]. Girls may require sex steroid replacement therapy to complete puberty, and it is known that infertility is a concern for girls and their parents [20]. The timing of POF in galactosaemia remains unknown. Levy et al. [21] reported normal folliculogenesis in a 5-day-old infant at autopsy. Kaufman et al. [22] demonstrated decreased or absent ovarian tissue on ultrasound examination in patients aged 9–29 years. Ovarian biopsy from two sisters with galactosaemia revealed true ovarian failure in one with unresponsive ovarian follicles in the other, suggesting that resistant ovary may precede true ovarian failure [23]. Contrasting results from animal studies have been unable to support the link between galactose metabolism and ovarian failure. Additionally, partially glycosylated circulating FSH has been hypothesised to cause aberrant function and subsequent POF. Heterozygotes show no evidence of ovarian insufficiency. In their study of 35 girls and women with galactosaemia, Sanders et al. [24] showed that across all age groups most female galactosaemia patients (>90%) demonstrate low levels of AMH. Additionally, bioactivity measurements of FSH were indistinguishable from that of age-matched controls suggesting that FSH is functionally normal in galactosaemia [12].

Blepharophimosis Syndrome Type 1 (BPES 1)
The association of blepharophimosis, ptosis, epicanthus inversus and telecanthus with premature ovarian failure is inherited in an autosomal-dominant manner, with de novo mutations in approximately 50% of the cases. BPES has been linked to the FOXL2 mutation. FOXL2 mutations are estimated to occur in 72% of individuals with a clinical diagnosis of BPES deletions involving FOXL2 vary in size from partial to whole-gene deletions, accounting for approximately 12% of all molecular defects in BPES [25]. Cytogenetic rearrangements involving 3q23 are estimated to occur in 2% of individuals with BPES [25]. Pelvic ultrasound imaging in these females shows a small hypoplastic uterus with streak ovaries.

Carbohydrate-Deficient Glycoprotein Syndrome Type 1 (CDG1)
CDG1 patients show a deficiency of phosphomannomutase (PMM), the enzyme responsible for conversion of mannose 6-phosphate to mannose 1-phosphate in the synthesis of GDP-mannose. PMM-1 is located on chromosome 22q13, PMM-2 on 16q13. These patients are affected by severe encephalopathy, psychomotor retardation, cerebellar hypoplasia and hypogonadism. There is significant mortality in early life due to severe infections, liver insufficiency or cardiomyopathy [26].

FSH Receptor
Several Finnish kindreds with an inactivating mutation of the FSH receptor (FSHR) associated with hypergonadotrophic ovarian failure in patients with XX gonadal dysgenesis have been described [27]. A locus for ovarian failure has been mapped to chromosome 2p where both the LH receptor and FSHR are located [28].

Clinical Assessment of Ovarian Function

Assessment of Ovarian Function

Given the obvious impracticality of direct assessment of ovarian reserve by biopsy and counting the number of NGFs, various proxy studies of ovarian reserve have been reported. These have largely been undertaken in the context of in vitro fertilisation treatments in a sub-fertile population of women [29]. It would be of considerable benefit to have a biochemical or biophysical marker of the number of NGF's in the ovary which would allow a more accurate assessment of age at menopause. There is, however, currently no reliable indicator of ovarian reserve in the healthy menstruating young woman. Nevertheless, a number of potential markers have been proposed and we discuss these in turn.

Menstrual History

Presence or absence of menstruation is an inaccurate assessment of ovarian function. In their study of 100 survivors of childhood cancer Larsen et al. [30] found significant ultrasound and endocrine changes indicative of impaired ovarian function even in the presence of normal cycles. Bath et al. [31] found subtle ovulatory disorders in the presence of normal menstrual cycles in women treated during childhood for leukaemia. In children before the onset of activation of the HPO axis at puberty, FSH cannot be used as a marker for impaired ovarian function. Many studies in adults use amenorrhoea as a surrogate for ovarian failure, with biochemical confirmation (i.e. elevated FSH concentration) in some. While amenorrhoea may have other causes than ovarian failure (e.g. weight loss or chronic illness), it would seem a reasonable surrogate for population based studies.

Reproductive Hormone Levels (Normal Ranges)

As a result of the decline in placental and gonadal steroids following birth, inhibition of gonadotroph production is reduced leading to activation of the hypothalamo-pituitary-gonadal axis, with increase in FSH, LH and oestradiol production over the first few weeks of life. This 'mini-puberty' exists for a variable duration over the first months of life, before returning to pre-pubertal levels reflecting relative quiescence of the HPA axis, which characterises this period of development. From their cohort of 473 female infants aged around 3 months, Chellakooty et al. [32] have derived normative data (summarised in table 2).

There is, however, large inter-individual variability in values especially FSH and inhibin-B. Most reproductive hormones were detectable except for inhibin-A. The median FSH level corresponded to the high levels observed later in childhood, however the LH levels were near to the lower detection limit of the fluoroimmunoassay (detection limit 0.05 IU/l) and comparable to levels seen in early puberty. FSH and inhibin-B levels were found to be similar to premenarchal girls at different pubertal stages, whereas low estradiol levels were more comparable to girls in early puberty [33].

Table 2. Reference ranges for infant girls aged 3 months (from Chellakooty et al. [32])

Hormone	n	Median	Lower limit	Upper limit	% below detection limit
Inhibin A, pg/ml	204	<7	<7	10	94
Inhibin B, pg/ml	324	82	<20	175	15
FSH, IU/l	325	3.8	1.2	18.8	0
LH, IU/l	324	0.07	<0.05	1.07	41
Oestradiol, pM	341	31	<18	83	15

Oestradiol

Increasingly, evidence suggests an important role for oestradiol in prepubertal girls, particularly with respect to its growth promoting effects and higher levels in girls compared to prepubertal boys may contribute to their earlier puberty.

Assay sensitivity has hampered the development of normative references for oestradiol levels in girls prior to puberty. Established immunoassays do not offer sufficient sensitivity to accurately measure low levels of circulating oestradiol and other sex steroids in prepubertal girls. Newer methodologies using gas chromatography tandem mass spectrometry offer much improved sensitivity [34] and a greater insight into the development of pubertal changes with understanding of biological roles at this stage of development. Using older methodologies, detection of circulating oestradiol implies more advanced pubertal development. Courant et al. [34] demonstrated significantly higher oestradiol levels in prepubertal girls compared to boys (median 9.6 vs. <3.7 pmol/l; p < 0.001) which may contribute to their earlier onset of puberty when compared to boys.

Inhibins

Later in childhood both inhibin A and B show marked variation with age and pubertal staging (tables 3, 4). In their study of 345 girls aged 0–18 years, Crofton et al. [35] provide age-related reference data. These data are largely consistent with earlier studies by Sehested et al. [33] whose observations were confined to girls older than 6 years of age. Inhibin B was undetectable in 65% of those less than 6 years of age; levels then rose slowly until 10 years of age increasing rapidly thereafter, and became detectable in all those over 11 years.

During the first 3 months of life inhibin A was detectable in most cases, thereafter becoming undetectable up to around 10 years of age. Inhibin B showed a wide range of values, however was detectable in all cases. This reflects the increased number of maturing follicles inhibin-B after 10 years of age. Similarly the increase in inhibin-A reflects the increasing number of larger follicles.

Table 3. Inhibins A and B (ng/l) in girls: reference data by age (from Crofton et al. [35])

Hormone	Age years	n	Median	Interquartile Interval	Mean (SD)	Undetectable n (%)	Reference range
Inhibin B	0–6	105	10.6	<8.0–18.6	1.1362 (0.2843)	37 (35)	<8.0–72.7
	6–10	80	20.8	13.1–32.7	1.3393 (0.2888)	5 (6)	<8.0–129.6
	10–11	20	37.1	33.2–60.3	1.5622 (0.2715)	1 (5)	<8.0–102.5*
	11–12	20	68.3	44.6–131.4	1.8427 (0.2846)	0	19.5–186.0*
	12–18	120	98.5	61.5–128.0	1.9196 (0.3111)	0	14.4–362.3
Inhibin-A	<0.25	14	5.9	3.9–6.6	0.7532 (0.2592)	1 (7)	<2.0–17.7 *
	0.25–10	160	<2.0	<2.0–<2.0	–	135 (84)	<2.0–5.3
	10–11	20	3.4	2.5–4.3	3.5 (1.2)	3 (15)	<2.0–5.4*
	11–14	60	16.8	10.4–22.2	1.1754 (0.3475)	2 (3)	<2.0–160.2
	14–18	77	28.6	18.1–53.8	1.5677 (0.4136)	0	9.9–248.7

Reference range values are 2.5–97.5th centiles, except where indicated *(range).

A rise in early follicular phase FSH with maintained oestrogen production is a well-recognised feature of the perimenopause. Unless significantly elevated, however, early follicular phase FSH is not useful on its own in the early recognition of impaired ovarian reserve and shows poor correlation with other markers of ovarian function such as AMH [36].

There are two biological forms of the glycoprotein hormone inhibin produced by the gonads – inhibin-A and inhibin-B. Earlier serum RIAs were unable to distinguish between these two forms; however, more recently two-site enzyme-linked immuno-sorbent assays specific for inhibin-A and inhibin-B have helped determine the function of each and their role in the regulation of the hypothalamic-pituitary-gonadal axis. Levels of inhibin-B are known to peak at around 3 months of age, reflecting activation of the hypothalamic-pituitary-gonadal axis with subsequent low levels by 2 years of age [37]. Thereafter, levels of gonadotrophins and sex steroids remain low until puberty, increasing to reflect the normal cyclical pattern through puberty.

Table 4. Inhibin A and B in premenarchal girls at different pubertal stages (from Crofton et al. [35])

Pubertal stage	n	Age years	Inhibin B ng/l	Inhibin A ng/l
BI	49	8.9 (7.3–9.9)	20.3 (12.0–36.4)	<2.0 (<2.0–<2.0)
B2	11	11.2 (9.9–12.3)	27.5 (19.4–34.4)	<2.0 (<2.0–<2.0)
B3–5	14	12.2 (11.7–13.1)	79.3 (60.8–126.9)	11.7 (9.6–23.3)

Sehested et al. [33] detailed the correlations between inhibin levels, FSH, LH and oestradiol levels with pubertal staging and stage of menstrual cycle.

The granulosa cells of small healthy follicles produce inhibin-B after cyclic recruitment during the early follicular phase of the menstrual cycle [38]. Levels of inhibin-B remain low until Tanner stage II when they rise sharply to stage III before declining through to stage V. However, inhibin-B does become detectable during Tanner stage I and increases as a function of age, indicating that follicular activity does begin prior to clinical evidence of pubertal development. Measurable oestradiol may also be detected although inhibin-B has the advantage that it is specific to the ovary, whereas oestradiol may be produced elsewhere, such as peripheral conversion of adrenal androgens [33].

Inhibin-A levels are undetectable in childhood and early puberty rising gradually through pubertal stages reaching maximum levels in adulthood. Levels greater than 19 pg/ml are only seen in postmenarchal girls and adult women, reflecting its source – the corpus luteum.

AMH is best characterized as a product of the fetal Sertoli cells, causing regression of the müllerian structures in the male. AMH (also known as müllerian-inhibiting substance) is a 140-kDa glycoprotein that belongs to the transforming growth factor-β family. It acts on its own type II receptor (AMHRII) [39]. The existence of AMH was first suggested by Alfred Jost in the 1940s and named with regard to the protein's role in foetal sexual differentiation. However, over the last 20 years attention has turned to the role of AMH in the female, specifically its involvement in the recruitment of NGFs and its potential as a marker of ovarian reserve.

The pattern of expression of AMH is sexually dimorphic. In the male, AMH production starts at roughly 8 weeks' gestation [40]. The hormone is produced in high concentrations [41], causing regression of the müllerian ducts and allowing male development. In the female, it was thought that expression did not start until after birth [42] but AMH has since been detected from 36 weeks' gestation [40]. Expression of AMH remains low throughout childhood [41] and only becomes reliably detected at puberty [42]. There is a lack of research regarding AMH concentration in children but the existing data suggests that AMH concentrations rise during childhood. Concentrations then decline throughout adult life and become undetectable after menopause [36, 43].

The expression pattern of AMH in the female suggests a role in follicle development. The main role of AMH in female mice is thought to be the inhibition of NGF recruitment. AMH *null* mice were born with a normal cohort of follicles, but by 4 months had significantly fewer than controls, due to increased recruitment [44]. These finding were confirmed by in vitro experiments, demonstrating that neonatal mouse ovaries cultured in the presence of AMH had 40% fewer growing follicles at 13 months compared to controls [45]. A second role for AMH is the inhibition of FSH-dependent follicle growth [46].

Gonadotrophins and the Gonadotrophin-Releasing Hormone Stimulation Test

GnRH is a decapeptide secreted by the hypothalamus and stimulates the production and secretion of LH and FSH by the anterior pituitary. The GnRH stimulation test is the dynamic function test most widely used in the evaluation of hypothalamo-pituitary-ovarian disease in delayed puberty including Turner syndrome, Prader-Willi and constitutional delay as well as the effects of cytotoxic chemotherapy and radiotherapy. In addition, it may be used to differentiate between central (e.g. hamartoma or craniopharyngioma) and gonadal (e.g. McCune-Albright syndrome) causes of precocious puberty.

A number of protocols are described; however, the most widely used is the 100-µg dose with basal hormone assessment at –15 and 0 min, followed by serial assays at 15, 30, 45, 60 and 90 min following bolus intravenous injection of GnRH. An average is taken of the baseline levels, and average of the three highest stimulated levels minimises the effects of slight variations in secretion and the laboratory. The normal response is dependent on age and pubertal development.

LH measurements are the most useful biochemical marker/assessment in the diagnosis of central precocious puberty. In contrast to boys, using traditional radioimmunoassay which lack sensitivity and specificity, prepubertal girls show significant overlap of basal hormone measurements with those of pubertal children [47]. In these circumstances, a GnRH stimulation test is required for further evaluation.

Newer immunochemiluminometric assays (ICMA) for LH and FSH when compared to older technologies offer improved sensitivity, specificity and reproducibility and improved cost-per-test [47]. In their comparison of ICMA and immunofluorometric assays (IFMA), Resende et al. [48] established basal and GnRH-stimulated gonadotrophin assay-specific reference values in normal girls at different stages of sexual development. ICMA was able to detect lower values of intra- and interassay coefficients of variation of less than 3.5%. They concluded ICMA was significantly more sensitive and precise than assays using IFMA. However, in many girls due to the overlap between pre-pubertal and pubertal basal assay results most marked in

Tanner stages I and II, GnRH stimulation tests were necessary to establish the maturity of the hypothalamo-pituitary-gonadal axis in precocious puberty. Basal LH levels in Tanner stage I are significantly lower when compared to Tanner stage III onward. Using ICMA, girls in Tanner stage III and beyond may not require a GnRH stimulation test to establish the differential diagnosis between central precocious puberty and premature thelarche or pubarche and LH greater than 0.2 IU/l suggest maturity of the HPG axis [48]. Using two third generation LH assays, Houk et al. [49] have demonstrated that a single LH measurement was sufficient to diagnose central precocious puberty in more than 90% of cases.

Potential of AMH as a Marker of Ovarian Reserve

AMH correlates with the NGF cohort in mice [50]. However, the method of taking blood samples, removing and fixing the ovaries and counting the NGFs is not feasible in women. Instead, researchers use indirect measures. These include the correlation of AMH with age, early follicular phase antral follicle count (AFC) and reproductive outcome.

There is a strong correlation between AMH and age. A prospective study in 2002 showed not only that AMH declined significantly with age (a mean decrease of 38% over 3 years) [36], but that it was the only marker to do so. Another team from the Netherlands found an average decrease in AMH of 58% over 4 years [51].

AMH is also strongly correlated with AFC, as shown on ultrasound [52]. Given that the number of growing follicles reflects the number of NGFs [50] gives support to the relationship between AMH and the ovarian reserve. Furthermore, AMH and AFC correlate with each other more strongly than age alone, suggesting their independence as ovarian reserve measures [53].

Clinical outcomes, such as oocyte retrieval for IVF, are also correlated with AMH. A retrospective analysis of women attending an IVF clinic demonstrated that women with 11 or more oocytes retrieved after hyperstimulation had a 2.5-fold greater mean serum concentration of AMH compared to women with fewer than 6 oocytes [54]. A prospective study showed serum AMH levels correlated positively with AFC and number of oocytes retrieved and negatively with poor ovarian response (<4 oocytes) [52]. A review used data from this study to calculate logistic regression and showed that AMH has a better predictive value of poor response after hyper-stimulation than FSH and inhibin B [55]. Many other studies have demonstrated the correlation between AMH and ovarian response to hyperstimulation before IVF.

Besides women attending infertility clinics, it is hoped that AMH measurements may be helpful to young women due to receive potentially gonadotoxic chemotherapy. AMH could be used to measure ovarian reserve before treatment in order to decide which patients have a smaller than average ovarian reserve and would most benefit from fertility preservation, such as ovarian cryopreservation. Measurements could also be used after treatment to give a more accurate assessment of the window of opportunity for fertility. This is particularly important as many cancer survivors still menstruate regularly, despite a severely reduced ovarian reserve [56]. AMH has been found to be the clearest indicator of ovarian reserve in childhood cancer survivors and has been shown to be the only endocrine marker to change after treatment [56, 57]. The decrease in AMH concentration is significant in women who received radiotherapy below the diaphragm [58].

Pelvic Ultrasound

In agreement with other studies as well as autopsy findings Badouraki et al. [59] described a continuous increase in size of ovaries and uterus from early childhood to puberty, and provided centile charts for reference in investigation of pubertal disorders Transvaginal ultrasound is a procedure free from radiation which is useful for assessing the pelvic organs in sexually experienced women. For children and young women who are not sexually active, the transabdominal approach may be helpful but less informative. Pelvic ultrasound examination of the uterus is used to measure longitudinal (A) and transverse (B) lengths, and the anteroposterior diameter. Uterine volume is then calculated using the ellipsoid volume formula (A × B × C × 0.52) [59, 60]. Debate exists concerning the appropriateness of this formula to calculate the uterine volume as the uterus is not shaped as an ellipse and it changes shape over time. Despite these concerns most studies of uterine volume use this formula.

Similarly, ovarian volume is calculated using the ellipsoid formula. In the early follicular phase of the menstrual cycle the AFC may be measured using trans-vaginal ultrasound. As with AMH, most data derive from the context of IVF/superovulation, with the number of oocytes recovered being the primary outcome rather than short or long-term fertility. Nevertheless, both antral follicle count (AFC; the number of follicles of 2–10 mm diameter) and to a lesser extent ovarian volume, have been explored as markers of ovarian damage during chemotherapy [61, 62]. In a prospective study of women undergoing chemotherapy for breast cancer, both AFC and ovarian volume decreased during treatment [61].

Normal Ultrasound Appearances Change with Age

In contrast to older observations [63] and the more recent work by de Vries and coworkers, most studies have shown that pelvic organs increase in size with age from early in life [59, 60]. The growth rate of the ovaries and uterus appears to be moderate during early childhood and then accelerate around the age of 8 years, most likely in association with gonadotrophin-dependent pubertal development.

Uterine volume is greater in children with thelarche when compared with those without thelarche (uterine volume 8.1 ± 6.6 cm^3 vs. 1.8 ± 1.2 cm^3/ovarian volume 1.7 ± 1.2 cm^3 vs. 0.5 ± 0.3 cm^3; $p < 0.0001$ [60]). Similar patterns are noted when comparing other uterine measurements alone including uterine length.

Ovaries consist of both stromal and gonadotrophin-dependent follicular components. Ovarian follicles are physiological and are seen at all stages of development. The presence of follicles appears to be related to elevated FSH levels and their presence in the neonatal period provides evidence that their development commences during prenatal life.

Conclusions

In conclusion, our understanding of normal ovarian function continues to improve (fig. 3) but our ability to assess ovarian reserve and predict the window of opportunity for fertility for individual women remains limited. Controversy still remains over whether there is a self-renewing stem cell population within the human ovary and more research is required. Most importantly, the pre-pubertal ovary is not a quiescent organ and is clearly susceptible to damage from potentially gonadotoxic treatment for cancer or chronic illness.

References

1 Baker TG: A quantitative and cytological study of germ cells in human ovaries. Proc Roy Soc Lond 1963;158:417–433.
2 Wallace WH, Kelsey TW: Human ovarian reserve from conception to the menopause. PLoS ONE 2010;5:e8772.
3 Johnson J, Canning J, Kaneko T, Pru JK, Tilly JL: Germline stem cells and follicular renewal in the postnatal mammalian ovary. Nature 2004;428:145–150.
4 Johnson J, Bagley J, Skaznik-Wikiel M, Lee HJ, Adams GB, Niikura Y, Tschudy KS, Tilly JC, Cortes ML, Forkert R, Spitzer T, Lacomini J, Scadden DT, Tilly JL: Oocyte generation in adult mammalian ovaries by putative germ cells in bone marrow and peripheral blood. Cell 2005;122:303–315.
5 Lee HJ, Selesniemi K, Niikura Y, Niikura T, Klein R, Dombkowski DM, Tilly JL: Bone marrow transplantation generates immature oocytes and rescues long-term fertility in a preclinical mouse model of chemotherapy-induced premature ovarian failure. J Clinical Oncol 2007;25:3198–3204.
6 de Vet A, Laven JS, de Jong FH, Themmen AP, Fauser BC: Antimullerian hormone serum levels: a putative marker for ovarian aging. Fertil Steril 2002;77:357–362.
7 Sklar CA, Mertens AC, Mitby P, Whitton J, Stovall M, Kasper C, Mulder J, Green D, Nicholson HS, Yasui Y, Robison LL: Premature menopause in survivors of childhood cancer: a report from the childhood cancer survivor study. J Natl Cancer Inst 2006;98:890–896.
8 Gosden RG, Wade JC, Fraser HM, Sandow J, Faddy MJ: Impact of congenital or experimental hypogonadotrophism on the radiation sensitivity of the mouse ovary. Hum Reprod 1997;12:2483–2488.
9 Meirow D, Lewis H, Nugent D, Epstein M: Subclinical depletion of primordial follicular reserve in mice treated with cyclophosphamide: clinical importance and proposed accurate investigative tool. Hum Reprod 1999;14:1903–1907.
10 Byrne J: Infertility and premature menopause in childhood cancer survivors. Med Pediatr Oncol 1999;33:24–28.
11 Wallace WH, Shalet SM, Crowne EC, Morris-Jones PH, Gattamaneni HR: Ovarian failure following abdominal irradiation in childhood: natural history and prognosis. Clinl Oncol 1989;1:75–79.
12 Sanders JE, Hawley J, Levy W, Gooley T, Buckner CD, Deeg HJ, Doney K, Storb R, Sullivan K, Witherspoon R, Appelbaum FR: Pregnancies following high-dose cyclophosphamide with or without high-dose busulfan or total-body irradiation and bone marrow transplantation. Blood 1996;87:3045–3052.

13 Wallace WH, Thomson AB, Saran F, Kelsey TW: Predicting age of ovarian failure after radiation to a field that includes the ovaries. Int J Radiat Oncol Biol Phys 2005;62:738–744.

14 Perheentupa J: Autoimmune polyendocrinopathy–candidiasis–ectodermal dystrophy (APECED). Horm Metab Res 1996;28:353–356.

15 Modi DN, Sane S, Bhartiya D: Accelerated germ cell apoptosis in sex chromosome aneuploid fetal human gonads. Mol Hum Reprod 2003;9:219–225.

16 Welt CK: Primary ovarian insufficiency: a more accurate term for premature ovarian failure. Clin Endocrinol 2008;68:499–509.

17 Allingham-Hawkins DJ, Babul-Hirji R, Chitayat D, et al: Fragile X premutation is a significant risk factor for premature ovarian failure: the International Collaborative POF in Fragile X study–preliminary data. Am J Med Genet 1999;83:322–325.

18 Sherman SL. Premature ovarian failure in the fragile X syndrome. Am J Med Genet 2000;97:189–194.

19 Murray A, Webb J, Grimley S, Conway G, Jacobs P: Studies of FRAXA and FRAXE in women with premature ovarian failure. J Med Genet 1998;35:637–640.

20 Bosch AM, Grootenhuis MA, Bakker HD, Heijmans HS, Wijburg FA, Last BF: Living with classical galactosemia: health-related quality of life consequences. Pediatrics 2004;113:e423–e428.

21 Levy HL, Driscoll SG, Porensky RS, Wender DF: Ovarian failure in galactosemia. N Engl J Med 1984; 310:50.

22 Kaufman FR, Kogut MD, Donnell GN, Goebelsmann U, March C, Koch R: Hypergonadotropic hypogonadism in female patients with galactosemia. N Engl J Med 1981;304:994–998.

23 Fraser IS, Russell P, Greco S, Robertson DM: Resistant ovary syndrome and premature ovarian failure in young women with galactosaemia. Clin Reprod Fertil 1986;4:133–138.

24 Sanders RD, Spencer JB, Epstein MP, Pollak SV, Vardhana PA, Lustbader JW, Fridovich-Keil JL: Biomarkers of ovarian function in girls and women with classic galactosemia. Fertil Steril 2009;92:344–351.

25 Beysen D, De Paepe A, De Baere E: FOXL2 mutations and genomic rearrangements in BPES. Hum Mutat 2009;30:158–169.

26 Matthijs G, Schollen E, Pardon E, Veiga-Da-Cunha M, Jaeken J, Cassiman JJ, Van Schaftingen E: Mutations in PMM2, a phosphomannomutase gene on chromosome 16p13, in carbohydrate-deficient glycoprotein type I syndrome (Jaeken syndrome) [erratum appears in Nat Genet 1997;16:316]. Nat Genet 1997;16:88–92.

27 Aittomaki K, Herva R, Stenman UH, Juntunen K, Ylostalo P, Hovatta O, de la Chapelle A: Clinical features of primary ovarian failure caused by a point mutation in the follicle-stimulating hormone receptor gene. J Clin Endocrinol Metabol 1996;81:3722–3726.

28 Rousseau-Merck MF, Atger M, Loosfelt H, Milgrom E, Berger R: The chromosomal localization of the human follicle-stimulating hormone receptor gene (FSHR) on 2p21-p16 is similar to that of the luteinizing hormone receptor gene. Genomics 1993; 15:222–224.

29 Broekmans FJ, Kwee J, Hendriks DJ, Mol BW, Lambalk CB: A systematic review of tests predicting ovarian reserve and IVF outcome. Hum Reprod Update 2006;12:685–718.

30 Larsen EC, Muller J, Rechnitzer C, Schmiegelow K, Andersen AN: Diminished ovarian reserve in female childhood cancer survivors with regular menstrual cycles and basal FSH <10 IU/l. Hum Reprod 2003;18:417–422.

31 Bath LE, Anderson RA, Critchley HO, Kelnar CJ, Wallace WH: Hypothalamic-pituitary-ovarian dysfunction after prepubertal chemotherapy and cranial irradiation for acute leukaemia. Hum Reprod 2001;16:1838–1844.

32 Chellakooty M, Schmidt IM, Haavisto AM, Boisen KA, Damgaard IN, Mau C, Petersen JH, Juul A, Skakkebaek NE, Main KM: Inhibin A, inhibin B, follicle-stimulating hormone, luteinizing hormone, estradiol, and sex hormone-binding globulin levels in 473 healthy infant girls. J Clin Endocrinol Metab 2003;88:3515–3520.

33 Sehested A, Juul AA, Andersson AM, Petersen JH, Jensen TK, Muller J, Skakkebaek NE: Serum inhibin A and inhibin B in healthy prepubertal, pubertal, and adolescent girls and adult women: relation to age, stage of puberty, menstrual cycle, follicle-stimulating hormone, luteinizing hormone, and estradiol levels. J Clin Endocrinol Metab 2000;85: 1634–1640.

34 Courant F, Aksglaede L, Antignac JP, Monteau F, Sorensen K, Andersson AM, Skakkebaek NE, Juul A, Bizec BL: Assessment of circulating sex steroid levels in prepubertal and pubertal boys and girls by a novel ultrasensitive gas chromatography-tandem mass spectrometry method. J Clin Endocrinol Metab 2010;95:82–92.

35 Crofton PM, Evans AE, Groome NP, Taylor MR, Holland CV, Kelnar CJ: Dimeric inhibins in girls from birth to adulthood: relationship with age, pubertal stage, FSH and oestradiol. Clin Endocrinol 2002;56:223–230.

36 de Vet A, Laven JS, de Jong FH, Themmen AP, Fauser BC: Antimullerian hormone serum levels: a putative marker for ovarian aging. Fertil Steril 2002;77:357–362.

37 Andersson AM, Muller J, Skakkebaek NE: Different roles of prepubertal and postpubertal germ cells and sertoli cells in the regulation of serum inhibin B levels. J Clin Endocrinol Metab 1998;83:4451–4458.

38 Fauser BC, Van Heusden AM: Manipulation of human ovarian function: physiological concepts and clinical consequences. Endocr Rev 1997;18:71–106.

39 Grootegoed JA, Baarends WM, Themmen AP: Welcome to the family: the anti-mullerian hormone receptor. Mol Cell Endocrinol 1994;100:29–34.

40 Rajpert-De Meyts E, Jorgensen N, Graem N, Muller J, Cate RL, Skakkebaek NE: Expression of anti-Mullerian hormone during normal and pathological gonadal development: association with differentiation of Sertoli and granulosa cells. J Clin Endocrinol Metab 1999;84:3836–3844.

41 Guibourdenche J, Lucidarme N, Chevenne D, Rigal O, Nicolas M, Luton D, Leger J, Porquet D, Noel M: Anti-mullerian hormone levels in serum from human foetuses and children: pattern and clinical interest. Mol Cell Endocrinol 2003;211:55–63.

42 Hudson PL, Dougas I, Donahoe PK, Cate RL, Epstein J, Pepinsky RB, MacLaughlin DT: An immunoassay to detect human mullerian inhibiting substance in males and females during normal development. J Clin Endocrinol Metabol 1990;70:16–22.

43 van Rooij IA, Tonkelaar I, Broekmans FJ, Looman CW, Scheffer GJ, de Jong FH, Themmen AP, te Velde ER: Anti-mullerian hormone is a promising predictor for the occurrence of the menopausal transition. Menopause 2004;11:601–606.

44 Durlinger AL, Kramer P, Karels B, de Jong FH, Uilenbroek JT, Grootegoed JA, Themmen AP: Control of primordial follicle recruitment by anti-Mullerian hormone in the mouse ovary. Endocrinology 1999;140:5789–5796.

45 Durlinger AL, Gruijters MJ, Kramer P, Karels B, Ingraham HA, Nachtigal MW, Uilenbroek JT, Grootegoed JA, Themmen AP: Anti-Mullerian hormone inhibits initiation of primordial follicle growth in the mouse ovary. Endocrinology 2002;143:1076–1084.

46 Durlinger AL, Gruijters MJ, Kramer P, Karels B, Kumar TR, Matzuk MM, Rose UM, de Jong FH, Uilenbroek JT, Grootegoed JA, Themmen AP: Anti-Mullerian hormone attenuates the effects of FSH on follicle development in the mouse ovary. Endocrinology 2001;142:4891–4999.

47 Neely EK, Hintz RL, Wilson DM, Lee PA, Gautier T, Argente J, Stene M: Normal ranges for immuno-chemiluminometric gonadotropin assays. J Pediatr 1995;127:40–46.

48 Resende EA, Lara BH, Reis JD, Ferreira BP, Pereira GA, Borges MF: Assessment of basal and gonadotropin-releasing hormone-stimulated gonadotropins by immunochemiluminometric and immunofluorometric assays in normal children. J Clin Endocrinol Metab 2007;92:1424–1429.

49 Houk CP, Kunselman AR, Lee PA: Adequacy of a single unstimulated luteinizing hormone level to diagnose central precocious puberty in girls. Pediatrics 2009;123:e1059–e1063.

50 Kevenaar ME, Meerasahib MF, Kramer P, van de Lang-Born BM, de Jong FH, Groome NP, Themmen AP, Visser JA: Serum anti-mullerian hormone levels reflect the size of the primordial follicle pool in mice. Endocrinology 2006;147:3228–3234.

51 van Rooij IA, Broekmans FJ, Scheffer GJ, Looman CW, Habbema JD, de Jong FH, Fauser BJ, Themmen AP, te Velde ER: Serum antimullerian hormone levels best reflect the reproductive decline with age in normal women with proven fertility: a longitudinal study. Fertil Steril 2005;83:979–987.

52 van Rooij IA, Broekmans FJ, te Velde ER, Fauser BC, Bancsi LF, de Jong FH, Themmen AP: Serum anti-Mullerian hormone levels: a novel measure of ovarian reserve. Hum Reprod 2002;17:3065–3071.

53 Nardo LG, Christodoulou D, Gould D, Roberts SA, Fitzgerald CT, Laing I: Anti-Müllerian hormone levels and antral follicle count in women enrolled in in vitro fertilization cycles: relationship to lifestyle factors, chronological age and reproductive history. Gynecol Endocrinol 2007;23:486–493.

54 Seifer DB, MacLaughlin DT, Christian BP, Feng B, Shelden RM: Early follicular serum mullerian-inhibiting substance levels are associated with ovarian response during assisted reproductive technology cycles. Fertil Steril 2002;77:468–471.

55 Visser JA, de Jong FH, Laven JS, Themmen AP: Anti-Mullerian hormone: a new marker for ovarian function. Reproduction 2006;131:1–9.

56 Bath LE, Wallace WH, Shaw MP, Fitzpatrick C, Anderson RA: Depletion of ovarian reserve in young women after treatment for cancer in childhood: detection by anti-Mullerian hormone, inhibin B and ovarian ultrasound. Hum Reprod 2003;18:2368–2374.

57 van Beek RD, van den Heuvel-Eibrink MM, Laven JS, de Jong FH, Themmen AP, Hakvoort-Cammel FG, van den Bos C, van den Berg H, Pieters R, de Munck Keizer-Schrama SM: Anti-mullerian hormone is a sensitive serum marker for gonadal function in women treated for Hodgkin's lymphoma during childhood. J Clin Endocrinol Metab 2007;92:3869–3874.

58 Lie Fong S, Laven JS, Hakvoort-Cammel FG, Schipper I, Visser JA, Themmen AP, de Jong FH, van den Heuvel-Eibrink MM: Assessment of ovarian reserve in adult childhood cancer survivors using anti-Mullerian hormone. Hum Reprod 2009; 24:982–990.

59 Badouraki M, Christoforidis A, Economou I, Dimitriadis AS, Katzos G: Sonographic assessment of uterine and ovarian development in normal girls aged 1 to 12 years. J Clin Ultrasound 2008;36:539–544.

60 Herter LD, Golendziner E, Flores JA, Becker E Jr, Spritzer PM: Ovarian and uterine sonography in healthy girls between 1 and 13 years old: correlation of findings with age and pubertal status. Am J Roentg 2002;178:1531–1536.

61 Anderson RA, Themmen AP, Al-Qahtani A, Groome NP, Cameron DA: The effects of chemotherapy and long-term gonadotrophin suppression on the ovarian reserve in premenopausal women with breast cancer. Hum Reprod 2006;21:2583–2592.

62 Lutchman Singh K, Muttukrishna S, Stein RC, McGarrigle HH, Patel A, Parikh B, Groome NP, Davies MC, Chatterjee R: Predictors of ovarian reserve in young women with breast cancer. Br J Cancer 2007;96:1808–1816.

63 Salardi S, Orsini LF, Cacciari E, Bovicelli L, Tassoni P, Reggiani A: Pelvic ultrasonography in premenarcheal girls: relation to puberty and sex hormone concentrations. Arch Dis Childh 1985;60:120–125.

Dr. W.H.B. Wallace
Department of Haematology/Oncology, Royal Hospital for Sick Children
17 Millerfield Place
Edinburgh EH9 1LW (UK)
Tel. +44 131 536 0420, Fax +44 131 536 0430, E-Mail Hamish.Wallace@nhs.net

Ranke MB, Mullis P-E (eds): Diagnostics of Endocrine Function in Children and Adolescents, ed 4.
Basel, Karger, 2011, pp 350–378

Assessing the Function of the Human Adrenal Cortex

Christa E. Flück

Pediatric Endocrinology and Diabetology, Department of Pediatrics and Department of Clinical Research,
University of Bern, Bern, Switzerland

The human adrenals consist of two organs which are located on top of the kidneys bilaterally. Each adrenal gland has a medulla and a cortex with three specific layers reflecting the distinct functions of the gland [1]. The medulla is part of the sympathetic nervous system and originates of the neuroectoderm. Thus, the medulla is a modified sympathetic ganglion and produces the catecholamines epinephrine and norepinephrine. By contrast, the adrenal cortex arises from a mesodermal anlage together with the kidneys and the gonads which separate and form the fetal adrenals at 8–9 weeks' gestation [2]. The fetal adrenal cortex consists of a small outer 'definitive' zone which appears steroidogenically quiescent until late gestation, and a larger inner 'fetal' zone which produces C19 steroids (adrenal androgens) throughout gestation; a 'transitional' zone between those two zones exists and produces cortisol towards the end of the fetal development. After birth, the large 'fetal' zone of the fetal adrenal involutes and disappears by 6 months of age. Simultaneously, the 'definitive' zone, maybe together with the 'transitional' zone, develops into the fully differentiated zonae glomerulosa and fasciculata. However, the third, innermost zona reticularis develops only slowly and may not be fully differentiated before the age of 15 years. The mature adrenal cortex produces mineralocorticoids in the zona glomerulosa for maintaining salt and water homeostasis of the body [3]. It produces glucocorticoids in the zona fasciculata for acute and chronic stress response maintaining energy balance, blood pressure and endurance. Finally, it produces C19 steroids (adrenal androgens, adrenal sex steroids) in the zona fasciculata to allow 'adrenarche' and 'adrenopause' to occur as physiologic events of unknown importance unique to humans and higher primates. Thus, this specific development of the human adrenals leads to a highly specific lifetime profile of normal adrenal hormone production (fig. 1) [4].

The production of all steroid hormones starts from cholesterol which is either synthesized by the cell or supplied from plasma low-density lipoproteins from dietary

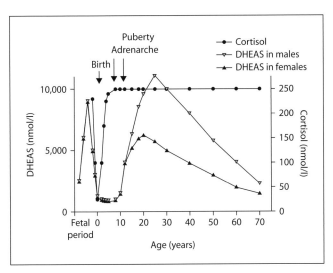

Fig. 1. Lifetime profile of mean plasma adrenal cortisol and DHEAS concentrations. DHEAS is produced abundantly by the fetal adrenal prenatally and declines with the involution of the fetal zone of the adrenal postnatally. DHEAS levels rise during adrenarche with the development of the zona reticularis and decrease during adrenopause after 30 years of age. Sex difference in circulating DHEAS concentrations reflects the secretion of the testes. By contrast, cortisol is produced in the fetal adrenal only during a short window during 5–12 weeks' gestation and thereafter in the third trimenon of pregnancy. Mean adult cortisol levels are reached shortly after birth and remain constant throughout life [4, 33].

intake [5]. Cholesterol is imported to the mitochondria by the help of steroidogenic acute regulatory protein (StAR) and converted to pregnenolone by the CYP11A1, side chain cleavage enzyme and ferredoxin-reductase co-factor system which is the first and rate-limiting step of all steroid hormone biosynthesis (fig. 2). Pregnenolone is then converted to the specific steroids through a cascade of specifically expressed steroidogenic enzymes, co-factors and intermediates in the three layers of the cortex as depicted in figure 2.

Steroid production of the adrenal cortex is controlled by feed forward and feedback loops (fig. 3). Glucocorticoid and adrenal androgen biosynthesis are principally regulated by the hypothalamus-pituitary-adrenal (HPA) axis through corticotropin-releasing hormone (CRH) and adrenocorticotropic hormone (ACTH) [1]. In addition, ACTH may be stimulated by antidiuretic hormone (vasopressin; AVP) directly. Specific regulators of adrenal androgen production may exist but remain elusive. Although ACTH has a permissive effect on mineralocorticoid production, the main regulators of aldosterone biosynthesis are the renin-angiotensin system and potassium. Detailed information on the regulation of mineralocorticoid production and specific diagnostic tests are included in the chapter on 'Diagnostic investigations in endocrine disorders of sodium regulation' by Paolo Ferrari and are therefore not discussed in this chapter. However, reference plasma concentrations of mineralocorticoids at

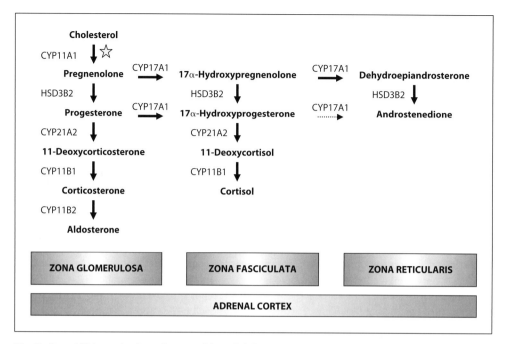

Fig. 2. Steroid biosynthetic pathways of the adult human adrenal cortex. Cholesterol is converted to pregnenolone through 20α-hydroxylation, 22-hydroxylation and scission of the C20–22 carbon bond by the mitochondrial cytochrome P450 side chain cleavage enzyme (CYP11A1) and cofactors NADPH, ferredoxin-reductase, ferredoxin. Δ5 steroids (pregnenolone (Preg), 17α-hydroxypregnenolone (17OHPreg) and dehydroepiandrosterone (DHEA)) are converted to Δ4 steroids (progesterone (Prog), 17α-hydroxyprogesterone (17OHP) and androstenedione (Δ4A)) by 3β-hydroxysteroid dehydrogenase type 2 (HSD3B2). P450c17–17α-hydroxylase activity (CYP17A1) converts Preg to 17OHPreg and Prog to 17OHP while P450c17–17,20 lyase activity (CYP17A1) converts 17OHPreg to DHEA and converts small amounts of 17OHP directly to Δ4A. 21-hydroxylation of Prog to 11-deoxycorticosterone (DOC) and of 17OHP to 11-deoxycortisol (11-DOC) is catalyzed by CYP21A2 (P450c21). 11-DOC is converted to cortisol by 11β-hydroxylation through CYP11B1 (P450c11β). DOC is converted to corticosterone by either 11-hydroxylase activity of CYP11B2 (P450c11AS) in the zona glomerulosa or of CYP11B1 in the zona fasciculata (P450c11β). CYP11B2 converts corticosterone in two steps (18-hydroxylation and 18-methyl-oxidation) to aldosterone. Note that steroidogenic activities of CYP17A1 and CYP21A2 (as well as of CYP19-aromatase activity) depend on co-factor P450 oxidoreductase (CYP OR). 'Star' sign indicates a role for steroidogenic acute regulatory protein (StAR) in the initial step of steroidogenesis.

different ages are given in table 1 together with average plasma cortisol concentrations [3].

Steroid production of the adrenals does not only show a life-time profile depending on the developmental stage of the organ but is also determined by the circadian rhythm modulating the HPA axis and thus leading to a diurnal variation of most adrenal steroids with the exception of dehydroepiandrosterone sulfate (DHEAS). A representative circadian profile of plasma ACTH and cortisol in a normal 10-year-old

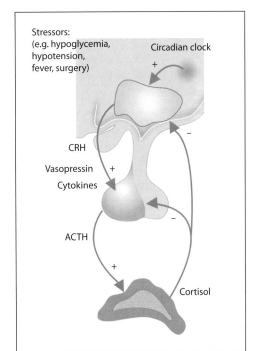

Fig. 3. The hypothalamus-pituitary-adrenal axis (HPA). ACTH is secreted from the pituitary gland under the stimulation of CRH and arginine vasopressin. CRH secretion of the hypothalamus is modulated by the biological clock (circadian rhythm) and by various stressors. ACTH is the principal stimulator of adrenal cortisol production. In turn, circulating cortisol exerts a negative feedback control on both CRH and ACTH secretion.

child is shown in figure 4 [6]. In addition, other stimuli including physical or emotional stress affect adrenal steroidogenesis (fig. 3).

Biochemical Assessment of Adrenal Steroids

Adrenal steroids may be measured from blood, urine or saliva. However, each choice of specimen and method of measurement has its own normative values and advantages and disadvantages that need to be taken into account when dealing with patient samples [7]. Urine assays are considered to measure most of the secretory activity of steroidogenesis but depend on completeness of the collection and a normal renal function, and they may reflect the contribution of not only adrenal steroidogenesis (e.g. the level of androstenedione is determined by production in the adrenals and the gonads). In addition, measurements from urine are time consuming and bear the inconvenience encountered in the collection of 24-hour urine. However, urine assays still have their place in the determination of free hormone, especially free cortisol.

Blood assays, on the other hand, have largely replaced urine assays for routine purposes as they are more convenient for both the laboratory and the patient. Immunoassays and chromatographic methods have been developed to determine virtually all steroids in the plasma that are clinically relevant [7]. Additionally, as

Table 1. Mean glucocorticoid and mineralocorticoid concentrations

		Cortisol nmol/l	DOC nmol/l	Cortico-sterone nmol/l	18OH cortico sterone nmol/l	Aldo-sterone nmol/l	Plasma renin activity mg/L/s
Age	Cord blood	360	5.5	19		2.4	50
	Premature babies	180			5.5	2.8	222
	Newborns	140		6.6	9.7	2.6	58
	Infants	250	0.6	16	2.2	0.8	33
	Children (08.00 h)						
	1–2 years	110–550			1.8	0.8	15
	2–10 years	as adults	0.3		1.2	0.3/0.8*	8.3
	10–15 years	as adults			0.7	0.1/0.6*	3.3
	Adults (08.00 h)	280–550	0.2	12	0.6	0.2/0.4*	2.8/4.0*
	Adults (16.00 h)	140–280		3.8			
Assay		RIA	RIA	RIA	RIA	RIA	RIA
Ref.		1	1	1	1	1	1

*Values in supine/upright posture.
Data are adapted from Endocrine Sciences, Tarzana, Calif., USA.

endocrine testing is founded on provocative testing (stimulation and suppression tests) blood samples for rapid dynamic tests are much more accurate than urine samples. However, plasma measurements also have their limitations because of the rapid fluctuations and pulsatility of hormonal levels (fig. 4). Thus a plasma steroid measurement reflects the hormonal level only at the exact time of sampling. Although there is no experimental evidence that steroid hormone levels are different in serum and plasma, rapid separation of red blood cells in the specimen is recommended as red blood cells can alter plasma concentrations of active steroid hormones such as cortisol which may be inactivated to cortisone [7].

Most steroids of clinical interest can also be measured from saliva. But normative values for measurements from saliva have not (yet) been fully established. For some steroids such as cortisol or progesterone, the salivary level appears to reflect the free (non-bound) steroid fraction in the blood providing similar information as derived from measurement of urinary free steroids. Salivary sampling protocols are advantageous for frequent and easy collection of samples by noninvasive, stress-free techniques.

Steroid assays measure the hormones either in a free state or the protein-bound state, or both [7, 8]. Measuring concentrations of free steroid hormones may be

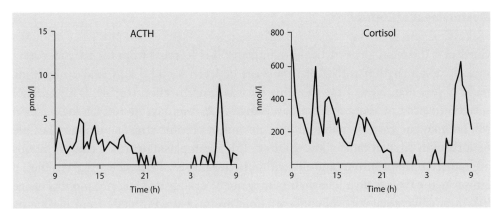

Fig. 4. Representative circadian profile of plasma ACTH and cortisol in a normal child. Measurements were performed from unextracted plasma using immunoassays [6].

preferable when suspecting alterations in the binding proteins in the circulation. Also, it is the free hormone that binds to the steroid receptor to elicit the biochemical effect; thus knowing the free hormone level is of interest in a number of clinical situations.

Steroid hormones can be measured directly from plasma by specific immunoassays which are generally rapid, easy to perform and therefore cheap; but immunoassays bear the disadvantage of not always being highly specific due to possible cross-reactivity or matrix effects [7, 8]. Alternatively, steroids may be identified highly specifically by chromatographic methods such as high-performance liquid chromatography (HPLC) or combined gas chromatography and mass spectrometry (GC/MS) which are more laborious and thus expensive techniques. GC/MS is currently not available for routine diagnostic in most centers. However, GC/MS is extremely specific and therefore regarded as the gold standard when evaluating steroid immunoassays for common use. Additionally to high specificity, those chromatographic techniques bear the advantage that they provide a full steroid profile with one measurement because they separate all steroids found in a sample which then may be identified according to internal standards provided for each method. The methodology of profiling steroids by GC/MS and its diagnostic value are described in great details in a separate chapter of this book by Wudy.

For routine steroid measurements, a large number of immunoassays have been developed using different types of antibodies, processing schemes, labels (isotopic or non-isotopic) and measurement principles, including beta and gamma counting, photometry, fluorometry and chemiluminescence [7, 8]. Thus, when looking at plasma steroid concentrations of a subject, it is crucial to know the reference values as well as specificity and sensitivity of the specific method with which the steroids were determined. This is of particular importance when looking at reference values given in all tables of this chapter.

Measurement of Cortisol

Cortisol is the main glucocorticoid in humans. It is secreted from the adrenal cortex in a circadian rhythm with a plasma surge between 4 and 8 a.m. and a nighttime nadir of less than 50% of the morning plasma concentration (fig. 4). Daily cortisol secretion rates are about 9.2 mg/day (range 8–25 mg/day; ~4.6–14.4 mg/m^2/day) [8], but may increase by manifold in acute and/or chronic stress situations. Half-life of cortisol in circulation is about 100 min [3]. Mean plasma cortisol concentrations are rather constant throughout life without relevant sex differences (fig. 1; table 1). However, the typical circadian rhythm may not be established before 6 months of age [9]. In practice, total cortisol concentrations are measured directly from plasma by various immunoassays, which are fast, easy to perform, quite specific and sensitive. Representative values of total cortisol (free and bound) in plasma measured by an immunoassay are given in table 1. Most immunoassays however detect cortisol and cortisone that are readily distinguishable by HPLC. This may be of importance when looking at plasma levels in newborns in the first few days of life as their plasma contains mainly cortisone rather than cortisol. Thus 'cortisol' measurement in a newborn will give higher values when measured by an immunoassay compared to HPLC and must not be mistaken for adenal insufficiency or excess.

Determination of the free, bioactive fraction of cortisol has been shown to be a useful screening for cortisol hypersecretion disorders [10]. Methods for estimating the free fraction in serum are not available for routine use [7, 8]. Measurement of free cortisol in urine reflects approximately 2% of the active cortisol and may be performed with most immunoassays. Appropriate extraction of the urine specimen is mandatory to avoid cross-reaction of cortisol metabolites and conjugates with the antibodies [7]. Clearly, chromatographic measurement techniques of urine free cortisol are more specific than immunoassays and are therefore preferable. Representative reference values for free cortisol from urine specimen are given in table 2 [7].

Measurement of free cortisol in saliva reflects the concentration of non-protein bound cortisol in blood accurately and is very convenient for both the laboratory and the patient. Most immunoassays can be used for salivary cortisol determination directly without extraction because saliva does not contain binding proteins or metabolites interfering with the assays. In adults reference values assessed by a representative radioimmunoassay are as follows: at 07.00 h 4–28 nmol/l (1.4–10.1 µg/dl) and at 22.00 h 2–6 nmol/l (0.7–2.2) [7].

Measurement of ACTH

Blood cortisol levels parallel ACTH concentrations with their circadian and episodic variability (fig. 4). ACTH is produced under stimulation of CRH of the hypothalamus

Table 2. Representative values for free cortisol excreted in urine

		nmol/day	µg/day	nmol/day	µg/day
Age	children				
	1–10 years	6–74	2–27		
	2–11 years			3–58	1–21
	11–20 years	14–152	5–55		
	12–16 years			6–105	2–38
	adults	55–248*	20–90*		
		207–745**	75–270**		
Assay		RIA	RIA	HPLC	HPLC

*Extracted.
**not Extracted.

and is the principal regulator of adrenal cortisol production (fig. 3). ACTH is a fragment of the precursor pro-opiomelanocortin (POMC) and is secreted in the circulation. However, ACTH is unstable in blood and has a short half-life (<10 min) making a proper pre-analytical handling very important for correct measurements. Samples must be drawn in plastic tubes containing heparin or EDTA and stored immediately on ice, as ACTH tends to adhere to glass and is quickly inactivated [7]. ACTH is usually measured by RIA but these measurements remain more difficult and variable than for other pituitary hormones. Elevated plasma ACTH levels may be informative but low or low-normal levels may not be measurable by most assays [8]. Therefore, interpretation of plasma ACTH levels must be done in the context of simultaneous plasma cortisol values [11]. In older children and adults with established circadian rhythm normal 08.00 h plasma ACTH levels rarely exceed 50 ng/l while 20.00 h concentrations are usually not detectable.

Measurement of Other Adrenal Steroid Hormones

All clinically relevant adrenal steroid hormones may be measured from blood by specific immunoassays or by chromatographic methods. Reference values for plasma progestins and adenal androgens are given in table 3 [9, 12].

Plasma levels of progestins (pregnenolone, progesterone, 17-hydroxyprogesterone, 17OHP) and androgens (dehydroepiandrosterone; DHEA), DHEA sulfate (DHEAS), androstenedione (Δ4A) vary with age and sex. For instance, at birth concentrations of

Table 3. Plasma concentrations of progestins and adrenal androgens according to sex and age

		Progesterone nmol/l	17OHP nmol/l	DHEAS nmol/l	DHEA nmol/l	Δ4A nmol/l
Birth						
Cord blood	M	1,540 ± 985	56.4 ± 31	3,415 ± 1,459	24.7 ± 6.6	3.0 ± 0.98
	F	254–1,780	70.8 ± 41	3,423 ± 1,817	20.6 ± 6.5	3.3 ± 1.3
Peripheral vein	M	12–32	12.7 ± 5.8	3,635 ± 3,200	24.7 ± 6.6	6.7 ± 3.2
	F	10–30	12.7 ± 5.8	3,533 ± 3,200	28.8 ± 6.5	6.1 ± 2.6
Infancy						
4–7 days	M	0-75–3.5	3.2 ± 1.8	691 ± 461	9.1 ± 7.4	1.22 ± 0.6
	F	0.2–1.2	2.9 ± 1.2	786 ± 512	10.0 ± 6.5	1.16 ± 0.6
1–2 months	M	0.09–1.1	6.1 ± 2.4	351 ± 282	6.4 ± 4.8	1.51 ± 0.45
	F	0.05–0.9	3.2 ± 1.5	256 ± 200	2.8 ± 1.6	0.66 ± 0.24
4–6 months	M	0.09–1.0	1.6 ± 1.0	151 ± 143	3.1 ± 2.6	0.75 ± 0.50
	F	0.1–0.8	1.6 ± 0.7	179 ± 161	4.4 ± 2.9	0.45 ± 0.25
7–9 months	M	0.09–0.5	0.88 ± 0.63	72 ± 61	3.1 ± 2.6	0.38 ± 0.09
	F	0.12–0.8	1.82 ± 1.27	77 ± 74	4.4 ± 2.9	0.38 ± 0.05
9–12 months	M	0.16–0.7	0.85 ± 0.66	72 ± 61	1.5 ± 1.4	0.38 ± 0.20
	F	0.11–0.8	1.3 ± 0.75	77 ± 74	2.7 ± 2.1	0.38 ± 0.15
Prepubertal						
1–2 years	M/F	0.1–0.5	0.7 ± 0.3	58 ± 43	0.87 ± 0.3	0.38 ± 0.20
3–5 years	M/F	0.1–0.5	0.8 ± 0.3	58 ± 43	0.87 ± 0.3	0.42 ± 0.20
6–8 years	M/F	0.1–0.8	1.0 ± 0.5	384 ± 61	3.4 ± 1.3	0.71 ± 0.40
Pubertal						
Tanner 1	M	<0.3–1.0	0.1–2.7	1,062 ± 836	7.12 ± 1.73	1.18 ± 0.61
	F	<0.3–1.0	0.1–2.5	1,103 ± 481	6.00 ± 2.36	1.08 ± 0.26
Tanner 2	M	<0.3–1.0	0.2–3.5	1,605 ± 1,027	10.62 ± 3.18	1.3 ± 0.56
	F	<0.3–1.7	0.3–3.0	1,252 ± 561	11.39 ± 2.08	1.86 ± 1.19
Tanner 3	M	<0.3–1.5	0.3–4.2	1,879 ± 1,249	13.95 ± 3.46	1.54 ± 0.15
	F	<0.3–14.3	0.3–4.7	1,826 ± 1,375	14.81 ± 5.58	2.40 ± 1.85
Tanner 4	M	<0.3–3.4	0.9–5.4	2,638 ± 1,426	13.02 ± 3.43	2.49 ± 1.11
	F	0.3–41.3	0.5–7.0	2,212 ± 1,237	17.02 ± 4.16	2.86 ± 1.65

Table 3. Continued

		Progesterone nmol/l	17OHP nmol/l	DHEAS nmol/l	DHEA nmol/l	Δ4A nmol/l
Tanner 5	M	0.7–2.6	0.7–5.3	3,158 ± 1,234	18.82 ± 3.91	2.92 ± 1.01
	F	0.3–30.2	0.6–8.0	3,083 ± 1,083	21.98 ± 9.36	3.22 ± 1.19
Adult						
Male	M	0-4–3.1	3.5 ± 1.2	5,735 ± 2,380	22.30 ± 3.9	3.7 ± 0.9
Female						
Follicular	F	1.8 ± 0.34	1.3 ± 0.25	3,540 ± 1,310	17.90 ± 3.7	2.7 ± 1.0
Luteal	F	43.0 ± 13.0	7.4 ± 2.0	3,540 ± 1,310	17.90 ± 3.7	5.2 ± 1.5

All data are given as range or mean ± SD.
Data are adapted from Forest [9].

adrenal steroids are elevated during the so-called hormonal surge. Thereafter, plasma concentrations of progesterone, 17OHP and 11-deoxycorticosterone (DOC) fall dramatically within the first 4 days of life. Therefore, measurement of 17OHP by RIA from blood spots collected on filter paper on day 4 of life has been established for screening newborn infants for congenital adrenal hyperplasia due to 21-hydroxylase (21OHase) deficiency [3]. This screening is effective in most European countries. RIAs used for screening are easy to perform and cheap, and have a very good sensitivity and a quite good specificity which may be improved by extracting steroids prior to analysis as performed in some laboratories [7]. Important, however, is that reference values depend not only on the specific method used and the exact day of life when the blood sample is drawn, but also on the gestational age of the newborn [9, 13]. Premature babies have generally higher 17OHP values on day 4 of life with much broader variability compared to term babies [13]. However these levels fall to normal levels within the first three months of life.

Adrenal androgens comprise DHEA, DHEAS and Δ4A [14]. DHEA is mostly the product of the adrenal cortex. More than 99% of DHEA is sulfated to DHEAS before it is secreted into the circulation. Plasma DHEA/DHEAS values vary considerably with age (fig. 1 and table 2). The rise in plasma DHEA/DHEAS around age 6–8 years is characteristic for the functional activation of the zona reticularis of the adrenal cortex which is called 'adrenarche' (fig. 1). 5–10% of adrenal DHEA is converted to Δ4A which is the immediate precursor for testosterone production. However, testosterone is not synthesized in the normal adrenal cortex, but Δ4A may be converted to it in the periphery. In children, plasma Δ4A originates predominantly from the adrenals. In adults, by contrast, approximately half of circulating Δ4A originates from the gonads in both sexes [9].

Dynamic Testing of the Adrenal Cortex Function

Because single measurements of plasma steroids often provide limited information for diagnosing adrenal disorders, functional stimulation and/or suppression tests may be used to assess adrenal steroid biosynthetic function. Depending on the functional disturbance that is suspected, different tests may be employed. Generally, disorders of the human adrenal cortex may be categorized in three groups at the functional level: adrenal insufficiency, adrenal excess and adrenal dysfunction. Testing of the HPA axis utilizes stimulating agents (e.g. ACTH or CRH) or suppressing agents (e.g. dexamethasone). Test interpretation must be made with reference values obtained from the specific agent and protocol used.

Tests to Assess Adrenal Glucocorticoid Insufficiency

In patients adrenal insufficiency may be suspected because of acute or chronic symptoms (weakness, fatigue, anorexia, GI symptoms, salt craving, dizziness, pain), clinical signs (weight loss, hyperpigmentation, low blood pressure, vitiligo) or laboratory findings such as electrolyte disturbances (low sodium, high potassium and calcium), azotemia and anemia. The etiology of adrenocortical insufficiency may be at the level of the adrenal cortex itself (primary) or at the level of the hypothalamus and/ or pituitary gland (secondary). A detailed list of possible causes of adrenocortical insufficiency is given in table 4. Generally, the biochemical confirmation of adrenal insufficiency requires the demonstration of inappropriately low cortisol production. Thus depending on the clinical state of the patient, the diagnostic strategy may vary. Basal cortisol and ACTH measurements may only be diagnostic in stressed patients presenting with an acute adrenal crisis (Addison's crisis). Blood samples for the measurements of ACTH and cortisol must be obtained before glucocorticoid therapy is initiated as otherwise ACTH levels may be suppressed. In unstressed patients randomly drawn cortisol and ACTH levels are of very limited diagnostic value and even 8.00 h morning levels show considerable overlap between adrenal insufficiency and normals [8, 11, 15]. Generally, plasma 8.00 h cortisol level less than 138 nmol/l are very suspect for adrenal insufficiency (salivary <5 nmol/l), while levels >550 nmol/l make the diagnosis unlikely (salivary >16 nmol/l) [8, 15]. However, only markedly elevated ACTH (>200 nmol/l) and very low cortisol levels are diagnostic for primary adrenal insufficiency [8, 15]. Therefore, in most situations dynamic tests of the HPA axis may be required to obtain greater diagnostic accuracy with respect to both sensitivity and specificity.

Table 4. Causes of adrenal insufficiency

Primary (Addison's disease)
Congenital adrenal hyperplasia (CAH)
Congenital adrenal hypoplasia (DAX1, SF1 mutations)
Familial ACTH resistance syndromes (MC2R, MRAP, Triple A)
X-linked adrenoleukodystrophy (ALD gene)
Adrenal hemorrhage or infarction
Autoimmune adrenalitis
– Isolated
– Part of autoimmune polyglandular syndromes type 1 (AIRE gene) or 2
Infectious (HIV, tuberculosis, fungi,CMV)
Bilateral adrenalectomy
Others, including
– Zellweger disease
– Wolman disease
– Primary xanthomatosis
– Smith-Lemli–Opitz syndrome
– IMAGe syndrome
– Idiopathic
Secondary
Exogenous glucocorticoid therapy
Hypopituitarism
Hypothalamic tumors
Irradiation of the CNS
Granulomatous disease of the brain (e.g. sarcoidosis, tuberculosis)
Isolated ACTH deficiency
– idiopathic
– lymphocytic hypophysitis
– TPIT gene mutation
– POMC gene mutation (or processing defect)

ACTH Stimulation Test

ACTH administration stimulates cortisol synthesis and secretion acutely and chronically. Acute stimulation with ACTH intravenously will not result in an appropriate increase in plasma cortisol levels in patients with primary and secondary adrenal insufficiency. This is because in secondary insufficiency loss of the trophic action of ACTH on the normal adrenal cortex leads to atrophy of the gland resulting in similarly inadequate tissue response to ACTH stimulation as seen in primary insufficiency [8]. For ACTH stimulation tests, a variety of doses and durations have been described with specific reference values. Today, usually synthetic ACTH (1–24) with full biologic potency of native ACTH (1–39) is employed [8]. Side effects are extremely rare. In clinical practice, short infusion tests are mostly performed for practical reasons [3, 9, 15]. By contrast, prolonged ACTH stimulation tests are seldom necessary because baseline plasma ACTH measurements used in conjunction with short ACTH stimulation mostly provide the required information.

Rapid (or Short), Standard (or High-Dose) ACTH Test

For the standard ACTH test the patient is ideally installed with a venous sampling catheter early morning. After an interval of about 30 min for stress release of the venipuncture a baseline blood sample is drawn at 08.00–09.00 h for plasma cortisol and ACTH measurements. If mineralocorticoid deficiency is also suspected, plasma renine activity, aldosterone and electrolytes should be checked at baseline. ACTH (1–24) is then administered intravenously as a bolus at a dose of 250 μg in adults, 250 μg/1.73 m^2 BSA in children. Plasma samples for cortisol measurements are then taken at 30 and/or 60 min after ACTH administration. The cortisol peak response is expected to exceed 500–550 nmol/l, although there is considerable variation among different assays [8, 9]. Normal cortisol response is also defined by a 2- to 3-fold rise in the cortisol level or by an absolute increase at any time of >190 nmol/l [9]. Maximal cortisol responses to ACTH are similar in all age groups except for the first 6 months of life where the rise in cortisol is higher [9].

Pitfalls of the Test
The major problem with short, standard ACTH tests is the poor sensitivity for secondary adrenal insufficiency, especially when it is partial or of recent onset [8, 9]. In this case, the atrophy of the adrenal cortex is limited allowing some response to ACTH stimulation. The more physiologic dose administered in the low-dose test is designed to improve sensitivity [8].

(Short) Low-Dose ACTH Test

Except for the dose of ACTH, the low-dose ACTH test is very similar to the standard ACTH test (see above). ACTH (1–24) is administered intravenously at an absolute dose of 1 μg or at 0.5 μg/m^2 BSA and cortisol measured at baseline and 20–60 min after ACTH administration. Generally, a plasma cortisol response >500 nmol/l is considered a normal response [15, 16], although some investigators set the cut-off level of cortisol at >600 nmol/l [9].

Clearly, the advantage of the low-dose test is the higher sensitivity to detect subtle secondary adrenal insufficiency, in particular when basal cortisol levels are still normal [17, 18]. Thus, this test is a useful, safe and inexpensive tool for initial assessment of the HPA axis in patients with hypothalamic-pituitary disorders. However, it cannot discriminate hypothalamic from pituitary disorders for which additional tests are available.

Metyrapone Test

Metyrapone inhibits the enzyme CYP11B1 (fig. 2) and therefore blocks the conversion of 11-deoxycortisol (11-DOC) to cortisol. Normally, a decrease in cortisol results in a reduction of the negative feedback to CRH and ACTH (fig. 3) prompting a stimulation of steroid biosynthesis up to the point of the blockade. Several protocols are available for this test. We describe the overnight, single dose test which seems reliable and convenient and is therefore most commonly used [8, 9, 16].

For the single dose test, 30 mg/kg (top dose 3.0 g) metyrapone is given at midnight with a snack to reduce gastrointestinal upset. Plasma 11-DOC, cortisol and ACTH are measured at 08.00 h the following morning. Blockade is regarded as sufficient when morning cortisol levels are <138 nmol/l. HPA axis is regarded as intact when plasma 11-DOC levels increase to >210 nmol/l [8]. Measurement of ACTH will distinguish primary from secondary adrenal insufficiency; normal response of ACTH is >75 ng/ml.

Pitfalls
Metyrapone testing is not without risk [8, 9]. It may trigger an acute adrenal crisis in a chronic glucocorticoid deficient patient and induces symptoms of glucocorticoid deficiency (nausea, vomiting, hypotension) even in healthy subjects. It is therefore not recommended to perform this test in the outpatient setting. In addition, false-positive results may be observed in patients taking glucocorticoids such as dexamethasone. Clearance of metyrapone is variable in man with 4% of the population being regarded as rapid metabolizers, and clearance can be induced by certain drugs (e.g. phenytoin, rifampicin) [8, 9].

Insulin-Induced Hypoglycemia Test

Hypoglycemia is a fast and potent stimulus of CRH secretion, which will in turn enhance ACTH secretion and thereafter cortisol production. Thus, a normal response to hypoglycemia requires integrity of the entire HPA axis. For this test the patient is kept in bed after an overnight fast and installed with a venous catheter [9]. Hypoglycemia of <2.2 mmol/l is induced by administering insulin at a dose of 0.05–0.15 U/kg BW [8, 9, 16]. Blood samples for measurements of glucose and cortisol (optionally ACTH) are obtained at baseline and at 15-min intervals up to 90–120 min after the insulin injection. Clinical symptoms of hypoglycemia such as sweating, tremor and nervousness are expected and indicate an effective challenge. However, more severe symptoms of hypoglycemia such as palpitations, loss of consciousness or seizure urge to interrupt the test by immediate intravenous glucose administration while further blood samples should be collected. Normally, insulin-induced hypoglycemia should result in a rise in plasma cortisol of >550 nmol/l [8, 9, 16].

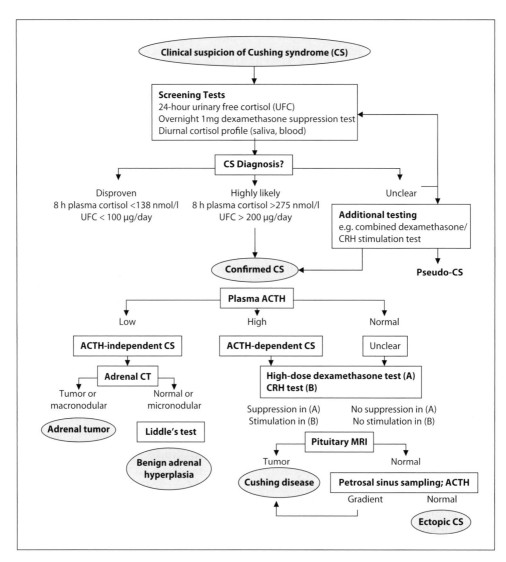

Fig. 5. Flow chart for the diagnostic evaluation of possible Cushing's syndrome.

The advantage of this test is that it allows simultaneous assessment of pituitary ACTH and growth hormone reserves. It has therefore been regarded as the gold standard for this assessment by some investigators [9]. However, the major disadvantage of this test relates to safety concerns especially in patients with high probability of pituitary disease which have poor counter-regulatory response to hypoglycemia [8]. Thus, most investigators use alternative tests to exclude HPA axis dysfunction. In patients with heart disease, cerebrovascular disease or seizure disorders, this test is absolutely contraindicated.

Glucagon Stimulation Test

An alternative to the insulin-induced hypoglycemia test in the evaluation of central adrenal insufficiency is the glucagon stimulation test. Glucagon requires endogenous ACTH to cause cortisol secretion. Glucagon is given at a dose of 0.1 mg/kg i.m. (top dose 1.0 mg) and blood for plasma cortisol measurement is obtained at baseline and every 30 min up to 180 min following glucagon injection. For a normal test response, peak plasma cortisol is expected to exceed 550 nmol/l.

CRH Stimulation Test

The CRH stimulation test assesses the ability of the pituitary gland to secrete ACTH for the stimulation of cortisol production (fig. 3). Generally, patients with pituitary ACTH deficiency have a decreased ACTH and cortisol response to CRH. In contrast, patients with hypothalamic disorders have an exaggerated and prolonged plasma ACTH response and a subnormal cortisol response. CRH test may also be used in combination with dexamethasone suppression tests for differential diagnosis of Cushing's syndromes as described below (fig. 5).

Synthetic ovine or human CRH is given as an intravenous bolus of 100 μg (or 1 μg/ kg BW) at 08.00–09.00 h to the patient after an overnight fast [8, 9, 16]. Baseline and stimulated plasma ACTH and cortisol levels are measured over the next 60–120 min at 15-min intervals. Flushing occurs in some patients. After administration of CRH, ACTH will peak rapidly within 15–30 min while cortisol peaks slightly later around 30–60 min after injection. Ovine CRH will prompt a greater and longer response than human CRH because of its lower metabolic clearance rate. As reported reference values vary considerably, normative values should be established for individual laboratories. While a 4-fold increase in mean plasma ACTH or cortisol concentrations has been observed in healthy individuals by some [19], others describe a normal response with a >34% increase in plasma ACTH and a >20% increase in plasma cortisol when compared to mean baseline values [20].

Tests to Assess Possible Glucocorticoid Excess Syndromes (Cushing Syndrome)

In children with Cushing syndrome, the classic cushingoid features are often not found at initial presentation. However, the earliest and most reliable signs of hypercotisolism in children are weight gain and growth arrest [3, 15]. Other findings in more than 50% of patients with Cushing include osteopenia, fatigue, hypertension and delayed or arrested pubertal development. Causes of hypercortisolism at the level of the adrenals include tumors (adenoma, carcinoma) or benign, nodular hyperplasia which is ACTH independent [15]. At the level of the pituitary gland, Cushing disease is caused by ACTH-producing tumors (adenoma, carcinoma). The role of the hypothalamus in central, ACTH-dependent Cushing disease is controversial [8]. By contrast, ACTH of nonpituitary origin causes the ectopic ACTH syndrome which is extremely rare in childhood but may be found in 15% of adults with Cushing syndrome [8, 15]. In addition, iatrogenic Cushing syndrome may be caused by administering supraphysiologic doses of glucocorticoids for various disorders principally aiming at modulating the immune system.

Similar to adrenal insufficiency, diagnosis of cortisol excess requires the demonstration of inappropriately high cortisol production. For initial screening three laboratory investigations have been recommended: (1) determination of the urinary free cortisol (UFC) excretion rate in a 24-hour urine collection (table 2), (2) circadian profiling of plasma or salivary cortisol concentrations, and (3) the low-dose or single dose dexamethasone suppression test [10, 15]. As the prevalence of cortisol excess syndromes is low, cut-off values of diagnostic tests aim for maximal sensitivity, thereby losing specificity. In a recent study looking at all three screening tests in 4,126 adults suspected for Cushing's syndrome, the overnight dexamethasone suppression test and the 24-hour UFC excretion rate showed the best performance (high sensitivity and specificity), while circadian rhythm (cortisol at midnight) was often false-positive (high sensitivity, low specificity) [21]. Also, as cortisol values vary considerably, tests may be repeated and/or more than one test may be performed on different days if clinical suspicion of Cushing's syndrome is high but not confirmed by testing immediately. If suspected hypercortisolism is confirmed, further evaluation of possible etiology requires functional testing and imaging studies (fig. 5).

In Cushing syndrome, the UFC excretion rate is usually grossly elevated and the normal circadian rhythm of plasma or salivary cortisol is lost; but 08.00 h values may still be found in the upper normal range [8, 15]. Mildly elevated UFC excretion rates may be found with obesity, depression and alcohol abuse; however, these problems are generally not an issue in children.

Dexamethasone Suppression Tests

Administration of glucocorticoids in supraphysiologic doses will normally result in an increase of the negative feedback to central CRH and ACTH production and suppress adrenal steroid biosynthesis promptly (fig. 3). In patients with ACTH-dependent Cushing syndrome this feedback loop is disturbed providing a possibility for diagnostic testing. Dexamethasone, a synthetic glucocorticoid which is not detected by cortisol assays is used for testing [8, 15]. It is characterized by a high glucocorticoid potency (30–80 times compared to cortisol) and a very long biological half-life of 36–54 h [3]. For dexamethasone suppression tests several protocols exist for specific clinical questions.

Overnight, Low-Dose (Single-Dose) Dexamethasone Test

This screening test involves giving 1 mg of dexamethasone at 23.00 h in the night and measuring plasma cortisol concentrations at 8.00 h in the morning before and after dexamethasone administration [3, 8, 9, 15]. In children, a dose adjustment to 0.3 mg/m^2 has been recommended by some investigators [22], but generally 1 mg is used for all age groups. The test cut-off for morning cortisol level is generally set at <138 nmol/l [8, 9, 15].

Pitfalls

This test is a screening test with reasonably good sensitivity but poor specificity and is therefore only informative when positive [8, 9]. However, false-positive results are quite frequently seen due to the following reasons: stress, malabsorption, fast metabolism of dexamethasone by P450-inducing drugs, estrogen treatment, renal failure or depression (in adults also with severe alcohol abuse). False-negative results are rare but possible in some patients with pituitary Cushing's disease or with intermittent, mild cases of hypercortisolism.

Standard Six-Day, Low-Dose, High-Dose Dexamethasone Suppression Test (Liddle Test)

The Liddle test has been the gold standard for the differential diagnosis of Cushing's syndrome for a long time. The classic protocol of this test requires 2 days of baseline urine collections (day 1 and day 2), then administration of 0.5 mg/1.73 m^2 (top dose 0.5 mg) dexamethasone every 6 h perorally starting at 06.00 h on day 3 for a total of 8 doses (low-dose phase), followed by 2 mg/1.73 m^2 (top dose 2 mg) dexamethasone every 6 h for 8 doses (days 5 and 6; high-dose phase) [15]. Urine is collected in 24-hour portions during the test and 1 day after the end of dexamethasone administration. UFC as well as 17-hydroxycorticosteroid (17-OHCS) secretion are measured; alternatively, plasma cortisol levels may be assessed. The normal response to the low-dose dexamethasone is defined as a decrease in UFC on day 4 to <50% of baseline, 17-OHCS to <3 mg/24 h (8.3 μmol/day) and/or a decrease in plasma cortisol to <138 nmol/l) [9, 15]. Normal response to the high-dose dexamethasone is defined as a decrease in UFC and 17-OHCS secretion at the end of the test to <90% of baseline values while plasma cortisol levels fall to <27 nmol/l. The low-dose phase of the test distinguishes reliably normal subjects from patients with Cushing syndrome which show no or incomplete suppression. The high dosage of dexamethasone will suppress cortisol in 90% of patients with pituitary Cushing disease, but will not suppress hypercortisolism in patients with adrenal adenoma or carcinoma and with ectopic ACTH-producing tumors [9].

Overnight, High-Dose (8 mg) Dexamethasone Suppression Test

This test has been introduced as a shorter, more cost-effective variant of the Liddle test for the differential diagnosis of Cushing's syndrome [9, 15]. Dexamethasone at a dose of 8 mg/1.73 m^2 (top dose 8 mg) is given at 23.00 h in the night and plasma cortisol and ACTH levels are measured at 08.00 h in the morning before and in the morning immediately after administration. Test sensitivity and specificity are reported to be similar to the classic Liddle test. In Cushing disease a >68% suppression of cortisol from baseline is seen, while a suppression of <50% is seen with adrenal or ectopic ACTH production [23].

Combined CRH Stimulation, Dexamethasone Suppression Test

This combination test is based on the fact that generally Cushing disease is more resistant to dexamethasone than pseudo-Cushing states but more sensitive to CRH stimulation [8]. The protocol for combined CRH-dexamethasone testing will start with a standard 2-day low-dose dexamethasone test (see Liddle test protocol), followed by intravenous administration of a bolus of 1 µg/kg synthetic CRH 2 h after the last dose of dexamethasone (see CRH test protocol). Plasma ACTH and cortisol measurements are recommended at the following time points: −15, 0, +5, +10, +15, +30, +45 and +60 min after CRH injection. Only few studies report cut-off values for this test [8]. However, with the criterion of a plasma cortisol of >38 nmol/l 15 min after CRH administration a 100% diagnostic accuracy has been reported [24].

Once classification of Cushing's syndrome is made by biochemical testing, further diagnostic evaluation is performed with specific imaging studies of the pituitary gland (MRI) or the adrenals (CT, MRI) (fig. 5). For imaging of the adrenal gland, CT is preferred over MRI for better delineation of cortex and medulla. Ultrasound studies are not sensitive and accurate enough for diagnostic evaluation [25].

Tests to Assess Biochemical Defects of Adrenal Steroidogenesis

The biochemical pathway of adrenal steroid hormone biosynthesis from cholesterol is long known and the genes involved well described (fig. 2). Human mutations for all genes encoding steroidogenic enzymes and some co-factors are reported [3, 5]. Generally, specific enzyme deficiency in the adrenal steroid biosynthetic pathway will result in accumulation of substrate(s) and loss of product(s) of this enzymatic step. However, as steroid biosynthesis is a cascade in which one substrate may be converted by more than one enzyme (e.g. progesterone to 17OHP by CYP17A1 or to DOC by HSD3B2) and products, in turn, are substrates for following enzymatic reactions, disruption of a single step will affect the whole adrenal steroid profile. In addition, genes encoding steroidogenic enzymes (and cofactors) essential for adrenal androgen biosynthesis (CYP11A1, StAR, CYP17A1, HSD3B2, HSD17B3, CYP OR) are also responsible for proper gonadal steroidogenesis. Therefore, mutations in these genes resulting in loss of enzyme activity will not only affect adrenal but also gonadal steroidogenesis leading to specific forms of disorders of sexual development (DSD), puberty disorders and/or infertility. Even mutations in genes not directly involved in sex steroid biosynthesis such as CYP21A2 and CYP11B1 may cause DSD and fertility problems as their loss of activity increases adrenal androgen secretion via diminished negative feedback of missing cortisol on ACTH production. For all these reasons, inborn errors of steroidogenesis affecting the adrenals and the gonads were named 'adrenogenital syndromes' in the pre-genetic era. Or they are summarized as congenital adrenal hyperplasias because ACTH is a potent growth factor for the adrenal cortex resulting in adrenal hyperplasia. For an overview of the clinical presentations and biochemical consequences of the different forms of CAH, see table 5.

By contrast, mutations in CYP11B2 for 18-hydroxylase and 18-methyl oxidase activities in the mineralocorticoid biosynthetic pathway (fig. 2) do not affect circulating sex hormone levels and will not result in ACTH mediated adrenal hyperplasia. They are therefore generally not regarded as forms of CAH. The biochemical consequences and diagnostic evaluation of these rare genetic disorders of mineralocorticoid synthesis are described in the chapter by Ferrari [this vol.] dealing with sodium regulation.

Overall, when studying consequences of mutations in genes of the steroid pathway, it is important to realize that enzyme activity of mutant proteins may not always be completely lost but only markedly diminished; usually to less than 50% for having clinical consequences. Thus, although patients with CAH present with characteristic changes in the steroid profile relating to their specific defect, different mutations in the same gene may cause subtle to severe biochemical alterations leading to a broad clinical spectrum of disease (e.g. classic versus late-onset CAH).

Baseline and ACTH Stimulated Steroid Measurements for Suspected CAH

As mentioned previously, most adrenal steroids (and metabolites) may be measured either directly from blood, saliva or urine (spot urine or 24-hour collection). Measurements may be made at baseline, timed and/or after ACTH stimulation. When using blood for diagnostic evaluation, a short, high-dose (standard) ACTH test (250 µg/1.73 m² BSA, top dose 250 µg) with steroid measurements at baseline and 60 min after ACTH administration is often necessary to stress the specific enzyme blockade revealing the characteristic changes in the steroid profile. Reference values for some plasma steroid concentrations at baseline and 60 min after ACTH stimulation

Table 5. Clinical and biochemical findings in the different forms of CAHs

Enyzmatic deficiency	Genetic defect	Clinical presentation	Laboratory findings
Lipoid CAH	StAR or CYP11A1	Salt-wasting crisis 46,XY DSD	Low levels of all steroid hormones Elevated ACTH and PRA Decreased/absent response to ACTH In 46,XY subjects: decreased or absent response of sex steroids to hCG
3βHSD	HSD3B2	Salt-wasting crisis 46,XY DSD 46,XX DSD	Elevated basal and ACTH stimulated Δ5 steroids (Preg, 17OHPreg, DHEA) Elevated ratio of Δ5/Δ4 steroids Elevated ACTH and PRA Suppression of elevated steroids after corticosteroid administration
21OHase	CYP21A2	Classic form: Salt wasting crisis 46,XX DSD Pre- and postnatal virilization Nonclassic form: Premature adrenarche Disordered puberty Menstrual irregularity, hirsutism, acne, infertility	Elevated basal and ACTH stimulated 17OHProg and pregnanetriol Elevated serum androgens and urinary metabolites Elevated ACTH and PRA Suppression of elevated steroids after corticosteroid administration
11β-Hydroxylase	CYP11B1	Classic form: 46,XX DSD Pre- and postnatal virilization Hypertension Nonclassic form: Premature adrenarche Disordered puberty Menstrual irregularity, hirsutism, acne, infertility	Elevated 11DOC and DOC basal and after ACTH stimulation Elevated serum androgens and urinary metabolites Elevated ACTH Suppressed PRA, low potassium Suppression of elevated steroids after glucocorticoid administration
Combined 17α-hydroxylase/17,20 lyase	CYP17A1	46,XY DSD Sexual infantilism Low renin hypertension	Elevated DOC, 18-OH DOC, corticosterone and 18-OH coticosterone Low 17α-hydroxylated steroids (androgens and estrogens) and poor response to ACTH Elevated ACTH Suppressed PRA, low potassium Suppression of elevated steroids after glucocorticoid administration In 46,XY subjects: poor response of sex steroids to hCG
Isolated 17,20 lyase	CYP17A1	46, XY DSD Sexual infantilism	Decreased androgens and estrogens

Table 5. Continued

Enyzmatic deficiency	Genetic defect	Clinical presentation	Laboratory findings
P450 oxidoreductase	CYP OR	46,XX and 46,XY DSD Antley-Bixler syndrome Infertility in adults	Elevated DOC, corticosterone Normal to elevated Prog and 17OHProg Normal or decreased cortisol Elevated 21-deoxycortisol Low DHEA, androstenedione, testosterone and estradiol Normal or elevated ACTH Normal electrolytes Poor response of cortisol and adrenal androgens to ACTH stimulation

CAH = Congenital adrenal hyperplasia; StAR = steroidogenic acute regulatory protein; DSD = disorder of sex development; ACTH = adrenocorticotropic hormone; PRA = plasma renin activity; hCG = human chorionic gonadotropin; 3βHSD = 3β-hydroxysteroid dehydrogenase; Preg = pregnenolone; 17OHPreg = 17-hydroxypregnenolone; DHEA = dehydroepi-androsterone; 17OHProg = 17-hydroxyprogesterone; 11DOC = 11-deoxycortisol; DOC = 11-deoxycorticosterone; Prog = progesterone.

are given in table 6 [5]. Similarly, when using 24-hour urine collections for evaluation, prolonged ACTH stimulation may be employed either by continuous intravenous administration of ACTH or by intramuscular injection of a depot preparation of ACTH [9]. However, for convenience and cost effectiveness, most centers use a short ACTH stimulation test, blood samples and direct immunoassays for steroid measurements for the biochemical work-up of suspected CAH. Chromatographic techniques such as GC/MS provide a very powerful tool for the diagnostic evaluation of multiple changes in the steroid profile obtained either from plasma or urine [see chapter by Wudy, this vol.]. These techniques are able to detect all extracted steroids with highest specificity and sensitivity in one measurement. However, these measurements are complex and expensive, and reference values are not generally available (especially not for children) limiting its use to few specialized laboratories.

Diagnostic Criteria for 21-Hydroxylase Deficiency

The commonest genetic defect in steroid hormone biosynthesis is 21OHase due to mutations in CYP21A2 (classic form in ~1:14,000). Loss of 21OHase activity leads to a blockade in the conversion of 17OHP to 11DOC and thus cortisol which will prompt an increase in pituitary ACTH secretion and stimulation of adrenal androgen production (DHEA, Δ4A). Simultaneously, loss of 21OHase leads also to a blockade in aldosterone production (low plasma sodium, high potassium) and thus a stimulation

Table 6. Average values for the adrenal steroid response to ACTH stimulation (0 and 60 min)

			17OHPreg nmol/l	17OHP nmol/l	DHEA nmol/l	11DOC nmol/l	Cortisol nmol/l	DOC nmol/l	Prog nmol/L
Age	infants	baseline	6.8	0.8	1.4	2.3	280	0.6	1.1
		stimulated		5.8			830	2.4	3.2
	prepubertal	baseline	1.7	1.5	2.4	1.8	360	0.2	1.1
		stimulated	9.6	5.8	4.3	5.8	830	1.7	4
	pubertal	baseline	3.6	1.8	9	1.7	280	0.2	1.9
		stimulated	24	4.8	19	4.9	690	1.7	4.8
Assay			RIA	RIA	RIA	RIA	RIA	RIA	RIA
Ref.			1	1	1	1	1	1	1

Data adapted from Endocrine Sciences, Tarzana, Calif., USA.

of the renin-angiotensin regulatory system. Thus, for 21OHase deficiency circulating 17OHP is the so-called marker steroid which is used for screening tests (whole blood) as well as for confirmation of the diagnosis (plasma). In the Swiss neonatal screening program, the cut-off value for 17OHP measured from whole blood, spotted on filter paper is currently set at 20 nmol/l for term newborns at 72–96 h of life (DELFIA Fluorescence Immunoassay, Wallac, Turcu, Finland; Dr. T. Toresani for the Swiss neonatal screening program [pers. commun.]). Likewise, a cut-off value for baseline plasma 17OHP of 6.1 nmol/l (2 ng/ml) (radioimmunoassay by Cis Bio, Gif-sur-Yvette, France) has been recently reported to predict late-onset CAH in children presenting with precocious pubarche (PP) with a 100% sensitivity and 99% specificity [26]. Therefore, as in children with PP the ACTH stimulation test reveals normal results in >80%, this test may be only necessary in children with baseline 17OHP levels >6.1 nmol/l. Similarly, for discriminating late-onset AGS from polycystic ovary syndrome (PCOS), several cohort studies in hyperandrogenic/hirsute adolescent and adult women recommend a threshold of baseline plasma 17OHP levels of 6–9 nmol/l for further diagnostic evaluation employing ACTH test and/or genetic analysis [27]. Figure 6 gives a diagnostic scheme for plasma 17OHP concentrations at baseline and following ACTH stimulation in normal subjects, heterozygote individuals as well as patients diagnosed with CYP21A2 mutations on both alleles resulting in non-classic (late-onset) or classic CAH (data are adapted from White et al. [28]). Measurement of plasma ACTH, cortisol, androgens, PRA, aldosterone and electrolytes will help in confirming the diagnosis and in estimating the severity of the impairment of the

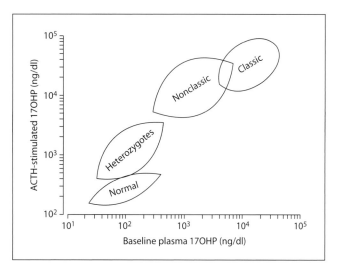

Fig. 6. Scheme providing reference ranges for baseline and ACTH-stimulated plasma 17OHP levels found in patients with 21OHase CAH (classic, nonclassic), carriers and normals. Conversion factor for 17OHP is 3.026 × ng/dl → nmol/l.

enzyme activity when characteristic changes are found. However, these measurements are not specific for 21OHase deficiency.

Diagnostic Criteria for the Rare Forms of CAH

Laboratory findings of the rare forms of CAH are summarized in table 5. Unlike for 21OHase deficiency, specific normative values for plasma steroid concentrations found in the rare forms of CAH do not exist. It is rather the overall pattern of observed changes in the steroid profile which is characteristic for the underlying defect. However, recent studies of smaller cohorts of patients with CYP11B1 and HSD3B2 mutations have revealed some diagnostic criteria which may be helpful when confronted with patients harboring rare forms of CAH.

Deficiency of 11β-hydroxylase is characterized by a marked increase in plasma 11-DOC and DOC, as well as an increase in the ratio of 11-DOC/cortisol and a decrease in PRA. An ACTH-stimulated plasma 11-DOC of ≥60 nmol/l is generally diagnostic.

Pitfalls
(1) Slightly elevated 17OHP plasma concentrations may be found with CYP11B1 deficiency [9]. Therefore, to distinguish CYP11B1 from CYP21A2 deficiency, the ratio of Δ4A/17OHP may be diagnostic. A value of Δ4A/17OHP >1 is typical for CYP11B1 deficiency (as normally Δ4A is inactivated to 11β-Δ4A by 11β-hydroxylase); by contrast, a ratio of Δ4A/17OHP ≤0.5 is found with 21OHase deficiency [9]. (2) In premature and young babies in the first 2 months of life, slightly elevated plasma 17OHP levels in combination with markedly elevated 11-DOC may be found due to cross-reactivity

of the 'usual' immunoassays with steroids secreted from the fetal adrenal zone which is still active. In these cases, more specific measurements and/or follow-up will reveal normal values with the involution of the fetal zone [Prof. Y. Morel, pers. commun.].

Deficiency of 3β-hydroxysteroid dehydrogenase type 2 causes an increase in all Δ5 steroids (pregnenolone, 17OHpregnenolone, DHEA) and a decrease in Δ4 steroids (progesterone, 17OHP and Δ4A). Accordingly, cohort studies of patients with genetically proven HSD3B2 mutations suggest that for the biochemical diagnosis of HSD3B2 deficiency basal and ACTH-stimulated 17OHpregnenolone (17OHPreg) and its ratio to cortisol have the best diagnostic value [29]. In patients presenting with premature pubarche due to genotype proven HSD3B2 deficiency basal and stimulated 17OHPreg were grossly elevated to ≥25 and ≥36 SD compared to control subjects. Ratios of 17OHPreg to cortisol were also immensely elevated to ≥29 SD at baseline and ≥52 SD after ACTH stimulation compared to controls.

Test to Assess 'Isolated' Androgen Excess

Signs of androgen excess in children include: (a) virilization at birth (e.g. 46,XX genital ambiguity) or later-on, (b) precocious puberty (premature pubarche, acne, advanced bone age), (c) decreased growth rate with obesity, male-pattern alopecia, abdominal masses, and (d) hirsutism and menstrual irregularities in adolescent females. In principal, plasma androgens originate from the adrenals or the gonads. However, occasionally androgen excess may be caused by either exogenous administration (e.g. drugs for doping in sports) or by increased peripheral production which is poorly understood (e.g. idiopathic hirsutism).

Diagnostic evaluation of the patient with 'isolated' androgen excess starts with measurements of plasma androgens (DHEA, DHEAS, Δ4A and free testosterone), luteinizing hormone, follicle-stimulating hormone, prolactin and assessment of possible concomitant hypercortisolism (screening tests) [9]. If cortisol is elevated, hyperandrogenism is part of a Cushing syndrome which will then be further evaluated with specific tests as described previously. If cortisol is normal, true central precocious puberty may be excluded by checking for clinical signs such as breast development and symmetrically enlarged testicles (≥Tanner 2) and by assessment of LH and FSH which should be in the normal range for age (baseline and/or stimulated).

Generally, a grossly elevated baseline plasma testosterone level in the adult male range (>12 nmol/l) before puberty or in females is indicative for a virilizing tumor while a level >7 nmol/l is suspicious [9]. Baseline DHEAS levels well above the adult range suggest an adrenal tumor in children. For moderately elevated plasma androgen levels, the differential diagnosis includes several forms of CAH (table 5) as well as precocious and/or exaggerated adrenarche. Those two conditions may be distinguished from each other by a short ACTH test revealing a typical change in the steroid profile for CAHs versus an excessive increase in Δ5 steroids in precocious adrenarche [9]. However, etiology of hyperandrogenemia remains unsolved in many patients and only recently three novel steroid disorders in patients with androgen excess have been described. In apparent cortisone reductase deficiency, mutations in the genes for 11β-hydroxysteroid dehydrogenase type 1 (HSD11B1) or its co-factor hexose-6-phosphate dehydrogenase (H6PDH) which are responsible for the conversion of inactive cortisone to active cortisol are found [26]. Both defects lead to impaired cortisol feedback to the HPA axis and an increase in ACTH secretion resulting in enhanced adrenal androgen production. Both disorders are diagnosed from urinary steroid profiles showing a typical reduction in the ratio of urine metabolites of cortisol to cortisone (THF+allo THF/ THE >0.05; normal 0.7–1.3) [26]. By contrast, mutations in the human PAPSS2 gene, a cofactor supporting the conversion of DHEA to DHEAS by sulfonyltransferase type 2 (SULT2A1) may be considered when the ratio of plasma DHEA to DHEAS is markedly elevated [30]. In addition, moderately elevated androgen levels may be the first finding in young girls presenting later with menstrual irregularities and/or polycystic ovaries consistent with the diagnosis of PCOS. PCOS, however, is still a diagnosis by exclusion as its etiology remains elusive [27].

Additional Tools for Diagnosing Adrenal Disorders

Assessment of Circulating Autoantibodies

The diagnosis of autoimmune adrenalitis is largely based on finding circulating antibodies directed against adrenal cells or adrenal cellular contents such as steroidogenic enzymes CYP21A2, CYP17A1, CYP11A1 or microsomes (ACA-IIF) [3, 9]. Autoantibodies against CYP21A2 are prevalent in most adult patients with autoimmune Addison's disease and are good predictive markers for future disease in children with other autoimmune endocrine disorders [9]. However, the titer of auto-antibodies is reported to decline over time, which probably arises due to progressive destruction of the target tissue.

Measurement of Very-Long-Chain Fatty Acids

In males manifesting with adrenal insufficiency circulating very-long-chain fatty acids (VLCFAs) should be assessed for possible diagnosis of adrenoleukodystrophy (ALD). In ALD peroxisomal β-oxidation of VLCFA is impaired due to mutations in the ALD gene coding for a defective peroxisomal membrane transport protein. Diagnosis is confirmed if circulating levels of VLCFAs (>C26) as well as ratios of C26 and C24 to C22 are elevated [3, 9].

Assessment of Chromosomal Sex

As described previously, disorders of steroidogenesis may cause genital ambiguity either by affecting biosynthesis of adrenal and gonadal sex steroid production directly or by secondary overstimulation of adrenal androgen production. Generally, impairment of androgen production will affect male sexual development (46,XY DSD), while androgen overproduction will affect female development (46,XX DSD), although some forms of CAH may cause both male undervirilization as well as female virilization (e.g. mutations in HSD3B3 or CYP OR). Thus determination of the chromosomal sex is one of the first investigations when dealing with a child with DSD ([see chapter by Holthrhus et al., this vol.]. Assessment of the karyotype from blood leukocytes (or other biomaterials, e.g. chorionic villus sample) is the gold standard but involves culturing the cells in a specialized laboratory and will take up to a week before the result may be available. Therefore, screening tests aiming at the detection of SRY material or other targets, which are only found on the Y chromosome, may provide results in less than 24 h. Different techniques and protocols exists employing either FISH or (quantitative) PCR [see also chapter by Pandey on genetics, this vol.]. Recently, fetal sexing may be even performed from circulating fetal DNA in maternal blood with high diagnostic accuracy [31]. To date this method is only established for routine diagnostic in a few laboratories. However, for the diagnostic evaluation of the fetus with possible 21OHase deficiency, this method has the potential to become the method of choice as it is able to provide accurate results as early as 6–7 weeks' gestation enabling to shorten (or even avoid) the prenatal treatment with dexamethasone in male fetuses [31].

Analysis of Specific Genes for Disease Causing Mutations
In the era of molecular medicine and international medical networking genetic tests for all known genetic disorders of the adrenal cortex are broadly available. It is conceivable that in the near future costs for genetic analysis performed by high-throughput methods [see chapter by Pandey on genetics, this vol.] in specialized laboratories may become cheaper than for many laborious biochemical tests. In addition, defining defects at the genetic level bears the advantage of being able to offer patients and their family diagnostic screening tests and exacter information on disease prognosis. Also, genetic diagnosis is mandatory when considering prenatal treatment and diagnosis for CAH [32]. Therefore, whenever possible, diagnostic evaluation of suspected genetic disorders of the adrenal cortex should include the genetic analysis of candidate genes.

Imaging Studies
Diagnostic evaluation of disorders of the HPA axis includes imaging studies, especially when looking for tumors [25]. MRI is the preferred method for the visualization of the hypothalamus and the anterior pituitary gland. Inferior petrosal sinus sampling may be needed for distinguishing pituitary from ectopic ACTH-dependent Cushing (fig. 5). For adrenal imaging both CT and MRI may be used although CT is the preferred method [15, 25]. Adrenal ultrasound plays a minor role in the imaging of adrenal disorders. Adrenal venous sampling as well as adrenal scintigraphy with specific radionuclide tracers [see also specific chapter by Reiners, this vol.] are

functional tests that are seldom used for the diagnostic evaluation of disorders of the adrenal cortex [25].

Acknowledgements

I would like to acknowledge Maguelon G. Forest, Lyon especially for all her invaluable data published in the 3rd edition of this book which form the 'backbone' of this revised chapter. This work is supported by the Swiss National Science Foundation grant 320000–116299.

References

1 Goodman HM: Basic Medical Endocrinology, ed 4. Burlington, Elsevier, 2009.

2 Kempna P, Flück CE: Adrenal gland development and defects; in Mullis P-E, Kiess W (eds): Fetal and Neonatal Endocrinolgy. Best Practice and Research in Clinical Endocrinology and Metabolism. Burlington, Elsevier, 2008, vol 22, pp 77–93.

3 Flück CE, Achermann JC, Miller WL: The adrenal cortex and its disorders; in Sperling MA (ed): Pediatric Endocrinology, ed 3. Philadelphia, Saunders, 2008.

4 Rainey WE, Carr BR, Sasano H, Suzuki T, Mason JI: Dissecting human adrenal androgen production. Trends Endocrinol Metab 2002;13:234–239.

5 Miller WL: Steroidogenic enzymes; in Flück CE, Miller WL (eds): Disorders of the Human Adrenal Cortex. Basel, Karger, 2008, pp 1–18.

6 Wallace WHB, Crowne EC, Shalet SM, et al: Episodic ACTH and cortisol secretion in normal children. Clin Endocrinol (Oxf) 1991;34:215–221.

7 Burtis CA, Ashwood ER: Tietz Textbook of Clinical Chemistry, ed 3. Philadelphia, Saunders, 1999.

8 Aron DC: Diagnostic implications of adrenal physiology and clinical epidemiology for evaluation of glucocorticoid excess and deficiency; in DeGroot LJ, Jameson JL (eds): Endocrinology, ed 4. Philadelphia, Saunders, 2001, pp 1655–1670.

9 Forest MG: Adrenal function tests; in Ranke MB (ed): Diagnostics of Endocrine Function in Children and Adolescents, ed 3. Basel, Karger, 2003, pp 372–426.

10 Society E: The diagnosis of Cushing's syndrome. J Clin Endocrinol Metab 2008;93:1526–1540.

11 Snow K, Jiang N, Kao P, Scheithauer B: Biochemical evaluation of adrenal dysfunction: the laboratory perspective. Mayo Clin Proc 1992;76:1055–1065.

12 de Peretti E, Mappus E: Pattern of plasma pregnenolone sulfate levels in humans from birth to adulthood. J Clin Endocrinol Metab 1983;57:550–556.

13 Linder N, Davidovitch N, Kogan A, et al: Longitudinal measurements of 17alpha-hydroxy-progesterone in premature infants during the first three months of life. Arch Dis Child Fetal Neonatal Ed 1999;81:F175–F178.

14 Miller WL: Androgen biosynthesis from cholesterol to DHEA. Mol Cell Endocrinol 2002;198:7–14.

15 Stratakis CA: Cushing syndrome caused by adrenocortical tumors and hyperplasias (corticotropin-independent Cushing syndrome). Endocr Dev 2008; 13:117–132.

16 Bethin KE, Muglia LJ: Adrenal insufficiency; in Radovick S, MacGillivray MH (eds): Pediatric Endocrinology. Totowa, Humana Press, 2003, pp 203–247.

17 Dickstein G, Shechner C, Nicholson WE, et al: Adrenocorticotropin stimulation test: effects of basal cortisol level, time of day, and suggested new sensitive low dose test. J Clin Endocrinol Metab 1991; 72:773–778.

18 Tordjman K, Jaffe A, Trostanetsky Y, Greenman Y, Limor R, Stern N: Low-dose (1 microgram) adrenocorticotrophin (ACTH) stimulation as a screening test for impaired hypothalamo-pituitary-adrenal axis function: sensitivity, specificity and accuracy in comparison with the high-dose (250 microgram) test. Clin Endocrinol (Oxf) 2000;52:633–640.

19 Lytras N, Grossman A, Perry L, et al: Corticotropin-releasing factor: Responses in normal subjects and patients with disorders of the hypothalamus and pituitary. Clin Endocrinol (Oxf) 1984;20:71–84.

20 Nieman LK, Oldfield EH, Wesley R, Chrousos GP, Loriaux DL, Cutler GBJ: A simplified morning ovine corticotropin-releasing hormone stimlation test for the differential diagnosis of adrenocorticotropin-dependent Cushing's syndrome. J Clin Endocrinol Metab 1993;77:1308–1312.

21 Pecori Giraldi F, Ambrogio AG, De Martin M, Fatti LM, Scacchi M, Cavagnini F: Specificity of first-line tests for the diagnosis of Cushing's syndrome: assessment in a large series. J Clin Endocrinol Metab 2007;92:4123–4129.

22 Hindmarsh PC, Brook CG: Single dose dexamethasone suppression test in children: dose relationship to body size. Clin Endocrinol (Oxf) 1985;23:67–70.

23 Dichek HL, Nieman LK, Oldfield EH, Pass HI, Malley JD, Cutler GB Jr: A comparison of the standard high dose dexamethasone suppression test and the overnight 8-mg dexamethasone suppression test for the differential diagnosis of adrenocorticotropin-dependent Cushing's syndrome. J Clin Endocrinol Metab 1994;78:418–422.

24 Yanovski JA, Cutler GB Jr, Chrousos GP, Nieman LK: Corticotropin-releasing hormone stimulation following low-dose dexamethasone administration: a new test to distinguish Cushing's syndrome from pseudo-Cushing's states. JAMA 1993;269:2232–2238.

25 Doppman JL: Adrenal imaging; in DeGroot LJ, Jameson JL (eds): Endocrinology, ed 4. Philadelphia, Saunders, 2001, pp 1747–1766.

26 Armengaud JB, Charkaluk ML, Trivin C, et al: Precocious pubarche: distinguishing late-onset congenital adrenal hyperplasia from premature adrenarche. J Clin Endocrinol Metab 2009;94:2835–2840.

27 Azziz R, Carmina E, Dewailly D, et al: The Androgen Excess and PCOS Society criteria for the polycystic ovary syndrome: the complete task force report. Fertil Steril 2009;91:456–488.

28 White PC, New MI, Dupont B: Congenital adrenal hyperplasia. Part 1. N Engl J Med 1987;316:1519–1524.

29 Mermejo LM, Elias LLK, Marui S, Moreira AC, Mendonca BB, de Castro M: Refining hormonal diagnosis of type II 3β-hydroxysteroid dehydrogenase deficiency in patients with premature pubarche and hirsutism based on HSD3B2 genotyping. J Clin Endocrinol Metab 2005;90:1287–1293.

30 Noordam C, Dhir V, McNelis JC, et al: Inactivating PAPSS2 mutations in a patient with premature pubarche. N Engl J Med 2009;360:2310–2318.

31 Avent ND, Chitty LS: Non-invasive dagnosis of fetal sex; utilisation of free fetal DNA in maternal plasma and ultrasound. Prenatal Diag 2006;26:598–603.

32 Speiser PW: Congenital adrenal hyperplasia. N Engl J Med 2003;349:776–788.

33 Goto M, Piper Hanley K, Marcos J, et al: In humans, early cortisol biosynthesis provides a mechanism to safeguard female sexual development. J Clin Invest 2006;116:953–960.

Christa E. Flück, MD
Pediatric Endocrinology and Diabetology, Department of Pediatrics and
Department of Clinical Research, University of Bern
Freiburgstrasse 15, Room G3 812, CH–3010 Bern (Switzerland)
Tel. +41 31 632 0499, Fax +41 31 632 8424, E-Mail christa.flueck@dkf.unibe.ch

Ranke MB, Mullis P-E (eds): Diagnostics of Endocrine Function in Children and Adolescents, ed 4.
Basel, Karger, 2011, pp 379–401

Mass Spectrometry in the Diagnosis of Steroid-Related Disorders: Clinical Applications

Stefan A. Wudy · Michaela F. Hartmann

Steroid Research and Mass Spectrometry Unit, Division of Pediatric Endocrinology and Diabetology, Center of Child and Adolescent Medicine, Justus-Liebig-University, Giessen, Germany

Up to now, routine steroid analysis has been primarily based on commercially available immunoassays. However, major analytical quality issues for steroid immunoassays such as lack of agreement between methods, poor specificity (antibody specificity, matrix effects), under-recovery of analyte, and the lack of agreement with reference methods have started a continuous debate on the accuracy of steroid immunoassays. Furthermore, individual immunoassays only allow determination of a single steroid at a time. Determination of rare steroids or identification of unknown steroids might not be possible due to the unavailability of specific kits for such unusual analytes.

Analytical methods based on mass spectrometry (MS) currently present the most specific qualitative and quantitative methods for steroid determination [1]. Combination with a chromatographic technique such as gas chromatography (GC) or liquid chromatography (LC) allows for the simultaneous determination of analytes ('profiling'). This chapter was written exclusively from a pediatric endocrinologist's point of view and concentrates on clinical applications of these techniques.

Since the mid-1980s gas chromatograpy-mass spectrometry (GC-MC) has proven to be a robust routine technique for the identification and quantification of steroids. In the case that stable isotope labeled analogs of the analytes were used as internal standards, reference methods presenting the 'gold standard' in steroid analysis were developed (isotope dilution/mass spectrometry, ID/MS) [2]. Stable isotope labeled internal standards have the advantage of showing practically the same chemical and chromatographic properties as their corresponding analytes and they allow procedural losses to be disregarded. Due to their different physical properties they can easily be distinguished from the unlabeled compounds in the mass spectrometer by monitoring different ions.

Table 1. Developmental milestones on the way to clinical steroid analysis by GC-MS

1908	Thompson	development of the mass spectrometer
1944	Cremer	development of gas chromatography
1960	Vanden Heuvel	separation of steroids by GC
1964	Ryhage and Sjövall	development of a robust interface permitting combination of MS and GC
1966	Horning	first comprehensive urinary steroid profile
1971	Völlmin	urinary steroid analysis on glass capillary columns
1978	Dandeneau	fused silica capillary
1980	Shackleton and Whitney	introduction of solid-phase extraction for steroids
1984	Hewlett Packard	first commercial mass selective detector
1985	Shackleton	clinical urinary steroid profiling by GC-MS
1992	Wudy and Shackleton	clinical plasma steroid profiling by ID/GC-MS
2008	Wudy and coworkers	noninvasive estimation of hormonal production rates

Meanwhile, the development of 'soft', i.e. nondisintegrating ionization techniques, has opened new avenues for the analysis of biomolecules by liquid chromatography-mass spectrometry (LC-MS). Therefore, an own section of this chapter will be devoted exclusively to this topic.

Profiling Steroids by GC-MS

Profiling Urinary Steroids by GC-MS
Methodological Aspects
Gas chromatography (GC) and MS have proven to be reliable tools in the delineation of steroid related disorders both in children and adults. Clinical analysis of steroids by GC and MS has received many – if not most – of its impetuses from pediatric endocrinology. This tight relationship is reflected by an often not only local but also 'spiritual' vicinity between laboratories spearheading analytical techniques in this field and several pediatric endocrine units. For methodological details the reader is referred to different reviews [1, 3, 4]. Important developmental milestones on the way to clinical GC-MS steroid analysis have been summarized in table 1.

Of all separating techniques GC bears the greatest potential for separating steroids and MS allows for highest specificity in determining steroid metabolites. Therefore, the potential of the 'hyphenated' technique of gas chromatography-mass spectrometry

Wudy · Hartmann

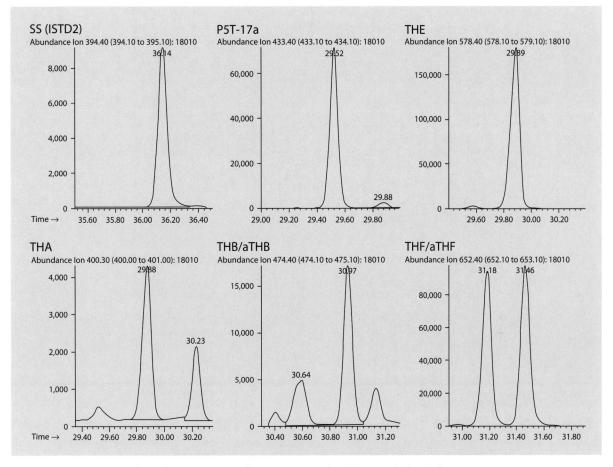

Fig. 1. Portions of ion chromatograms of a urinary steroid profile recorded with the mass spectrometer run in the selected ion monitoring mode (Agilent 6890 series GC coupled with an Agilent 5973N mass selective detector). For abbreviations, see table 2. The peaks at typical retention times (t_r) represent the following compounds: SS (internal standard, ion m/z 394.40, retention time t_r 36.14 min); P5T-17α (m/z 433.40, t_r 29.52 min); THE (m/z 578.40, t_r 29.89); THA (m/z 400.30, t_r 30.23 min); THB (m/z 474.40, t_r 30.64 min); aTHB (m/z 474.40, t_r 30.97 min); THF (m/z 652.40, t_r 31.18 min); aTHF (m/z 652.40; t_r 31.46 min).

in determining a multitude of steroid metabolites simultaneously in a single 'steroid profile' with highest specificity is still unsurpassed.

Urinary steroid analysis by GC with flame ionisation detector or GC-MS using repetitive scanning mode are nonselective techniques for the quantitative determination of excreted steroid metabolites of adrenocortical and gonadal origin. The result of this multicomponent chromatographic analysis is the urinary steroid profile (fig. 1, 2). The major urinary steroids of healthy individuals are conjugated metabolites of dehydroepiandrosterone sulphate, progesterone, corticosterone and cortisol (table 2).

		Data file name:	1201001.D			
		Date acquired:	05/15/01 10:47			
		Acq. method file:	USIM			
		Sample name:	PH			

NO.	Name	Retention time	Signal resp	M I	Amount	Units
1	*AD-ISTD1*	*17.89*	*60578*	*0*	*625.00*	*µg/day*
2	AN	19.62	1117801	0	2,359.25	µg/day
3	ET	19.98	589051	0	1,280.92	µg/day
4	A5-3β,17α	20.50	10178	0	58.53	µg/day
5	16α-OH-DHEA	21.06	22566	0	233.43	µg/day
6	A5-3β,17β	21.46	24412	0	147.10	µg/day
7	11-O-AN	21.91	4665	0	36.94	µg/day
6	11-OH-AN	23.79	181023	0	659.34	µg/day
7	11-OH-ET	24.16	6846	0	49.48	µg/day
8	16α-OH-DHEA	24.62	81476	0	660.45	µg/day
9	PD	25.30	2575	0	47.40	µg/day
10	PT	25.97	373636	0	597.35	µg/day
11	P5D	26.64	7886	0	117.36	µg/day
12	A5T-16α	27.05	88903	0	598.86	µg/day
13	THS	27.56	7937	0	51.96	µg/day
14	11-O-PT	28.59	5372	0	12.21	µg/day
15	*SS-ISTD2*	*36.26*	*26493*	*0*	*625.00*	*µg/day*
16	P5T-17α	29.62	136811	0	446.14	µg/day
17	THE	29.98	437627	0	3,785.46	µg/day
18	THA	30.33	4285	0	171.41	µg/day
19	THB	30.73	14140	1	255.64	µg/day
20	aTHB	31.07	43014	0	583.73	µg/day
24	THF	31.27	214799	0	1,528.63	µg/day
21	aTHF	31.56	259077	0	1,768.51	µg/day
25	α-Cl	31.88	556337	0	1,372.56	µg/day
26	β-C	32.46	96381	1	1,124.93	µg/day
27	β-Cl	32.57	420178	0	1,286.98	µg/day
28	α-C	33.48	31019	0	315.69	µg/day
29	F	36.94	1812	1	86.63	µg/day
30	6β-OH-F	37.83	1253	0	196.13	µg/day
31	20α-DHF	38.60	1280	0	40.09	µg/day

Fig. 2. Report sheet of a selected ion monitoring run producing a urinary steroid profile. For abbreviations, see table 2. AD and SS are internal standards.

A scheme of human steroid biosynthesis is depicted in figure 3. Catabolism of steroid hormones consists of a series of reductions and hydroxylations, and the steroids are finally conjugated either with glucuronic or sulfuric acid. The compounds thus formed are eliminated for the most part in urine, with a minor quantity passing into the feces. The polycyclic carbon ring of steroid hormones is not degraded during metabolism. Table 2 informs about important steroid hormones and their principal urinary metabolites. The complexity of steroid metabolism requires specialist steroid biochemical knowledge and expertise to correctly interpret steroid profiles.

The measurement of steroid excretion rates in a 24-hour urine sample (quantitative urinary steroid profile) represents a noninvasive approach to estimate the integrated output of adrenocortical and gonadal steroid production [5, 6]. The identification of

Table 2. Abbreviations and origin of excreted urinary steroid metabolites.

	Abbreviation	Trivial name	Origin of urinary steroid
1	AN	androsterone	DHEA, androstenedione, testosterone
2	ET	etiocholanalone	DHEA, androstenedione, testosterone
3	DHEA	dehydroepiandrosterone	DHEA-S
4	A5-3β,17β	5-androstene-3β,17β-diol	DHEA
5	11-O-An	11-oxo-androsterone	cortisol, 11-hydroxy-androstenedione
6	11-OH-AN	11-hydroxy-androsterone	cortisol, 11-hydroxy-androstenedione
7	17-OH-PO	17-hydroxypregnanolone	17-hydroxyprogesterone
8	11-OH-ET	11-hydroxy-etiocholanolone	cortisol, 11-hydroxy-androstenedione
9	16α-OH-DHEA	16α-hydroxy-DHEA	DHEA-S
10	PD	pregnanediol	progesterone
11	PT	pregnanetriol	17-hydroxyprogesterone
12	P^5D	pregnenediol	pregnenolone
13	A^5T-16α	5-androstene-3β,16α,17β-triol	DHEA-S
14	THS	tetrahydro-11-deoxycortisol	11-deoxycortisol
15	11-O-PT	11-oxo-pregnanetriol	21-deoxycortisol
16	P^5T-17α	5-pregnene-3β-17α,20α-triol	17-hydroxypregnenolone
17	THE	tetrahydrocortisone	cortisone
18	THA	tetrahydro-11-dehydro-corticosterone	corticosterone
19	THB	tetrahydrocorticosterone	corticosterone
20	aTHB	5α-tetrahydrocorticosterone	corticosterone
21	THF	tetrahydrocortisol	cortisol
22	aTHF	5α-tetrahydrocortisol	cortisol
23	α-CL	α-cortolone	cortisone
24	β-CL	β-cortolone	cortisone
25	α-C	α-cortol	cortisol
26	F	cortisol	cortisol
27	6β-OH-F	6β-hydroxycortisol	cortisol
28	20α-DHF	20α-dihydrocortisol	cortisol

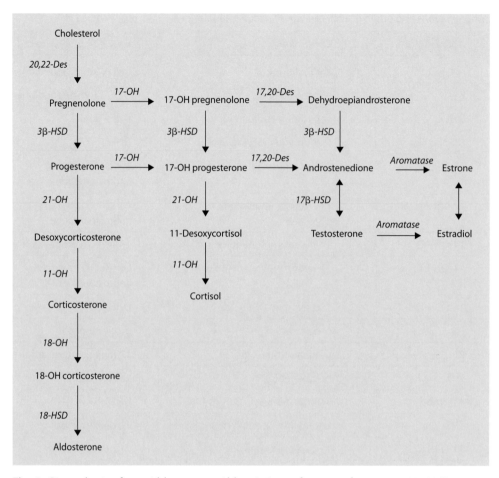

Fig. 3. Biosynthesis of steroid hormones. Abbreviations of names of enzymes: 20, 22-Des = 20, 22-desmolase; 17, 20-Des = 17, 20-desmolase; 3β-HSD = 3β-hydroxysteroid dehydrogenase; 17β-HSD = 17β-hydroxysteroiddehydrogenase; 18-HSD = 18-hydroxysteroiddehydrogenase; 17-OH = 17α-hydroxylase; 21-OH = 21-hydroxylase; 11-OH = 11β-hydroxylase; 18-OH = 18-hydroxylase.

steroids using mass spectrometry is more specific than relying solely upon the retention time of a peak recorded during GC analysis with flame ionization detection (FID). Quantitative urinary steroid profiling permits detection of the different types of congenital adrenal hyperplasia (CAH), adrenal or gonadal tumors, Cushing syndromes and states of adrenal insufficiency or suppression. GC-MS urinary steroid profiling from spot urine samples allows us to diagnose inborn errors of steroid biosynthesis by identifying characteristic steroid metabolites and by calculating ratios between precursor metabolites and product metabolites. Quantitative urinary steroid profiling by GC/MS using selected ion monitoring provides much higher sensitivity but is a more selective approach. It enables to further determine aldosterone

Table 3. Potential of GC-MS in clinical urinary steroid profiling.

Clinical finding	Diagnostic of	Not diagnostic of
Ambiguous genitalia	21-hydroxylase defect 11β-hydroxylase defect 3β-hydroxysteroid- dehydrogenase defect 17α-hydroxylase defect 5α-reductase defefect lipoid adrenal hyperplasia P450 oxidoreductase defect	mixed gonadal dysgenesis true hermaphroditism XX male leydig cell hypoplasia androgen receptor defects 17β-hydroxysteroid dehydrogenase defect
Sodium-losing states	21-hydroxylase defect 3β-hydroxysteroid- dehydrogenase defect lipoid adrenal hyperplasia 18-hydroxylase defect 18-hydroxysteroid- dehydrogenase defect adrenal insufficiency pseudohypoaldosteronism	renal insufficiency hypoaldosteronism
Precocious pseudopuberty	21-hydroxylase defect (simple virilizing, late onset) 11β-hydroxylase defect adrenal tumors gonadal tumors	McCune-Albright's syndrome testotoxicosis β-hCG excess
Premature pubarche, hirsutism, virilization	21-hydroxylase defect (simple virilizing, late onset) 11β-hydroxylase defect 3β-hydroxysteroid dehydrogenase defect adrenal tumors gonadal tumors polycystic ovaries cortisone reductase deficiency	idiopathic hirsutism
Hypertension, hypokalemia	11β-hydroxylase defect 17α-hydroxylase defect apparent mineralocorticoid excess (AME) type I and II Cushing's disease adrenal tumors	renal hypertension phaeochromocytoma
Hypoglycemia	adrenal insufficiency	islet-cell hyperplasia nesidioblastosis

and 18-hydroxylated cortisol metabolites in hypertension research [7] and in the diagnosis of different steroid enzyme deficiencies of aldosterone synthetase [3].

Usually 5–20 ml of urine shipped by regular mail are needed for urinary steroid profiling. Addition of preservatives or transport on dry ice are not necessary in case the sample is received at the laboratory within 2–3 days. For diagnostic purposes only spot urine is sufficient. Collection of 24-hour specimens is necessary in case excretion rates should be determined (e.g. diagnosis of adrenal insufficiency or Cushing syndrome) or for therapeutic monitoring. In brief, the method for urinary steroid profiling comprises solid phase extraction of steroids, enzymatic hydrolysis, reextraction, addition of internal standard, derivatisation (formation of methyloxime-trimethylsilyl esters), purification by gel chromatography and instrumental analysis either by GC or GC-MS.

Diagnostic Potential of GC-MS Urinary Steroid Profiling

A wide range of clinical symptoms like ambiguous genitalia, sodium-loosing states, precocious pseudopuberty, hirsutism, virilization, arterial hypertension, hypokalemia, truncal obesity, primary amenorrhea and hypoglycemia are the most important clinical indications for the use of urinary steroid profiling for diagnostic purposes (table 3). Urinary steroid profiling is also useful to monitor treatment and compliance in CAH due to enzyme deficiencies and after surgery of adrenal or gonadal tumors. The advantages of the method are nonselectivity and independence of circadian rhythm of the most steroid hormones secreted. Another advantage, which bears special importance for pediatric endocrinology, is that the procedure is noninvasive, i.e. the analytical sample can easily be obtained. Normative data of excretion rates in children adolescents and adults are summarized in table 4.

21-Hydroxylase Deficiency. In newborns, the urinary steroid profile with salt-losing CAH is dominated by 17-hydroxpregnanolones, pregnanetriol, 11-oxo-pregnanetriol and 15ß-hydroxypregnanolone [8]. In simple virilizing and late-onset CAH additional detectable or low amounts of cortisol metabolites are excreted.

11β-Hydroxylase Deficiency. In newborns, characteristically 6-hydroxy-tetrahydro-11-deoxycortisol (6-OH-THS) is excreted. Later, excretion of metabolites of 11-deoxycortisol is increased, while excretion of cortisol metabolites is low or absent [9].

3β-Hydroxysteroid Dehydrogenase Deficiency. In the salt-losing form, dehydroepiandrosterone (DHEA), 16-hydroxy-DHEA, pregnanetriol and 17-hydroxypregnenetriol are the major excreted steroids by virtually absent or very low excretion of cortisol metabolites. Patients with simultaneous elevation of post-ACTH serum 17-hydroxypregnenolone to 17-hydroxprogesterone ratio and basal urinary 5-ene steroid excretion have mild 3β-HSD deficiency [10].

17-Hydroxylase/17,20-Lyase Deficiency. The urinary steroid profile is dominated by metabolites of corticosterone and its precursors, cortisol metabolites are lacking [11, 12].

Wudy · Hartmann

P450 Oxidorecuctase Deficiency. This variant of CAH is caused by inactivation of P450 oxidoreductase, an enzyme providing electrons to both 21-hydroxylase and 17-hydroxylase/17,20-lyase. The diagnosis is readily established with GC-MS providing metabolic evidence of both impaired 17-hydroxylase and 21-hydroxylase activity [13, 14].

18-Hydroxylase Deficiency. Characteristically, corticosterone and metabolites of corticosterone are excreted in increased amounts, while 18-hydroxylated corticosterone metabolites are absent or very low. The excretion of cortisol metabolites is normal.

18-Hydroxysteroid Dehydrogenase Deficiency. In addition to high amounts of corticosterone metabolites, the urinary steroid profile shows also 18-hydroxylated corticosterone metabolites (18-OH-THA, 18-OH-THB) [15].

Pseudohypoaldosteronism, another condition associated with severe salt-wasting, can be detected by profiling urinary steroids [16].

Adrenal Insufficiency. Low excretion of glucocorticoid metabolites and adrenal androgen metabolites are characteristic. Different causes (Addison's disease, lipoid adrenal hyperplasia, congenital adrenal hypoplasia) cannot be differentiated using urinary steroid profiling, however.

11β-Hydroxysteroid Dehydrogenase Deficiency-Type 2 (Cortisol Oxidase Deficiency, Apparent Mineralocorticoid Excess. The excretion of tetrahydrocortisone (THE) is much too low compared to high tetrahydrocortisol (THF), 5α-THF and free cortisol excretion.

11β-Hydroxysteroid Dehydrogenase Deficiency-Type 1 (Cortisone Reductase Deficiency). The urinary steroid profile is characterized by very high secretion of THE, cortolones and adrenal androgens and low excretion of THF and 5α-THF.

5α-Reductase Deficiency. Extremely low excretion of 5α-THF in young infants and additional low excretion of androsterone and 11β-hydroxyandrosterone in older children indicate 5α-reductase deficiency [17].

Polycystic Ovary Syndrome. The urinary steroid profile is dominated by adrenal androgens as well as high excretion of androsterone and 5α-THF. Among urinary steroid metabolites, the 5α/5β ratio is significantly increased.

Cushing's Syndrome. Irrespective of the underlying cause, the urinary steroid profile is characterized by increased excretion of THF and free cortisol, 6β-hydroxycortisol and 20-dihydrocortisol.

Adrenocortical Tumors. In children with adrenocortical carcinoma, the urinary steroid profile reveals excessively high amounts of DHEA and other 3β-hydroxy-5-ene steroids, but similar profiles can also be produced by adrenal adenoma. Elevated 11β-hydroxyandrosterone excretion alone or in combination with high excretion of cortisol metabolites or 3β-hydroxy-5-ene steroids are characteristic of adrenocortical adenomas [18]. In adults suffering from adrenocortical carcinoma, the elevated excretion of 3β-hydroxy-5-ene steroids and/or high amounts of tetrahydro-11-deoxycortisol (THS) and cortisol metabolites (THF) are the major characteristics of the urinary steroid profile.

Table 4. Excretion rates (µg/24 h) of urinary steroids in healthy children, adolescents and adults

	0.5–1 year		>1 year		>2 years	
	girls, n = 3	boys, n = 6	girls, n = 7	boys, n = 3	girls, n = 7	boys, n = 1
AN	0 (0–11)	0 (0–32)	7 (0–70)	16 (0–89)	8 (0–129)	7 (–)
ET	0 (0–0)	0 (0–27)	0 (0–162)	49 (0–52)	22 (0–55)	95 (–)
A5-3ß,17α	0 (0–0)	0 (0–16)	0 (0–11)	0 (0–26)	0 (0–0)	0 (–)
DHEA	0 (0–0)	0 (0–0)	0 (0–16)	0 (0–39)	0 (0–5)	7 (–)
A5-3ß, 17ß	0 (0–0)	0 (0–0)	0 (0–0)	0 (0–0)	0 (0–27)	0 (–)
11-O-An	0 (0–41)	0 (0–0)	0 (0–72)	0 (0–41)	0 (0–121)	0 (–)
11-OH-AN+17-OH-PO	26 (0–29)	52 (16–62)	23 (0–81)	70 (39–118)	60 (26–138)	36 (–)
11-OH-ET	0 (0–0)	0 (0–16)	11 (0–54)	0 (0–45)	0 (0–89)	36 (–)
16α-OH-DHEA	0 (0–0)	0 (0–0)	0 (0–0)	0 (0–0)	0 (0–110)	0 (–)
PD	0 (0–0)	0 (0–101)	0 (0–18)	0 (0–8)	0 (0–55)	7 (–)
PT	0 (0–17)	26 (0–42)	36 (8–93)	52 (45–356)	37 (23–267)	44 (–)
P⁵D	17 (0–20)	8 (0–30)	0 (0–50)	45 (0–65)	30 (0–68)	36 (–)
A⁵T-16α	0 (0–0)	0 (0–39)	0 (0–27)	13 (0–24)	0 (0–43)	0 (–)
11-O-PT	0 (0–36)	0 (0–0)	0 (0–0)	0 (0–0)	0 (0–55)	0 (–)
P⁵T	0 (0–0)	4 (0–56)	0 (0–93)	52 (20–148)	0 (0–55)	14 (–)
THE	364 (361–534)	473 (186–628)	456 (246–1,229)	758 (623–955)	878 (671–1,787)	840 (–)
THA	67 (0–92)	20 (0–91)	62 (0–234)	39 (0–144)	122 (0–243)	162 (–)
THB	0 (0–0)	54 (0–100)	30 (0–245)	52 (0–152)	177 (0–300)	0 (–)
5α-THB	85 (57–209)	221 (105–281)	137 (54–351)	237 (118–403)	157 (0–687)	316 (–)
THF	64 (0–104)	193 (107–314)	127 (62–342)	391 (267–589)	336 (156–495)	427 (–)
5α-THF	135 (128–384)	457 (360–664)	309 (104–837)	392 (383–860)	490 (218–962)	272 (–)
α-Cl	46 (42–52)	95 (45–140)	129 (75–351)	196 (118–304)	225 (119–365)	235 (–)
ß-Cl, ß-C	93 (92–130)	115 (28–154)	116 (60–225)	148 (105–197)	240 (156–412)	184 (–)
α-C	0 (0–29)	85 (61–210)	40 (0–69)	123 (59–144)	64 (0–124)	58 (–)
THS	0 (0–0)	0 (0–25)	0 (0–8)	0 (0–41)	26 (0–69)	29 (–)
F	0 (0–0)	0 (0–0)	0 (0–0)	0 (0–0)	0 (0–67)	0 (–)
6ß-OH-F	0 (0–0)	0 (0–265)	0 (0–0)	0 (0–329)	0 (0–147)	0 (–)
20α-OH-F	0 (0–0)	0 (0–0)	0 (0–0)	0 (0–0)	0 (0–0)	0 (–)

	> 3 years		> 4 years		> 5 years		> 6 years	
	girls, n = 2	boys, n = 3	girls, n = 8	boys, n = 3	girls, n = 11	boys, n = 4	girls, n = 13	boys, n = 4
AN	36 (28–43)	52 (14–202)	20 (0–70)	30 (15–424)	57 (0–106)	38 (13–149)	82 (0–164)	30 (18–256)
ET	9 (0–17)	21 (0–101)	0 (0–93)	53 (0–172)	26 (0–175)	64 (0–118)	35 (0–106)	87 (18–205)
A5-3ß,17α	0 (0–0)	0 (0–0)	0 (0–17)	0 (0–0)	0 (0–0)	0 (0–0)	0 (0–18)	0 (0–0)
DHEA	0 (0–0)	0 (0–43)	0 (0–15)	0 (0–22)	0 (0–45)	13 (0–31)	0 (0–53)	0 (0–65)
A5-3ß, 17ß	0 (0–0)	0 (0–21)	0 (0–22)	0 (0–0)	0 (0–0)	0 (0–0)	0 (0–70)	0 (0–0)
11-O-An	0 (0–0)	42 (0–58)	0 (0–23)	0 (0–0)	0 (0–0)	0 (0–84)	0 (0–164)	74 (0–117)
11-OH-AN+17-OH-PO	54 (48–60)	36 (0–87)	62 (38–175)	60 (45–106)	96 (0–210)	81 (58–201)	140 (14–249)	136 (83–256)
11-OH-ET	0 (0–0)	21 (0–94)	31 (0–38)	0 (0–37)	39 (0–225)	37 (0–78)	21 (0–54)	61 (51–68)
16α-OH-DHEA	0 (0–0)	0 (0–0)	0 (0–0)	0 (0–0)	0 (0–0)	0 (0–0)	0 (0–0)	0 (0–0)
PD	9 (0–17)	0 (0–21)	6 (0–36)	10 (0–15)	17 (0–76)	10 (0–39)	14 (0–117)	53 (18–112)
PT	41 (34–48)	50 (26–303)	36 (22–150)	45 (20–53)	69 (0–173)	73 (39–97)	93 (21–346)	63 (37–85)
P⁵D	41 (34–48)	14 (0–26)	8 (0–34)	0 (0–22)	24 (0–85)	16 (0–39)	24 (0–141)	56 (26–136)
A⁵T-16α	0 (0–0)	0 (0–21)	0 (0–33)	0 (0–0)	0 (0–270)	12 (0–28)	0 (0–94)	13 (0–37)
11-O-PT	0 (0–0)	0 (0–0)	0 (0–0)	0 (0–0)	0 (0–56)	0 (0–0)	0 (0–73)	0 (0–35)
P⁵T	14 (0–28)	0 (0–14)	0 (0–25)	0 (0–0)	0 (0–61)	39 (0–78)	43 (0–116)	10 (0–119)
THE	812 (513–1,110)	1,073 (759–1,107)	767 (348–1,925)	1,093 (640–1,462)	1,291 (543–3,031)	1,341 (728–1,635)	1,452 (674–3,395)	1,435 (610–2,119)
THA	43 (0–85)	105 (0–268)	71 (0–251)	60 (0–106)	85 (0–308)	134 (65–337)	79 (0–282)	90 (0–428)
THB	33 (0–66)	120 (0–166)	40 (0–110)	120 (50–265)	0 (0–251)	95 (0–130)	96 (0–581)	70 (45–222)
5α-THB	189 (111–266)	337 (210–362)	232 (0–400)	212 (187–215)	234 (0–637)	173 (110–403)	275 (0–821)	164 (117–307)
THF	207 (94–320)	368 (252–435)	317 (153–665)	403 (260–427)	365 (148–791)	410 (357–691)	387 (175–1,040)	461 (286–585)
5α-THF	270 (257–283)	337 (204–819)	384 (281–1,125)	490 (187–722)	532 (126–817)	323 (168–539)	378 (175–1,423)	254 (222–849)
α-Cl	270 (197–343)	194 (168–348)	260 (125–575)	307 (205–350)	276 (132–695)	393 (299–449)	318 (159–1046)	351 (166–479)
ß-Cl, ß-C	218 (170–266)	199 (168–326)	227 (139–700)	225 (110–297)	315 (66–811)	287 (236–325)	387 (118–1163)	269 (175–286)
α-C	46 (32–60)	42 (0–123)	67 (44–150)	37 (0–55)	64 (0–193)	92 (39–110)	59 (0–232)	58 (0–163)
THS	0 (0–0)	0 (0–31)	13 (0–44)	0 (0–75)	0 (0–60)	22 (0–47)	0 (0–182)	54 (45–68)
F	0 (0–0)	0 (0–0)	0 (0–0)	0 (0–0)	0 (0–85)	0 (0–0)	0 (0–0)	0 (0–76)
6ß-OH-F	0 (0–0)	0 (0–0)	0 (0–0)	0 (0–0)	0 (0–90)	0 (0–0)	0 (0–0)	0 (0–102)
20α-OH-F	0 (0–0)	0 (0–0)	0 (0–0)	0 (0–0)	0 (0–120)	0 (0–0)	0 (0–84)	0 (0–0)

Table 4. Continued

	> 7 years		> 8 years		> 9 years		> 10 years	
	girls, n = 13	boys, n = 7	girls, n = 19	boys, n = 10	girls, n = 18	boys, n = 15	girls, n = 10	boys, n = 11
AN	88 (0–714)	131 (28–350)	157 (0–609)	81 (30–260)	315 (17–817)	302 (24–598)	219 (0–502)	357 (0–697)
ET	52 (0–191)	110 (0–262)	130 (0–421)	68 (0–159)	182 (0–449)	162 (28–312)	168 (57–890)	202 (0–322)
A5-3ß,17α	0 (0–0)	0 (0–78)	0 (0–56)	0 (0–31)	0 (0–95)	0 (0–59)	0 (0–0)	0 (0–0)
DHEA	0 (0–40)	0 (0–167)	32 (0–195)	16 (0–120)	0 (0–114)	16 (0–125)	47 (0–168)	39 (0–172)
A5-3ß,17ß	0 (0–13)	0 (0–70)	0 (0–56)	0 (0–32)	0 (0–123)	0 (0–63)	0 (0–59)	0 (0–30)
11-O-An	0 (0–209)	0 (0–68)	0 (0–401)	31 (0–231)	14 (0–292)	0 (0–406)	0 (0–312)	0 (0–262)
11-OH-AN+17-OH-PO	150 (66–322)	168 (119–276)	281 (78–656)	160 (75–492)	271 (35–525)	230 (140–687)	305 (120–1,442)	332 (105–724)
11-OH-ET	50 (0–122)	39 (0–157)	87 (0–254)	64 (0–602)	117 (46–244)	101 (0–312)	141 (0–327)	78 (0–260)
16α-OH-DHEA	0 (0–44)	0 (0–78)	0 (0–130)	0 (0–90)	0 (0–135)	0 (0–162)	0 (0–126)	0 (0–237)
PD	40 (0–103)	23 (0–69)	41 (0–231)	17 (0–146)	55 (0–217)	62 (0–195)	64 (0–176)	37 (0–227)
PT	90 (46–193)	70 (0–140)	203 (42–655)	121 (52–365)	150 (17–290)	147 (27–425)	124 (48–515)	135 (50–316)
P⁵D	32 (0–112)	52 (0–227)	31 (0–87)	52 (0–162)	49 (0–225)	67 (0–324)	50 (0–170)	40 (0–150)
A⁵T-16α	0 (0–75)	0 (0–39)	15 (0–112)	46 (0–182)	27 (0–670)	27 (0–105)	41 (0–106)	31 (0–260)
11-O-PT	0 (0–0)	0 (0–0)	0 (0–75)	0 (0–180)	0 (0–22)	0 (0–270)	0 (0–97)	0 (0–30)
P⁵T	48 (0–125)	41 (0–78)	61 (0–601)	32 (0–127)	75 (0–168)	45 (0–250)	70 (0–140)	73 (0–135)
THE	1,295 (562–2,975)	1,706 (871–2,694)	1,637 (383–4,025)	1,075 (0–1,956)	1,476 (496–2,912)	1,471 (0–2,671)	1,279 (0–2,604)	2,322 (437–4,615)
THA	80 (0–230)	252 (0–632)	37 (0–382)	37 (0–1,245)	94 (0–507)	36 (0–1,998)	42 (0–1,522)	131 (0–520)
THB	95 (0–297)	102 (0–280)	81 (0–296)	99 (0–304)	144 (0–371)	70 (0–219)	114 (0–543)	56 (0–342)
5α-THB	230 (0–537)	244 (117–525)	224 (0–453)	213 (0–608)	258 (0–540)	165 (0–690)	177 (0–342)	252 (0–650)
THF	336 (202–1,335)	448 (215–700)	544 (0–1,421)	391 (195–879)	476 (144–1,171)	470 (192–811)	406 (144–1,171)	580 (127–1,105)
5α-THF	365 (218–847)	469 (352–917)	412 (38–1,042)	492 (210–755)	460 (179–1,252)	568 (124–918)	401 (176–1,855)	614 (175–812)
α-Cl	411 (230–905)	471 (131–540)	524 (105–765)	429 (150–581)	408 (157–922)	529 (234–977)	430 (104–890)	546 (110–1,625)
ß-Cl, ß-C	332 (207–565)	420 (205–591)	442 (94–1,177)	326 (175–575)	381 (79–938)	419 (206–684)	381 (104–721)	405 (145–1,625)
α-C	58 (0–175)	85 (65–157)	85 (15–217)	114 (57–315)	108 (42–187)	125 (56–486)	105 (0–462)	120 (0–189)
THS	0 (0–162)	0 (0–88)	0 (0–93)	16 (0–109)	0 (0–70)	0 (0–108)	0 (0–97)	0 (0–67)
F	0 (0–0)	0 (0–0)	0 (0–48)	0 (0–57)	0 (0–0)	0 (0–0)	0 (0–39)	0 (0–46)
6ß-OH-F	0 (0–0)	0 (0–0)	0 (0–0)	0 (0–0)	0 (0–0)	0 (0–0)	0 (0–0)	0 (0–0)
20α-OH-F	0 (0–0)	0 (0–0)	0 (0–73)	0 (0–0)	0 (0–0)	0 (0–0)	0 (0–0)	0 (0–0)

	> 11 years		> 12 years		> 13 years	
	girls, n = 10	boys, n = 16	girls, n = 13	boys, n = 10	girls, n = 13	boys, n = 12
AN	445 (137–1,181)	376 (79–1,056)	517 (301–961)	650 (67–1,665)	681 (81–2,256)	1,114 (109–1,827)
ET	222 (112–596)	221 (106–843)	299 (157–595)	401 (56–975)	405 (146–1,849)	582 (109–1,313)
A5-3ß,17α	0 (0–0)	0 (0–50)	0 (0–42)	0 (0–190)	0 (0–91)	0 (0–80)
DHEA	52 (0–112)	77 (0–1,286)	30 (0–99)	82 (0–356)	48 (0–215)	147 (0–429)
A5-3ß, 17ß	0 (0–82)	0 (0–131)	0 (0–75)	0 (0–142)	0 (0–223)	34 (0–220)
11-O-An	38 (0–247)	78 (0–375)	0 (0–300)	0 (0–337)	0 (0–984)	86 (0–525)
11-OH-AN+17-OH-PO	322 (0–562)	359 (173–850)	360 (0–498)	438 (101–857)	472 (65–1,049)	605 (141–1,029)
11-OH-ET	69 (0–328)	94 (0–276)	100 (0–150)	80 (0–665)	136 (0–616)	138 (0–502)
16α-OH-DHEA	13 (0–168)	146 (0–412)	0 (0–130)	0 (0–300)	0 (0–826)	153 (0–340)
PD	45 (0–450)	47 (0–390)	80 (0–125)	64 (0–190)	85 (0–1,300)	130 (0–263)
PT	160 (90–259)	212 (79–475)	230 (135–375)	335 (67–632)	363 (0–1,275)	349 (0–1,968)
P^{5}D	53 (0–143)	99 (0–356)	60 (0–127)	96 (0–273)	72 (0–212)	118 (0–400)
A^{5}T-16α	0 (0–61)	103 (0–356)	29 (0–250)	131 (0–285)	36 (0–787)	155 (0–421)
11-O-PT	0 (0–0)	0 (0–437)	0 (0–0)	0 (0–0)	0 (0–49)	0 (0–196)
P^{5}T	70 (0–140)	166 (0–437)	119 (0–227)	156 (0–332)	185 (54–275)	252 (88–421)
THE	1,258 (937–2,357)	1,950 (920–3,787)	1,620 (847–2,921)	2,089 (585–4,167)	2,380 (666–5,050)	2,802 (683–4,301)
THA	19 (0–292)	0 (0–411)	86 (0–208)	118 (0–270)	0 (0–303)	117 (0–540)
THB	24 (0–241)	82 (0–319)	54 (0–356)	62 (0–300)	0 (0–351)	215 (0–375)
5α-THB	206 (63–358)	228 (94–515)	195 (0–416)	185 (52–470)	283 (0–934)	284 (0–660)
THF	452 (177–762)	706 (379–1,275)	501 (229–727)	574 (223–1163)	784 (162–1,237)	840 (149–1,109)
5α-THF	352 (177–562)	537 (205–1,083)	434 (140–967)	515 (157–934)	562 (165–1,590)	812 (273–1,540)
α-Cl	448 (190–846)	527 (308–901)	607 (210–937)	696 (171–1,540)	816 (216–1,787)	752 (364–2,205)
ß-Cl, ß-C	342 (190–517)	453 (165–797)	408 (190–855)	560 (118–1,035)	625 (162–1,675)	605 (227–2,540)
α-C	86 (0–169)	117 (0–219)	90 (40–180)	121 (37–472)	127 (54–454)	259 (92–351)
THS	0 (0–5)	0 (0–61)	0 (0–90)	0 (0–100)	0 (0–176)	0 (0–120)
F	0 (0–0)	0 (0–85)	0 (0–0)	0 (0–0)	0 (0–0)	0 (0–0)
6ß-OH-F	0 (0–0)	0 (0–0)	0 (0–0)	0 (0–0)	0 (0–0)	0 (0–0)
20α-OH-F	0 (0–0)	0 (0–0)	0 (0–0)	0 (0–0)	0 (0–0)	0 (0–0)

Table 4. Continued

	> 14 years		> 15 years		> 16 years	
	girls, n = 8	boys, n = 12	girls, n = 10	boys, n = 11	girls, n = 3	boys, n = 4
AN	931 (247–2,389)	1060 (537–1,638)	1397 (502–2,300)	1,400 (568–2,337)	1,141(973–1,485)	1,516 (1,015–2,372)
ET	587 (130–1695)	612 (215–1,120)	878 (355–1,794)	883 (305–1,225)	696 (582–1,380)	746 (393–889)
A5-3ß,17α	0 (0–68)	0 (0–115)	0 (0–63)	0 (0–90)	0 (0–46)	0 (0–42)
DHEA	73 (0–121)	51 (0–240)	90 (0–227)	137 (0–2,213)	0 (0–158)	85 (33–148)
A5-3ß, 17ß	0 (0–60)	0 (0–120)	0 (0–259)	34 (0–426)	0 (0–46)	0 (0–52)
11-O-An	0 (0–260)	75 (0–472)	0 (0–211)	79 (0–596)	0 (0–112)	0 (0–1,381)
11-OH-AN+17-OH-PO	592 (188–984)	606 (245–1,662)	530 (126–1,721)	964 (262–1,483)	663 (383–1,160)	551 (0–854)
11-OH-ET	222 (19–334)	147 (0–540)	171 (65–455)	225 (0–451)	92 (0–185)	163 (55–425)
16α-OH-DHEA	0 (0–638)	303 (0–1,175)	121 (0–406)	0 (0–577)	185 (178–232)	0 (0–78)
PD	222 (140–839)	104 (0–638)	188 (87–750)	122 (0–375)	86 (0–261)	119 (70–170)
PT	583 (123–942)	387 (215–977)	523 (250–1,015)	495 (227–1,169)	663 (205–1,021)	785 (306–918)
P^{5}D	69 (0–203)	109 (0–268)	54 (0–163)	140 (0–338)	109 (52–1,624)	44 (0–170)
A^{5}T-16α	95 (0–468)	260 (0–764)	123 (0–439)	200 (0–495)	0 (0–132)	129 (0–382)
11-O-PT	0 (0–111)	0 (0–0)	0 (0–0)	0 (0–0)	0 (0–0)	0 (0–0)
P^{5}T	172 (0–402)	166 (0–684)	222 (61–568)	187 (78–742)	141 (0–198)	291 (166–467)
THE	3,030 (767–4,776)	2,155 (918–4,992)	2,138 (892–5,075)	2,748 (1,958–5,212)	1,529 (0–3,718)	1,896 (908–3,463)
THA	166 (0–362)	75 (0–402)	0 (0–211)	201 (0–974)	130 (112–2,146)	111 (0–425)
THB	170 (0–319)	102 (0–230)	33 (0–270)	240 (0–673)	145 (0–207)	73 (0–467)
5α-THB	315 (84–1,034)	294 (0–780)	232 (51–703)	338 (0–783)	196 (0–264)	331 (0–637)
THF	927 (227–2,135)	701 (318–2,184)	706 (240–2,236)	855 (659–1,760)	562 (0–837)	1,034 (485–1,868)
5α-THF	761 (260–1,114)	814 (350–2,235)	604 (257–1,502)	708 (450–1,430)	402 (251–717)	913 (692–1,168)
α-Cl	867 (130–1,477)	778 (577–1,725)	634 (129–1,691)	1,196 (607–1,827)	464 (311–957)	827 (712–1,360)
ß-Cl, ß-C	701 (117–1,517)	726 (370–1,955)	540 (133–1,123)	675 (362–1,695)	580 (483–1,000)	574 (291–1,020)
α-C	164 (45–232)	179 (116–360)	167 (0–374)	194 (90–394)	239 (72–580)	178 (145–212)
THS	0 (0–0)	0 (0–216)	0 (0–121)	0 (0–135)	0 (0–0)	18 (0–77)
F	0 (0–0)	0 (0–0)	0 (0–0)	0 (0–0)	0 (0–0)	0 (0–0)
6ß-OH-F	0 (0–0)	0 (0–0)	0 (0–0)	0 (0–0)	0 (0–0)	0 (0–0)
20α-OH-F	0 (0–0)	0 (0–0)	0 (0–0)	0 (0–0)	0 (0–0)	0 (0–0)

	> 17 years		> 18 years	
	girls, n = 2	boys, n = 1	girls, n = 14	boys, n = 7
AN	1,560 (1,275–1,845)	2,436 (–)	1,275 (840–2,193)	1,231 (800–2,715)
ET	950 (573–1,327)	2,155 (–)	925 (0–1,290)	630 (480–1,200)
A5-3ß,17α	23 (0–45)	0 (–)	0 (0–455)	0 (0–92)
DHEA	292 (212–371)	78 (–)	244 (0–750)	92 (50–1,995)
A5-3ß, 17ß	56 (0–112)	109 (–)	41 (0–262)	0 (0–225)
11-O-An	169 (0–337)	171 (–)	0 (0–700)	0 (0–115)
11-OH-AN+17-OH-PO	1264 (1,147–1,381)	1,046 (–)	788 (280–1,740)	843 (415–1,665)
11-OH-ET	187 (148–225)	593 (–)	244 (0–1,020)	202 (150–1,510)
16α-OH-DHEA	614 (531–697)	0 (–)	278 (0–600)	0 (0–254)
PD	206 (157–255)	437 (–)	169 (0–1,600)	92 (33–175)
PT	526 (467–585)	1,296 (–)	505 (175–1,200)	590 (343–1,267)
P^5D	119 (67–170)	0 (–)	79 (0–218)	96 (0–162)
A^5T-16α	214 (0–427)	312 (–)	0 (0–393)	0 (0–292)
11-O-PT	0 (0–0)	0 (0–0)	0 (0–175)	0 (0–0)
P^5T	319 (255–382)	374 (–)	304 (0–2,030)	253 (137–555)
THE	2,653 (2,257–3,048)	2,343 (–)	1,349 (0–3,450)	1,931 (820–3,099)
THA	354 (0–708)	328 (–)	0 (0–416)	0 (0–0)
THB	298 (0–596)	0 (–)	41 (0–455)	0 (0–462)
5α-THB	264 (0–528)	312 (–)	41 (0–1,050)	462 (0–794)
THF	1,504 (1,462–1,545)	1,452 (–)	1,089 (560–1,620)	1,107 (642–2,039)
5α-THF	1,070 (900–1,239)	671 (–)	666 (250–1,380)	1,462 (546–2,227)
α-Cl	1,522 (1,097–1,946)	952 (–)	632 (333–1,980)	744 (543–1,937)
ß-Cl, ß-C	978 (708–1,248)	796 (–)	373 (175–900)	520 (400–1,278)
α-C	297 (177–416)	281 (–)	128 (0–304)	200 (124–421)
THS	0 (0–0)	156 (–)	0 (0–157)	0 (0–125)
F	0 (0–0)	0 (–)	0 (0–0)	0 (0–0)
6ß-OH-F	0 (0–0)	0 (–)	0 (0–0)	0 (0–0)
20α-OH-F	0 (0–0)	0 (–)	0 (0–0)	0 (0–0)

Smith-Lemli-Opitz Syndrome. Patients with this disease have impaired ability to synthesize cholesterol due to attenuated activity of 7-dehydrosterol-Δ^7-reductase. Metabolically these patients are characterized by Δ^7 and Δ^8 unsaturated steroids [19].

Profiling Plasma Steroids by Stable Isotope Dilution/Gas Chromatography-Mass Spectrometry

Methodological Aspects

The early attempts to measure plasma steroids by GC-MS were rapidly surpassed by the introduction of immunoassay techniques with which mass spectrometry could not compete especially with respect to analytical run time and cost. However, it was not until recently that it was realized that the lacking specificity of immunoassays might initiate a renaissance for clinical mass spectrometric techniques in steroid analysis.

Currently, most methods for the determination of steroid hormones in human plasma are based on immunoassays. Immunoassays are rapid and easy to perform. However, for a number of reasons, the hormone concentrations measured in the same sample may vary considerably dependent on the kit used thus questioning their reliability. Severe problems due to cross-reactivity or matrix effects are likely to arise, e.g. in neonatal plasma, plasma from hyperandrogenic women or follicular fluid.

Because of its high specificity, stable isotope dilution GC-MS seems to be especially suited to circumvent these analytical problems. The technique is currently regarded as the 'gold standard' for the evaluation of steroid immunoassays. So far, isotope dilution GC-MS has not been utilized in a routine clinical setting for plasma steroid analysis. In contrast to immunoassays, where only a single steroid can be measured at a time, GC-MS offers the advantageous potential of determining a whole spectrum of plasma steroid hormones simultaneously in a profile. In our attempt to evaluate disorders of androgen metabolism – they belong to the most common endocrinopathies –, a specific, accurate and sensitive method for the assessment of androgen metabolism was needed. By our ID/GC-MS assay it is meanwhile possible to simultaneously determine 8 different steroid hormones in a single plasma sample. The main steps of our ID/GC-MS method [20] for plasma steroid hormone profiling are incubation of plasma (0.1–1.0 ml) with an internal standard cocktail (stable isotope labeled analogs of the analytes), solvent extraction, a short clean up step by gel chromatography, derivatization (perfluoracylation) and analysis by GC-MS using selected ion monitoring. Portions of typical selected ion chromatograms are shown in figure 4.

Diagnostic Potential of ID/GC-MS Plasma Steroid Profiling

The many clinical indications of steroid hormone analysis by ID/GC-MS are at best demonstrated by explaining the diagnostic significance of the respective steroid hormones.

17α-Hydroxyprogesterone is the most valuable hormonal plasma parameter for the diagnosis and monitoring of 21-hydroxylase deficiency, i.e. the most frequent enzyme defect in steroid hormone biosynthesis leading to hyperandrogenism. The first mass spectrometric concentrations of plasma 17-hydroxyprogesterone in neonates,

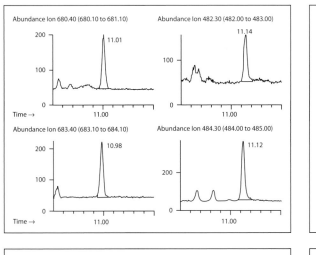

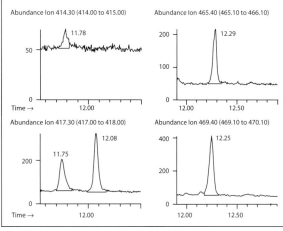

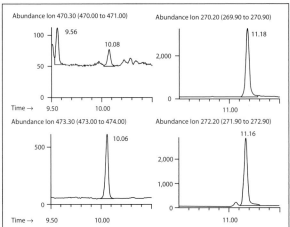

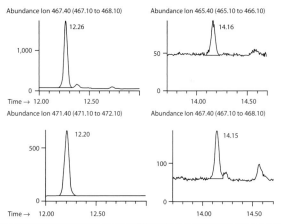

Fig. 4. Selected ion monitoring of 8 steroid hormones profiled of a plasma sample (total of 0.5 ml of plasma analyzed) of a male neonate to which 1 ng of the corresponding deuterated internal standard has been added. An aliquot of 1/100 of the extract has been analyzed by GC-MS (Agilent 6890 series GC coupled with an Agilent 5973N mass selective detector). Corresponding ion traces of analyte and respective internal standard are superposed: testosterone (m/z 680.40, t_r 11.01 min, 1.38 ng/ml), [16,16,17–^{2}H$_3$]testosterone (m/z 683.40, t_r 10.98 min), 4-androstenedione (m/z 482.30, t_r 11.14 min, 0.58 ng/ml), [7,7–^{2}H$_2$] 4-androstenedione (m/z 484.30, t_r 11.12 min), 5α-androstane-3α,17β-diol (m/z 470.30, t_r 10.08 min, 0.12 ng/ml), [16,16,17–^{2}H$_3$]5α-androstane-3α,17β-diol (m/z 473.30, t_r 10.06 min), dehydroepiandrosterone (m/z 270.20, t_r 11.18 min, 8.82 ng/ml), [7,7–^{2}H$_2$]dehydroepiandrosterone (m/z 272.20, t_r 11.16 min), 5α-dihydrotestosterone (m/z 414.30, t_r 11.78 min, 0.22 ng/ml), [16,16,17–^{2}H$_3$] 5α-dihydrotestosterone (m/z 417.30, t_r 11.75 min), 17α-hydroxyprogesterone (m/z 465.40, t_r 12.29 min, 0.80 ng/ml), [11,11,12,12–^{2}H$_4$]17α-hydroxyprogesterone (m/z 469.40, t_r 12.25 min), 17α-hydroxypregnenolone (m/z 467.40, t_r 12.26 min, 6.38 ng/ml), [2,2,4,4,21,21,21–^{2}H$_7$]17α-hydroxypregnenolone (m/z 471.40, t_r 12.20 min), 11-deoxycortisol (m/z 465.40, t_r 14.16 min, 1.00 ng/ml) and [1α,2α-^{2}H$_2$]11-deoxycortisol (m/z 467.40, t_r 14.15 min).

children and adolescents have been published by our group [21–23]. In amniotic fluid, 17-hydroxyprogesterone is a highly valuable parameter in the hormonal prenatal diagnosis of 21-hydroxylase deficiency [24].

11-Deoxycortisol presents the leading hormonal plasma marker of 11-hydroxylase deficiency [25].

4-Androstenedione is the most important precursor hormone of androgens in females. Plasma levels are often increased in hirsute women. Besides 17α-hydroxyprogesterone, it is an important diagnostic parameter of 21-hydroxylase deficiency in plasma and amniotic fluid [24]. A decreased ratio between testosterone and androstenedione is indicative of 17-hydroxysteroiddehydrogenase deficiency [21, 22].

In men, 80% of testosterone is produced by the testes. In women, testosterone is produced by the ovaries, the adrenals and in peripheral tissue. Plasma testosterone is an indicator of endocrine testis function. It serves as a marker for androgen-producing tumors or is elevated in female hirsutism [21, 22].

17α-Hydroxypregnenolone is the marker hormone of the adrenal enzyme defect 3ß-hydroxysteroid dehydrogenase deficiency. It can be elevated in 21-hydroxylase deficiency as well.

Dehydroepiandrosterone (DHEA) and its conjugate dehydroepiandrosterone-sulfate (DHEA-S) are almost exclusively of adrenal origin. In contrast to DHEA, the plasma concentration of DHEA-S is about 500-fold higher and does not reveal a circadian rhythm. Considered the leading marker of adrenal androgen secretion, plasma DHEA-S is an important parameter for the evaluation of adrenal androgen production. Both metabolites are indicative of 3β-hydroxysteroid dehydrogenase deficiency. DHEA-S serves as marker for adrenal androgen producing tumors. It can further be elevated in hirsutism. Furthermore, it has been suggested to be an indicator of ACTH secretion and a tumor marker in women with breast cancer [20, 22, 26].

5α-Dihydrotestosterone is the most potent human androgen. Its production is decreased in 5α-reductase deficiency and this condition is diagnosed by an increased ratio between testosterone and 5α-dihydrotestosterone [20, 22].

Androstandediol and androstanediol glucuronide are end metabolites of 5α-dihydrotestosterone. We have analyzed the developmental patterns of androstanediol and androstanediol glucuronide in children and adults as well as their role in idiopathic hirsutism [22, 27].

Profiling Steroids by LC-MS(-MS)

Methodological Aspects
The introduction of fast atom bombardment (FAB) and related techniques allowed the analysis of steroids without derivatisation. Shortly after, the introduction of first soft ionization methods, such as Thermospray, permitted the introduction of LC-MS. In LC-MS, the effluent from LC is led through a capillary to the source of the mass

spectrometer. In Thermospray, the temperature of the capillary is adjusted to a level where the solvent is partially vaporized, charged droplets are generated and finally ions of the analyte which can be analyzed in the MS are expelled. The Thermospray technique in combination with stable isotope dilution was used in a pioneering project for the development of the first LC-MS assay for a clinically most important plasma steroid: dehydroepiandrosterone sulfate (DHEA-S) [28]. It was interesting that the values we obtained for DHEA-S estimation by LC-MS were generally approximately one-half those obtained by measurement with radioimmunoassay when the same serum samples were analyzed. While we described the method for DHEA-S analysis, we simultaneously suggested it as technique suitable for routine clinical use because of the short sample work up and the short chromatography time. The method permitted analysis of a new sample every 5 min.

Currently, electrospray ionization (ESI) and atmospheric pressure chemical ionization (APCI) are the most widely applied soft ionization techniques. Introduction of tandem mass spectrometry (MS-MS) represented a further break through in LC-MS since this technique compensates for the rather poor chromatographic capacity of LC. Tandem MS is a combination of three mass spectrometers (MS-1, collision cell (MS-2), MS-3) to improve analytical potential. It permits sequential filtration, fragmentation and focussing of ions. The collision cell is similar to the quadrupole analyzers MS-1 and MS-3, thus the term triple quad is also applied. In each MS, specific ions can be selected or a mass range can be scanned to record ion spectra. For quantitative MS, multiple reaction monitoring (MRM) is used.

Our group demonstrated the applicability of bench top LC-MS-MS to clinical steroid analysis by developing the first stable isotope dilution LC-(APCI) MS-MS assay for 17-hydroxyprogesterone, the most important indicator of 21-hydroxylase deficiency in human plasma [23].

Clinical Steroid Analysis by LC-MS(-MS)
Our publications on ID/LC-(Thermospray)MS analysis of plasma DHEA-S as well as on ID/LC-(APCI)MS-MS determination of plasma 17-hydroxyprogesterone heralded a revolutionary development in the field of clinical analysis of steroid hormones (table 5). The fulfillment of our anticipation of LC-MS(-MS) being suitable for routine steroid analysis has been shown by consecutive developments: LC-MS(-MS) has meanwhile come of age with dramatic improvements in sensitivity, specificity, and automation and has led to the replacement of immunoassays in many routine laboratories by now.

Using LC-MS(-MS) steroids can be measured singly in specimens or as a profile. Minimal sample preparation is an important advantage saving time and money. However, most of the LC-MS(-MS) methods are currently at the in-house stage; therefore, results need to be interpreted carefully. Manufacturers are just about to start providing kits for analyses and profiles. This will contribute to assay standardization.

Table 5. Developmental milestones on the way to clinical steroid analysis by liquid chromatography-mass spectrometry (LC-MS)

1982	Shackleton and Straub	analysis of intact steroid conjugates by FAB (fast atom bombardement)
1987	Liberato and Shackleton	LC-MS of intact steroid conjugates
1990	Shackleton, Wudy and Pratt	first stable isotope dilution LC-(Thermospray)MS assay for serum DHEA-S
1990	Esteban	cortisol production rates measured by LC-MS
2000	Wudy, Hartmann and Svoboda	first stable isotope dilution benchtop LC-MS-MS assay for 17-hydroxyprogesterone
2001	Kao and coworkers	steroid profiling by LC-MS-MS

It has to be kept in mind that despite the apparent simplicity of LC-MS(-MS) methods, the technique is prone to MS matrix effects such as ion suppression and ion enhancement. Disturbing influences from isomeric and/or isobaric steroids have to be excluded. Further sources of interference have been reported such as phospholipids, drugs and other compounds. The level of methodological robustness does not yet seem to be comparable to that known from GC-MS [29].

In LC-MS(-MS) one can only determine compounds for which retention times and transitions are known and recorded. Steroid determinations have been carried out in plasma (serum), urine and saliva. Concerning application of LC-MS-MS in plasma steroid analysis, profiles including the clinically most important steroid hormones have been reported [30, 31]. Reference ranges for steroids determined by LC-MS-MS have been reported, e.g. pediatric reference intervals for aldosterone, 17α-hydroxyprogesterone, dehydroepiandrosterone (DHEA), testosterone and 25-hydroxyvitamin D_3 [32] or for testosterone and dihydrotestosterone [33, 34].

Clinical Steroid Analysis by MS: Significance and Perspective

Steroid analysis in pediatric endocrinology is much more challenging than in adult endocrinology. This is due to the many changes in the endocrine environment of the developing organism, e.g. the neonatal period with the high amounts of 5-ene steroids from the fetal zone of the adrenals, adrenarche with its increase in DHEA production in the zona reticularis, or puberty with the maturation of gonads and increase in production of sex steroids.

Due to uncritical efforts of saving money in the biomedical disciplines, steroid determination in children has mostly been carried out using commercially available immunoassays which have never been developed for or tested in children. Therefore, steroid determination by – mostly direct – immunoassays has faced considerable loss of reliability. In this context, it is a pleasing development that MS-based steroid determination has made significant progress during the last decade.

Steroid determination by GC-MS entered clinical routine earlier than LC-MS(-MS). Urinary steroid profiling using GC-MS is a nonselective (nontargeted) multicomponent analysis of very high diagnostic potential. The technique is noninvasive and rapid. The constellation of urinary steroid metabolites allows the diagnosis of most steroid-related disorders from spot urine samples, whereas determination of excretion rates of steroid metabolites requires 24-hour urinary samples (e.g. for monitoring patients with Addison's disease, CAH or for noninvasive determination of hormonal production rates). In patients with steroid-secreting tumors unusual steroids are produced for which specific serum assays are not available but their metabolites can be monitored by urinary profiling. Furthermore, the technique is excellently suited as confirmatory technique after positive screening values in neonatal screening for 21-hydroxylase deficiency.

In case GC-MS instrumentation is available – besides its role as reference methodology ('gold standard') – quantitative plasma steroid analysis by ID/GC-MS could be set up as a complementary analytical technique with highest specificity whenever problems from matrix effects or cross-reactivity are likely to arise or suspicious results need to be rechecked. To keep costs at a reasonable limit, we suggest to set up priorities for urinary and plasma steroid analysis by GC-MS. Thus, steroid analyses are at best carried out in a small number of highly specialized supraregional laboratories (referral centers) equipped with the analytical instrumentation and where support from specialist biochemists or clinicians is available.

Lately, LC-MS-MS has become more attractive as a routine tool in clinical steroid analysis. The technique enables relatively shorter time for sample preparation or instrumental analysis. However, while LC-MS-MS is often regarded as reference technology, concern has lately arisen that it might not yet meet the higher precision standards achieved with GC-MS. With LC-MS-MS often lower results are obtained, but significant performance variation due to lack of skill, time pressure or calibration differences exists [29].

To conclude, great progress has been obtained in the field of clinical steroid analysis by the introduction of MS-based analytical techniques. These developments will lead to improved specificity in clinical steroid determination though at higher costs than the hitherto applied immunoassays. However, especially in pediatric endocrinology, improvement in the reliability of steroid hormone-based diagnostics is desperately needed. Therefore, it still has to be realized that quality is not equivalent to luxury.

References

1 Wudy SA, Hartmann M: Gas chromatography-mass spectrometry profiling of steroids in times of molecular biology. Horm Metab Res 2004;36:415–422.

2 Wudy SA: Synthetic procedures for the preparation of deuterium-labeled analogs of naturally occurring steroids. Steroids 1990;55:463–471.

3 Shackleton CHL, Merdinck J, Lawson AM: Steroid and bile acid analyses; in McEwen CN, Larsen BS (eds): Mass Spectrometry of Biological Materials. New York, Marcel Dekker, 1990, pp 297–378.

4 Honour JW: Steroid profiling. Ann Clin Biochem 1997;34:32–44.

5 Heckmann M, Hartmann MF, Kampschulte B, Gack H, Bödeker RH, Gortner L, Wudy SA: Cortisol production rates in preterm infants in relation to growth and illness: a noninvasive prospective study using gas chromatography-mass spectrometry. J Clin Endocrinol Metab 2005;90:5737–5741.

6 Wudy SA, Harmann M, Remer T: Sexual dimorphism in cortisol secretion starts after age 10 in healthy children: urinary cortisol exretion rates during growth. Am J Physiol Endocrinol Metab 2007;293:E970–E976.

7 Shackleton CHL: Mass spectrometry in the diagnosis of steroid-related disorders and in hypertension research. J Steroid Biochem Mol Biol 1993;45:127–140.

8 Wudy SA, Hartmann M, Homoki J: Hormonal diagnosis of 21-hydroxylase deficiency in plasma and urine of neonates using bench top gas chromatography-mass spectrometry. J Endocrinol 2000;165:679–683.

9 Wudy SA, Homoki J, Wachter UA, Teller WM: Diagnosis of the adrenogenital syndrome caused by 11ß-hydroxylase deficiency using gas chromatographic-mass spectrometric analysis of the urinary steroid profile. Dtsch Med Wochenschr 1997;122:3–10.

10 Sólyom J, Halasz Z, Hosszú E, Glaz E, Vihko R, Orava M, Homoki J, Wudy SA, Teller WM: Serum and urinary steroids in girls with precocious pubarche and/or hirsutism due to mild 3ß-hydroxysteroiddehydrogenase deficiency. Horm Res 1995;44:133–141.

11 Tisano D, Knopf C, Koren H, Levanon N, Hartmann MF, Hochberg Z, Wudy SA: Metabolic evidence for impaired 17α-hydroxylase activity in a kindred bearing the E305 G mutation for isoloate 17,20-lyase activity. Eur J Endocrinol 2008;158:385–392.

12 Tisano D, Navon R, Flor O, Knopf C, Harmann MF, Wudy SA, Yakhini Z, Hochberg Z: A steroid metabolomic approach to 17α-hydroxylase/17,20 lyase deficiency. Metabolomics 2010;epub ahead of print.

13 Wudy SA, Hartmann MF, Draper N, Stewart P, Arlt W: A male twin infant with skull deformity and elevated neonatal 17-hydroxyprogesterone: a prismatic case of P450 oxidoreductase deficiency. Endocr Res 2004;30:957–964.

14 Hershkovitz E, Parvari R, Wudy SA, Hartmann MF, Gomes LG, Loewental N, Miller WL: Homozygous mutation G539R in the gene for P450 oxidoreductase in a family previously diagnosed as having 17,20 lyase deficiency. J Clin Endocrinol Metab 2008;93:3584–3588.

15 Nguyen HH, Hannemann F, Hartmann MF, Wudy SA, Bernhardt R: Aldosterone synthase deficiency caused by homozygous L45/F mutation in the CYP11B2 gene. Mol Genet Metab 2008;93:458–467.

16 Akin L, Kurtoglu S, Kendirci M, Akin MA, Hartmann MF, Wudy SA: Hook effect: a pitfall leading to misdiagnosis of hypoaldosteronism in an infant with pseudohypoaldosteronism. Horm Res Paediatr 2010;74:72–75.

17 Walter KN, Kienzle FB, Frankenschmidt A, Hiort O, Wudy SA, van der Werf-Grohmann N, Superti-Furga A, Schwab KO: Difficulties in diagnosis and treatment of 5α-reductase type 2 deficiency in a newborn with 46,XY DSD. Horm Res Paediatr 2010;74:67–71.

18 Malunowicz EM, Ginalska-Malinowska M, Romer TE, Ruszczynska-Wolska A, Dura M: Heterogeneity of urinary steroid profiles in children with adrenocortical tumors. Horm Res 1995;44:182–188.

19 Shackleton CHL, Roitman E, GuoL-W, Wilson WK, Porter FD: Identification of 7(8) and 8(9) unsaturated adrenal steroid metabolites produced by patients with 7-dehydrosterol-Δ^7-reductase deficiency (Smith-Lemli-Opitz syndrome). J Steroid Biochem Mol Biol 2002;82:225–232.

20 Wudy SA, Wachter UA, Homoki J, Teller WM, Shackleton CHL: Androgen metabolism assessment by routine gas chromatography/mass spectrometry profiling of plasma steroids. 1. Unconjugated steroids. Steroids 1992;57:319–324.

21 Wudy SA, Wachter UA, Homoki J, Teller WM: 17α-Hydroxyprogesterone, 4-androstenedione, and testosterone profiled by stable isotope dilution/gas chromatography-mass spectrometry in plasma of children. Pediatr Res 1995;38:76–80.

22 Wudy SA, Hartmann M, Solleder C, Wachter UA, Homoki J: Clinical steroid hormone analysis by stable isotope dilution/gas chromatography-mass spectrometry; in Heys JR, Melillo DG (eds): Synthesis and Applications of Isotopically Labelled Compounds 1997. Chichester, Wiley, 1998, pp 575–579.

23 Wudy SA, Harmann M, Svoboda M: Determination of 17α-hydroxyprogesterone in plasma by stable isotope dilution/bench top liquid chromatography-tandem mass spectrometry. Horm Res 2000;53:68–71.

24 Wudy SA, Dörr HG, Solleder C, Homoki J: Profiling steroid hormones in amniotic fluid of midpregnancy by routine stable isotope gas chromatography-mass spectrometry: reference values and concentrations in fetuses at risk for 21-hydroxylase deficiency. J Clin Endocrinol Metab 1999;84:2724–2728.

25 Wudy SA, Hartmann M, Homoki J: Determination of 11-deoxycortisol (Reichstein's compound S) in human plasma by clinical isotope dilution mass spectrometry using bench top gas chromatography-mass selective detection. Steroids 2002;67:851–857.

26 Wudy SA, Wachter UA, Homoki J, Teller WM: Determination of dehydroepiandrosterone sulfate in human plasma by gas chromatography/mass spectrometry using a deuterated internal standard: a method suitable for routine clinical use. Horm Res 1993;39:235–240.

27 Wudy SA, Wachter UA, Homoki J, Teller WM: 5α-androstane-3α,17ß-diol and 5α-androstane-3α,17ß-diol-glucuronide in plasma of normal children, adults and patients with idiopathic hirsutism: a mass spectrometric study. Eur J Endocrinol 1996;134:87–92.

28 Shackleton CHL, Kletke C, Wudy SA, Pratt JH: Dehydroepiandrosterone sulfate quantification in serum using high-performance liquid chromatography/mass spectrometry and deuterated internal standard: a technique suitable for routine use or as a reference method. Steroids 1990;55:472–478.

29 Honour JW: Steroid assays in paediatric endocrinology. J Clin Res Pediatr Endocrinol 2010;2:1–16.

30 Kao PC, Machacek DA, Magera MJ, Lacey JM, Rinaldo P: Diagnosis of adrenocortical dysfunction by liquid chromatography-tandem mass spectrometry. Ann Clin Lab Sci 2001;31:199–204.

31 Ceglarek U, Kortz L, Leichtle A, Fiedler GM, Krazsch J, Thiery J: Rapid quantification of steroid patterns in human serum by on-line solid phase extraction combined with liquid chromatography – triple quadrupole linear ion trap mass spectrometry. Clin Chim Acta 2009;401:114–118.

32 Soldin OP, Sharma H, Husted L, Soldin SJ: Pediatric reference intervals for aldosterone, 17α-hydroxyprogesterone, dehydroepiandrosterone, testosterone and 25-hydroxyvitamin D_3 using tandem mass spectrometry. Clin Biochem 2009;42:823–827.

33 Shiraishi S, Lee PW, Leung A, Goh VH, Serdloff RS, Wang C: Simultaneous measurement of serum testosterone and dihydrotestosterone by liquid chromatography-tandem mass spectrometry. Clin Chem 2008;54:1855–1863.

34 Kulle AE, Riepe FG, Melchior D, Hirot O, Holterhus PM: A novel ultraprssure liquid chromatography tandem mass spectrometry method for the simultaneous determination of androsteronedione, testosterone, and dihydrotestosterone in pediatric blood samples: age- and sex-specific reference data. J Clin Endocrionol Metab 2010;95:2399–2409.

Prof. Dr. Stefan A. Wudy
Steroid Research and Mass Spectrometry Unit, Pediatric Endocrinology and Diabetology
Justus-Liebig University, Feulgenstrasse 12
DE–35392 Giessen (Germany)
Tel. +49 641 99 434 00, Fax +49 641 99 434 59, E-Mail stefan.wudy@paediat.med.uni-giessen.de

Ranke MB, Mullis P-E (eds): Diagnostics of Endocrine Function in Children and Adolescents, ed 4.
Basel, Karger, 2011, pp 402–428

Assessing Endocrine Function in the Newborn Baby

A.L. Ogilvy-Stuart

Neonatal Unit, Rosie Hospital, Cambridge University Hospitals NHS Trust, Cambridge, UK

Endocrine disease in the newborn is uncommon, but may be life threatening or have profound long-term consequences if not diagnosed and treated promptly. Endocrine dysfunction, however, is not uncommon, particularly in the sick and preterm baby. The hormonal milieu is influenced by the mother and placenta and in addition, abrupt changes occur with parturition and interpretation of results needs to take this into account. In the baby born prematurely the situation is even more complex than the term baby. As the baby should be in utero, there are no truly 'normative' data with which to compare the results of a baby suspected of endocrine dysfunction.

Endocrine dysfunction may be suspected because of an anomaly found on examination including: (a) dysmorphic features, in particular, midline defects (central cleft palate and/or lip, hypotelorism, hypertelorism) which might suggest an abnormality of the hypothalamic-pituitary axis or features of a recognisable syndrome associated with endocrine dysfunction (table 1); (b) ambiguous genitalia or micropenis suggesting a disorder of sex development, hypopituitarism or a specific syndrome; (c) cryptorchidism which may be associated with a disorder of sex development and is a feature of several syndromes; (d) a pigmented scrotum; whilst the usual reason for a pigmented scrotum is racial or familial, it is a feature of excess adrenocorticotrophic hormone (ACTH); (e) large for gestational age, which is a feature of Beckwith Wiedemann syndrome (particularly if associated with exomphalos, abnormal ear creases and hypoglycaemia), or (f) symmetrical growth retardation.

Endocrine disease may also be suspected if there is cardiovascular collapse, hypotension (which might be picked up on 'routine' monitoring) particularly if associated with dehydration (excessive weight loss), electrolyte abnormalities, hypoglycaemia, or a history of birth asphyxia. There may also be a family history of similarly affected family members or sudden neonatal deaths.

Prolonged jaundice, both unconjugated and conjugated may be the presenting feature of adrenal or thyroid insufficiency (both primary and secondary).

Many of the symptoms and signs of endocrine dysfunction are non-specific and need to be considered in the differential diagnosis. These include poor feeding, jitteriness, irritability, hypotonia, hypertonia and convulsions. Particularly in the preterm baby, who is being monitored because of its prematurity, abnormalities may be picked up on 'routine' blood tests. Finally, screening tests specifically for endocrine abnormalities (hypothyroidism and congenital adrenal hyperplasia) may diagnose disease in an asymptomatic baby.

Neonatal Thyroid Function

When a baby is delivered at term, in response to a fall in the ambient temperature, there is an abrupt increase in both TRH and TSH with levels of TSH peaking at about 30 min of age to about 70 mU/l, before decreasing to normal infant levels by 3–5 days of age. This is accompanied by a brisk two- to sixfold increase in both T4 and T3 levels peaking at 2–3 days. Serum total and free T4 levels remain elevated for several weeks but are still higher at 6 months in term babies than they are in older children and adults [1]. T3 levels increase both in response to the TSH surge and secondary to increased conversion of T4 to the more metabolically active T3 by increased type 1 iodothyronine deiodinase activity in newborn tissues. In addition, placental separation decreases deiodination of T3 to inactive T2 which contributes to the high T3 levels [2]. TBG and prealbumin levels remain unchanged during this period. Levels of rT3 are high at birth and decrease to adult values over the first 2–3 weeks [3]. The healthy newborn baby is thus in a hyperthyroid state immediately after birth having been in a relatively hypothyroid state before delivery.

In the preterm infant born after 30 weeks' gestation, there is a similar but attenuated surge in TSH, T4 and T3 after birth. T4 and fT4 peak between 12 and 72 h and decline in a similar pattern to that seen in the term baby. In these babies, T4 and fT4 levels increase over the next 4–8 weeks to levels comparable to those of babies born at term [4–7]. In the baby born before 30 weeks' gestation and those with very low birth weight (<1,500 g), the TSH and T4 surge is limited or absent [7–12]. In babies born between 28 and 30 weeks' gestation, although the postnatal elevation in T4 is absent, the levels are similar to cord blood levels of babies of equivalent gestation at 7–14 days. FT4 levels are higher at 7–14 days than cord levels of equivalent gestational age cord samples. In contrast, the T4 levels at 7–14 days in babies born between 23 and 27 weeks' gestation fall compared with cord blood levels, and are lower than those of gestation matched cord blood levels. FT4 levels in this 23- to 27-week gestation group, however, remain within cord levels of those of equivalent gestational age. TSH levels in these preterm babies were higher in cord blood compared with days 7–28. TBG levels in all preterm babies (23–34 weeks' gestation), remain within gestation-matched cord levels over the first 28 days of life. TSH levels are similar in all gestational age groups when measured in cord blood, at 7, 14 and 28 days, being highest

Table 1. Dysmorphic syndromes associated with endocrine disease

Syndrome	Features	Endocrine disease	Gene mutations
Antley-Bixler syndrome	Craniosynostosis, midface hypoplasia, proptosis, choanal stenosis/atresia, humeroradial synostosis, bowing of the femora and ulnas, long bone fractures, long slender fingers with camptodactyly, cardiac and renal malformations	About 50% associated with ambiguous genitalia and adrenal dysfunction – may represent a distinct disorder caused by mutations in cytochrome P450 oxidoreductase (POR) gene In POR deficiency females may be virilized, and males undervirilized, and cortisol synthesis impaired	Can be caused by mutations in fibroblast growth factor receptor 2 gene (FGFR2)
Beckwith-Wiedemann syndrome	Ear creases, macroglossia, exomphalos, visceromegaly, hyperinsulinism Usually large for gestational age, with a large placenta and long umbilical cord Polyhydramnios may be present Increased incidence of Wilms' tumour, adrenal carcinoma, nephroblastoma, hepatoblastoma, and rhabdomyosarcoma	Transient hyperinsulinism	Caused by a mutation in the chromosome 11p15.5 region, with imprinting
Denys Drash syndrome	Genital ambiguity, congenital nephropathy and Wilms' tumour	Genital ambiguity	Caused by mutations in the Wilms' tumor suppressor (WT1) gene
DiGeorge syndrome	Outflow tract defects of heart Ear and eye anomailies, short philtrum, small mouth, micrognathia, cleft lip and deafness Short stature and mild-to-moderate learning difficulties Thymic hypoplasia	Hypocalcemia (parathyroid hypoplasia), hypothyroidism	Most cases result from a deletion of chromosome 22q11.2
Ectrodactyly, ectodermal dysaplasia, and cleft lip/palate (EEC) syndrome	Ectrodactyly of hands and feet, ectodermal dysplasia with severe keratitis Cleft lip/palate Maxillary hypoplasia, short philtrum, and broad nasal tip Choanal atresia	Associated with growth hormone deficiency and/or genital anomalies secondary to developmental defects of the hypothalamus	

Table 1. Continued

Syndrome	Features	Endocrine disease	Gene mutations
Fanconi anaemia	Cardiac, renal, and limb malformations skin pigmentary changes All marrow elements usually affected, resulting in anaemia, leucopenia, and thrombocytopenia Haematological abnormalities may not be manifest in the neonatal period	Genital anomalies are common in males, and there may be hypergonadotrophic hypogonadism	
Frasier syndrome	Genital ambiguity and renal failure	Streak gonads, genital ambiguity	Caused by mutation in the WT1
Hypoparathy-roidism-retardation-dysmorphism (HRD) (Sanjad-Sakati)	Dysmorphism (deep-set eyes, depressed nasal bridge with beaked nose, long philtrum, thin upper lip, micrognathia, and large floppy earlobes), growth retardation and developmental delay Medullary stenosis and other skeletal defects Reduced numbers of T cell subsets	Hypoparathyroidism: hypocalcaemia is associated with hyperphosphatemia and low concentrations of immunoreactive parathyroid hormone	
IMAGE (X chromo some)	Intrauterine growth retardation, genital anomalies (bilateral cryptorchidism, small penis), metaphyseal dysplasia, mild dysmorphic features	CAH, genital anomalies, hypogonadotropic hypogonadism hypercalciuria and/or hypercalcaemia	CAH presents most often either as an isolated abnormality, caused by mutations in the DAX1 gene
Kallman syndrome	Anosmia Small penis, cryptorchidism Choanal atresia and cleft lip or palate May represent the least severe form of the holoprosencephaly-hypopituitarism complex	Hypogonadotrophic hypogonadism Absent postnatal rise in LH and testosterone, with blunted response to GnRH and hCG	
Meacham syndrome	Sex reversal (XY males have undervirilization of the external genitalia, retention of müllerian structures and double vagina) Diaphragmatic hernia with hypoplastic or dysplastic lungs, and complex congenital heart disease	Ambiguous genitalia	Now thought that this syndrome may be associated with WT1 mutations

Table 1. Continued

Syndrome	Features	Endocrine disease	Gene mutations
Mullerian derivatives, persistence of, with lymphangiectasia and postaxial polydactyly (Urioste syndrome)	Prenatal growth deficiency, hypertrophied alveolar ridges, redundant nuchal skin, and postaxial polydactyly XY karyotype with cryptorchidism, small penis, and internal Müllerian duct remnants Renal anomalies Lymphangiectasia, protein-losing enteropathy Early death	Prenatal growth deficiency Male undervirilization	
Pallister-Hall syndrome	Neonatally lethal malformation syndrome Polydactyly, imperforate anus, laryngeal cleft, bifid epiglottis, abnormal lung lobation, renal agenesis or dysplasia, short 4th metacarpals, nail dysplasia, multiple buccal frenula, microphallus, congenital heart defect, and intrauterine growth retardation Dysmorphic facial features	Hypothalamic hamartoblastoma, hypopituitarism, hypoadrenalism	
Robinow syndrome	Characteristic facial features, cleft lip/palate, shortened tongue with midline indentation Hypoplastic genitalia, hypospadias or cryptorchidism, renal abnormalities Webbed digits/broad or bifid thumb Mesomelic bachymelia/short stature (may give the impression of achondroplasia, but distinguished by radiological features), vertebral anomalies Hip dislocation Intelligence may be normal	Hypoplastic genitalia, hypospadias or cryptorchidism Adult males show partial primary hypogonadism, whereas gonadal function and fertility in females seems to be normal	Inheritance can be autosomal-recessive (ROR2 gene on chromosme 9q22 affecting cartilage and bone formation) or dominant The autosomal-recessive form has been shown to be caused by homozygous mutations in the ROR2 gene Heterozygous mutations in the same gene cause autosomal-dominant brachydactyly B The recessive Robinow syndrome tends to be more severe

Table 1. Continued

Syndrome	Features	Endocrine disease	Gene mutations
Short rib-polydactyly (SRPS) type II (Majewski syndrome)	Median cleft lip, pre- and postaxial polysyndactyly, short ribs and limbs, anomalies of epiglottis and viscera Hydrops, malformation of the larynx, pulmonary hypoplasia, glomerular and renal tubular cysts or polycystic kidneys, ambiguous genitalia Death occurs perinatally	Ambiguous genitalia	
Smith-Lemli-Opitz syndrome	Clinical and biochemical spectrum of severity Small for gestational age, microcephaly, epicanthic folds, ptosis, broad nasal tip with anteverted nostrils, micrognathia, slanted or low-set ears Post-axial polydactyly, syndactyly of 2nd and 3rd toes Cataracts, cleft palate, congenital heart disease, pulmonary abnormalities Renal hypoplasia, hypospadias or cryptorchidism or sex reversal May be hyotonic, distinctive shrill cry	Hypospadias or cryptorchidism or sex reversal (i.e. XY with female phenotype) Plasma cholesterol is low and 7-dehydrocholesterol elevated	Caused by mutations in the sterol delta-7-reductase gene, which maps to 11q12-q13
Velocardiofacial (Shprintzen) syndrome	Cleft palate, cardiac anomalies, dysmorphic facies (narrow almond-shaped palpebral fissures, prominent tubular nose, slightly retruded mandible, myopathic facies, and small open mouth) Learning disabilities Hypernasal speech	Neonatal hypocalcaemia	Velocardiofacial syndrome and DiGeorge syndrome may result from mutations in the same genes (chromosome 22q11)
Williams' syndrome	Elfin facies with hypercalcaemia, supravalvular aortic stenosis , multiple peripheral pulmonary arterial stenoses Mild-to-moderate mental retardation with disproportionately strong language skills Dental malformations		95–98% have a deletion on band 7q11.23 near the elastin gene Most cases are sporadic, but some are autosomal dominant
Wilms' tumour WT1 'WAGR'	Susceptibility to Wilms' tumour, aniridia, genitourinary abnormalities, mental retardation, hemihypertrophy Gonadoblastoma	Genital anomalies	A constitutional deletion on chromosome 11p13 affects several contiguous genes, resulting in a constellation of defects

in the cord sample and constant from 7 days. T3 levels in all preterm babies rise in the 4 weeks after birth compared with cord levels and remain above gestation equivalent cord samples. Conversely, rT3 levels fall after birth and are lower than gestation equivalent cord samples [12].

Although the more preterm the baby, the more marked the hypothyroxinaemia, T4 levels also reflect the severity of the neonatal illness, with the sickest babies having the lowest T4 levels. A number of factors probably contribute to the aetiology of the hypothyroxinaemia, including loss of the contribution of maternal T4 from placental transfer, immaturity of the hypothalamic-pituitary-thyroid axis, immaturity of peripheral tissue deiodination and negative iodine balance in the first few weeks after birth. This may be compounded by the use of drugs which reduce the pituitary secretion of TSH (such as dopamine and glucocorticoids), the use of iodine-containing antiseptic and contrast media, and iodine deficiency in areas of the world with low environmental iodine. The hypothyroxinaemia may be a feature of non-thyroidal illness (sick euthyroid syndrome) and an adaptive response to illness, resulting in a reduced metabolic rate.

Hypothyroxinaemia of Prematurity

Whilst hypothyroxinaemia is associated with an increased mortality and morbidity (including prolonged need for mechanical ventilation and oxygen supplementation, prolonged hospital stay, an increase in intraventricular haemorrhage and white matter echolucencies, a reduction in IQ and cerebral palsy) [13–19], supplementation with thyroid hormones does not appear to improve outcome [20, 21].

Interpreting Thyroid Function in Babies of Mothers with Autoimmune Thyroid Disease
Foetal and neonatal thyroid function can be affected by maternal autoimmune thyroid disease (Hashimoto's thyroiditis or Graves' disease). The TSH receptor antibodies which block or stimulate the maternal thyroid gland may cross the placenta and block or stimulate the foetal (and after delivery, neonatal) thyroid gland. These antibodies may still be present and affect foetal (and then neonatal) thyroid function even after treatment of maternal thyrotoxicosis with surgery or radioiodine. Thionamides used in the treatment of maternal thyrotoxicosis may also cross the placenta and render the foetus hypothyroid. TSH receptor antibody levels from the mother in the third trimester correlate well with the likelihood of the baby developing thyroid dysfunction.

If the maternal TRH receptor antibody level is within normal limits in the third trimester, and the mother not taking anti-thyroid treatment, no specific investigations are required for the baby after birth except routine screening for congenital hypothyroidism.

If the TSH receptor antibody levels are high or unknown, the baby is at risk of transient hypo- or hyperthyroidism. The assays used do not differentiate stimulating from blocking antibodies, and both may co-exist. Indeed, postnatal hypothyroidism secondary to blocking antibodies may be followed by hyperthyroidism. Generally, foetal and neonatal thyroid function is unaffected unless the antibody levels are in excess of 3–5 times the upper limit of the normal range of the assay [22].

Babies at high risk of hyperthyroidism should be followed carefully. A cord blood sample for a TSH level and TSH receptor antibody level can be helpful. If the TSH level is already suppressed on the cord blood sample, thyrotoxicosis should be suspected.

Careful clinical and biochemical review of both TSH and fT4 over the first 2 weeks is recommended for high-risk babies. Thyroid function does need to be interpreted in line with the expected normal value for day of life; in particular, T4 levels will normally be high as described above.

Adrenal Function in the Newborn

Plasma cortisol in well term babies rises after birth to about 200–300 nmol/l and then falls to around 100–200 nmol/l by day 7 and can fall below 100 nmol/l in the second week of life [23, 24].

Cortisol levels in preterm babies are higher than well term babies (but similar to sick term babies) [25–28]. Cortisol rises after birth to about 300–400 nmol/l in preterm babies, falling to about 280 nmol/l by day 7 and falling further thereafter. Normal cortisol levels may be as low as 28–55 nmol/l [26]. Cortisol is released in a pulsatile manner with 5 secretory bursts in 6 h and the cortisol production rate is around 8 mg/m^2/day in term babies and 21 ± 11 mg/m^2/day in preterm babies. Diurnal variation in cortisol develops at 8–12 weeks of age in term infants [29, 30]. Preterm infants >31 weeks' gestation develop diurnal variation at a similar postnatal age in the home environment, but hospitalized infants below this gestation do not [31].

Although cortisol production rates in preterm infants are not low, differences in hypothalamic-pituitary-adrenal response to stimulation have been associated with differences in clinical course suggesting that preterm babies may not produce sufficient cortisol for their requirements, i.e. they have relative adrenal insufficiency. This may contribute to the aetiology of inotrope unresponsive hypotension, which often has a prompt response to hydrocortisone treatment [32]. Attempts to link random cortisol levels with clinical outcome/illness severity have been largely unsuccessful; however, a reduced cortisol response to ACTH in preterm infants in the first week of life has been associated with an increased incidence of chronic lung disease, and similar findings have been reported with CRH testing [33]. There are no truly 'normative' cortisol levels in the preterm baby. Levels are influenced by glucocorticoids administered to the mother because of the imminent preterm delivery [34].

Adrenal dysfunction may be suspected in the baby with ambiguous genitalia, particularly if there is excessive pigmentation. The latter, which is commonly but not exclusively scrotal, may be a feature of adrenal insufficiency without genital ambiguity. Abnormities in electrolytes (high potassium levels and low sodium levels) may also suggest adrenal dysfunction; however, in practice, fluid overload and renal impairment are more likely, particularly in the preterm and sick newborn baby. Adrenal insufficiency may also present as hypotension or cardiovascular collapse.

In the baby in whom adrenal failure is suspected, a history of asphyxia may point to a diagnosis of bilateral adrenal haemorrhage. A history of maternal steroid excess (Cushing's syndrome or therapeutic administration) may result in adrenal suppression. These, however, usually have little effect on the baby as the enzyme 11β-hydroxysteroid dehydrogenase 2 in placental and foetal tissues will inactivate 80% of maternal cortisol. However, synthetic glucocorticoids such as dexamethasone are a poor substrate for this enzyme and so reach the foetus to exert pharmacological effects.

Assessment of the baby should include a measurement of blood pressure, assessment of the degree of hydration, a blood glucose level and serum electrolytes.

Causes of primary adrenal failure are given in the chapter by Flück [this vol.].

Investigation of Suspected Adrenal Insufficiency

A detailed description of the investigation of adrenal insufficiency is covered in the chapter by Flück [this vol.]. This includes a discussion on ACTH levels which may be helpful in differentiating primary adrenal insufficiency from abnormalities of the hypothalamic-pituitary axis, and the methodology of the standard ACTH test. The dose of ACTH in the newborn is dependent on local protocol (e.g. 36 µg/kg or a standard dose of 62.5 µm i.v. or i.m.). The response will be poor but not absent in chronic ACTH deficiency. An absent response is seen in familial glucocorticoid deficiency. The depot preparations are contraindicated in neonates.

Specific points in the newborn:

(1) Equivocal cortisol results after ACTH administration are sometimes obtained in the neonatal period.

(2) Low-dose ACTH tests in the newborn: Whilst the standard test involves a supramaximal dose, much smaller doses have been used to assess the response of the adrenal gland to a more physiological stimulus (doses as low as 500 ng/1.73 m²), usually on a research basis in preterm infants. It has the advantage that it may be more sensitive at picking up subtle abnormalities of adrenal function, but it does make a 'sub-optimal' response difficult to interpret. What constitutes a normal response to such a low stimulus in the preterm infant has yet to be determined. The 10th centile cortisol response 30 min after a 1 µg/kg dose in extremely low birth weight infants has been reported to be 469 nmol/l [35].

(3) It may be helpful in investigating the newborn with suspected adrenal insufficiency to include at least 3 random cortisol measurements before performing an ACTH test. Single samples are difficult to interpret because of the pulsatile manner of cortisol secretion, so taking three samples makes it less likely that all three will fall in a nadir.

(4) Infants mount a poor cortisol response to hypoglycaemia (usually measured as part of a 'hypoglycaemia screen' on a baby found to clinically or incidentally hypoglycaemic) and is not a reliable way of excluding adrenal insufficiency in the newborn [36].

(5) A urine steroid profile will determine the site of block in adrenal hormone synthesis in congenital adrenal hyperplasia (CAH). A 24-hour sample is not usually obtained but the ratio of the different metabolites in the collected random sample is used.

(6) An adrenal ultrasound scan can be useful to determine if there is bilateral adrenal haemorrhage or hypertrophy (seen in CAH).

Genetic Analysis

The transcription factors DAX1 and SF1 have an important role in differentiation and development of the adreno-gonadal primordium, which gives rise to both the adrenal cortex and the gonads. SF1 is the major gene with an important role in regulation of steroidogenesis, reproduction and male sexual differentiation. Nuclear localisation of DAX1 is tightly coupled with that of SF, and DAX1 is thought to be a transcriptional repressor of SF1 action. DAX1 is expressed in adrenal cortex, testis, ovary, anterior pituitary and hypothalamus.

DAX1 mutations cause adrenal hypoplasia congenita, an X-linked disorder causing adrenal insufficiency and hypogonadotropic hypogonadism and impaired spermatogenesis.

SF1 mutations can be dominantly or recessively inherited and are associated with adrenal failure and XY sex reversal with the presence of müllerian structures. The developing testes appear to be more SF1 dose-dependent than the adrenals and so not all have adrenal failure.

StAR (steroidogenic acute regulatory protein) mutations cause congenital lipoid adrenal hyperplasia (large adrenals full of cholesterol esters). Absence of aldosterone production causes salt loss, but presenting later than infants with 21-hydroxylase deficiency. Lack of testosterone production by Leydig cells leads to XY sex reversal.

Specific genetic tests for these mutations may be helpful if the clinical picture suggests a mutation may be possible.

Assessment of Ambiguous Genitalia

The history may be informative. It should include details of the pregnancy, including the use of drugs which may virilize a female foetus or previous neonatal deaths (which might point to an undiagnosed adrenal crisis). A history of virilization of the mother may suggest an androgen-secreting tumour or aromatase deficiency. The family history may reveal consanguinity (increasing the probability of an autosomal-recessive condition) or a history of genital ambiguity in other family members (which might point towards an X-linked recessive disorder such as androgen insensitivity).

Examination should assess whether there are dysmorphic features as a number of syndromes are associated with genital ambiguity (table 1). The state of hydration and blood pressure should be assessed as various forms of CAH can be associated with salt loss and hypertension, although cardiovascular collapse does not usually occur until after the 4th day of life. Examination of the external genitalia will determine the degree of virilization (Prader stages 1–5; fig. 1) and whether the gonads are palpable.

The initial investigations ascertain whether the baby is an undervirilised male or a virilised female and from these a differential diagnosis is established and further investigations planned (fig. 2). An urgent karyotype should be sent. Rapid FISH studies using probes specific for the X (DX1) and Y (SRY) chromosomes are useful although a full karyotype is required for confirmation and exclusion of mosaicism.

Genital Ambiguity with a 46XX Karyotype Indicates a Virilised Female

The female foetus with ovaries and normal internal genitalia has been exposed to excessive testosterone, and hence dihydrotestosterone (by conversion of testosterone by 5α-reductase) which virilises the external genitalia. The androgens may be derived from the foetal adrenal gland (CAH and placental aromatase deficiency), foetal gonad (the testis or ovotestis in true hermaphroditism), or rarely, exogenously via transplacental passage from the mother (adrenal or ovarian tumours).

Absence of palpable gonads in association with otherwise apparently male genitalia should always alert one to the possibility of a virilised female. By far the commonest cause of this is CAH. Of the enzyme defects that cause virilization in female foetuses, 21-hydroxylase deficiency is the most frequent (accounting for 90–95%, UK incidence 1:15–20,000). Diagnosis is made on an elevated serum 17-hydroxyprogesterone (17-OHP) level. This level may be elevated in the first 48 h in normal babies, and may be significantly elevated in sick and preterm babies in the absence of CAH. Hence, the sample should be delayed until after the first 48 h. Although the 17-OHP levels are usually extremely high with CAH, if there is doubt a synacthen test should be performed (see below). The other enzyme defects that can cause virilization of female foetuses are 11β-hydroxylase deficiency (where the 11-deoxycortisol levels will be elevated) and less commonly 3β-hydroxysteroid dehydrogenase deficiency (diagnosed by elevated 17-hydroxypregnenolone and dehydroepiandrosterone).

If CAH is confirmed, the electrolytes need to be watched closely as salt wasting occurs in 70% of cases of 21-hydroxylase deficiency, usually between days 4 and 15. Mineralocorticoid deficiency induces a rise in serum potassium levels (usually the first sign of salt-wasting) and sodium levels fall. Urinary sodium levels will be inappropriately high. Further confirmatory tests for CAH are DHEA, androstenedione, testosterone, ACTH and plasma renin activity, all of which may be elevated. From day 3 of life, the ratio of urinary steroid metabolites will be altered depending upon the site of the block, and is very helpful in the diagnosis of 21-OHD and the rarer forms

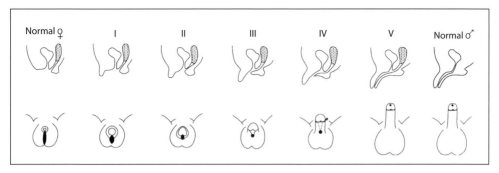

Fig. 1. Prader staging of the internal and external genitalia.

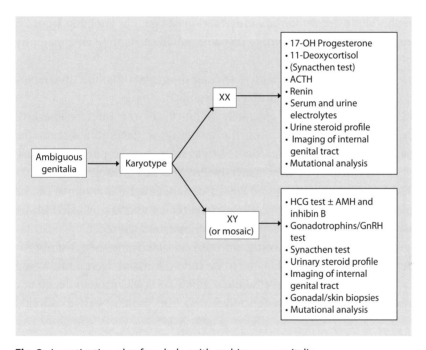

Fig. 2. Investigation plan for a baby with ambiguous genitalia.

of CAH. A skilled ultrasound examination will show normal internal genitalia, but an examination under anaesthesia may be required to confirm the presence of normal müllerian structures, and to demonstrate the level of entry of the vagina into the urogenital sinus, in the case of a single perineal opening.

The excessive androgen may be gonadal in origin – usually from an ovotestis or testis in a true hermaphrodite. Whilst the commonest karyotype of the true hermaphrodite is 46XX (70.6%), the next commonest karyotype is a chromosomal mosaicism containing a Y chromosome (usually 46XX/46XY) (20.2%) [37]. It is important to check fibroblast and or gonadal genotype in these babies which may contain a mosaic cell line.

Transplacental transfer of androgen may rarely occur if the mother has androgen-secreting tumour (she may be virilised as a result) or from drugs given during pregnancy. Placental aromatase deficiency, by inhibiting the conversion of androgens to oestrogens, may cause virilization of a female foetus, and, in addition, maternal virilization occurs from placental transfer of the excessive foetal androgens [38].

Conditions that cause virilization of a female foetus are listed in table 2.

Genital Ambiguity with a 46XY Karyotype Indicates an Undervirilised Male
A genetically XY male is a male with two testes, but whose genital tract fails to differentiate normally. There are numerous presentations of genital anomaly from an apparently normal female (Prader 1) with a palpable gonad through to an apparently normal male with hypospadias (Prader IV).

The three main diagnostic categories are testicular dysgenesis/malfunction, a biosynthetic defect and end-organ unresponsiveness (table 2).

If the gonads are palpable, they are likely to be testes (or rarely ovotestes). Investigations are directed at determining the anatomy of the internal genitalia, and establishing whether the testicular tissue is capable of producing androgens. Investigations that may help with the former include pelvic ultrasound, examination under anaesthetic with cystoscopy and laparoscopy. Genital skin biopsies can be taken at the time of endoscopies. Occasionally, urogenital sinogram or MRI can be helpful. Laparoscopy/laparotomy and gonadal biopsy may be required.

The principal aims of the initial investigations are to determine the most appropriate sex of rearing and in a genetic female, to exclude CAH and avert a salt losing crisis. Rarer forms of CAH (steroidogenic acute regulatory; StAR) protein deficiency and 3β-hydroxysteroid dehydrogenase deficiency may also present with an adrenal crisis.

Determination of the Internal Anatomy
The degree of virilization of the internal genital tracts is defined by Prader stages 1–5 (fig. 1). Ultrasound may determine the anatomy of the vagina or a urogenital sinus and uterus, locate inguinal gonads (although is not sensitive for intra-abdominal gonads), visualize the adrenal glands and exclude associated renal anomalies particularly if Denys-Drash syndrome is suspected or proven.

Ultrasound sensitivity and accuracy depends on probe resolution and requires an experienced ultrasonographer.

Further delineation of anatomy may require an examination under anaethetic/cystoscopy, urogenital sonogram, MRI, or laparoscopy. MRI or laparoscopy may also be required to identify the gonads. Gonadal and genital skin biopsies can be performed at the time of laparoscopy.

Table 2. Disorders of sex differentiation

Virilisation of XX females
Increased foetal adrenal androgen production
    Congenital adrenal hyperplasia (3β-hydroxysteroid dehydrogenase deficiency,
    21-hydroxylasedeficiency, 11β-hydroxylase deficiency)
    Androgen secreting tumour
    Placental aromatase deficiency

Foetal gonadal androgen production
    True hermaphrodite with both testicular and ovarian tissue

---

Transplacental passage of maternal androgens
    Drugs administered during pregnancy, e.g. progesterone, danazole
    Maternal androgen secreting tumour, luteoma of pregnancy

Other causes
    Dysmorphic syndromes
    Prematurity – prominent clitoris

Bisexual gonads
    Hermaphroditism; usual genotype 46XX

Undervirilisation of XY males

Testicular dysgenesis/malfunction
    Pure XY gonadal dysgenesis
    Mixed gonadal dysgenesis – 45X/46XY; may be associated with gene mutations
    on SRY, SOX9, or WT1 genes
    Dysgenetic testis
    Testicular regression syndromes
        True agonadism, rudimentary testis syndrome

Biosynthetic defect – decreased foetal androgen biosynthesis

Leydig cell hypoplasia (LH deficiency or LH receptor defect)

    Testosterone biosynthesis (non-virilising CAH): (StAR, 3b-HSD, 17α-OHD/17–20 lyase,
    Smith-Lemli-Opitz syndrome)
    5a-reductase deficiency
    Deficient synthesis or action of AMH – persistent müllerian duct syndrome; may be due to
    mutations in AMH or AMH receptor gene or SF1 gene

End organ unresponsiveness
    Androgen receptor and post-receptor defects (complete and incomplete
    androgen insensitivity syndrome)

Others
    Urogenital malformations
    Dysmorphic syndromes
    Exogenous maternal oestrogens

Testosterone Response to Human Chorionic Gonadotrophin (hCG)

To determine if functioning Leydig cells are present (i.e. capable of producing testosterone in response to LH), an hCG stimulation test is undertaken. This is also used to delineate a block in testosterone biosynthesis from androstenedione (17β-hydroxysteroid dehydrogenase deficiency) or conversion of testosterone to DHT (5α-reductase deficiency). There are a variety of protocols for the hCG test, but essentially it involves taking baseline samples for testosterone and its precursors dehydroepiandrosterone [DHEA] (or DHEA sulphate [DHEAS]) and androstenedione and its metabolite (DHT). One to three intramuscular injections of high-dose hCG (500–1,500 IU) are given at 24-hour intervals and repeat androgen samples are taken at 72 or 24 h after the last injection. The neonatal gonad is more active than at anytime in childhood until puberty reaching a peak at about 6–8 weeks of age. A balance needs to be reached between performing the hCG test when the gonad is normally most active (testosterone secretion normally rises in the fourth week of life, peaking at 1–3 months [39–41]) and proceeding with the investigations as promptly as possible. Whilst some would advocate this test is deferred beyond 2 weeks of age, this may not be necessary.

Interpretation of Results

- In the neonatal period, testosterone would be expected to reach adult levels after hCG with a two- to threefold increase from basal levels.
- If testicular function is poor, the response is blunted.
- An absent response with elevated gonadotrophins suggests primary gonadal failure.
- An absent response with elevation of testosterone precursors suggests a block in testosterone biosynthesis.
- A rise in testosterone with no rise in DHT suggests 5α-reductase deficiency.

The hCG test can be extended to a 3-week test if the 3-day hCG test is inconclusive. The same dose of hCG is administered twice weekly for 3 weeks and testosterone, DHT and androstenedione are taken 24 h after the last hCG injection. The clinical response in terms of testicular descent and change in the size of the phallus and frequency of erections should be documented. Photographs before and after hCG administration may be helpful.

Anti-Müllerian Hormone and Inhibin B Levels

Whilst hCG stimulation tests the function of the Leydig cells, both anti-müllerian hormone (AMH) and inhibin B are secreted by the Sertoli cells. Inhibin B is detectable for the first 6 months, rising again at puberty. AMH levels are high in human male serum postnatally for several years before declining during the peripubertal period, but AMH is undetectable in female serum until the onset of puberty. AMH may prove to be a more sensitive marker for the presence of testicular tissue than serum testosterone levels, both before and after the neonatal androgen surge, and, consequently, may obviate the need for hCG stimulation in the evaluation of certain intersex disorders [42]. Similarly, basal inhibin B has been shown to predict the testosterone response to hCG in boys and therefore may give reliable information about both the presence and function of the testes. Furthermore, inhibin B levels have been shown to demonstrate specific alterations in patients with genital ambiguity which may aid the differential diagnosis of male undervirilization [43]. However, these assays are not routinely available.

Assessment of Gonadotrophins
Assessment of the gonadotrophins may give useful information. Elevated basal gonadotrophins are consistent with primary gonadal failure. The gonadotrophin response to GnRH is difficult to interpret in the prepubertal child unless exaggerated, which is consistent with gonadal failure but adds little to the basal levels alone. Pituitary failure would give a flat response but is not diagnostic and hypothalamic abnormalities such as Kallmann's syndrome are not excluded by a 'normal' response The optimal time to assess this is within the first 6 months of life when there is a gonadal surge in both sexes (girls greater than boys), and the axis is hence maximally responsive.

Assessment of Adrenal Function

Urine Steroid Profile
Output of adrenal steroids will be low in adrenal insufficiency. In CAH, specific ratios of metabolites will be altered depending on the level of the enzyme block.

Synacthen Test
A standard short synacthen is useful in the following situations:
1 Suspected CAH where a peak 17-OHP of 100–200 nmol/l is suggestive of 21-hydroxylase deficiency (higher reference ranges for preterm infants).
2 Suspected CAH to assess adrenal cortical reserve (measurement of cortisol levels).

Interpretation of Results
Adrenal Function – Cortisol
See chapter by Flück [this vol.].

Note: A normal basal cortisol value, or even a normal stimulated response does not exclude the evolution of adrenal insufficiency, and may need to be repeated depending upon clinical suspicion. A basal ACTH level may be helpful but in most laboratories the turnaround time is slower than for cortisol.

Interpretation in 21-Hydroxylase Deficiency
With a block in cortisol synthesis, the 17-OHP level will rise after synacthen but there will be little increase in cortisol.

Skin and Gonadal Biopsies

Genital skin biopsies (2–4 mm) collected at the time of EUA or genitoplasty are useful to establish cell lines for androgen receptor-binding assays and analysis of 5α-reductase activity. The cell line is also a source of genomic DNA and RNA and/or subsequent molecular and functional studies. Karyotype analysis for the presence of mosaicism may be indicated. Gonadal biopsies are essential when considering diagnostic categories such as dysgenesis and true hermaphroditism. A detailed histopathological report is essential. As special treatment of the samples may be required, prior discussion with the pathologist or genetics laboratory should take place.

Reaching a Diagnosis in Male Undervirilisation

Testicular Dysgenesis/Malfunction

A 46 XY karyotype, with low basal and hCG-stimulated testosterone and low testosterone precursors suggests either gonadal dysgenesis (which may require laparoscopy and testicular biopsy) or lipoid CAH (caused by an abnormality in the StAR protein). In the latter condition, total adrenal failure is confirmed on synacthen test, electrolytes and urinary steroids. Because of the other associated gene defects, there may be other anomalies such as bony dysplasias or renal anomalies, which should be looked for.

The poorly functioning testicular tissue is likely to give a subnormal testosterone response to hCG and basal gonadotrophins will usually be elevated, consistent with primary gonadal failure. In addition, the dysgenetic testes may secrete inadequate amounts of anti-müllerian hormone, and müullerian structures may be present (although often hypoplastic) in children with gonadal dysgenesis and a 46XY karyotype.

A mosaic karyotype, e.g. 45,X/46,XY suggests gonadal dysgenesis. There is a very variable phenotype both in terms of internal and external genitalia, which is not dependent on the percentage of each karyotype as determined by lymphocyte analysis. Over 90% of individuals with a prenatally diagnosed 45,X/46,XY karyotype have a normal male phenotype suggesting that most individuals with this karyotype escape detection and an ascertainment bias exists toward those with clinically evident abnormalities [44, 45].

Biosynthetic Defect

A 46XY karyotype, low basal and peak testosterone level on hCG testing, often with elevated gonadotrophins, suggests a diagnosis of an inactivating mutation of the LH receptor (Leydig cell hypoplasia).

This condition is associated with a variable phenotype from a completely phenotypic female to undervirilisation of varying degrees [46].

A 46XY karyotype with normal or elevated basal and peak testosterone on hCG test, and an elevated T:DHT ratio is seen in 5α-reductase deficiency. DHT-dependent virilization of the external genitalia is deficient, resulting in a small phallus and perineal hypospadias. Wolffian structures are normal but spermatogenesis is usually impaired [47]. This condition is rare in the UK, but recognized in the Dominican Republic where individuals are often raised as female and convert to male in puberty when their body habitus and psychosexual orientation becomes male. Virilization improves but is incomplete.

A biochemical diagnosis is made by demonstrating a ratio of T:DHT >30 after puberty or following hCG stimulation before puberty, and the ratio of 5α:5β metabolites in a urine steroid profile will be elevated after 6 months of age. The urinary 5α:5β metabolites can also be used if the gonads have been removed. The diagnosis is confirmed by screening for mutations in the 5α-reductase type II gene (5RD5A2).

A 46XY karyotype, low basal and hCG-stimulated testosterone levels with elevated testosterone precursors indicates a testosterone biosynthetic defect.

Those forms of CAH that cause undervirilization of male genitalia include 17α-hydroxylase/17,20 lyase deficiency and 3β-hydroxysteroid dehydrogenase deficiency.

The conversion of androstenedione to testosterone occurs predominantly in the gonad and a post-hCG stimulated ratio of androstenedione to testosterone of >20:1 suggests 17β-hydroxysteroid dehydrogenase deficiency. A urine steroid profile is generally not helpful in this diagnosis before puberty. Molecular analysis of the HSD III gene (HSD17B3) is sought as confirmation of the diagnosis.

End Organ Unresponsiveness

A 46XY karyotype with genital ambiguity, normal or elevated basal and peak testosterone on hCG test, and a normal T:DHT ratio points to partial androgen insensitivity.

There is a variable phenotype, and sex of rearing depends upon the degree of phallic development, and sometimes cultural considerations. The child may benefit from a trial of topical DHT cream or intramuscular testosterone (e.g. using 12.5–25 mg monthly for 3 months) on penile growth to help anticipate response in puberty.

The diagnosis is suggested by demonstrating an abnormality in androgen binding in genital skin fibroblasts and subsequently demonstrating a mutation in the androgen receptor gene. This requires DNA and a genital skin biopsy taken at the time of EUA or genital surgery. Despite clear evidence of a phenotype consistent with partial androgen PAIS and normal production and metabolism of androgens, only a minority of patients are found to have an androgen receptor gene mutation. The likelihood of finding a mutation is increased if there is a family history consistent with X-linkage.

The majority of XY infants with undervirilisation remain unexplained.

DNA Analysis

Many of the causes of genital ambiguity have a genetic basis, and in these cases genetic counselling will be required. For example, androgen insensitivity syndrome is X-linked recessive and CAH is autosomal recessive. In addition, identification and characterization of a number of mutations of the genes involved in sexual differentiation has resulted in DNA tests which can be used in prenatal diagnosis. Identification of carriers will facilitate genetic counselling.

Congenital Adrenal Hyperplasia

Several laboratories undertake DNA analysis for this condition. Once the diagnosis has been made, a DNA sample should be taken from the proband. If a gene mutation is identified, the carrier status of the parents may be determined and the family should be counselled about the possibility of antenatal screening of subsequent pregnancies and of steroid treatment of the mother in an attempt to reduce virilization of a subsequent affected female foetus.

Androgen Insensitivity

DNA analysis may be performed in suspected cases where clinical, biochemical and histological data are consistent with an androgen-insensitive pathophysiology.

DNA samples in patients with suspected 5α-reductase deficiency and 17β-hydroxy-steroid dehydrogenase may also help in the diagnosis.

Mutations of developmental genes such as DAX1, SOX9 and WT1 may account for rarer cases of sexual ambiguity. Samples should be taken and DNA extracted and either stored or forwarded to the relevant laboratories depending upon clinical suspicion.

Investigation of Hypercalcaemia and Hypocalcaemia in the Newborn

The foetus is entirely dependent on the mother for the calcium and phosphorus required for skeletal development and tissue growth and function. From 15 weeks' gestation both total and ionized concentrations are higher in the foetus than in the mother due to active transport across the placenta, stimulated by parathyroid hormone (PTH)-related peptide (PTHrP) produced in the foetal parathyroid glands, the placenta, the chorion and amnion and augmented by vitamin D from the foetal kidney and placenta [48]. Calcium levels are independent of maternal calcium levels.

The most rapid accretion of calcium in the foetus occurs in the third trimester, with 30–35 g/day actively transported across the placenta. About 200 mg of calcium is added to the foetal skeleton at the end of pregnancy [49]. Whole body bone mineral density is related to gestation as well as body length and weight [49].

While PTHrP levels are high in the foetus, PTH levels are low. PTH does not stimulate placental calcium transport but is secreted from foetal parathyroid glands in response to hypocalcaemia, and suppressed in response to hypercalcaemia.

At birth, cord blood levels correlate with gestational age and are about 0.25–0.5 mmol/l higher than maternal levels. With clamping of the cord, calcium levels fall rapidly in the first 6 h, ionized calcium reaching a nadir of 1.2–1.45 mmol/l at 24 h [48, 50]. The newborn baby is now dependent on parathyroid PTH secretion, dietary calcium, renal calcium reabsorption, skeletal calcium stores and vitamin D. PTH levels increase on the first day of life in response to the fall in serum calcium levels peaking at 48 h. However, there is a nadir in serum calcium levels within the first 2 days of life. Calcitriol levels also rise. In the first 2–4 weeks after birth, there is increased efficiency of intestinal absorption of calcium [48]. Renal tubular handling matures over this period. Accretion of bone calcium continues at a rate of 150 mg/kg/day for several months after birth.

Serum phosphate levels are maximal in the neonate as there is decreased glomerular filtration and increased tubular reabsorption.

Hypocalcaemia

This is defined as a total calcium <2.2 mmol/l or ionized calcium <1.2 mmol/l. Ionized calcium level should be measured in the preterm baby as the normal relationship with total calcium is atypical. Physiological hypocalcaemia occurs after birth as the transplacental calcium supply is cut, there is insufficient supply from the GI tract and insufficient release of PTH from the immature parathyroid gland. Total calcium levels drop to about 2 mmol/l and ionized to about 1.2 mmol/l with the nadir in calcium level occurring within the first 48 h [51, 52].

Hypocalcaemia is common, it is usually physiological, or an exaggeration of the normal physiological response, or iatrogenic and short lasting. Other causes of hypocalcaemia are rare and aetiologies are conventionally grouped according to the time of onset. Early hypocalcaemia (occurring within 72 from birth) is caused by an exaggeration of normal fall in serum calcium. Late hypocalcaemia (after 72 h of age) is considered to be a manifestation of relative resistance of the immature kidney to PTH resulting in retention of phosphate levels and loss of calcium.

The usual presentation is incidental asymptomatic hypocalcaemia on 'routine' blood samples. Symptoms include neuromuscular irritability (myoclonic jerks, jitteriness, exaggerated startle responses, seizures), apnoea, cyanosis, tachypnoea, vomiting, laryngospasm, or cardiac symptoms and signs (tachycardia, heart failure, prolonged Q-T interval on electrocardiogram, decreased contractility). Severe vitamin D deficiency may present with cardiomyopathy. There may be the dysmorphic features of DiGeorge syndrome/CATCH-22 (table 1). History may reveal that the baby is preterm, birth depression, infant of a diabetic mother, or an abnormality in maternal calcium metabolism.

It is important to exclude other differential diagnoses of common non-specific symptoms (above) (including sepsis, meningitis, hypoglycaemia, hypomagnesaemia, intracranial haemorrhage).

Early Onset (First 72 h). In the preterm baby and delivery following pre-eclampsia, hypocalcaemia after birth is common. Possible mechanisms include a blunted

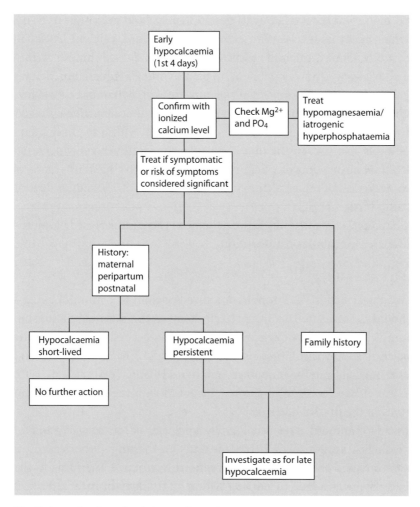

Fig. 3. Investigation of early hypocalcaemia.

increase in PTH, a prolonged increase in calcitonin, rapid accretion of skeletal calcium and relative resistance to vitamin D-induced resorption of bone and absorption of calcium from the gut. Hypocalcaemia also commonly occurs in asphyxiated babies and infants of diabetic mothers. In the former, increased phosphate load from cellular injury and reduced calcium intake contribute. In the latter, reduced placental transfer of calcium, decreased PTH and elevated calcitonin levels and hypomagnesaemia levels contribute. Early-onset hypocalcaemia may also be caused by maternal hyperparathyroidism (where intrauterine hypercalcaemia suppresses parathyroid activity in the foetus, resulting in impaired parathyroid responsiveness to hypocalcaemia after birth). Hypocalcaemia in this case may be severe and prolonged.

Late Onset (>72 h). This is usually iatrogenic and caused by excessive intake of phosphate, the use of citrated blood products, lipid infusions, bicarbonate therapy, loop and thiazide diuretics, glucocorticoids and historically high phosphate-containing milk feeds, e.g. cow's milk.

Other causes include vitamin D deficiency (usually secondary to maternal vitamin D deficiency). This may be associated with maternal anticonvulsant use (phenobaritone or phenytoin), malabsorption of calcium or vitamin D, hypomagnesaemia, transient hypoparathyroidism, transient PTH resistance, renal failure, alkalosis, and congenital hypoparathyroidism.

Congenital hypoparathyroidism may be part of DiGeorge sequence/CATCH 22/ velocardiofacial syndrome where the hypoparathyroidism may be transient, with resolution during infancy, but may be exacerbated by the use of loop diuretics for heart failure. It may also be caused by activating mutations in Ca^{2+} sensing receptor (mild variant of hypoparathyroidism, autosomal-dominant hypocalcaemia), agenesis of parathyroid glands or part of a number of metabolic syndromes including Kenny-Caffey syndrome, mitochondrial trifunctional protein deficiency, long-chain fatty acyl CoA dehydrogenase deficiency, and Kearns-Sayre syndrome.

Investigation of Hypocalcaemia

Blood samples should be taken for calcium level (ideally ionized calcium), phosphate, magnesium, alkaline phosphatase, albumin, pH, creatinine and electrolytes, PTH level and vitamin D level. A sample may be sent to the cytogenetics laboratory for processing for further investigation if necessary (mutational analysis).

A urine sample should be collected for calcium, phosphate, creatinine, glucose, amino acids, cAMP and the urinary calcium:creatinine ratio, and urinary PO_4 excretion (tubular reabsorption of phosphate) to be determined.

As the maternal calcium concentration and vitamin D status during pregnancy influences vitamin D levels and parathyroid function in the foetus, investigation of hypercalcaemia and unexplained hypocalcaemia should include an analysis of calcium metabolism in the mother. If defects in the calcium-sensing receptor are suspected, calcium levels in the father and siblings should be assessed.

Other investigations include an X-ray of the wrist for evidence of rickets or osteopenia and an assessment of maternal mineral metabolism status.

For diagnosis, see figures 4 and 5.

Hypercalcaemia in the Newborn

Hypercalcaemia is defined as a total calcium >2.82 mmol/l, or ionized calcium >1.4 mmol/l. In the neonatal unit, hypercalcaemia may be picked up incidentally on 'routine' blood tests. Mild hypercalcaemia (2.74–3.2) mmol/l is usually asymptomatic. Moderate-to-severe hypercalcaemia: (>3.2 mmol/l) may present with anorexia, gastro-oesophageal reflux, vomiting, constipation (rarely diarrhoea).

Other symptoms and signs include polyuria (which may result in dehydration), hypertension (secondary to vasoconstrictive effect of hypercalcaemia), shortened ST segment and heart block (secondary to direct effect on cardiac conduction) and CNS

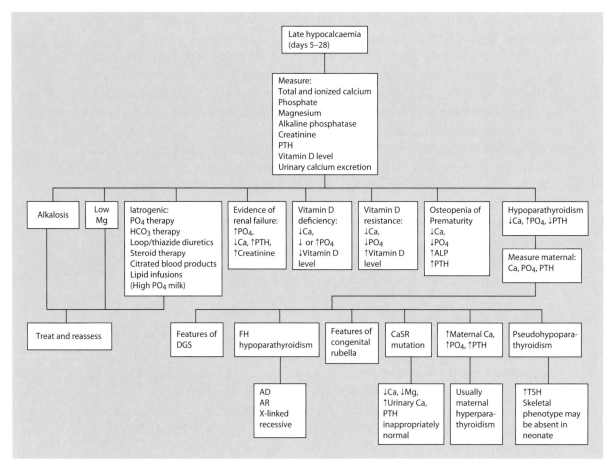

Fig. 4. Investigation of late hypocalcaemia.

symptoms: irritability, hypotonia, drowsiness, seizures, stupor and coma. Chronic hypercalcaemia usually presents with failure to thrive [51, 52].

Hyperparathyroidism may be associated with bone deformities or fractures (inadequate mineralization), respiratory difficulties (if the ribcage is affected), hepatosplenomegaly and anaemia.

If hypercalcaemia is present, the history may reveal birth trauma or perinatal asphyxia and signs of subcutaneous fat necrosis. There may be a family history hypocalciuric hypercalcaemia. Examination may reveal the dysmorphic features of Williams' syndrome with murmur of supravalvular aortic or peripheral pulmonary branch stenosis.

An assessment of calcium and phosphate intake in the baby should be made, especially in preterm infants receiving breast milk without supplementation of phosphate and infants on prolonged low phosphate-containing parenteral nutrition. The vitamin D intake should be assessed (by checking the milk formulation and vitamin D

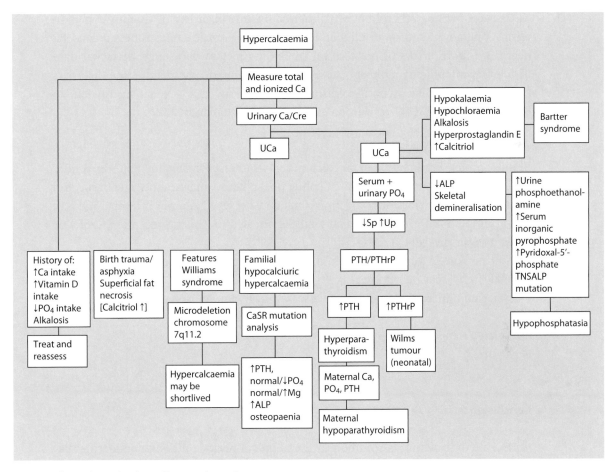

Fig. 5. Investigation of hypercalcaemia.

supplementation). There should be an assessment of maternal mineral metabolism (calcium concentration and vitamin D status) and therefore parathyroid status.

The causes of hypercalcaemia include iatrogenic causes (hypophosphataemia, vitamin A or D excess, excessive calcium supplements, extra-corporeal membrane oxygenation and thiazide diuretics), functional hyperparathyroidism, and nonparathyroid hypercalcaemia.

Functional hyperparathyroidism (where PTH and serum Ca^{2+} levels are raised, with low PO_4 levels and normal or raised alkaline phosphatase levels). Causes include maternal hypocalcaemia (secondary to pseudohypoparathyroidism, renal tubular acidosis); congenital parathyroid hyperplasia, inactivating mutations in the calcium-sensing receptor gene (either familial hypocalciuric hypercalcaemia (heterozygous manifestation) or neonatal severe hyperparathyroidism – (homozygous manifestation); Jansen's metaphyseal chondrodysplasia (caused by constitutive mutation in the PTH/PTH-related peptide (PTHrP) receptor) or persistent parathyroid hormone-related peptide.

Causes of nonparathyroid hypercalcaemia include disorders of vitamin D metabolism; Williams' syndrome; idiopathic infantile hypercalcaemia; subcutaneous fat necrosis; inborn errors of metabolism (including lactase deficiency, disaccharidase deficiency, infantile hypophosphatasia, blue diaper syndrome); endocrine disorders (including congenital hypothyroidism, thyrotoxicosis, and adrenal insufficiency); Down syndrome; IMAGe syndrome (table 1) and malignancy.

Investigation of Hypercalcaemia
Blood samples should be taken for calcium (either total, corrected for albumin, or ideally, ionized), phosphate, albumin, alkaline phosphatase, magnesium, creatinine and electrolytes. Other blood investigations include PTH level, vitamin D level (25OHD), and a sample for DNA (mutational analysis of calcium sensing receptor (CaSR) or Williams (elastin) gene, 1,25(OH)$_2$D).

A urine sample for urinary calcium, phosphate, and creatinine should be taken. A skeletal survey may be helpful.

Maternal mineral status should be assessed (calcium, phosphate, PTH).

Interpretation of Results
See figure 5.

Conclusions

Endocrine dysfunction is common in the neonatal period, although endocrine disease is rare. Both may be picked up incidentally by abnormalities found on newborn examination or 'routine' blood samples or non-specific symptoms exhibited by the baby. Endocrine disease may also be picked up before any symptoms are obvious on screening tests.

Because of the hormonal changes that occur with parturition, results need to be interpreted accordingly. In the preterm baby, there are no truly normative hormonal levels as these babies should still be in utero, and often treatment (particularly for adrenal dysfunction) needs to be given empirically if dysfunction is suspected.

References

1 Fisher DA, Nelson JC, Carlton EI, Wilcox RB: Maturation of human hypothalamic-pituitary-thyroid function and control. Thyroid 2000;10:229–234.

2 Santini F, Chiovato L, Ghirri P, Lapi P, Mammoli C, Montanelli L, Scartabelli G, Ceccarini G, Coccoli L, Chopra IJ, Boldrini A, Pinchera A: Serum iodothyronines in the human fetus and the newborn: evidence for an important role of placenta in fetal thyroid hormone homeostasis. J Clin Endocrinol Metab 1999;84:493–498.

3 Delange F, Fisher DA: The thyroid gland; in Brook GD (ed): Clinical Paediatric Endocrinology, ed 3. Oxford, Blackwell Science, 1995, pp 397–433.

4 Cuestas RA: Thyroid function in healthy premature infants. J Pediatr 1978;92:963–967.

5 Fisher DA: Thyroid function in premature infants. Clin Perinatol 1998;25:999–1014.

6 Fuse Y, Shimizu M, Uga N, et al: Maturation of the feedback control of thyrotropin in premature infants. J Dev Physiol 1990;14:17–22.

7 Ares S, Escobar-Morreale HF, Quero J, et al: Neonatal hypothyroxinaemia: effects of iodine intake and premature birth. J Clin Endocrinol Metab 1997;82:1704–1712.

8 Van Wassenaer AG, Kok JH, Dekker FW, De Vijlder JJM: Thyroid function in very preterm infants: influences of gestational age and disease. Pediatr Res 1997;42:812–818.

9 Rooman RP, Du Caju MVL, Op De Beeck L, et al: Low thyroxinaemia occurs in the majority of very preterm newborns. Eur J Pediatr 1996;155:211–215.

10 Frank JE, Faix JE, Hermos RJ, et al: Thyroid function in very low birth weight infants: effects on neonatal hypothyroidism screening. J Pediatr 1996;128:548–554.

11 Biswas S, Buffery J, Enoch H, Bland JM, Walters D, Markiewicz M: A longitudinal assessment of thyroid hormone concentrations in preterm infants younger than 30 weeks' gestation during the first 2 weeks of life and their relationship to outcome. Pediatrics 2002;109:222–227.

12 Williams FL, Simpson J, Delahunty C, Ogston SA, Bongers-Schokking JJ, Murphy N, van Toor H, Wu SY, Visser TJ, Hume R, Collaboration from the Scottish Preterm Thyroid Group: Developmental trends in cord and postpartum serum thyroid hormones in preterm infants. J Clin Endocrinol Metab 2004;89:5314–5320.

13 Reuss ML, Paneth N, Lorenz JM, et al: Correlates of low thyroxine values at newborn screening among infants born before 32 weeks gestation. Early Hum Dev 1997;28:821–827.

14 Paul DA, Leef KH, Stefano J, et al: Low serum thyroxine on initial newborn screening is associated with intraventricular hemorrhage and death in very low birthweight infants. Pediatrics 1998;101:903–907.

15 Levington A, Paneth N, Reuss ML, et al: Hypothyroxinaemia of prematurity and risk of cerebral white matter damage. J Pediatr 1999;134:706–711.

16 Reuss ML, Paneth N, Pinto-Marin JA, et al: The relationship of transient hypothyroxinemia in preterm infants to neurologic development at two years of age. N Engl J Med 1996;28:821–827.

17 Den Ouden AL, Kok JH, Verkerk P, et al: The relation between neonatal thyroxine levels and neurodevelopmental outcome at 5 and 9 years in a notional cohort of very preterm and/or very low birth weight infants. Pediatr Res 1996;39:142–145.

18 Meijer WJ, Verloove-Vanhorick SP, Brand R, et al: Transient hypothyroxinaemia associated with developmental delay in very preterm infants. Arch Dis Child 1992;67:944–947.

19 Lucas A, Rennie J, Baker BA, et al: Low plasma triiodothyronine concentrations and outcome in preterm infants. Arch Dis Child 1988;63:1201–1206.

20 Osborn DA, Hunt RW: Prophylactic postnatal thyroid hormones for prevention of morbidity and mortality in preterm infants. Cochrane Database Syst Rev 2007:CD005948.

21 Osborn DA, Hunt RW: Postnatal thyroid hormones for preterm infants with transient hypothyroxinaemia. Cochrane Database Syst Rev 2007:CD005945.

22 Peleg D, Cada S, Peleg A, Ben-Ami M: The relationship between maternal serum thyroid-stimulating immunoglobulin and fetal and neonatal thyrotoxicosis. Obstet Gynecol 2002;99:1040–1043.

23 Sippell WG, Becker H, Versmold HT, Bidlingmaier F, Knorr D: Longitudinal studies of plasma aldosterone, corticosterone, deoxycorticosterone, progesterone, 17-hydroxyprogesterone, cortisol, and cortisone determined simultaneously in mother and child at birth and during the early neonatal period. I. Spontaneous delivery. J Clin Endocrinol Metab 1978;46:971–985.

24 Kraiem Z, Sack J, Brish M: Serum cortisol levels: the first 10 days in full-term and preterm infants. Isr J Med Sci 1985;21:170–172.

25 Doerr HG, Sippell WG, Versmold HT, Bildingmaier F, Knorr D: Plasma mineralocorticoids, glucocorticoids, and progestins in premature infants: longitudinal study during the first week of life. Pediatr Res 1988;23:525–529.

26 Midgley PC, Holownia P, Smith J, Moore M, Russell K, Oates N, Shaw JC, Honour JW: Plasma cortisol, cortisone and urinary glucocorticoid metabolites in preterm infants. Biol Neonate 2001;79:79–86.

27 Hingre RV, Gross SJ, Hingre KS, Mayes DM, Richman RA: Adrenal steroidogenesis in very low birth weight preterm infants. J Clin Endocrinol Metab 1994;78:266–270.

28 Jett PL, Samuels MH, McDaniel PA, Benda GI, Lafranchi SH, Reynolds JW, Hanna CE: Variability of plasma cortisol levels in extremely low birth weight infants. J Clin Endocrinol Metab 1997;82:2921–2925.

29 Santiago LB, Jorge SM, Moreira AC: Longitudinal evaluation of the development of salivary cortisol circadian rhythm in infancy. Clin Endocrinol (Oxf) 1996;44:157–161.

30 Vermes I, Dohanics J, Tóth G, Pongrácz J: Maturation of the circadian rhythm of the adrenocortical functions in human neonates and infants. Horm Res 1980;12:237–244.

31 Kidd S, Midgley P, Nicol M, Smith J, McIntosh N: Lack of adult-type salivary cortisol circadian rhythm in hospitalized preterm infants. Horm Res 2005;64: 20–27.

32 Seri I, Tan R, Evans J: Cardiovascular effects of hydrocortisone in preterm infants with pressor-resistant hypotension. Pediatrics 2001;107:1070–1074.

33 Watterberg KL, Scott SM: Evidence of early adrenal insufficiency in babies who develop bronchopulmonary dysplasia. Pediatrics 1995;95:120–125.

34 Ng PC, Wong GW, Lam CW, Lee CH, Wong MY, Fok TF, Wong W, Chan DC: Pituitary-adrenal response in preterm very low birth weight infants after treatment with antenatal corticosteroids. J Clin Endocrinol Metab 1997;82:3548–3552.

35 Watterberg KL, Shaffer ML, Garland JS, Thilo EH, Mammel MC, Couser RJ, Aucott SW, Leach CL, Cole CH, Gerdes JS, Rozycki HJ, Backstrom C: Effect of dose on response to adrenocorticotropin in extremely low birth weight infants. J Clin Endocrinol Metab 2005;90:6380–6385.

36 Crofton PM, Midgley PC: Cortisol and growth hormone responses to spontaneous hypoglycaemia in infants and children. Arch Dis Child 2004;89:472–478.

37 Krob G, Braun A, Kuhnle U: True hermaphroditism: geographical distribution, clinical findings, chromosomes and gonadal histology. Eur J Pediatr 1994;153:2–10.

38 Shozu M, Akasofu K, Harada T, Kubota Y: A new cause of female pseudohermaphroditism: placental aromatase deficiency. J Clin Endocrinol Metab 1991;72:560–566.

39 Winter JS, Hughes IA, Reyes FI, Faiman C: Pituitary-gonadal relations in infancy: 2. Patterns of serum gonadal steroid concentrations in man from birth to two years of age. J Clin Endocrinol Metab 1976;42: 679–686.

40 Ng KL, Ahmed SF, Hughes IA: Pituitary-gonadal axis in male under masculinisation. Arch Dis Child 2000;82:54–58.

41 Davenport M, Brain C, Vandenberg C, Zappala S, Duffy P, Ransley PG, Grant D: The use of the hCG stimulation test in the endocrine evaluation of cryptorchidism. Br J Urol 1995;76:790–794.

42 Rey RA, Belville C, Nihoul-Fekete C, et al: Evaluation of gonadal function in 107 intersex patients by means of serum antimullerian hormone measurement. J Clin Endocrinol Metab 1999;84: 627–631.

43 Kubini K, Zachmann M, Albers N, Hiort O, Bettendorf M, Wolfle J, Bidlingmaier F, Klingmuller D: Basal inhibin B and the testosterone response to human chorionic gonadotropin correlate in prepubertal boys. J Clin Endocrinol Metab 2000;85:134–138.

44 Chang HJ, Clark RD, Bachman H: Chromosome mosaicism in 6,000 amniocenteses. Am J Med Genet 1989;32:506–513.

45 Wilson MG, Lin MS, Fujimoto A, Herbert W, Kaplan FM: The phenotype of 45,X/46,XY mosaicism: an analysis of 92 prenatally diagnosed cases. Am J Hum Genet 1990;46:156–167.

46 Laue L, Wu S-M, Kudo M, Hsueh AJ, Cutler GB, Griffin JE, Wilson JD, Brain C, Berry AC, Grant DB, Chan W-Y: A nonsense mutation of the human luteinizing hormone receptor gene in Leydig cell hypoplasia. Hum Mol Genet 1995;4:1429–1433.

47 Hochberg Z, Chayen R, Reiss N, Falik Z, Makler A, Munichor M, Farkas A, Goldfarb H, Ohana N, Hiort O: Clinical, biochemical, and genetic findings in a large pedigree of male and female patients with 5 alpha-reductase 2 deficiency. J Clin Endocrinol Metab 1996;81:2821–2827.

48 Kovacs CS, Kronenberg HM: Maternal-fetal calcium and bone metabolism during pregnancy, puerperium, and lactation. Endocr Rev 1997;18:832–872.

49 Rigo J, De Curtis M, Pieltain C, Picaud JC, Salle BL, Senterre J: Bone mineral metabolism in the micropremie. Clin Perinatol 2000;27:147–170.

50 Loughead JL, Mimouni F, Tsang RC: Serum ionized calcium concentrations in normal neonates. Am J Dis Child 1988;142:516–518.

51 Hsu SC, Levine MA: Perinatal calcium metabolism: physiology and pathophysiology. Semin Neonatol 2004;9:23–36.

52 Diamond FB, Root AW: Disorders of calcium metabolism in the newborn and infant; in Sperling MA (ed): Pediatric Endocrinology, ed 2. Philadelphia, Saunders, 2002, pp 97–110.

Dr. A.L. Ogilvy-Stuart
Neonatal Unit, Rosie Hospital
Cambridge University Hospitals NHS Trust
Cambridge, CB2 2SW (UK)
Tel. +44 01223 245 151, Fax +44 01223 217 064, E-Mail amanda.ogilvy-stuart@addenbrookes.nhs.uk

Ranke MB, Mullis P-E (eds): Diagnostics of Endocrine Function in Children and Adolescents, ed 4.
Basel, Karger, 2011, pp 429–447

Bone Metabolites

Patricia M. Crofton

Royal Hospital for Sick Children, Edinburgh, UK

In children, as in adults, bone is a metabolically active tissue in a constant state of turnover called remodelling. Remodelling is a tightly coupled process involving sequential resorption of bone by osteoclasts, followed by bone formation by osteoblasts. It fulfils a maintenance role, repairing micro-defects in bone and preserving bone strength. However, unlike adults, children are also growing. Skeletal growth involves not only longitudinal growth by chondrocytes at the epiphyseal growth plate, with subsequent mineralisation by osteoblasts, but also growth in bone width and reshaping of bone to optimise bone strength in response to the forces imposed by growing muscles. This latter process is called modelling. In the long bones, increase in bone width is achieved by teams of osteoblasts creating new bone on the outer bone surface of newly synthesised osteoid while simultaneously teams of osteoclasts resorb bone from the inner surface of the bone cortex, increasing the bone marrow cavity. These processes are not coupled but work independently. The net effect is an increase in the amount of bone tissue.

Type I collagen is the predominant collagen in bone and soft tissue. It is formed from a precursor procollagen molecule which undergoes extracellular processing to remove the bulky C-terminal and smaller N-terminal propeptides, allowing assembly of the collagen triple helices into fibrils that provide much of the tensile strength of bone. Mature type I collagen in bone subsequently forms intermolecular cross-links at the N-terminal and C-terminal telopeptide regions, helping to stabilise the fibrillar structure. However, the main structural strength of bone derives from its mineral component: hydroxyapatite, a crystalline form of calcium phosphate, that slots into specific grooves formed by the neatly staggered array of collagen molecules within fibrils.

There are a number of biochemical markers of bone formation and bone resorption that reflect these dynamic processes (table 1). Bone formation markers are all measured in serum or plasma. Bone resorption markers may be measured in serum, plasma or urine, depending on the marker and the assay. Figure 1 shows a schematic representation of the synthesis and clearance of most of the commonly measured bone markers.

Table 1. Biochemical markers of bone turnover

Marker	Abbre-viation	Marker of	Sample type	Measurement principle
Bone formation				
Procollagen type I C-terminal propeptide	PICP	type I collagen synthesis - mainly bone osteoblast – early proliferative phase	plasma/ serum	RIA
Procollagen type I N-terminal propeptide	PINP	type I collagen synthesis - mainly bone osteoblast – early proliferative phase	plasma/ serum	RIA
Bone alkaline phosphatase	bone ALP	osteoblast – maturation phase matrix vesicles (bone mineralisation) hypertrophic chondrocytes (epiphyseal growth plate)	serum plasma/ serum plasma/ serum	IRMA or ELISA or lectin affinity electrophoresis
Osteocalcin		osteoblast – mineralisation phase hypertrophic chondrocytes (epiphyseal growth plate)	plasma/ serum	RIA or IRMA or ELISA
Bone resorption				
Hydroxyproline		collagen turnover (bone and skin)	urine	HPLC
Pyridinium crosslinks				
– Pyridinoline (free + peptide-bound)	Pyd	breakdown of mature collagen	urine	HPLC
– Deoxypyridinoline (free + peptide-bound)	Dpd	breakdown of mature bone collagen	urine	HPLC
– Free deoxypyridinoline	free Dpd	breakdown of mature bone collagen	urine	ELISA
Galactosyl-hydroxylysine	Gal-Hyl	breakdown of collagen – mainly bone	urine	HPLC
N-terminal telopeptide of type I collagen	NTX	breakdown of mature type I collagen	urine plasma/ serum	ELISA ELISA
C-terminal telopeptide of type I collagen	CTX	breakdown of mature type I collagen	urine plasma/ serum	ELISA ELISA
Cross-linked telopeptide of type I collagen	ICTP	breakdown of mature type I collagen	plasma/ serum	RIA
Tartrate-resistant acid phosphatase, isoenzyme 5b	TRAP5b	osteoclast activity (ruffled border)	plasma/ serum	ELISA
Receptor activator of nuclear factors kB	RANKL	inducer of osteoclastic bone resorption	plasma/ serum	ELISA
Osteoprotegerin	OPG	decoy receptor – binds RANKL to prevent RANKL-induced bone resorption	plasma/ serum	ELISA

Crofton

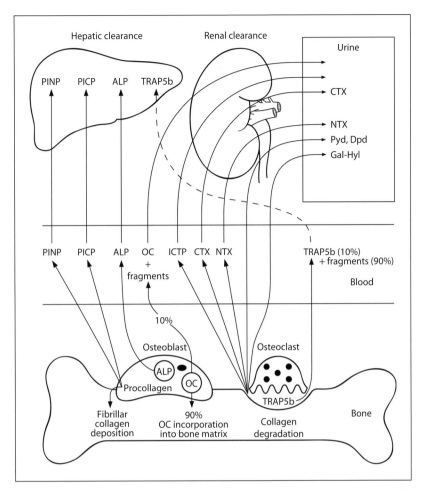

Fig. 1. Schematic representation of synthesis and clearance of bone markers. Bone formation markers: PICP and PINP enter the circulation during the synthesis of type I collagen and are cleared by hepatic endothelial cells. Bone ALP is a large molecule synthesised by the mature osteoblast and also cleared by hepatic uptake. Osteocalcin (OC) is synthesised by the mature osteoblast and approximately 90% is incorporated into bone matrix. Only about 10% reaches the blood where it circulates as a mixture of intact osteocalcin and various fragments. Osteocalcin is mainly cleared by the kidney. Bone resorption markers: osteoclasts secrete proteases which release heterogeneous collagen fragments of varying size into the circulation. Some contain galactosyl-hydroxylysine (Gal-Hyl), pyridinium (Pyd) or deoxypyridinium (Dpd) cross-links, or the specific structures and/or amino acid sequences in the C-terminal (ICTP, CTX) or N-terminal (NTX) telopeptide regions of the type I collagen molecule that form the cross-links which characterise mature type I collagen. Larger collagen fragments may be further metabolised by the kidney (and possibly liver) until they are small enough to be excreted in urine. TRAP5b is synthesised in the ruffled border of the osteoclast and is released into the circulation where it reflects osteoclast activity. Only 10% circulates as the intact, enzymatically active molecule. Over time, TRAP5b is degraded to inactive fragments that are cleared by the liver.

Bone Formation Markers

Type I Collagen Propeptides
The C-terminal (PICP) and N-terminal (PINP) propeptides of type I collagen are released into the circulation in equimolar amounts during the synthesis of type I collagen and quantitatively reflect type I collagen formation [1]. They are produced by the osteoblast during its early proliferative phase. Although type I collagen is not exclusive to bone, bone is nevertheless the main source of these circulating propeptides. PICP is cleared by mannose receptors and PINP by scavenger receptors in liver endothelial cells. The clearance of PICP appears to be influenced by the hormonal milieu but that of PINP is not. PINP is therefore less susceptible to confounding variables affecting clearance.

Alkaline Phosphatase
Alkaline phosphatase (ALP) exists as several different isoenzymes coded for by separate genes [1]. The main circulating isoforms are liver and bone ALP, both products of the same gene and differing only as a result of post-translational modification of their sugar moieties. In growing children, bone ALP generally predominates. Bone ALP is produced both by the mature osteoblast and by the hypertrophic chondrocytes of the epiphyseal growth plate. In children, it therefore reflects both osteoblast function and longitudinal growth. In bone, its function is to permit mineralisation by removing pyrophosphate, a strong inhibitor of hydroxyapatite formation [2]. Bone ALP is cleared by hepatic uptake via the galactose receptor.

Osteocalcin
Osteocalcin (also known as bone gla protein) is the most abundant noncollagenous protein in bone and is produced by mature osteoblasts during the mineralisation phase, with small amounts also being produced by hypertrophic chondrocytes in the epiphyseal growth plate [1]. It carries three vitamin K-dependent carboxylated glutamic acid residues which mediate strong binding of osteocalcin to hydroxyapatite in the bone matrix. However, some newly synthesised osteocalcin is released into the circulation where its concentration reflects bone formation. It also circulates as a variety of fragments some of which may derive from bone itself following osteoclastic degradation. Osteocalcin is mainly cleared by the kidney. The intact molecule accounts for approximately 40% of total osteocalcin in healthy individuals but a smaller proportion in patients with impaired renal function.

Bone Resorption Markers

Urine Bone Resorption Markers
Historically, until recently markers of bone resorption have been measured in urine (table 1). The earliest of these markers was hydroxyproline but this suffers from a

number of major disadvantages. It reflects collagen turnover in both bone and skin, is affected by dietary ingestion of collagen, is extensively metabolised by the liver and only about 10% is excreted unchanged in urine [1]. It is therefore now considered to be an obsolete test. The other urinary markers listed in table 1 are better markers of bone resorption because they are unaffected by dietary intake, are not taken up by the liver and are excreted quantitatively in urine [1]. Most of them reflect degradation products of mature cross-linked collagen. The urinary markers currently considered most specific for bone collagen breakdown are the N-terminal (NTX) and C-terminal (CTX) telopeptides of type I collagen.

Although collection of urine is non-invasive, it suffers from a number of disadvantages. Within-individual biological variation of urinary markers is high, approximately 30%. Timed urine collections are difficult and often incomplete in small children. First or second morning void or random urine samples are therefore often used, expressing results as a ratio to creatinine to compensate for variations in urine flow. However, creatinine excretion itself is influenced by muscle mass, age, gender and puberty. Results expressed as ratios to creatinine may be particularly misleading in precocious or delayed puberty, and in conditions affecting muscle mass such as some chronic diseases, or tissue catabolism, for example in patients with infection.

Plasma/Serum Bone Resorption Markers
A few markers of bone resorption can be measured in plasma or serum (table 1), facilitating direct comparisons with markers of bone formation and eliminating the problems associated with collecting urine and interpreting results. These include NTX, CTX and another marker of the C-terminal telopeptide region of type I collagen, ICTP. ICTP and CTX fragments, although nominally both from the same region of the type I collagen molecule, are generated by different collagenolytic pathways, namely metalloproteinase and cathepsin K, respectively. Although in some clinical contexts they have been shown to be tightly correlated, in others their relative abundance may vary depending on the bone pathology. Only one plasma/serum marker of osteoclast activity is currently available: tartrate-resistant acid phosphatase isoenzyme 5b (TRAP5b), an enzyme involved in bone matrix degradation [3]. The enzyme is produced in the osteoclast ruffled border and is released into the circulation during the resorption process itself or after detachment of the osteoclast from the bone surface. Only the intact, enzymatically active form (approximately 10% of the total) reflects recent osteoclast activity. Over time, intact TRAP5b is degraded to inactive fragments that are cleared by the liver.

Osteoprotegerin and RANKL
Osteoprotegerin (OPG) is synthesised by osteoblasts and acts as a decoy receptor by binding the receptor activator of nuclear factors kB (RANKL), thereby preventing RANKL-induced osteoclastic bone resorption [4]. Many hormonal and other

modulators of osteoclastogenesis exert their effects in bone by regulating OPG and/or RANKL production and their ratio. However, it is doubtful to what extent circulating levels of OPG and RANKL reflect the bone microenvironment.

Methods for Measuring Bone Metabolites

Bone Formation Markers

PICP and PINP are both measured by radioimmunoassay (RIA) and commercial kits are available (table 1).

Bone-specific ALP may be measured by immunoradiometric assay (IRMA), enzyme-linked immunosorbent assay (ELISA) or wheat-germ lectin affinity electrophoresis. Both the IRMA and ELISA methods show 5–10% cross-reactivity with liver ALP. This is negligible in most clinical contexts as liver ALP forms only a small proportion of total ALP in growing children, but may result in significant positive interference in patients with cholestasis.

There are several different commercial assays (RIA, IRMA and ELISA) for osteocalcin, recognising different epitopes, using different standards and giving different numerical results. Ideally, an osteocalcin assay should be specific for the intact osteocalcin produced by the osteoblast. However, in practice many assays cross-react with osteocalcin fragments in the circulation and give discordant results in different clinical conditions, especially in renal failure when these fragments accumulate [5]. Intact osteocalcin itself is unstable both at room temperature and at 4°C. Blood samples must therefore be centrifuged within 1–2 h of collection and the serum stored frozen before analysis, with avoidance of freeze-thaw cycles. In vitro breakdown of intact osteocalcin may even occur during the course of the assay. This requirement for special handling limits the usefulness of osteocalcin assays.

Bone Resorption Markers

Several of the urinary markers of bone collagen resorption were originally measured by high-performance liquid chromatography (HPLC): hydroxyproline, total pyridinoline (Pyd), total deoxypyridinoline (Dpd) and galactosyl-hydroxylysine (Gal-Hyl). These more cumbersome methods have now largely been abandoned. Later, commercial immunoassay kits were developed for free Dpd in urine (ELISA), urine and plasma/serum NTX (ELISA), urine and plasma/serum CTX (ELISA), ICTP (RIA) and intact TRAP5b (ELISA). Serum osteoprotegerin and RANKL can also be measured by sensitive commercial ELISA assays but their use remains highly experimental and confined to research.

All of these assays are expensive and are not widely available in many routine laboratories.

Biological Variation

Most markers of bone turnover show between 5 and 30% circadian variation in children, with higher values at night than during the day. The exception is bone ALP which shows negligible circadian variation. To minimise the effects of such variation when assessing children longitudinally, the time of day when samples are collected should ideally be standardised. Within-individual day-to-day variation of the urinary markers may also be considerable. Between-individual biological variation is relatively wide for all markers in all paediatric age groups (see below), particularly during adolescence. Single measurements therefore have limited diagnostic value unless they are very aberrant.

Factors Influencing Markers of Bone Turnover

For most bone markers, concentrations in plasma mirror the paediatric growth curve, with highest values in infancy, decreasing in childhood, then increasing again during puberty, before decreasing to much lower adult values (see fig. 2 for PINP as an example [6]). Girls have an earlier pubertal increase and post-pubertal decrease in bone markers compared to boys, reflecting their earlier growth spurt and post-menarche decline in bone mineral accrual rates. Urinary markers of bone degradation tend to show less marked changes during puberty when expressed as ratios to creatinine, owing to the blunting effect of the rise of creatinine excretion during puberty. OPG and RANKL concentrations in plasma show no relationship with the paediatric growth curve. Although OPG concentrations are slightly higher in children younger than 4 years, older children have similar values to those observed in adults, with no pubertal increase [7]. Serum RANKL levels in children do not differ significantly from adults [7].

Bone marker concentrations in plasma are influenced by height velocity, sex and Tanner stage. A recent study has demonstrated that these factors, together with whole-body bone mineral content (BMC) and BMC accrual, together explain about 80% of the variability of serum bone ALP and urine Dpd [8]. However, most studies in children have shown no, or only weak associations between bone markers and areal bone mineral density (BMD, g/cm^2) gain, measured by dual energy X-ray absorptiometry.

Paediatric Reference Ranges

It is essential that bone markers are interpreted in relation to appropriate paediatric normative data for the assay in question. This is particularly true of osteocalcin which shows large inter-assay differences and bone ALP which may be reported in activity

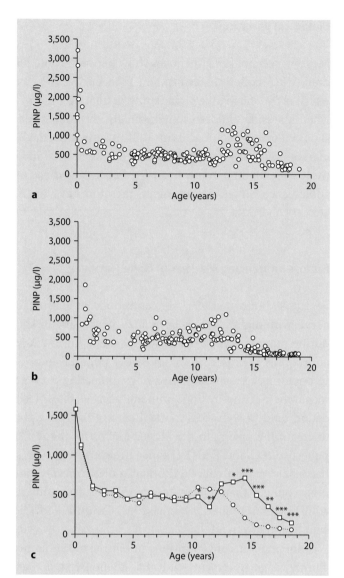

Fig. 2. PINP concentrations in 327 healthy children in relation to age and gender. **a** Individual boys (n = 163). **b** Individual girls (n = 164). **c** Geometric means (defined as the arithmetic mean of log-transformed PINP concentrations, raised to the power of 10). Squares = Boys; circles = girls. Geometric means for each age band are plotted at the midpoint of that age band. Unpaired t tests between age-matched boys and girls: * p <0.05; ** p <0.01; *** p <0.001. Data reproduced from Crofton et al. [6], with permission.

or mass units, depending on the method. It should also be noted that most bone markers have a non-Gaussian distribution, so that logarithmic or other transformations are required to calculate reference intervals. Paediatric age- and sex-related reference data have been reported for a number of bone markers in a variety of formats (table 2, fig. 3). Several authors have also attempted to provide reference data that will allow calculation of SD scores. Use of SD scores allows amalgamation and interpretation of data from boys and girls of varying age, in a manner analogous to the use of height or weight SD scores in clinical paediatrics.

Table 2. Paediatric reference data for selected markers of bone formation and resorption in plasma or serum

Marker	Sex	Age years	n	* Mean (SD) or $ log-transformed mean (SD) or # median	§ 2.5th to 97.5th or¶ 25th to 75th percentiles	Units	Assay
Bone ALP	M	5–9	23	* 95 (26)	§ 43–147	U/l	ELISA
		10–14	16	* 124 (38)	§ 48–200		(Metra
		15–19	5	* 22 (5.6)	§ 11–33		Biosystems) [3]
	F	5–9	23	* 95 (26)	§ 43–147		
		10–14	31	* 87 (36)	§ 15–159		
		15–19	33	* 23 (11)	§ 1–45		
PINP	M/F	<1	11	$ 3.046 (0.209)	§ 424–2,916	µg/l	RIA
		1–9	147	$ 2.679 (0.119)	§ 277–824		(Orion
	M	10–11	20	$ 2.611 (0.115)	§ 240–693		Diagnostica) [6]
		12–14	30	$ 2.828 (0.189)	§ 282–1,604		
		15	10	$ 2.695 (0.174)	§ 223–1,103		
		16	6	$ 2.552 (0.338)	§ 75–1,690		
		17–18	14	$ 2.294 (0.192)	§ 81–476		
	F	10–12	30	$ 2.756 (0.161)	§ 272–1,194		
		13	10	$ 2.575 (0.208)	§ 144–980		
		14	10	$ 2.328 (0.169)	§ 98–462		
		15–16	20	$ 2.059 (0.220)	§ 42–316		
		17–18	19	$ 1.866 (0.128)	§ 41–133		
PICP	M/F	1	12	$ 3.2081 (0.1181)	§ 935–2,783	µg/l	RIA
		2–3	29	$ 2.6069 (0.1152)	§ 238–688		(Orion
	M	4–16	141	$ 2.5699 (0.1424)	§ 193–716		Diagnostica)
		17–18	15	$ 2.3377 (0.1587)	§ 105–452		[10, 11]
	F	4–12	84	$ 2.5910 (0.1194)	§ 225–676		
		13–14	20	$ 2.3921 (0.1806)	§ 108–567		
		15–18	41	$ 2.1854 (0.1345)	§ 82–285		
Osteocalcin (intact)	M	1	43	# 63	¶ 52–63	µg/l	IRMA
		2	24	# 68	¶ 64–70		(CIS-Bio

Table 2. Continued

Marker	Sex	Age years	n	* Mean (SD) or $ log-transformed mean (SD) or # median	§ 2.5th to 97.5th or¶ 25th to 75th percentiles	Units	Assay
Osteocalcin (intact)		3	39	# 60	¶ 54–70		International)
		4	43	# 68	¶ 53–90		[12]
		5	55	# 67	¶ 52–83		
		6	59	# 63	¶ 51–84		
		7	51	# 67	¶ 49–104		
		8	66	# 65	¶ 51–80		
		9	70	# 75	¶ 62–83		
		10	86	# 73	¶ 58–88		
		11	78	# 69	¶ 56–80		
		12	41	# 74	¶ 68–80		
		13	47	# 88	¶ 74–98		
		14	55	# 87	¶ 66–102		
		15	49	# 87	¶ 61–105		
		16	27	# 45	¶ 36–50		
	F	1	31	# 58	¶ 48–79		
		2	31	# 70	¶ 61–88		
		3	35	# 69	¶ 44–93		
		4	47	# 78	¶ 51–98		
		5	49	# 78	¶ 66–88		
		6	66	# 79	¶ 65–96		
		7	42	# 73	¶ 53–97		
		8	78	# 71	¶ 50–89		
		9	57	# 70	¶ 61–78		
		10	82	# 79	¶ 65–96		
		11	69	# 62	¶ 36–93		
		12	39	# 89	¶ 74–99		
		13	35	# 55	¶ 42–75		
		14	51	# 33	¶ 25–43		
		15	50	# 44	¶ 35–59		

Table 2. Continued

Marker	Sex	Age years	n	* Mean (SD) or $ log-transformed mean (SD) or # median	§ 2.5th to 97.5th or¶ 25th to 75th percentiles	Units	Assay
		16	39	# 39	¶ 27–47		
ICTP	M/F	<1	16	$ 1.7391 (0.2316)	§ 18.9–159.3	µg/l	RIA
		1–4	41	$ 1.1397 (0.1213)	§ 7.9–24.1		(Orion
	M	4–11	83	$ 0.9693 (0.1310)	§ 5.1–17.0		Diagnostica)
		12–16	52	$ 1.1169 (0.1200)	§ 7.5–22.8		[10, 11]
		17–18	14	$ 0.8066 (0.1896)	§ 2.7–15.3		
	F	4–8	44	$ 0.9631 (0.1055)	§ 5.7–14.9		
		9–13	50	$ 1.0803 (0.1102)	§ 7.2–20.0		
		14–15	20	$ 0.8706 (0.1272)	§ 4.1–13.3		
		16–18	30	$ 0.6977 (0.1149)	§ 2.9–8.5		

* Mean (SD) of untransformed concentrations/activity. To calculate an SD score for bone ALP, SD score = (x – mean)/SD for the appropriate age/sex from the Table, where x = measured activity in U/l.

$ Mean (SD) of log-transformed concentrations. To calculate an SD score for PINP, PICP or ICTP, SD score = $(\log_{10}x - mean)/SD$ for the appropriate age/sex from the table, where x = measured concentration in µg/l.

#, ¶ Data provided do not allow calculation of SD scores or 2.5th to 97.5th percentile reference intervals.

§ 2.5th to 97.5th percentile reference interval is calculated as the mean ± 2 SD for bone ALP, or the arithmetic mean of log-transformed data ±2 SD, raised to the power of 10 (i.e. back-transformed) for PINP, PICP and ICTP.

Clinical Applications of Bone Metabolite Measurements

Diagnosis of Inherited Bone Disorders
A few inherited disorders of bone are caused by a genetic defect affecting a specific bone metabolite.

Hypophosphatasia
Hypophosphatasia is caused by mutations in the gene encoding the tissue non-specific isoenzyme of ALP [2]. It is genetically very heterogeneous, with most cases being compound heterozygotes, and there is a corresponding wide clinical spectrum with presentation at any age from neonatal to adult. The clinical manifestations are caused by a functional deficiency of bone ALP resulting in impaired bone mineralisation. Because liver ALP is also deficient, there is no need to measure bone-specific ALP:

total ALP will suffice provided it is interpreted in relation to well-validated paediatric (not adult) reference ranges. However, low ALP may also occur in other disorders affecting growth and bone turnover (see below). On the other hand, in some cases of hypophosphatasia total ALP may overlap the lower end of the age-appropriate reference range. Confirmation of the diagnosis is therefore required by demonstrating increased urinary excretion of phosphoethanolamine and/or increased serum pyridoxal phosphate [2].

Osteogenesis Imperfecta

Osteogenesis imperfecta (OI) is associated with mutations in the genes that encode the chains of type I collagen. In non-lethal forms of OI, PICP is decreased compared with controls or unaffected relatives, although there is some overlap. Patients with types I and III OI tend to have lower PICP levels than patients with type IV, and those patients with mild OI and a quantitative collagen defect have lower PICP levels than those with more severe OI and a qualitative collagen defect [14]. PINP appears to be less discriminatory. Measurement of PICP may therefore provide supporting evidence for OI, particularly among relatives of known OI patients, or to differentiate mild OI from child abuse.

Several studies have reported that treatment of OI types I, III and IV with cyclical intravenous pamidronate results in relief of pain, improved mobility, improved BMD and a reduction in markers of both bone resorption and bone formation, indicating suppression of bone turnover [15]. However, these changes in bone metabolites do not appear to predict changes in bone mass or size. Routine measurement of bone turnover markers to monitor response to therapy is therefore of doubtful benefit.

Juvenile Paget's Disease

Juvenile Paget's disease (also known as hereditary hyperphosphatasia) is a rare disorder characterised by rapid and continual remodelling of woven bone, resulting in osteopenia, fractures and progressive skeletal deformity. It is caused by a defect in the gene encoding OPG (TNFRSF11B) and serum OPG levels have been reported to be undetectable in two unrelated patients with the disorder [16].

Fig. 3. Reference curves for osteocalcin (**a**), bone ALP (**b**), ICTP (**c**), CTX (**d**) and TRAP5b (**e**) in boys and girls. Solid lines represent 50th percentiles and dotted lines represent 3rd and 97th percentiles, obtained by mathematical modelling of results obtained in 300 boys and 272 girls. Assay methods were: IRMA for intact osteocalcin (Active Human Osteocalcin, Diagnostic Systems Laboratories, ng/ml), IRMA for bone ALP (Tandem-R-Ostase, Hybritech, μg/l), RIA for ICTP (Orion Diagnostica, μg/l), ELISA for CTX (CrossLaps, Osteometer, ng/l), ELISA for TRAP5b (Bone TRAP, Medac, U/l). To calculate SD scores, refer to Rauchenzauner et al. [13]. Redrawn from Rauchenzauner et al. [13].

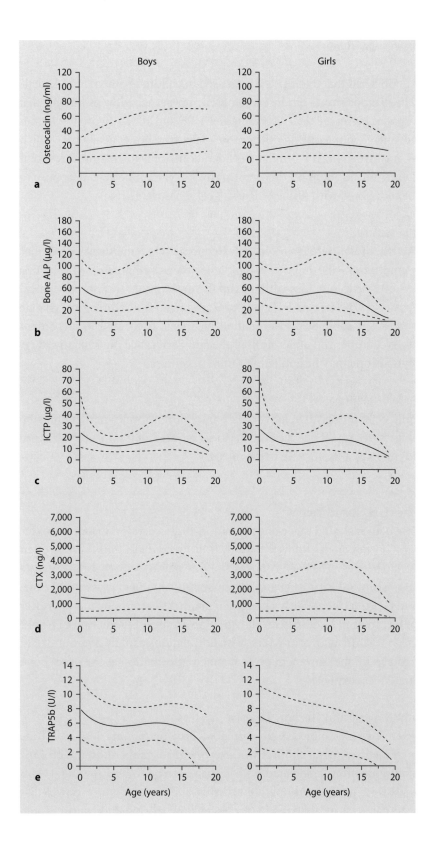

Other Disorders Affecting Bone
Rickets
It has long been established that total ALP is increased in children with vitamin D deficiency rickets. The diagnosis rests on the radiological appearances, low or low-normal calcium and phosphate, increased total ALP, increased PTH and low 25-hydroxy-vitamin D. There is no advantage in measuring other, more expensive, bone metabolites which are generally less sensitive than ALP. Similar considerations apply to vitamin D resistant rickets due to defects in the vitamin D receptor or hydroxylation defects. Response to treatment may be monitored with serial ALP and PTH measurements.

Osteopenia of Prematurity
Total ALP is also the most useful marker for osteopenia of prematurity. A number of studies have emphasised the importance of serial measurements of ALP in this context, as peak ALP rarely coincides with maximal bone demineralisation or clinical or radiological rickets [17]. Peak ALP usually precedes maximal radiological change by two to four weeks. Radiological examination has been advocated in any infant whose ALP exceeds six times the upper limit of the adult reference range at any stage, although different cut-offs may be applied in different centres.

Idiopathic Juvenile Osteoporosis
Idiopathic juvenile osteoporosis is relatively rare in children. Bone markers may be low, normal or high, presumably depending on the stage and aetiology of the disease and therefore do not have a useful role in diagnosis.

Growth Disorders
Growth Hormone (GH) Insufficiency
Many studies have demonstrated that bone formation and resorption markers are statistically lower in GH-deficient children than in healthy controls, but there is often considerable overlap between the two groups [18]. Bone markers are therefore of little value in the diagnosis of GH insufficiency. Their main value lies in assessing individual response to GH treatment. Early changes in many different bone markers after 1 to 3 months of GH treatment have been shown to give a useful prediction of height velocity response to treatment after one year, with correlations usually of around 0.6–0.8 [18]. Again, total ALP measurement gives as much information as the other bone markers and is much less expensive.

Impaired Growth in Acute and Chronic Disease
Total ALP is often low in children with impaired growth for any reason. These include patients in intensive care, children with severe burns and children with cancer. Chronic conditions often associated with impaired growth and low total ALP for age include asthma, juvenile idiopathic arthritis and inflammatory bowel disease. This may be particularly obvious in adolescence when patients with chronic

disease may have delayed puberty and hence a delayed growth spurt. Low ALP may indicate impaired growth when antecedent height measurements are unavailable. Measurement of other bone markers is not required.

Use of Bone Turnover Markers in Research

With the exception of total ALP and the specific disorders of bone and growth described above, the main use of bone turnover marker measurements has been in research where they complement the outcome measures of BMD and height velocity, giving insight into mechanisms. Bone turnover markers are particularly valuable in predicting response to treatment because they respond rapidly to therapeutic interventions and give information on dynamic processes of bone turnover long before any change in BMD or height velocity can be detected. Their limitation is that they cannot give information on particular bone sites, nor can they definitively separate out multifactorial influences on bone.

In research, it is important to measure a panel of markers of both bone formation and resorption as otherwise interpretation may be difficult. Of the bone formation markers, PINP or PICP provide the most rapid responses to changes in clinical state or treatment interventions but are not entirely bone specific. Osteocalcin is bone specific but is an unstable analyte and there may be cross-reaction with breakdown fragments in some assays. Bone ALP responds more slowly than PINP or PICP but is bone-specific (at least in the absence of cholestatic liver disease) and shows less within-individual variation than the other markers. Of the bone resorption markers, it is recommended that the newer serum markers are measured (serum NTX, CTX or ICTP) to avoid the complications of urine collection and the confounding variable of creatinine excretion. There is insufficient information to recommend which of these three serum markers of bone resorption is preferable.

Ideally, markers should be expressed as SD scores for age and sex to eliminate these confounding variables (see above). However, the confounding effects of puberty and its timing in individual adolescents should also be born in mind. Because of wide inter-individual variation in bone markers, longitudinal studies are often the most informative, allowing individuals to act as their own controls.

Malnutrition Disorders
Young children with severe malnutrition have low PICP and bone ALP and high ICTP and CTX levels, indicating low bone formation rates and high bone degradation rates [19]. Refeeding results in full or partial normalisation of these markers.

Similarly, children with untreated coeliac disease have low markers of bone formation and high urine NTX excretion, expressed as a ratio to creatinine [20]. However, care is required in interpreting NTX excretion in this context as muscle mass and creatinine excretion may be low. Introduction of a gluten-free diet results in marked increases in markers of bone formation but little change in urinary NTX:creatinine ratio.

Some [21], but not all [22], studies of adolescent girls with anorexia nervosa have also demonstrated low levels of markers of bone formation and high levels of markers of bone degradation in relation to normative data for age, sex and Tanner stage, although in this group, many of whom have amenorrhoea, oestrogen status is a powerful confounding variable.

Overall, the evidence is that malnutrition of any cause in children is associated with low rates of bone formation and high rates of bone resorption.

Other Chronic Childhood Diseases

Many chronic childhood disorders may result in reduced BMD and increased fracture rates. The reasons are often multifactorial, including the disease process itself, poor nutrition, immobility and inflammation. Cytokines released during inflammation (especially interleukin-6 and tumour necrosis factor-α) stimulate osteoclastic bone resorption and inhibit osteoblast function. Glucocorticoids are used in the treatment of many childhood diseases, including asthma and inflammatory bowel disease. However, they suppress growth and are associated with decreased calcium absorption, increased calcium excretion, impaired osteoblast function, increased osteoblast apoptosis and muscle atrophy and weakness [23]. All of these factors increase the risk of developing osteopenia and fracture.

Asthma

Children with asthma may have poor growth associated with the disease itself, but also as a result of growth suppression by glucocorticoids. Several studies have demonstrated that both systemic and (to a lesser extent) inhaled glucocorticoids suppress PICP, osteocalcin, ICTP and urinary Pyd and Dpd, indicating suppression of both bone formation and bone resorption [24].

Juvenile Idiopathic Arthritis (JIA)

Many children with JIA have problems with poor growth, osteopenia and fractures, which may be multifactorial in origin. Children with active disease have been shown to have low BMC, and low bone ALP, osteocalcin and TRAP5b compared with those with inactive disease or healthy controls, indicating a low bone turnover state [25]. Remission of the disease resulted in improved BMC and increased osteocalcin, whereas those whose disease became or remained active had decreased or unchanged low osteocalcin and BMC [26]. There are conflicting data on serum RANKL/OPG ratios in JIA. As previously indicated, serum levels of these markers may not reflect what is happening in bone and should be interpreted with caution.

Cystic Fibrosis

In cystic fibrosis, there is a high prevalence of osteopenia and an increased fracture rate. Markers of bone resorption are high and markers of bone formation tend to be low, possibly related to a combination of inflammation and nutritional factors [27].

Inflammatory Bowel Disease

Children with inflammatory bowel disease are similarly at risk of osteopenia. A recent study demonstrated that, at diagnosis children with Crohn's disease and ulcerative colitis had low levels of bone formation markers (bone ALP and PICP) with a tendency also to relatively low levels of urinary markers of bone degradation (NTX and CTX, expressed as ratios to creatinine) [28]. Clinical improvement and improved nutrition coincided with an increase in bone formation markers over time, but no change in bone resorption markers.

Acute Lymphoblastic Leukaemia

At diagnosis, a high proportion of children with acute lymphoblastic leukemia have radiographic abnormalities in bone, with 10% showing evidence of fractures. Bone formation markers are low or very low but the data on bone resorption markers are conflicting, with some reporting low and some normal levels. Insulin-like growth factor 1 (IGF-1) and GH-binding protein are low and urinary GH is high [29]. Taken together, the evidence suggests that children with acute lymphoblastic leukemia are in a GH-resistant state resulting in markedly reduced bone formation that, depending on timescale, may result in a modest reduction in BMD at diagnosis and increased fracture risk due to the disease process itself.

It has been reported that up to 40% children may develop fractures during acute lymphoblastic leukemia chemotherapy using modern intensive protocols, associated with declining lumbar spine BMD SD scores. However, BMD measurements can only be done at intervals of 6 months or more. Bone markers give insight into the dynamic processes affecting bone during chemotherapy. During induction and intensification chemotherapy, bone formation markers are further suppressed, with a lesser suppression of markers of bone resorption, resulting in negative bone balance [29]. These effects are independent of circulating IGF-1 (which returns to normal during this period), suggesting a direct effect on bone. The likely culprit is prednisolone (or dexamethasone, depending on the protocol). After prednisolone is discontinued, there is a rebound increase in bone ALP and collagen markers, with modulation by high-dose intravenous methotrexate treatment, which impairs bone formation and enhances bone resorption. During less-intensive continuing chemotherapy, collagen markers return to normal but bone ALP remains low, indicating a continuing adverse effect on osteoblast function; bone ALP only returns to normal after completion of treatment [10]. This illustrates how longitudinal studies of bone markers can complement BMD measurements and give insight into dynamic processes and mechanisms of the effects of successive treatments on bone.

Conclusions

Commercial assays for a range of biochemical markers of bone formation and bone resorption are now available. These bone metabolites reflect the dynamic processes of bone collagen synthesis, osteoblast activity, bone collagen degradation and osteoclastic activity. Markers that can be measured in serum are preferred to urinary markers to avoid the confounding effect of variations in creatinine excretion. With the exception of OPG and RANKL, the relationship of bone metabolites with age and sex generally mirrors the paediatric growth curve. It is essential that bone metabolites are interpreted in relation to appropriate paediatric age- and sex-related reference ranges for the assay used. For a few inherited bone disorders, measurement of a single specific bone metabolite is of diagnostic value. In other bone disorders, and in growth disorders, measurement of total ALP probably gives as much information as the newer bone metabolites, at least in the absence of liver disease. Total ALP has the advantage of being universally available in routine laboratories and is a much cheaper test for which same-day results are produced, unlike the newer bone metabolites which must be stored and analysed in batches. However, the newer bone metabolites come into their own in research where they complement outcome measures such as BMC, BMD and height velocity and give insight into mechanisms. In research, it is important that markers of both bone formation and resorption are analysed, as both sides of the equation are required for proper interpretation. Single measurements are of limited value unless they are very aberrant owing to the relatively wide paediatric reference ranges. Serial measurements are often the most informative, allowing assessment of the impact of treatment interventions on bone dynamics. At this stage of our knowledge, it is doubtful whether measurements of OPG and RANKL in serum reflect the bone micro-environment: the limited research that has been carried out on serum OPG and RANKL in children has produced conflicting and contradictory data.

References

1 Calvo MS, Eyre DR, Gundberg CM: Molecular basis and clinical application of biological markers of bone turnover. Endocr Rev 1996;17:333.

2 Whyte MP: Hypophosphatasia and the role of alkaline phosphatase in skeletal mineralization. Endocr Rev 1994;15:439.

3 Halleen J: Tartate-resistant acid phosphatase 5b (TRACP 5b) as a marker of bone resorption. Immunodiagnostic Systems Rev Ser 2006;3:1.

4 Khosla S: Minireview: the OPG/RANKL/RANK system. Endocrinology 2001;142:5050.

5 Diego EMD, Guerrero R, Piedra C: Six osteocalcin assays compared. Clin Chem 1994;40; 2071.

6 Crofton PM, Evans N, Taylor MRH, Holland CV: Procollagen type I amino-terminal propeptide: pediatric reference data and relationship with procollagen type I carboxyl-terminal propeptide. Clin Chem 2004;50:2173.

7 Buzi F, Maccarinelli G, Guaragni B, Ruggeri F, Radetti G, Meini A, Mazzolari E, Cocchi D: Serum osteoprotegerin and receptor activator of nuclear factors kB (RANKL) concentrations in normal children and in children with pubertal precocity, Turner's syndrome and rheumatoid arthritis. Clin Endocrinol (Oxf) 2004;60:87.

8 Tuchman S, Thayu M, Shults J, Zemel BS, Burnham JM, Leonard MB: Interpretation of biomarkers of bone metabolism in children: impact of growth velocity and body size in healthy children and chronic disease. J Pediatr 2008;153:484.

9 Rauch F, Middelmann B, Cagnoli M, Keller KM, Schonau E: Comparison of total alkaline phosphatase and three assays for bone-specific alkaline phosphatase in childhood and adolescence. Acta Paediatr 1997;86:583.

10 Crofton PM, Ahmed SF, Wade JC, Elmlinger MW, Ranke MB, Kelnar CJH, Wallace WHB: Bone turnover and growth during and after continuing chemotherapy in children with acute lymphoblastic leukemia. Pediatr Res 2000;48:490.

11 Crofton PM, Wade JC, Taylor MRH, Holland CV: Serum concentrations of carboxyl-terminal propeptide of type I procollagen, amino-terminal propeptide of type III procollagen, cross-linked carboxyl-terminal telopeptide of type I collagen, and their interrelationships in schoolchildren. Clin Chem 1997;43:1577.

12 Cioffi M, Molinari AM, Gazzerro P, Di Finizio B, Fratta M, Deufemia A, Puca GA: Serum osteocalcin in 1634 healthy children. Clin Chem 1997;43:543.

13 Rauchenzauner M, Schmid A, Heinz-Erian P, Kapelari K, Falkensammer G, Greismacher A, Finkenstedt G, Hogler W: Sex- and age-specific reference curves for serum markers of bone turnover in healthy children from 2 months to 18 years. J Clin Endocrinol Metab 2007;92:443.

14 Lund AM, Hansen M, Kollerup G, Juul A, Teisner B, Skovby F: Collagen-derived markers of bone metabolism in osteogenesis imperfecta. Acta Paediatr 1998;87:1131.

15 Arikoski P, Silverwood B, Tillmann V, Bishop NJ: Intravenous pamidronate treatment in children with moderate to severe osteogenesis imperfecta: assessment of indices of dual-energy X-ray absorptiometry and bone metabolite markers during the first year of therapy. Bone 2004;34:539.

16 Whyte MP, Obrecht SE, Finnegan PM, Jones JL, Podgornik MN, McAlister WH, Mumm S: Osteoprotegerin deficiency and juvenile Paget's disease. N Engl J Med 2002;347:175.

17 Kovar I, Mayne P, Barltrop D: Plasma alkaline phosphatase activity: a screening test for rickets in preterm neonates. Lancet 1982;i:308.

18 Crofton PM, Kelnar CJH: Bone and collagen markers in paediatric practice. Int J Clin Pract 1998; 52:557.

19 Doherty CP, Crofton PM, Sarkar MAK, Shakur MS, Wade JC, Kelnar CJH, Elmlinger MW, Ranke MB, Cutting WA: Malnutrition, zinc supplementation and catch-up growth: changes in insulin-like growth factor I, its binding proteins, bone formation and collagen turnover. Clin Endocrinol (Oxf) 2002; 57:391.

20 Mora S: Celiac disease in children: impact on bone health. Rev Endocr Metab Disord 2008;9:123.

21 Oswiecimska J, Ziora K, Pluskiewicz W, Geisler G, Broll-waska K, Karasek D, Dyduch A: Skeletal status and laboratory investigations in adolescent girls with anorexia nervosa. Bone 2007;41:103.

22 Calero JA, Munoz MT, Argente J, Traba ML, Mendez-Davila C, Garcia-Moreno C, de la Piedra C: A variation in bone alkaline phosphatase levels that correlates positively with bone loss and normal levels of amino-terminal propeptide of collagen I in girls with anorexia nervosa. Clin Chim Acta 1999; 285:121.

23 Ward LM: Osteoporosis due to glucocorticoid use in children with chronic illness. Horm Res 2005; 64:209.

24 Kannisto S, Korppi M, Arikoski P, Remes K, Voutilainen R: Biochemical markers of bone metabolism in relation to adrenocortical and growth suppression during the initiation phase of inhaled steroid therapy. Pediatr Res 2002;52:258.

25 Hillman L, Cassidy JT, Johnson L, Allen SH: Vitamin D metabolism and bone mineralization in children with juvenile rheumatoid arthritis. J Pediatr 1994; 124:910.

26 Reed AM, Haugen M, Pachman LM, Langman CB: Repair of osteopenia in children with juvenile rheumatoid arthritis. J Pediatr 1993;122:693.

27 Baroncelli GI, de Luca F, Magazzu G, Arrigo T, Sferlazzas C, Catena C, Bertelloni S, Saggese G: Bone demineralization in cystic fibrosis: evidence of imbalance between bone formation and degradation. Pediatr Res 1997;41:397.

28 Sylvester FA, Wyzga N, Hyams JS, Davis PM, Trudy Lere T, Vance K, Hawker G, Griffiths AM: Natural history of bone metabolism and bone mineral density in children with inflammatory bowel disease. Inflamm Bowel Dis 2007;13:42.

29 Crofton PM, Ahmed SF, Wade JC, Stephen R, Elmlinger MW, Ranke MB, Kelnar CJH, Wallace WHB: Effects of intensive chemotherapy on bone and collagen turnover and the growth hormone axis in children with acute lymphoblastic leukemia. J Clin Endocrinol Metab 1998;83:3121.

Dr. P.M. Crofton
Department of Paediatric Biochemistry
Royal Hospital for Sick Children, Sciennes Road
Edinburgh EH9 1LF (UK)
Tel. +44 131 536 0403, Fax +44 131 536 0410, E-Mail patricia.crofton@luht.scot.nhs.uk

Ranke MB, Mullis P-E (eds): Diagnostics of Endocrine Function in Children and Adolescents, ed 4.
Basel, Karger, 2011, pp 448–464

Quantification of Densitometric Bone Parameters and Muscle Function

Eckhard Schoenau · Oliver Fricke

Children's Hospital, University of Cologne, Cologne, Germany

Densitometric quantification of bone mass and density has gained considerable importance in pediatric endocrinology. The methodic concepts of osteodensitometry were primarily developed for the diagnosis and follow-up of adult bone disorders, in particular postmenopausal and senile osteoporosis. Osteodensitometric analyses are associated with specific methodic problems in pediatric patients, which have to be solved to avoid the misinterpretation of diagnostic results. The last 15 years in pediatric osteology were coined by the functional relationship between bone and muscle development. Thereby, the concept of the 'Mechanostat' was a useful theoretical concept to develop hypotheses on the interaction between bone and muscle function. The present chapter aims to provide a framework for the evaluation of bone densitometric parameters and muscle function and focuses especially on the diagnostic evaluation of the muscle-bone interaction.

Bone densitometry is still an essential tool in pediatrics. There is currently only limited proof that the information yielded by densitometric devices leads to improved clinical management and outcome. Nevertheless, many clinicians may feel that bone densitometry should be included in a work-up of children and adolescents who have sustained factures without adequate trauma or who have radiological evidence for inadequate bone mass. Densitometry is also used in treatment studies to document the effect of drugs that are suspected to have an effect on bone physiology. Primarily, it has to be emphasized that pediatric reference data have to be available whatever densitometric method is used. This basic prerequisite is often neglected leading to not interpretable results.

What Is Quantified in Osteodensitometric Analyses?

Bone densitometry refers to an arsenal of diagnostic methods pursuing to quantify bone mineral density (BMD) or bone mineral mass. The terms 'bone density' and

Table 1. Densitometric parameters and their definitions

Parameter	Abbreviation	Unit	Definition
Bone mineral content	BMC	g	mineral mass
Bone mineral content	BMC	g/cm	mineral mass per unit bone length
Areal bone mineral density	aBMD	g/cm^2	mineral mass per unit projection area
Volumetric bone mineral density	vBMD	g/cm^3	mineral mass per unit volume

'bone mass' are often used instead of 'bone mineral density' and 'bone mineral mass', which is not completely correct because the mineral components of the bone primarily contribute to these parameters. Therefore, organic substances are usually not considered in bone densitometry.

Even though density and mass are different in physics, the terms mass and density are often used interchangeably in the densitometric literature. The likely explanation for this disregard of physics is the fact that changes in bone mass are usually related to changes in bone density in adults, because bone size is a relatively stable variable in adulthood. This fact is obviously different in growing individuals because in the growing skeleton bone mass can increase despite a decrease of density due to bone growth. Therefore, a decrease in bone density does not necessarily reflect a decreased bone mineral substance, e.g. in children with short stature.

Densitometric Parameters

The most commonly used densitometric parameters are shown in table 1 and figure 1 [38].

Bone Mineral Content (BMC). The term 'BMC' is used to denote two different physical conditions – either the mineral mass of bone in its physical sense (unit: g), or the mineral mass per unit bone length (unit: g/cm). Although the same term 'BMC' is used for these two measures, they reflect different aspects. Consider two bones of different lengths, with all other properties being identical. The longer bone has a higher BMC expressed in g, whereas BMC in g/cm is not different between bones of different lengths. Therefore, the user of a densitometric device has to know, which type of BMC is indicated by the machine.

Bone Mineral Density. The term 'density' has an unequivocal meaning in physics. This uniqueness does not exist in osteodensitometrics. There are two different types of density, which are not always clearly separated from each other. On the one hand, the density is defined by Archimedes' law (volumetric density), and on the other hand mass is referred to bone area (areal density).

Areal BMD (aBMD). aBMD is defined as the mass of mineral per unit area of the projection image of the skeletal element, as judged by the attenuation of the radiation beam. Thus, aBMD does not only reflect the mineral density, but also the path length

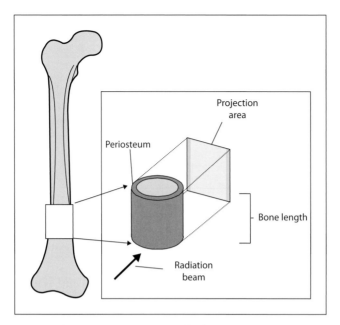

Fig. 1. Schematic representation of a long bone to demonstrate densitometric parameters. BMC measured in grams primarily corresponds with the mineral mass of the bone. BMC measured in grams/centimeter is the mineral mass of a piece of bone in relation to the length of the measured piece. aBMD is the mass of mineral in the piece of bone in relation to the projection area. Total vBMD corresponds to with the mineral mass of the piece of bone in relation to the volume enclosed by the periosteum. Trabecular vBMD is the mineral mass of the trabecular compartment in relation to its volume. Cortical vBMD is the mineral mass of the cortical compartment related to its volume.

of the radiation beam through the skeletal element. This path length depends on bone size and on the position of the skeletal element relatively to the direction of the radiation beam, because the skeletal element does not have a perfect circular shape. For example, the aBMD of a lumbar spine measured in the posterior-anterior direction is different from aBMD of the same lumbar spine measured in a lateral position [62].

Volumetric BMD (vBMD). vBMD is defined as mineral mass per volume and represents a density analogous to the physical definition of the term 'density'. Since bone is a heterogeneous material down to the microscopic level, vBMD is a mean value of a continuum of density values. Three different types of vBMD can be measured with current noninvasive densitometric devices – total, cortical and trabecular vBMD. These densities reflect the mean mineral density of the entire bone (or a cross-section of the bone), of the cortical compartment or of the trabecular compartment, respectively.

Structural Correlates of Densitometric Parameters
Table 2 displays the structural characteristics which are indicated by densitometric parameters. BMC measured in g increases or decreases whenever bone mineral is

Schoenau · Fricke

Table 2. Structural correlates of densitometric parameters

	BMC g	BMC g/cm	aBMC g/cm²	Total vBMD g/cm³	Trabecular vBMD g/cm³	Cortical vBMD g/cm³
Bone size and geometry						
Bone length	+	–	–	–	–	–
Cross-sectional bone size	+	+	+	–	–	–
Cortical thickness (relative cortical area)	+	+	+	+	–	–
Mineral density of the cortical compartment						
Cortical porosity	+	+	+	+	–	+
Material density of cortical bone	+	+	+	+	–	+
Mineral density of the trabecular compartment						
Number of trabeculae	+	+	+	+	+	–
Thickness of trabeculae	+	+	+	+	+	–
Material density of trabeculae	+	+	+	+	+	–

+ = Parameter is influenced by this structural featuer; – no influence.

added or removed from bone, either in longitudinal direction or in the cross-section of the skeletal element. BMC measured in g/cm is not primarily influenced by alterations of the length of the bone. This parameter also increases with longitudinal growth because skeletal elements also increase in the vertical direction their size in longitudinal growth. The parameter aBMD is influenced by similar aspects as vBMD measured in g/cm, but it dependence on bone size is lower because of its normalization on bone length and width. In contrast, vBMD is not dependent on bone size because of its normalization on three dimensions – length, width and depth. Trabecular and cortical vBMD reflect two parts of total vBMD. Trabecular vBMD is characterized by the number, thickness and material density of trabeculae. Cortical vBMD is dependent on cortical porosity and cortical material density.

How Is Bone Quantified?

Single Photon and Single X-Ray Absorptiometry (SPA and SXA)
SPA was introduced for the evaluation of bone at appendicular sites in 1969. A photon beam of radionucleotide source (SPA) or a small X-ray tube (SXA) is used for the measurement of attenuation after irradiation of the skeletal element [23]. The technical drawback of SPA and SXA is the invalidity of single energy measurements at sites with widely varying soft tissue thickness and tissue composition, such as the spine or hip.

Dual Photon and Dual X-ray Absorptiometry (DPA and DXA)
DPA was introduced to measure at sites which are inaccessible for SPA or SXA. The influence of overlying soft tissue is canceled out by using a radionucleotide source with tow effective energy levels [23]. DXA uses the same principle of measurement as DPA, but the radionucleotide source is replaced by an X-ray tube. DXA is the most frequently used densitometric method.

Quantitative Computed Tomography (QCT)
QCT measurements are obtainable at any skeletal site with a standard clinical CT scanner using and external bone mineral reference phantom for calibration [23]. Because the exposure to radiation is relatively high, this method has limited use in pediatrics. In order to avoid the high exposure to radiation, special high-resolution scanners for the peripheral skeleton were developed and are called peripheral QCT (pQCT). This procedure allows to measure bone density and to characterize bone geometry in a high resolution with minimal radiation exposure. Therefore, pQCT is suitable for the assessment of bone density, mass and geometry in pediatrics. Usually, pQCT analyses are performed at the radius or tibia.

Ultrasonic Methods
Ultrasound-based methods are often classified under the label of 'bone densitometry', although these methods do not measure parameters of bone density or mass in the same definition as for the 'classical densitometric' methods described above. Typical parameters of ultrasonographic measurements are 'speed of sound' (SOS) and broadband ultrasound attenuation (BUA). The speed of ultrasound transmission through a homogeneous substance depends on a variety of properties including density, microstructure and elastic modulus (a physical parameter reflecting stiffness) [48]. The situation of transmission speed is even more complex in a heterogeneous tissue such as bone tissue. Ultrasound parameters reflect a mixture of structural properties, such as size of the skeletal element and the marrow cavity, cortical thickness, orientation of trabeculae and also the thickness and composition of the overlying soft tissue. Therefore, the interpretation of ultrasonographic results is vague in individual pediatric patients (table 3).

Pediatric Reference Data of Osteodensitometric Measurements

Densitometric parameters show markedly different changes at different sites of measurement during the normal skeletal development. This is not surprising because different biological characteristics of the bone are reflected. It is also important to recognize that reference ranges for a given parameter at a specific skeletal region depend on sex, age, ethnic origin of the study population, densitometric method, measurement procedures and software version used for quantification of the sampled images. Therefore, the presentation of a simple set of densitometric reference data is not

Table 3. Methods for the measurement of densitometric parameters

	BMC g	BMC g/cm	aBMC g/cm^2	Total vBMD g/cm^3	Trabecular vBMD g/cm^3	Cortical vBMD g/cm^3
Single photon absorptiometry (SPA)	–	+	+	(+)	–	–
Dual energy X-ray absorptiometry (DXA)	+	+	+	(+)	–	(+)
Peripheral quantitative computed tomography (pQCT)	–	+	–	+	+	(+)

+ = Parameter is measured by this method; – = cannot be measured.

possible. The reader is referred to recent articles providing reference material for a variety of devices and skeletal locations, as listed in table 4. Even if the advantage of pQCT analyses and the disadvantage of DXA in the diagnostics of bone diseases in children and adolescents become clear theoretically, the actual recommendations of the PDCs report on the ISCD recommendations state that the actual reference data are not sufficient for the clinical use of pQCT for fracture prediction or diagnosis of low bone mass [9]. Therefore, the PDCs report recommends DXA measurements as the preferred method for assessing BMC and areal BMD in children and adolescents [31].

Mechanostat: Concept and Relevance for Bone Diagnostics

Mechanostat
Harold Frost recognized the relevance of Wolff's 'Transformationsgesetz' for bone health and the correct treatment of bone diseases (osteoporosis, accidental fractures and malpositions of skeletal elements) [22]. Figure 2 illustrates Frost's concept of the 'Mechanostat' that bone strength is adapted due to regulation of bone mass and geometry which are the controlled variables of the feedback loop. Currently, the network of osteocytes is recognized to be responsible for the measurement of bone strain due to mechanical stimuli [58]. Thereby, high forces induce the apposition of bone on the outer cortex of the skeletal element (modeling). This process is carried out by osteoblasts. In the meanwhile, osteoclasts work on the inner circumference of the cortical bone to shape its surface to achieve sufficiently adapted bone strength with a minimum of bone material. Figure 3 illustrates that with the same amount of bone material higher bone strength is accomplished when the cortex is thinner, the cross-sectional cortical area is equivalent, but the perimeter of the skeletal element

Table 4. Reference values for bone and muscle parameters in children and adolescents (age in years)

Device	Origin of population	Age range	n	Site of measurement	Ref. no.
SPA/SXA					
Norland Cameron 178	Belgium	3–25	202	radius (proximal and distal)	24
Norland Cameron 278O	Japan	0–12	229	radius (distal third)	57
Osteometer DT 100	Denmark	5–17	527	radius plus ulna ('distal' and 'ultradistal')	25
Lunar SP2	UK	4–10	420	radius (one-third distal site)	8
DPA/DXA					
Novo BMC Lab 22a	Belgium	3–25	202	lumbar spine (L2 to L4)	24
Lunar DP4	Belgium	3–25	88	whole body	24
Norland XR-26 HS	Argentina	2–20	778	whole body, femoral neck, trochanter, Ward's triangle, lumbar spine postero-anterior (L2 to L4) and laterial (L3 to L4), radius	62
Norland XR-26 HS	Argentina	2–20	433 (girls)	lumbar spine postero-anterior (L2 to L4) and laterial (L2 to L3)	37
Lunar DPX 3.6z	USA	8–18	148	whole body and subregions (head, arms, spine, pelvis, legs)	33
Lunar DPXL/PED	Netherlands	4–20	500	whole body, lumbar spine	9
Hologic QDR 1000	USA	1–19	218	lumbar spine (L1 to L4)	56
Hologic QDR 1000	UK	5–13	132	lumbar spine (L2 to L4), femoral neck, Ward's triangle	10
Hologic QDR 1000/W	UK	6–17	58	whole body, lumbar spine (L1 to L4), total hip and subregions (femoral neck, trochanteric region, intertrochanteric region)	61
Hologic QDR 1000/W	Switzerland	9–20	198	lumbar spine (L2 to L4), femoral neck, midfemoral shaft	13
Hologic QDR 1000/W	Denmark	5–19	343	whole body	34
Hologic QDR 2000	Canada	8–17	977	whole body and subregions (head, upper limbs, lower limbs, trunk, pelvis)	12
pQCT					
Stratec XCT 2000	Germany	6–40	377	distal and proximal radius	35,36, 50

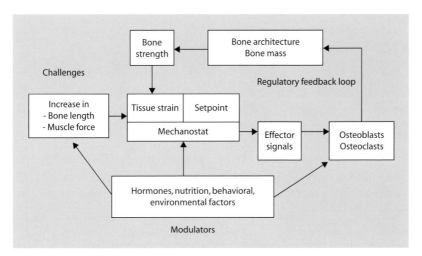

Fig. 2. The Mechanostat. The feedback loop between bone deformation (tissue strain) and bone strength is the essential mechanism of bone regulation. This homeostatic system is continually forced to adapt to external challenges during growth. Factors shown below modulate various aspects of the central regulatory system.

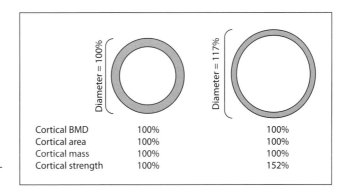

Fig. 3. Effect of bone geometry on bone strength.

is enlarged. Bone strength is measured with the Strength Strain Index (SSI, often also called Bone Strength Index, BSI), which is a variable describing the mechanical strength of an object due to applied torsion forces [29, 50].

Concept of the 'Functional Muscle-Bone Unit'

BMC increases with age, height and muscle mass (assessed by the correspondent cross-sectional muscle area) in children and adolescents [52]. In contrast, BMD is a material constant in healthy individuals without any significant association to age (adjusted for height) and muscle mass [52]. In contrast, bone strength (strength strain index, SSI) is significantly associated with age and muscle mass. Analyses

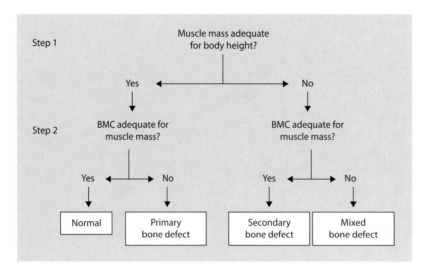

Fig. 4. Algorithm for diagnostics of pediatric bone diseases based on the FMBU.

have given clear evidence that the relationship between bone strength and age is mainly explained by the increase of muscle force in childhood and adolescence [50]. This functional relationship is described by the term 'functional muscle-bone unit' (FMBU). The FMBU may serve as a diagnostic pathway to classify bone diseases in primary and secondary diseases (fig. 4). Harold Frost developed the consideration that estrogens could change the relationship between bone and muscle mass in pubertal females for the additional storage of calcium for later episodes of gestation and lactation. The re-analysis of already published data and results from the DONALD study were consistent with this hypothesis [14, 47, 49]. In conclusion, the analysis of the FMBU has always to include gender and puberty to accomplish a correct and proper description of the musculoskeletal interaction. The FMBU concept was given evidence in the development of long bones of the extremities (in children and adolescents the radius) [36, 50]. Theoretically, there is not any relevant explanation why the basic principles of the cellular bone physiology should be different at other anatomical locations. But actually, because of lacking empirical data in children and adolescents, clear evidence for the truth of the FMBU concept is still missing for anatomical locations such as the vertebra which is a typical fracture location in osteoporosis in children.

Osteodensitometric Measurement of Corresponding Muscle and Bone Mass

The mechanostat concept of bone physiology describes the close functional relationship between muscle force and bone strength. Because peak muscle force corresponds with muscle mass, the measurement of surrogate parameters of peak muscle force is reasonable for the assessment of the muscle-bone interaction. In children and adolescents, reference values of bone mass and geometry area available for pQCT at the forearm. The corresponding measurement muscular parameter as surrogate for the peak muscle force is the cross-sectional muscle area at the 65% distance of the forearm length from the ulnar styloid process. The 65% measurement site indicates the peak of the cross-sectional circumference of the forearm which has a close relationship to the peak muscle force. When parameters of bone mass and geometry are measured at the tibia, the corresponding scan position is 66% of the bone length from the distal tibia. When total BMC is assessed in measurements with DXA, lean body mass is a reasonable parameter to describe total muscle mass. Reference values of cross-sectional muscle area are available in the literature for pediatric populations (table 5).

Dynamometric and Kinetic Analyses of Muscle Function in Pediatrics

The quantitative approach to characterize muscle function may be performed in two different ways: the description of a mass centre in the space (kinematics) and the measurement of forces (kinetics) [16]. When time is also recorded during the measurement of forces the calculation of related parameters such as velocity, energy and power is possible. Because bone metabolism depends on bone strain, especially maximal forces, due to applied muscle forces, the approach of kinetic analyses is more reasonable than the kinematic description of movement. An easy approach is the measurement of dynamometric forces such as 'maximal isometric grip force' (MIGF) [39]. This procedure is easy, cheap and has a high reliability in children and adolescents. The disadvantage of this method is the relatively low correspondence with daily activities of children and adolescents today. Therefore, the choice of a method based on an optimized movement with the occurrence of maximal forces should be preferred. A possible alternative to the measurement of MIGF is the kinetic description of a target-oriented movement by the goal-directed counter-movement jump (GDCMJ) which has a good reliability in children and adolescents beginning with 6 years of age [17]. The methodic background of this method is the measurement of ground-reaction forces with a force plate over the time to obtain peak jump force (PJF), peak jump power (PJP), maximal velocity of the center of gravity (v_{max}), jump height and energy. Thereby, PJF of the one-leg jump has a higher correspondence to the cross-sectional muscle area (MA) of the calf than the counter-movement jump when the one-leg jump is performed in adolescents and adults. The kinetic analysis of the GDCMJ may also serve as a useful tool to characterize the impaired muscle function in detail. Individuals with a conditioned but force-reduced muscular system are characterized by the production of low maximal forces with correspondent low maximal power. In contrast, the unconditioned neuromuscular system has a typical pattern of power generation. The maximal force produces

Table 5. Pediatric reference values and studies on muscle mass and function

Device	Population/disease	Age, years	Number of individuals	Site of measurement/test of muscle function	Ref. no.
Leonardo Force Plate	multiethnic	12–14	99 girls	1-LJ (PJF) 2-LJ (v_{max}, PJP, JH, time, EFI)	60
Leonardo Force Plate	Caucasian, reference values	6–19	312 (177 girls)	2-LJ (PJF, PJP)	17
Leonardo Force Plate	Caucasian	19–88	58 (33 women)	2-LJ (PJP)	42
Leonardo Force Plate	Caucasian	18–88	258 (169 women)	2-LJ (PJF, PJP)	45
Leonardo Force Plate, Dynamometer	preterm birth	7	45 (23 girls)	2-LJ (PJF, PJP, V_{max}), MIGF	21
Leonardo Force Plate, Dynamometer	diabetes mellitus	6–18	40 (20 girls)	2-LJ (PJF, PJP), MIGF	19
Leonardo Force Plate, Dynamometer	congenital heart disease	14–23	29 (15 girls)	2-LJ, PJF, PJP, V_{max}), MIGF	18
pQCT	juvenile idiopathic arthritis	17.7 + 2.6	12 (7 girls)	forearm CSMA (65%)	5
pQCT	small for gestational age	Mean 7.1	74	forearm CSMA (65%)	54
pQCT	juvenile idiopathic arthritis	9–24	25 (17 girls)	forearm CSMA (65%)	44
pQCT	juvenile idiopathic arthritis	4-20	57 (34 girls)	forearm CSMA (65%)	43
pQCT	inflammatory bowel disease	13.9 + 3.5	143	forearm CSMA (65%)	6
pQCT	diabetes mellitus	11.7 ± 3.0	88 (42 girls)	forearm CSMA (65%)	4
pQCT	rheumatic diseases	13.4 ± 2.9	94 (23 girls)	forearm CSMA (65%)	3
pQCT	Turner syndrome	19.5 ± 2.3	21	forearm CSMA (65%)	1
pQCT	juvenile idiopathic arthritis	15.3 ± 2.5	34 (18 girls)	forearm CSMA (65%)	2
pQCT	small for gestational age, growth hormone deficiency	4–12	91 (32 girls	forearm CSMA (65%)	32
pQCT	small for gestational age	7.3 ± 2.6	34 (11 girls)	forearm CSMA (65%)	55
DXA	healthy individuals	6–25	145 (94 girls)	femoral MA	28
DXA	idiopathic short stature	3–17	77	BMC in relation to lean mass	27

Table 5. Continued

Device	Population/disease	Age, years	Number of individuals	Site of measurement/test of muscle function	Ref. no.
DXA	Turner syndrome	4–24	83	BMC in relation to lean mass	26
pQCT	Caucasian, reference population	6–40	469 (184 girls)	forearm CSMA (65%)	40
Dynamometer	osteogenesis imperfecta	0.5–15.7	59 (30 girls)	MIGF	30
Dynamometer	glycogen storage disease	children	19	MIGF	53
Dynamometer	Caucasian, reference population	6–19	315 (157 girls)	MIGF	39
pQCT	Caucasian, reference population	6–19	349 (183 girls)	forearm CSMA (65%)	51
Dynamometer	renal disease	children	30	MIGF	59
Dynamometer	anticonvulsive therapy	6–19	39 (18 girls)	MIGF	41
pQCT	Caucasian, prediction of muscle mass by birth weight	5–19	284 (145 girls)	forearm CSMA (65%)	20
Dynamometer	eating disorder	11–18	25 girls	MIGF	15
pQCT, Leonardo Force Plate	healthy individuals	6–16	105 (51 girls)	tibial CSMA (66%), 2-LJ (PJF, PJP)	7

1-LJ = 1-Leg jump; 2-LJ = 2-leg jump; PJF = peak jump force; PJP = peak jump power; V_{max} = maximal velocity; JH = jump height; MIGF = maximal isometric grip force; CSMA = cross-sectional muscle area; BMC = bone mineral content.

a relatively low maximal power [18]. This pattern is easily understandable when the expression 'power = force × velocity' is considered. The result of a relatively low force is caused by the production of a relatively low v_{max} which is a characteristic of an impaired inter- and intramuscular coordination (low efficiency of movement). The analysis of kinetic parameters may also serve as useful clinical tool in pediatric osteology because of a second reason despite the assessment of maximal forces. The occurrence of fractures depends on bone strength (associated with maximal forces) in accidental falls, whereas the occurrence of falls depends on coordinative skills and of the risk behavior of the individual. Thus, mechanographic analyses may describe two of the three main pathogenetic factors for the occurrence of fractures. Reference values dependent on sex, age, weight and height are available for pediatric populations in the literature (table 6). Studies on muscle function were performed in different pediatric diseases (table 6).

Table 6. Reference values of muscle function, muscle mass and its relation to bone mass in children and adolescents

Age	Peak jump force (2-LJ in N on force plate)[1]		Peak jump power (2-LJ in W on force plate)[1]	
	male	female	male	female
6 years		597±126		750±136
7 years	677±119	660±149	895±159	853±204
8 years	723±115	807±198	1,116±218	1,092±220
9 years	799±190	793±187	1,300±251	1,171±230
10 years	970±172	957±296	1,510±258	1,409±352
11 years	1,206±414	1,130±210	1,697±282	1,629±305
12 years	1,120+233	1,266±294	1,996±513	1,944±417
13 years	1,470±235	1,217±190	2,781±722	2,157±479
14 years	1,601±393	1,298±160	2,986±675	2,268±400
15 years	1,660±248	1,493±292	3,389±512	2,358±495
16 years	1627±406	1,559±363	3,298±454	2,638±507
17 years	1,718±413	1,275±304	3,980±753	2,425±460
18 years	1,923±121	1,675±352	3,950±53	2,978±528
19 years	2,018±564	1,300±123	4,123±486	2,482±119

Cross-sectional MA is used as surrogate of muscle mass and BMC is used as surrogate of bone mass. MA and BMC were measured with pQCT. Individuals with body height differing from the reference should be referred to body height or for peak jump power to body weight and not to age.

[1] Reference values of peak jump force and peak jump power were published in Fricke et al. [17].

[2] Reference values of maximal isometric grip force were published in Neu et al. Am J Physiol Endocrinol Metab 2002;283:E103–E107and based on height were published by Rauch et al. [39].

[3] Reference values of the relationship between Bone Mineral Content (BMC) and Cross-sectional Muscle Area (CSMA) were published in Schoenau et al. [51].

* The age range comprises 18–23 years [39].

Maximal isometric grip force (N)[2]		MA (at 65% site in cm^2)[2]		Ratio between BMC (mg/mm) and MA (cm^2) at 65% site[3]	
male	female	male	female	male	female
90±20	77±20	16.6±1.9	15.5±1.9	2.54±0.34	2.59±0.29
119±28	106±31	20.4±3.3	18.1+2.7	2.55±0.31	2.62+0.38
175±43	168±43	22.6±3.4	21.9±3.6	2.58±0.30	2.59±0.35
211±58	209±55	25.9±4.7	25.0±4.3	2.47±0.43	2.64±0.40
317±82	246±40	33.3±5.7	27.0±3.2	2.39±0.32	2.90±0.35
387±79	283±47	39.2±5.9	28.0±2.8	2.36±0.26	2.91±0.31
448±74*	278±48*	45.0±6.6*	28.3±3.6*	2.44±0.26	2.96±0.36

References

1 Bechthold S, Rauch F, Noelle V, Donhauser S, Neu CM, Schoenau E, Schwarz HP: Musculoskeletal analyses of the forearm in young women with Turner syndrome: a study using peripheral quantitative computed tomography. J Clin Endocrinol Metab 2001;86:5819–5823.

2 Bechthold S, Ripperger P, Dalla Pozza R, Schmidt H, Haefner R, Schwarz HP: Musculoskeletal and functional muscle-bone analysis in children with rheumatic disease using peripheral quantitative computed tomography. Osteoporos Int 2005;16: 757–763.

3 Bechthold S, Ripperger P, Bonfig W, Dalla Pozza R, Haefner R, Schwarz HP: Growth hormone changes bone geometry and body composition in patients with juvenile idiopathic arthritis requiring glucocorticoid treatment: a controlled study using peripheral quantitative computed tomography. J Clin Endocrinol Metab 2005;90:3168–3173.

4 Bechthold S, Dirlenbach I, Raile K, Noelle V, Bonfig W, Schwarz HP: Early manifestation of type I diabetes in children is a risk factor for changed bone geometry: data using peripheral quantitative computed tomography. Pediatrics 2006;118: e627–e634.

5 Bechthold S, Ripperger P, Dalla Pozza R, Roth J, Haefner R, Michels H, Schwarz HP: Dynamics of body composton and bone in patients with juvenile idiopathic arthritis treated with growth hormone. J Clin Endocrinol Metab 2010;95:178–185.

6 Bechthold S, Alberer M, Arenz T, Putzker S, Filipiak-Pittroff B, Schwarz HP, Koletzko S: Reduced muscle mass and bone size in pediatric patients with inflammatory bowel disease. Inflamm Bowel Dis 2010;16:216–225.

7 Binkley TL, Specker BL: Muscle-bone relationships in the lower leg of healthy pre-pubertal females and males. J Musculoskelet Neuronal Interact 2008;8: 239–243.

8 Bishop NJ, dePriester JA, Cole TJ, Lucas A: Reference values for radial bone width and mineral content using single photon absorptiometry in healthy children aged 4 to 10 years. Acta Paediatr 1992;81:463–468.

9 Boot AM, de Ridder MAJ, Pols HAP, Krenning EP, de Muinck Keizer-Schrama S: Bone mineral density in children and adolescents: relation to puberty, calcium intake and physical activity. J Clin Endocrinol Metab 1997;82:57–62.

10 Davie MW, Haddaway MJ: Bone mineral content and density in healthy subjects and in osteogenesis imperfecta. Arch Dis Child 1994;70:331–334.

11 Faulkner RA, Bailey DA, Drinkwater DT, Wilkinson AA, Houston CS, McKay HA: Regional and total body bone mineral content, bone mineral density, and total body tissue composition in children 8–16 years of age. Calcif Tissue Int 1993;53:7–12.

12 Faulkner RA, Bailey DA, Drinkwater DT, McKay HA, Arnold C, Wilkinson AA: Bone densitometry in Canadian children 8–17 years of age. Calcif Tissue Int 1996;59:344–351.

13 Fournier PE, Rizzoli R, Slosman DO, Theintz G, Bonjour JP: Asynchrony between the rates of standing height gain and bone mass accumulation during puberty. Osteoporos Int 1997;7:525–532.

14 Ferretti JL, Capozza RF, Cointry GR, et al: Gender-related differences in the relationship between densitometric values of whole-body bone mineral content and lean body mass in humans between 2 and 87 years of age. Bone 1998;22:683–690.

15 Fricke O, Tutlewski B, Stabrey A, Lehmkuhl G, Schoenau E: A cybernetic approach to osteoporosis in anorexia nervosa. J Musculoskelet Neuronal Interact 2005;5:155–161.

16 Fricke O, Schoenau E: Examining the developing skeletal muscle: why, what and how? J Musculoskelet Neuronal Interact 2005;5:225–231.

17 Fricke O, Weidler J, Tutlewski B, Schoenau E: Mechanography: a new device for the assessment of muscle function in pediatrics. Pediatr Res 2006;59: 46–49.

18 Fricke O, Witzel C, Schickendantz S, Sreeram N, Brockmeier K, Schoenau E: Mechanographic charcteristics of adolescents and young adults with congenital heart disease. Eur J Pediatr 2008;167: 331–336.

19 Fricke O, Seewi O, Semler O, Tutlewski B, Stabrey A, Schoenau E: The influence of auxology and long-term glycemic control on muscle function in children and adolescents with type 1 diabetes mellitus. J Musculoskelet Neuronal Interact 2008;8:188–195.

20 Fricke O, Semler O, Stabrey A, Tutlewski B, Remer T, Herkenrath P, Schoenau E: High and low birth weight and its implication for growth and bone development in childhood and adolescence. J Pediatr Endocrinol Metab 2009;22:19–30.

21 Fricke O, Roedder D, Kribs A, Tutlewski B, von Kleist-Retzow JC, Herkenrath P, Roth B, Schoenau E: Relationship of muscle function to auxology in preterm born children at the age of seven years. Horm Res Paediatr. 2010;73:390–397.

22 Frost HM: Changing concepts in skeletal physiology: Wolff's Law, the Mechanostat and the 'Utah Paradigm'. J Hum Biol 1998;10:599–605.

23 Genant HK, Engelke K, Fuerst T, Gluer CC, Grampp S, Harris ST, Jergas M, Lang T, Lu Y, Majumdar S, Mathur A, Takada M: Noninvasive assessment of bone mineral and structure: state of the art. J Bone Miner Res 1996;11:707–730.

24 Geusens P, Cantatore F, Nijs J, Proesmans W, Emma F, Dequeker J: Heterogeneity of growth of bone in children at the spine, radius and total skeleton. Growth Dev Aging 1991;55:249–256.

25 Gunnes M: Bone mineral density in the cortical and trabecular distal forearm in healthy children and adolescents. Acta Paediatr 1994;83:463–467.

26 Hoegler W, Briody J, Moore B, Garnett S, Lu PW, Cowell CT: Importance of estrogen on bone health in Turner syndrome: a cross-sectional and longitudinal study using dual-energy X-ray absorptiometry. J Clin Endocrinol Metab 2004;89:193–199.

27 Hoegler W, Briody J, Lu PW, Cowell CT: Effect of growth hormone therapy and puberty on bone and body composition in children with idiopathic short stature and growth hormone deficiency. Bone 2005;37:642–650.

28 Hoegler W, Blimkie CJ, Cowell CT, Inglis D, Rauch F, Kemp AF, Wiebe P, Duncan CS, Farpour-Lambert N, Woodhead HJ: Sex-specific developmental changes in muscle size and bone geometry at the femoral shaft. Bone 2008;42:982–989.

29 Kokoroghiannis C, Charopoulos I, Lyritis G, Raptou P, Karachalios T, Papaioannou N: Correlation of pQCT bone strength index with mechanical testing in distraction osteogenesis. Bone 2009;45:512–516.

30 Land C, Rauch F, Montpetit K, Ruck-Gibis J, Glorieux FH: Effect of intravenous pamidronate therapy on functional abilities and level of ambulation in children with osteogenesis imperfecta. J Pediatr 2006;148:456–460.

31 Liewiecki EM, Gordon CM, Baim S, Binkley N, Bilezikian JP, Kendler DL, Hand DB, Silverman S, Bishop NJ, Leonard MB, Bianchi ML, Kalkwarf HJ, Langman CB, Plotkin H, Rauch F, Zemel BS: Special report on the 2007 adult and pediatric Position Development Conferences of the International Society for Clinical Densitometry. Osteoporos Int 2008;19:1369–1378.

32 Martin DD, Schweizer R, Schoenau E, Binder G, Ranke MB: Growth hormone-induced increases in skeletal muscle mass alleviates the associated insulin resistance in short children born small for gestational age, but not with growth hormone deficiency. Horm Res 2009;72:38–45.

33 Maynard LM, Guo SS, Chumlea WC, Roche AF, Wisemandle WA, Zeller CM, Towne B, Siervogel RM: Total-body and regional bone mineral content and areal bone mineral density in children aged 8–18 years: the Fels Longitudinal Study. Am J Clin Nutr 1998;68:1111–1117.

34 Molgaard C, Thomsen BL, Prentice A, Cole TJ, Michaelsen KF: Whole body bone mineral content in healthy children and adolescents. Arch Dis Child 1997;76:9–15.

35 Neu C, Manz F, Rauch F, Schoenau E: Modeling of cross-sectional bone size and geometry at the proximal radius: a study of normal bone development using peripheral quantitative computed tomography. Osteoporos Int 2001;12:538–547.

36 Neu CM, Manz F, Rauch F, et al: Bone densities and bone size at the distal radius in healthy children and adolescents: a study using peripheral quantitative computed tomography. Bone 2001;28:227–232.

37 Plotkin H, Nùñez M, Alvarez Filgueira ML, Zanchetta JR: Lumbar spine bone density in Argentine children. Calcif Tissue Int 1996;58:144–149.

38 Rauch F, Schoenau E: The developing bone: slave or master of its cells and molecules? Pediatr Res 2001;50:309–314.

39 Rauch F, Neu CM, Wassmer G, Beck B, Rieger-Wettengl G, Rietschel E, Manz F, Schoenau E: Muscle analysis by measurement of maximal isometric grip force: new reference data and clinical applications in pediatrics. Pediatr Res 2002;51:505–510.

40 Rauch F, Schoenau E: Peripheral quantitative computed tomography of the proximal radius in young subjects: new reference data and interpretation of results. J Musculoskelet Neuronal Interact 2008;8:217–226.

41 Rieger-Wettengl G, Tutlewski B, Stabrey A, Rauch F, Herkenrath P, Schauseil-Zipf U, Schoenau E: Analysis of the musculoskeletal system in children and adolescents receiving anticonvulsant monotherapy with valproic acid or carbamazepine. Pediatrics 2001;108:E107.

42 Rittweger J, Schiessl H, Felsenberg D, Runge M: Reproducibility of the jumping mechanogarphy as a test of mechanical power output in physically competent adult and elderly subjects. J Am Geriatr Soc 2004;52:128–131.

43 Roth J, Palm C, Scheunemann I, Ranke MB, Schweizer R, Dannecker GE: Musculoskeletal abnormalities of the forearm in patients with juvenile idiopathic arthritis relate mainly to bone geometry. Arthritis Rheum 2004;50:1277–1285.

44 Roth J, Linge M, Tzaribachev N, Schweizer R, Kuemmerle-Deschner J: Musculoskeletal abnormalities in juvenile idiopathic arthritis: a 4-year longitudinal study. Rheumatology 2007;46:1180–1184.

45 Runge M, Rittweger J, Russo CR, Schiessl H, Felsenberg D: Is muscle power output a key factor in the age-related decline in physical performance? A comparison of muscle cross section, chair-rising test and jumping power. Clin Physiol Funct Imaging 2004;24:335–340.

46 Rueth E-M, Weber LT, Schoenau E, Wunsch R, Seibel MJ, Feneberg R, Mehls O, Toenshoff B: Analysis of the functional muscle-bone unit of the forearm in pediatric renal transplant recipients. Kidney Int 2004;66:1694–1706.

47 Schiessl H, Frost HM, Jee WS: Estrogen and bone-muscle strength and mass relationships. Bone 1998;22:1–6.

48 Schoenau E: Problems of bone analysis in childhood and adolescence. Pediatr Nephrol 1998;12:420–429.

49 Schoenau E, Neu CM, Mokov E, et al: Influence of puberty on muscle area and cortical bone area of the forearm in boys and girls. J Clin Endocrinol Metab 2000;85:1095–1098.

50 Schoenau E, Neu CM, Rauch F, Manz F: The development of bone strength at the proximal radius during childhood and adolescence. J Clin Endocrinol Metab 2001;86:613–618.

51 Schoenau E, Neu CM, Beck B, Manz F, Rauch F: Bone mineral content per muscle cross-sectional area as an index of the functional muscle-bone unit. J Bone Miner Res 2002;17:1095–1101.

52 Schoenau E: From mechanostat theory to development of the 'functional muscle–bone-unit'. J Musculoskelet Neuronal Interact 2005 ;5:232–238.

53 Schwahn B, Rauch F, Wendel U, Schoenau E: Low bone mass in glycogen storage disease type 1 is associated with reduced muscle force and poor metabolic control. J Pediatr 2002;141:350–356.

54 Schweizer R, Martin DD, Haase M, Roth J, Trebar B, Binder G, Schwarze CP, Ranke MB: Similar effects of long-term exogenous growth hormone (GH) on bone and muscle parameters: a pQCT study of GH-deficient and small-for-gestational-age (SGA) children. Bone 2007;41:875–881.

55 Schweizer R, Martin DD, Schoenau E, Ranke MB: Muscle function improves during growth hormone therapy in short children born small for gestational age: results of a peripheral quantitative computed tomography study on body composition. J Clin Endocrinol Metab 2008;93:2978–2983.

56 Southard RN, Morris JD, Mahan JD, Hayes JR, Torch MA, Sommer A, Zipf WB: Bone mass in healthy children: measurement with quantitative DXA. Radiology 1991;179:735–738.

57 Sugimoto T, Nishino M, Tsunenari T, Kawakatsu M, Shimogaki K, Fujii Y, Negishi H, Tsutsumi M, Fukase M, Chihara K: Radial bone mineral content of normal Japanese infants and prepubertal children: influence of age, sex and body size. Bone Miner 1994;24:189–200.

58 Taylor AF, Saunders AM, Shingle DL, Cimbala JM, Zhou Z, Donahue HJ: Mechanically stimulated osteocytes regulate osteoblastic activity via gap junctions. Am J Physiol Cell Physiol 2007;292:545–552.

59 Tenbrock K, Kruppa S, Mokov E, Querfeld U, Michalk D, Schoenau E: Analysis of muscle strength and bone structure in children with renal disease. Pediatr Nephrol 2000;14:669–672.

60 Ward KA, Das G, Berry JL, Roberts SA, Rawer R,Adams JE, Mughal Z: Vitamin D status and muscle function in post-menarchal adolescent girls. J Clin Endocrinol Metab 2009;94:559–563.

61 Warner JT, Cowan FJ, Dunstan FD, Evans WD, Webb DK, Gregory JW: Measured and predicted bone mineral content in healthy boys and girls aged 6–18 years: adjustment for body size and puberty. Acta Paediatr 1998;87:244–249.

62 Zanchetta JR, Plotkin H, Alvarez Filgueira ML: Bone mass in children: normative values for the 2- to 20-year-old population. Bone 1995;16:393S–399S.

Prof. Dr. med. Eckhard Schoenau
Children's Hospital, University of Cologne
Kerpener Strasse 62
DE–50924 Cologne (Germany)
Tel. +49 221 478 4360, Fax +49 221 478 4635, E-Mail eckhard.schoenau@uk-koeln.de

Ranke MB, Mullis P-E (eds): Diagnostics of Endocrine Function in Children and Adolescents, ed 4.
Basel, Karger, 2011, pp 465–482

Body Composition Assessment in Children and Adolescents

Jonathan C.K. Wells

MRC Childhood Nutrition Research Centre, Institute of Child Health, London, UK

Recent research is increasingly emphasising the benefits of information on body composition in paediatric research and clinical practice. Almost all paediatric diseases adversely affect body composition, and treatments can influence and sometimes reverse such changes. Many such effects are too subtle to be inferred from changes in weight, leading to growing interest in the measurement of body composition itself. Whilst the recent emergence of an epidemic of childhood obesity has drawn attention to high levels of body fat, in many diseases lean mass (used here synonymously with fat-free mass) is also affected. Both fat mass and lean mass are important health outcomes. High levels of body fat impact adversely on health during childhood [1] and predispose to cardiovascular disease and diabetes in later life [2], while low levels of lean mass tend to be associated with poorer physiological function.

Due to the ease with which weight and height can be measured in most contexts, weight-for-height or body mass index (BMI) has long comprised the primary body composition outcome in paediatric clinical practice. With the growing interest in body composition has come increasing recognition that BMI is insufficient for this purpose. This chapter will first highlight the limitations of BMI as a measure of childhood body composition, and then discuss other approaches with greater accuracy.

Body Mass Index and Body Composition

The statistical rationale of BMI is that it adjusts weight (WT, in kg) for variability in height (HT, in m^2):

$$BMI = WT/HT^2 \tag{1}$$

Ideally, BMI should have zero correlation with stature and hence rank individuals in terms of their relative weight. Several studies have demonstrated its success in this

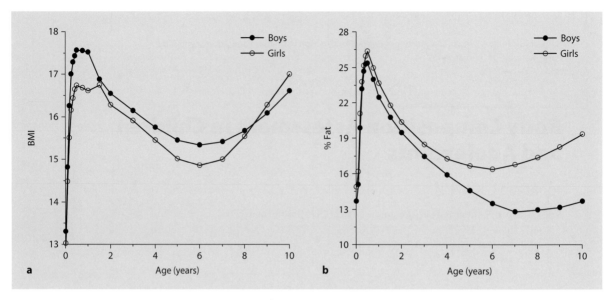

Fig. 1. Associations between indices of body composition and age. **a** Body mass index. **b** Percentage fat (calculated as [fat mass/weight] · 100). Data are taken from the reference child [6].

context [3, 4], and even though at some ages (e.g. early infancy, puberty) a small residual correlation remains between weight and stature, this has negligible effect on ranking. Thus from a statistical point of view BMI successfully adjusts weight for height. The critical question is what information is actually conveyed by relative weight?

As demonstrated in numerous studies [5, 6], BMI has a characteristic relationship with age as shown in figure 1a. Values rise rapidly during infancy, decline to a nadir in mid-childhood and then increase again towards adult values. These patterns appear to have consistency with indices of adiposity such as skinfold thicknesses [7] or percent fat [6] (although note that the sexual dimorphism in BMI is the reverse of that for the other two outcomes). Thus, figure 1b illustrates the age-related development of percentage fat for comparison. The increase in BMI during mid-childhood has been referred to as the 'adiposity rebound' [8] and the time of its occurrence has been proposed to be an important factor in the risk of developing obesity. It is also clear that within any given age group, a group of individuals with very high BMI is likely to have high levels of body fat [9]. Collectively, this has led to a general perception that BMI is a useful index of adiposity in individuals, reflecting the approach adopted for adults.

In adults BMI is used to categorise nutritional status across the entire spectrum of body weight. The World Health Organisation categorises chronic energy deficiency as BMI <18.5 [10], while Garrow and Webster [11] proposed that normal weight be categorised as BMI 20–25, overweight as BMI 25–30, and obesity as BMI >30. This classification remains widely used despite evidence that central obesity (as indicated

Wells

Table 1. Body mass index cut-offs for thinness, overweight and obesity, based on international data aiming to link paediatric data with adult cut-offs of 18.5, 25 and 30, respectively

Age	Thin (BMI 18.5)		Overweight (BMI 25)		Obese (BMI 30)	
	M	F	M	F	M	F
2 years	15.14	14.83	18.41	18.02	20.09	19.81
3 years	14.74	14.47	17.89	17.56	19.57	19.36
4 years	14.43	14.19	17.55	17.28	19.29	19.15
5 years	14.21	13.94	17.42	17.15	19.30	19.17
6 years	14.07	13.82	17.55	17.34	19.78	19.65
7 years	14.04	13.86	17.92	17.75	20.63	20.51
8 years	14.15	14.02	18.44	18.35	21.60	21.57
9 years	14.35	14.28	19.10	19.07	22.77	22.81
10 years	14.64	14.61	19.84	19.86	24.00	24.11
11 years	14.97	15.05	20.55	20.74	25.10	25.42
12 years	15.35	15.62	21.22	21.68	26.02	26.67
13 years	15.84	16.26	21.91	22.58	26.84	27.76
14 years	16.41	16.88	22.62	23.34	27.63	28.57
15 years	16.98	17.45	23.29	23.94	28.30	29.11
16 years	17.54	17.91	23.90	24.37	28.88	29.43
17 years	18.05	18.25	24.46	24.70	29.41	29.69
18 years	18.50	18.50	25.00	25.00	30.00	30.00

Data from Cole et al. [14, 15].

by waist circumference) varies widely for a given BMI value [12] and that waist circumference is a stronger predictor of cardiovascular risk factors [13]. In children, BMI values change with age [5], hence the approach used in adults cannot be adopted directly. Instead, individual children are ranked in terms of BMI standard deviation score (SDS), with centile cut-offs used to identify childhood overweight and obesity. Currently, these cut-offs are based on the back extrapolation of adult values of 25 (overweight) and 30 (obese) to equivalent values at earlier ages [14]. A similar approach subsequently provided cut-offs to define thinness, again equivalent to the adult value of 18.5 [15]. BMI values defining thinness and overweight/obesity over the age range 2–18 years are given in table 1.

The hypothesis that individual variability in childhood BMI is proportional to variability in body fat is not well supported by evidence. Although some studies have reported relatively high correlations between BMI and percent fat [16, 17], this apparent level of agreement is an artefact of the wide range of body weights and percent fat studied. In the middle part of the range, where the majority of the population lie, the agreement between these variables is very poor. Furthermore, the use of percent fat as the reference index of adiposity in such analyses is also problematic. Percent fat refers to the proportion of fat in body weight. Since in all individuals percent fat and percent lean must add up to 100%, it can be seen that percent fat is not an independent index of adiposity, but is influenced by the relative amount of lean mass [18]. There are also statistical problems with the index, given that fat mass is present in both the numerator and the denominator (weight) [19].

These problems can be resolved by adopting a more sophisticated approach to the expression of body composition data. The simplest model of body composition divides weight (WT) into fat mass (FM) and lean mass (LM) components, hence:

$$WT = LM + FM \qquad (2)$$

Although a variety of more complex body composition models have been used, for example distinguishing the mineral, protein and water in lean mass, or the distribution of fat in different regional depots, the two component model described in equation 2 is adequate for many purposes. Van Itallie et al. [20] proposed that equations 1 and 2 could be combined in order to divide BMI into its fat and lean components:

$$BMI = LM/HT^2 + FM/HT^2 \qquad (3)$$

These two terms, known as the lean mass index and the fat mass index, represent separate indices adjusting both lean mass and fat mass for height. They are therefore intended to be independent both of height and each other, and allow investigation of two body composition outcomes. However, it is not inevitable that the power by which height should be raised, in order to adjust both lean mass and fat mass for it, will always be 2. An analysis of this issue in eight year old children found that whereas LM/HT^2 did adjust successfully for height, the optimal index for fat mass was FM/HT^6 [18]. This difference can be attributed to inconsistency in the degree of variability in the three terms HT, LM and FM, with FM having greater between-individual variability than the other two terms. Nevertheless, the index FM/HT^2 retains only a moderate correlation with height, such that <2% of the variability in it can be attributed to the effect of height [18]. Thus, the two indices derived from equation 3 are adequate for most purposes, and will be problematic only when comparing two individuals or two groups differing markedly in height. The great advantage of LMI and FMI is that they are presented in the same units as BMI and hence facilitate analyses.

For example, Hattori et al. [21] devised a graph plotting FMI on the y-axis against LMI on the x-axis. Since in any individual FMI and LMI must add up to BMI, the

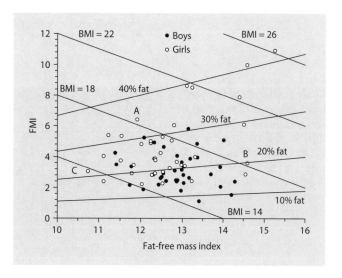

Fig. 2. Hattori chart plotting fat mass adjusted for height on the y-axis against lean mass adjusted for height on the x-axis. The data represent 75 healthy UK children aged 8 years of age. The data points labelled A and B represent 2 girls with identical BMI but very different % fat, while those labelled B and C represent 2 girls with identical % fat but very different BMI.

graph also shows diagonal lines of constant BMI value, and it is possible to add further nonparallel lines of constant percent fat value. These Hattori graphs elegantly illustrate the limitations of BMI as an index of adiposity in individuals. Figure 2 illustrates data from a sample of 75 normal healthy children aged eight years. It can be seen that individual children of the same age and sex may vary up to twofold in percentage fat for a given BMI value, which can be attributed to the fact that children vary substantially in their LMI as well as their FMI [22]. This variability is apparent from early infancy onwards [22], and remains present at the extremes of nutritional status.

The same graphs illustrate the limitations of BMI as an indicator of the developmental patterns of body composition. Figure 3 plots LMI and FMI data from a sample of healthy UK children measured using the criterion 4-component model (see on). At puberty, average FMI remains relatively stable in boys whereas LMI increases from around 13 to 18. In contrast, in girls average LMI increases only from 13 to 15, whereas FMI increases from 5 to 7 [23]. Studies of individual children are broadly consistent with these descriptions of average children, with the majority of increasing BMI attributable to lean mass [24]. Collectively, these data demonstrate the fallacy of the concept of a generic adiposity rebound expressed by increasing BMI. It has also been pointed out that the time of BMI rebound (the nadir in BMI value) is an artefact of BMI centile, such that heavier individuals tend for statistical, rather than biological, reasons to increase in BMI earlier [25]. Normative data for LMI and FMI, in the form of sex-specific centiles based on the data presented in figure 3, will be published in the near future.

In addition to the above limitations as an index of body fat in individuals, BMI is also confounded by population differences. In adults, for example, ethnic groups

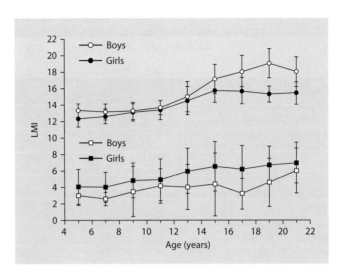

Fig. 3. Changes in LMI (circles, upper lines) and FMI (squares, lower lines) with age in boys and girls from 4 to 21 years. Boys show larger increments in LMI and girls larger increments in FMI, illustrating the limitations of BMI for assessing age changes in adiposity during development. Reprinted with permission from Cambridge University Press [23].

differ in the average body fat content for a given BMI value [26]. This has led to the derivation of ethnic-specific BMI cut-offs for defining overweight and obesity [27]. The same scenario is apparent in childhood [28, 29]. At any given BMI value, Asian children tend to have a higher level of body fat. These ethnic differences in body composition are of considerable importance given the central role of obesity, especially central obesity, in the aetiology of the metabolic syndrome, and ethnic variability in adiposity is believed to represent one of the mechanisms underlying the greater vulnerability to cardiovascular disease of some populations compared to others [30].

There is also some indication that the relationship between BMI and body fat alters over time. This issue remains difficult to investigate reliably due to the lack of high-quality data on children's body composition from prior decades. Nevertheless, several data sets indicate that secular increases in adiposity indices are greater than secular increases in BMI [31–33], an inconsistency that would imply a secular decrease in lean mass [30]. Such a decrease is highly plausible if children's activity levels have indeed declined as is widely hypothesised. Exercise is an established stimulant of lean mass deposition during childhood [34], hence it remains plausible that changes in lifestyle have predisposed to both increasing levels of adiposity and lower levels of lean mass in contemporary children compared to those of previous decades. This hypothesis merits further attention, because it would indicate that the health consequences of high BMI could be worse in the current generation compared to previous generations of children [31].

BMI may be particularly misleading as an index of body fat in disease states where both fat mass and the lean mass have been influenced. In some patients, growth of lean mass is constrained. Often dieticians feed such patients on the assumption that the weight gain improves health; however, the weight gain may be entirely fat. In two patients with a rare condition called myofibromatosis, BMI z-scores were around −3, but measurements of body composition demonstrated 40% fat [35]. Thus, the low weight of these patients could be attributed to very low lean mass, and energy intake could not be assumed to be constraining growth. Similarly, a recent clinical trial evaluating provision of a gastrostomy to paediatric patients with cerebral palsy found that the additional weight gained by those receiving a gastrostomy was primarily fat [36].

A second area where BMI is particularly problematic as an outcome is the association between early growth and later body composition. Many studies have reported a positive correlation between birth weight and later BMI [37], which has often been interpreted as indicating that fat neonates have a higher risk of obesity in later life. A recent systematic review identified both high birth weight and rapid infant weight gain as risk factors for high childhood BMI [38]. More detailed studies have, however, found that birth weight has inconsistent associations with later fat mass, and has a much more consistent association with later lean mass [39]. Three studies undertaken in developing countries have extended these observations to weight gain in infancy, demonstrating that greater weight gain in the first few months of life is associated with greater lean mass but not fat mass in later childhood [40–42]. However, similar studies in industrialised populations have suggested that infant weight gain may also predict later body fat [43, 44]. This issue remains in need of further research, as the studies have differed in the period of infancy investigated. There is much greater consistency between populations for later developmental periods, with high levels of weight gain in childhood being more strongly associated with later adiposity [40, 42, 45].

BMI is highly correlated with all the major components of body weight, including fat mass, lean mass and skeletal mineral mass. It is because it is correlated with each of these variables that it acts as a reliable proxy of none of them – for example, its capacity to index variability in adiposity is confounded by its association with lean mass. There is no doubt that BMI remains an important tool for the paediatrician, enabling a simple, rapid and convenient evaluation of nutritional status. Rapid increases in BMI indicate excess weight gain in individuals, since any child rapidly increasing in BMI SDS is likely to be gaining primarily fat and at risk of obesity. For the epidemiologist, BMI may reveal broad trends within and between populations in relative weight, and varying associations with variables such as socioeconomic status [46]. BMI also remains the current approach for categorising obesity, although its specificity for this task is better than its sensitivity, and waist circumference is increasingly used as a more sensitive index of central adiposity [47]. However, as an index of body composition in individuals, the limitations of BMI are unresolvable.

Body Composition in Different Contexts

Body composition itself is of interest in a number of different contexts. First, in order to guide clinical practice, clinicians require an evidence base derived from epidemiological studies and clinical trials [48]. In such studies, the requirement is for a practical method capable of discerning the desired outcome with a relatively consistent level of error. Outcomes may range from global assessments of whole-body fat or lean masses to specific regional evaluations of muscle mass or visceral fat mass. Second, clinicians require methods capable of guiding the treatment of individual children in routine clinical practice [48]. Once again the optimal methods will depend on the outcome of interest.

A recent review of body composition techniques highlighted a wide variety of methods capable of contributing to these varied requirements [48]. The accuracy of any method requires evaluation against a reference method. The gold standard for body composition is cadaver dissection; hence, all in vivo methods are imperfect and rely on assumptions. Currently, the most accurate in vivo techniques are multi-component models for the chemical composition of the body, and MRI for regional tissue distributions. Where possible, other technique should be evaluated against these references and the literature increasingly reflects this ideal.

Simple Anthropometric Markers

Humans store fat largely in peripheral subcutaneous depots, which can be evaluated using skinfold calipers or girth measurements. Measurements of skinfold thicknesses have been used in paediatric clinical practice and research for decades, and are well tolerated by children aged 4+ years. The imprecision of skinfold measurements derives from two factors: first, inconsistency in locating the site to be measured, and second, inconsistency in the style of measurement. In obese children this error is significant, and it is often hard to identify an appropriate skinfold to measure, hence they are less useful in this condition. In the vast majority of other scenarios, however, variability between individuals is substantially greater than inter-observer error, and the technique is worthwhile.

Skinfold thickness data are of greatest value if left in their raw state. In this form they provide accurate evaluations of specific subcutaneous fat depots. The main difficulty is in interpreting the data. Centile charts for children were published several decades ago [49] but are unlikely to be representative of contemporary children given the recent obesity epidemic. There is, therefore, a need for updated reference data against which individual measurements can be evaluated. With such data, already collected and currently being analysed in the UK, skinfold measurements represent a highly convenient and reliable assessment of subcutaneous adiposity, also suitable for longitudinal monitoring.

It is often assumed that skinfold data are of greatest benefit if incorporated into equations which predict whole body fat mass, and hence, by difference with weight, lean mass [50, 51]. However, such equations suffer from a major limitation, common to all predictive techniques, in assuming that all individuals have the *average*

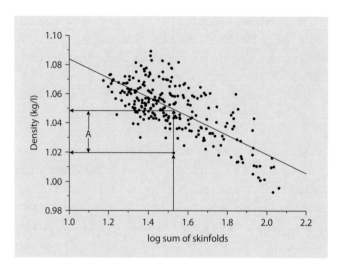

Fig. 4. The relationship between two variables in a predictive method, where the variable on the x-axis is used to predict the outcome on the y-axis. Here, log sum of skinfolds is used to predict body density, from which fat mass is calculated using Archimedes' principle [64]. The regression slope describes the best-fit relationship between the variables, however the individual data points are scattered around this line. Use of the regression equation therefore assumes all individuals have the average y value for a given x value, resulting in a significant difference (A) between the actual and predicted y values.

relationship between the raw data and the predicted outcome. Figure 4 illustrates the generic scenario for a predictive method, showing the relationship between raw data on the x-axis (e.g. sum of four skinfolds) and outcome (e.g. body density) on the y-axis. Using the empirically-determined regression line, all individuals are treated as if their values lie along the regression line, whereas in reality as shown in the plot the individual data points are scattered around the line. The slope of the regression line also tends to differ between populations. Predictive equations therefore introduce significant error to both individuals' and groups' data [52], and predicted values have substantially greater inaccuracy than the raw data. Finally, it is worth emphasising that regional data on adiposity may be much more informative than a single whole-body value.

The one limitation of skinfold thickness measurements is that they are unable directly to address intra-abdominal adipose tissue, the depot most strongly associated with adverse outcomes. The gold standard for measuring internal adiposity is magnetic resonance imaging (MRI) as discussed below. However, waist circumference has been shown to be a robust and valid index of abdominal adiposity in children [53], and a recent study found that waist circumference explained 65% of the variability in visceral adipose tissue [54]. These studies therefore indicate an important role for waist circumference in monitoring abdominal adiposity, as increasingly advocated [47]. The availability of reference data [55] is also a major benefit for this outcome. The waist-height ratio adjusts the girth for height, and has also been developed as an obesity index [56], but whether it has greater sensitivity for monitoring obesity or cardiovascular risk than waist girth alone remains to be established.

Despite the profusion of more sophisticated techniques discussed below, anthropometry deserves to maintain a central role in the paediatrician's toolkit. Anthropometric techniques are convenient, cheap, portable, non-invasive and can be repeated at regular intervals. As with all techniques they are of greatest value when used with high-quality reference data. The combination of raw skinfold thickness measurements and waist circumference SD score offers a highly informative assessment of adiposity in individuals, arguably only bettered by MRI. However anthropometry cannot address lean mass satisfactorily, hence the value of two-component techniques.

Two-Component Techniques

A variety of techniques are now available for differentiating the fat and lean components of body weight. These include isotope dilution for measurement of TBW, dual energy X-ray absorptiometry (DXA), and densitometry. Each technique has its pros and cons, along with a specific theoretical basis which limits the context in which the technique will be accurate.

The principle of isotope dilution measurements is that isotopes of water (^{2}H or ^{18}O) can be used to dilute and hence quantify TBW [57]. These isotopes are non-toxic, non-radioactive and naturally occurring, and hence present no ethical issues. Making assumptions about the hydration of lean tissue, TBW can therefore be used to estimate lean mass, using the following equation:

Lean mass (kg) = total body water (kg)/hydration fraction

where age- and sex-specific values for hydration are available for infants [6] and children aged 5+ years [58]. Of all the body composition techniques isotope dilution is the most versatile, being practical in virtually all contexts, age groups and disease states. The measurement requires only collection of body fluid samples (saliva, urine or blood) before and after administration of a dose of labelled water. The dose can be given as fruit juice or milk in younger age groups, and in patients through a gastrostomy tube, or if suitably sterilised, through a parenteral nutrition line. The technique is robust for determining body water, though if the subject has oedema it is necessary to adopt a more sophisticated protocol for sample collection. The main factor limiting its application is the validity of the assumption that lean mass has a known water content. In healthy subjects, hydration is tightly regulated and variability is within ±1.5% [52], though varying in relation to age and sex. New reference data for the hydration of lean tissue will aid apply this technique more widely [58] (fig. 5).

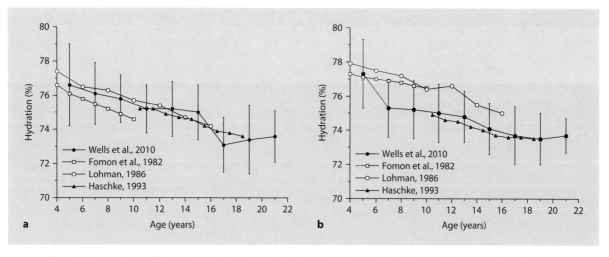

Fig. 5. Comparison of the published modelled values of Lohman, Haschke and colleagues for the hydration of lean tissue with empirical values obtained in healthy UK boys (**a**) and girls (**b**) using the 4-component model [58]. Mean values and SD.

However, some disease states exert further effects on hydration. In some diseases the alteration is of modest magnitude and similar in all individuals. For example, in young female patients with cystic fibrosis mean hydration is significantly different from that of healthy children, due to delayed puberty, but the variability is similar, allowing a disease-specific correction factor to be applied [Williams, Wells and Fewtrell, unpubl. data]. In these circumstances, isotope dilution remains a relatively accurate approach for assessment of body composition, particularly if an appropriate correction factor can be applied. Where fluid distribution is altered, and the extent of this alteration varies between individuals, isotope dilution needs to be combined with other techniques as discussed below.

DXA is increasingly available in hospitals and in some countries, especially the US, is now regarded as a gold standard body composition technique. The method relies on the differential attenuation of X-rays by bone, fat and lean tissue in order to distinguish these three components of body weight [59]. The technique has high precision but its accuracy is poorer than is often assumed, and varies according to instrumentation. The method first distinguishes pixels with and without bone. In those pixels lacking bone, the method then distinguishes fat and lean tissue. This information is then used to infer soft tissue composition of those pixels containing bone. Thus the technique only measures soft tissue directly in non-bone pixels, and in the trunk much of the data is an estimation rather than a measurement. Studies comparing DXA against multi-component models have generally reported good agreement; however, most of these studies have been conducted in healthy adults within the normal range of weight. Recent evaluations have incorporated a

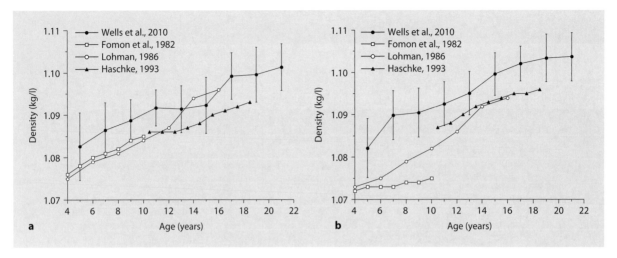

Fig. 6. Comparison of the published modelled values of Lohman, Haschke and colleagues for the density of lean tissue with empirical values obtained in healthy UK boys (**a**) and girls (**b**) using the 4-component model [58]. Mean values and SD.

wide range of age, body size and adiposity, and have also considered disease states. These studies demonstrated that the bias of DXA varies systematically in relation to adiposity, size, gender and disease state [60, 61]. Its accuracy for both cross-sectional and longitudinal assessments in obese children has also been quantified [62]. On this basis, DXA cannot be considered optimal for case-control studies, or for longitudinal evaluations, since the bias will tend to differ between groups or time points. Nevertheless DXA is capable of contributing to routine patient care, in particular because of its capacity to estimate both total and regional lean mass. Of all the techniques currently available it remains the most practical for this purpose in routine care. For example, measurements by DXA have recently been used to estimate the total body water for the calculation of dialysis dosages [63]. This approach proved substantially more accurate than the conventional alternative of predicting body water from weight and height.

Densitometry is one of the older approaches to body composition, relying on the theoretical basis that fat and lean tissues have predictable densities [64]. Using Archimedes' principle, measurement of whole body density can then be used to calculate the proportion of fat and lean in body weight. Fat has a constant density in all age groups, but in children, as for lean mass hydration, age- and sex-specific values for lean mass density are required. The generic equation is as follows:

% fat = (C1/body density) – C2,

where C1 and C2 refer to age- and sex-specific values that address the density of fat and lean tissue with again, new reference data having recently been published [58] (fig. 6). Whole-body air displacement plethysmography [65, 66] has replaced the cumbersome method of underwater weighing, and makes densitometry a readily applied technique in most paediatric populations. The technique involves the subject sitting in a small chamber (the Bodpod®) for a couple of minutes while changes in air pressure and temperature are monitored in order to estimate body volume. The technique is well tolerated by children of 4 years upwards, has been validated in children [66, 67], and is increasingly widely used in research studies. However, further analyses have identified significant variability, both within populations and between disease states, in the density of lean tissue, due to variability in the water and mineral content [68, 69]. This variability confounds the use of Archimedes principle for distinguishing fat and lean masses, and increases both individual error and also group accuracy in any given disease state. As a clinical technique, therefore, the accuracy of densitometry remains dependent on the accuracy of assumptions about lean mass density. It can be used to evaluate broad trends and may be useful in monitoring broad changes in obese patients, since changes in their gross body composition are likely to be of considerably greater magnitude than changes in their lean tissue composition. Furthermore, as with isotope probes, disease-specific values for the density of lean mass may be obtained from empirical research and used in subsequent applications to improve accuracy. However, the greatest value of plethysmography is its role in multi-component techniques (see below).

Regional body composition can be measured by radiographic techniques such as computerized tomography (CT) scanning or magnetic resonance imaging (MRI). The former technique is unsuitable for whole-body paediatric use due to the high radiation exposure. Recently, however, a peripheral version (PQCT) has emerged. CT scans use multiple cross-sectional X-rays to construct a 3-dimensional volumetric model of bone, muscle and fat tissue. PQCT is designed to scan only specific limb sites such as the radius or tibia. Measurements are made during a 1- to 2-min period, and the radiation dose is acceptable for children at <2 µSV. Focusing on the limbs, the technique represents a significant contribution to the capacity to measure muscle mass [70], although measurements refer to cross-sectional area within a given location (similar to arm anthropometry) rather than total limb lean mass as provided by DXA. Reference data now exist for children [71]; however, care is needed with respect to differences between types of instrumentation [72].

MRI scanning does not involve radiation and measures instead the alignment of hydrogen nuclei in a magnetic field. Variability in the density of hydrogen nuclei is proportional to the water content of the tissue, allowing the technique to discriminate tissues of different water content. Raw data are obtained in transverse 'slices', which can be summed in order to provide regional or whole-body volumes. In contrast to the techniques described above, MRI differentiates with high accuracy the location of different tissue types. Alone of all the acceptable techniques it can quantify intra-abdominal adipose tissue, in particular the visceral fat depot [73] which is most strongly associated with adverse health outcome. It is also the most accurate technique for measurement of regional muscle mass [74], and can be used to quantify specific organ volumes. However, it should be noted that adipose tissue is not equivalent to fat mass, hence the technique measures a different adiposity outcome to the other methods discussed above. Again, the technique is only available in specialised centres and is expensive, but it provides the most accurate data on regional body composition and tissue composition in research studies and is a key source of evidence.

Multi-Component Models

In healthy individuals, two-component techniques generally offer sufficient accuracy for the measurement of whole-body lean and fat mass. In disease states where the composition of tissues, and hence tissue properties, are altered, it is ideal to combine techniques in order to achieve acceptable accuracy.

Many diseases influence the composition of lean mass, for example altering the mineral or water content. Such changes can be addressed by three- or four-component models, which provide information both on the composition of lean tissue and also properties such as the hydration or density of lean tissue. The three-component model requires measurements of body weight, body volume and body water, by plethysmography and isotope dilution, respectively. These data allow differentiation of fat mass, water mass, and the mass of fat-free dry tissue (containing mineral, protein, glycogen and free amino acids) [52]. The four-component model further incorporates measurement of bone mineral mass by DXA, and hence separates the mineral and protein components of fat-free dry tissue [52]. The application of the four-component model in obese children has highlighted many effects of this condition on tissue composition, with obese children having an increased water content and decreased mineral content of lean mass, and hence a lower density of lean tissue [9]. The four-component model represents the most accurate in vivo technique for differentiation of fat and lean tissue, and is increasingly used in research studies.

An alternative multi-component approach involves addressing water distribution. In healthy individuals there is a predictable relationship between intracellular and extracellular water. Many disease states perturb this relationship, for example in obesity the extracellular space expands [75]. Water distribution can be evaluated by combining two probes, one for the estimation of total body water and the other for the estimation of extra-cellular water, allowing calculation of intra-cellular water by difference. Extra-cellular water can be quantified by sodium bromide dilution [76], though multi-frequency bio-electrical impedance analysis may also contribute in this context. Unlike deuterium dilution, bromide dilution requires blood samples pre-dose and after equilibration. The calculation of extra-cellular water is also more difficult than that for total body water, requiring several correction factors and assumptions to be applied [76]. However, this approach is merited in research on critically ill children.

Conclusions

This review has described a variety of body composition methodologies that can be used in paediatric research and clinical practice. Different techniques are appropriate for different functions and applications [48], but any technique becomes much more valuable for paediatric application if appropriate reference data are available. It is inevitable that routine clinical care will favour simpler, cheaper and more portable techniques; however, it is also clear from rapidly accumulating research studies that body composition is an important indication of health, that it predicts future risk or outcome, and that it therefore merits increased attention.

References

1 Reilly JJ, Methven E, McDowell ZC, Hacking B, Alexander D, Stewart L, Kelnar CJ: Health consequences of obesity. Arch Dis Child 2003;88:748–752.

2 Power C, Lake JK, Cole TJ: Measurement and long-term health risks of child and adolescent fatness. Int J Obesity 1997;21:507–526.

3 Cole TJ: Weight/height^p compared to weight/height^2 for assessing adiposity in childhood: influence of age and bone age on p during puberty. Ann Hum Biol 1986;13:433–451.

4 Gasser T, Ziegler P, Seifert B, Prader A, Molinari L, Largo R: Measures of body mass and of obesity from infancy to adulthood and their appropriate transformation. Ann Hum Biol 1994;21:111–125.

5 Cole TJ, Freeman JV, Preece MA: Body mass index reference curves for the UK, 1990. Arch Dis Child 1995;73:25–29.

6 Fomon SJ, Haschke F, Ziegler EE, Nelson SE: Body composition of reference children from birth to age 10 years. Am J Clin Nutr 1982;35:1169–1175.

7 Rolland-Cachera MF, Deheeger M, Guilloud-Bataille M, Avons P, Patois E, Sempé M: Tracking the development of adiposity from one month of age to adulthood. Ann Hum Biol 1987;14:219–229.

8 Rolland-Cachera M-F, Deheeger M, Bellisle F, Sempé M, Guilloud-Bataille M, Patois E: Adiposity rebound in children: a simple indicator for predicting obesity. Am J Clin Nutr 1984;39:129–135.

9 Wells JC, Fewtrell MS, Williams JE, Haroun D, Lawson MS, Cole TJ: Body composition in normal weight, overweight and obese children: matched case-control analyses of total and regional tissue masses, and body composition trends in relation to relative weight. Int J Obes 2006;30:1506–1513.

10 James WPT, Ferro-Luzzi A, Waterlow JC: Definition of chronic energy deficiency in adults. Eur J Clin Nutr 1994;42:969–981.

11 Garrow JS, Webster J: Quetelet's index (W/H2) as a measure of fatness. Int J Obes 1985;9:147–153.

12 Wells JCK, Treleaven P, Cole TJ: BMI compared with 3D body shape The UK National Sizing Survey. Am J Clin Nutr 2007;85:419–425.

13 Savva SC, Tornaritis M, Savva ME, Kourides Y, Panagi A, Silikiotou N, Georgiou C, Kafatos A: Waist circumference and waist-to-height ratio are better predictors of cardiovascular disease risk factors in children than body mass index. Int J Obes 2000;24:1453–1458.

14 Cole TJ, Bellizzi MC, Flegal KM, Dietz WH: Establishing a standard definition for child overweight and obesity worldwide: international survey. BMJ 2000;320:1240–1243.

15 Cole TJ, Flegal KM, Nicholls D, Jackson AA: Body mass index cut offs to define thinness in children and adolescents: international survey. BMJ 2007;335: 194–201.

16 Pietrobelli A, Faith MS, Allison DB, Gallagher D, Chiumello G, Heymsfield SB: Body mass index as a measure of adiposity among children and adolescents: a validation. J Pediatr 1998;132:204–210.

17 Chan YL, Leung SSF, Lam WWM, Peng XM, Metrewli C: Body fat estimation in children by magnetic resonance imaging, bioelectrical impedance, skinfold and body mass index: a pilot study. J Paediatr Child Health 1998;34:22–28.

18 Wells JCK, Cole TJ, ALSPAC Study Team: Adjustment of fat-free mass and fat mass for height in children aged 8 years. Int J Obes 2002;26:947–952.

19 Wells JCK, Victora CG: Indices of whole-body and central adiposity for evaluating the metabolic load of obesity. Int J Obes 2005;29:483–489.

20 Van Itallie TB, Yang M-U, Heymsfield SB, Funk RC, Boileau RA: Height-normalised indices of the body's fat-free mass and fat mass: potentially useful indicators of nutritional status. Am J Clin Nutr 1990;52:953–959.

21 Hattori K, Tatsumi N, Tanaka S: Assessment of body composition by using a new chart method. Am J Hum Biol 1997;9:573–578.

22 Wells JCK: A Hattori chart analysis of body mass index in infancy and childhood. Int J Obesity 2000;24:325–329.

23 Wells JCK: The Evolutionary Biology of Human Body Fatness: Thrift and Control. Cambridge, Cambridge University Press, 2009.

24 Maynard LM, Wisemandle W, Roche AF, Chumlea WC, Guo SS, Siervogel RM: Childhood body composition in relation to body mass index. Pediatrics 2001;107:344–350.

25 Cole TJ: Children grow and horses race: is the adiposity rebound a critical period for later obesity? BMC Pediatr 2004;12:4–6.

26 Deurenberg P, Yap M, van Staveren WA: Body mass index and percent body fat: a meta-analysis among different ethnic groups. Int J Obes 1998;22:1164–1171.

27 Wang J, Thornton JC, Russell M, et al: Asians have lower body mass index (BMI) but higher percent body fat than do whites: comparisons of anthropometric measurements. Am J Clin Nutr 1994;60:23–28.

28 Deurenberg P, Deurenberg-Yap M, Foo LF, Schmidt G, Wang J: Differences in body composition between Singapore Chinese, Beijing Chinese and Dutch children. Eur J Clin Nutr 2003;57:405–409.

29 Eckhardt CL, Adair LS, Caballero B, Avila J, Kon IY, Wang J, Popkin BM: Estimating body fat from anthropometry and isotopic dilution: a four-country comparison. Obes Res 2003;11:1553–1562.

30 Whincup PH, Gilg J, Papacosta O, Seymour C, Miller GJ, Alberti KGM, Cook DG: Early evidence of ethnic differences in cardiovascular risk: cross sectional comparison of British South Asian and white children. Br Med J 2002;324:635–638.

31 Wells JCK, Coward WA, Cole TJ, Davies PSW: The contribution of fat and fat-free tissue to body mass index in contemporary children and the reference child. It J Obes 2002;26:1323–1328.

32 Flegal KM: Defining obesity in children and adolescents: epidemiologic approaches. Crit Rev Food Sci Nutr 1993;33:307–312.

33 Moreno LA, Fleta J, Sarria A, Rodriguez G, Gil C, Bueno M: Secular changes in body fat patterning in children and adolescents of Zaragoza (Spain), 1980–1995. Int J Obes 2001;25:1656–1660.

34 Torun B, Viteri FE: Influence of exercise on linear growth. Eur J Clin Nutr 1994;48(suppl 1):S186–S189.

35 Wells JCK, Mok Q, Johnson AW: Nutritional status in children. Lancet 2001;357:1293.

36 Sullivan PB, Alder N, Bachlett AME, Grant H, Juszczak E, Henry J, Vernon-Roberts A, Warner J, Wells JCK: Gastrostomy feeding in cerebral palsy – too much of a good thing? Dev Med Child Neurol 2006;48:877–882.

37 Parsons TJ, Power C, Logan S, Summerbell CD: Childhood predictors of adult obesity: a systematic review. Int J Obes 1999;(suppl 8):S1-S107.

38 Baird J, Fisher D, Lucas P, Kleijnen J, Roberts H, Law C: Being big or growing fast: systematic review of size and growth in infancy and later obesity. BMJ 2005;331:929–934.

39 Wells JCK, Chomtho S, Fewtrell MS: Programming of body composition by early growth and nutrition. Proc Nutr Soc 2007;66:423–434.

40 Wells JCK, Hallal PC, Wright A, Singhal A, Victora CG: Fetal, infant and childhood growth: relationships with body composition in Brazilian boys aged 9 years. Int J Obes 2005;29:1192–1198.

41 Sachdev HS, Fall CH, Osmond C, Lakshmy R, Dey Biswas SK, Leary SD, Reddy KS, Barker DJ, Bhargava SK: Anthropometric indicators of body composition in young adults: relation to size at birth and serial measurements of body mass index in childhood in the New Delhi birth cohort. Am J Clin Nutr 2005;82:456–466.

42 Li H, Stein AD, Barnhart HX, Ramakrishnan U, Martorell R: Associations between prenatal and postnatal growth and adult body size and composition. Am J Clin Nutr 2003;77:1498–1505.

43 Ekelund U, Ong K, Linne Y, Neovius M, Brage S, Dunger DB, Wareham NJ, Rossner S: Upward weight percentile crossing in infancy and early childhood independently predicts fat mass in young adults: the Stockholm Weight Development Study (SWEDES). Am J Clin Nutr 2006;83:324–330.

44 Chomtho S, Wells JC, Williams JE, Davies PS, Lucas A, Fewtrell MS: Infant growth and later body composition: evidence from the 4-component model. Am J Clin Nutr 2008;87:1776–1784.

45 Botton J, Heude B, Maccario J, Ducimetière P, Charles MA, FLVS Study Group: Postnatal weight and height growth velocities at different ages between birth and 5 y and body composition in adolescent boys and girls. Am J Clin Nutr 2008;87:1760–1768.

46 Wang Y: Cross-national comparison of childhood obesity: the epidemic and the relationship between obesity and socioeconomic status. Int J Epidemiol 2001;30:1129–1136.

47 McCarthy HD, Ashwell M: A study of central fatness using waist-to-height ratios in UK children and adolescents over two decades supports the simple message – 'keep your waist circumference to less than half your height'. Int J Obes 2006;30:988–992.

48 Wells JCK, Fewtrell MS: Measuring body composition. Arch Dis Child 2006;91:612–617.

49 Tanner JM, Whitehouse RH: Revised standards for triceps and subscapular skinfolds in British children. Arch Dis Child 1975;50:142–145.

50 Slaughter MH, Lohman TG, Boileau RA, Horswill CA, Stillman RJ, van Loan MD, Bemben DA: Skinfold equations for estimation of body fatness in children and youth. Hum Biol 1988;60:709–723.

51 Brook CGD: Determination of body composition of children from skinfold measurements. Arch Dis Child 1971;46:182–184.

52 Wells JCK, Fuller NJ, Dewit O, Fewtrell MS, Elia M, Cole TJ: Four-component model of body composition in children: density and hydration of fat-free mass and comparison with simpler models. Am J Clin Nutr 1999;69:904–912.

53 Owens S, Litaker M, Allison J, Riggs S, Ferguson M, Gutin B: Prediction of visceral adipose tissue from simple anthropometric measurements in youths with obesity. Obes Res 1999;7:16–22.

54 Brambilla P, Bedogni G, Moreno LA, Goran MI, Gutin B, Fox KR, Peters DM, Barbeau P, De Simone M, Pietrobelli A: Cross-validation of anthropometry against magnetic resonance imaging for the assessment of visceral and subcutaneous adipose tissue in children. Int J Obes 2006;30:23–30.

55 McCarthy HD, Jarrett KV, Crawley HF: The development of waist circumference percentiles in British children aged 5.0–16.9 y. Eur J Clin Nutr 2001;55:902–907.

56 Nambiar S, Hughes I, Davies PS: Developing waist-to-height ratio cut-offs to define overweight and obesity in children and adolescents. Public Health Nutr 2010;13:1566–1574.

57 Wells JC, Fewtrell MS, Davies PS, Williams JE, Coward WA, Cole TJ: Prediction of total body water in infants and children. Arch Dis Child 2005;90:965–971.

58 Wells JC, Williams JE, Chomtho S, Darch T, Grijalva-Eternod C, Kennedy K, Haroun D, Wilson C, Cole TJ, Fewtrell MS: New pediatric reference data for lean tissue properties: density and hydration from age 5 to 20 y. Am J Clin Nutr 2010;91:610–618.

59 Mazess RB, Barden HS, Bisek JP, Hanson J: Dual-energy x-ray absorptiometry for total-body and regional bone-mineral and soft-tissue composition. Am J Clin Nutr 1990;51:1106–1112.

60 Williams JE, Wells JCK, Wilson CM, Haroun D, Lucas A, Fewtrell MS: Evaluation of Lunar Prodigy dual-energy X-ray absorptiometry for assessing body composition in healthy individuals and patients by comparison with the criterion four-component model. Am J Clin Nutr 2006;83:1047–1054.

61 Wong WW, Hergenroeder AC, Stuff JE, Butte NF, Smith EO, Ellis KJ: Evaluating body fat in girls and female adolescents: advantages and disadvantages of dual-energy X-ray absorptiometry. Am J Clin Nutr 2002;76:384–389.

62 Wells JC, Haroun D, Williams JE, Wilson C, Darch T, Viner RM, Eaton S, Fewtrell MS: Evaluation of DXA against the four-component model of body composition in obese children and adolescents aged 5–21 years. Int J Obes 2010;34:649–655.

63 Mendley SR, Majkowski NL, Schoeller DA: Validation of estimates of total body water in pediatric dialysis patients by deuterium dilution. Kidney Int 2005;67:2056–2062.

64 Siri WE: Body composition from fluid spaces and density: analysis of methods; in Brozek J, Henschel A (eds): Techniques for Measuring Body Composition. Washington, National Academy of Sciences, NRC, 1961, pp 223–244.

65 Dempster P, Aitkens S: A new air displacement method for the determination of human body composition. Med Sci Sports Exerc 1995;27:1692–1697.

66 Dewit O, Fuller NJ, Fewtrell MS, Elia M, Wells JCK: Whole-body air-displacement plethysmography compared to hydrodensitometry for body composition analysis. Arch Dis Child 2000;82:159–164.

67 Wells JCK, Fuller NJ, Wright A, Fewtrell MS, Cole TJ: Evaluation of air-displacement plethysmography in children aged 5–7 years using a three-component model of body composition. Br J Nutr 2003;90:699–707.

68 Haroun D, Wells JCK, Williams JE, Fuller NJ, Fewtrell MS, Lawson MS: Composition of the fat-free mass in obese and non-obese children: matched case-control analyses. Int J Obes 2005;29:29–36.

69 Murphy AJ, Wells JC, Williams JE, Fewtrell MS, Davies PS, Webb DK: Body composition in children in remission from acute lymphoblastic leukemia. Am J Clin Nutr 2006;83:70–74.

70 Schoenau E, Neu CM, Mokov E, Wassmer G, Manz F: Influence of puberty on muscle area and cortical bone area of the forearm in boys and girls. J Clin Endocrinol Metab 2000;85:1095–1098.

71 Rauch F, Schoenau E: Peripheral quantitative computed tomography of the distal radius in young subjects – new reference data and interpretation of results. J Musculoskelet Neuronal Interact 2005;5:119–126.

72   Rauch F, Tutlewski B, Schoenau E: Peripheral quantitative computed tomography at the distal radius: cross-calibration between two scanners. J Musculoskelet Neuronal Interact 2001;2:153–155.

73   Fox K, Peters D, Armstrong N, Sharpe P, Bell M: Abdominal fat deposition in 11-year-old children. Int J Obes 1993;17:11–16.

74   Mitsipoulos N, Baumgartner RN, Heymsfield SB, Lyons W, Gallagher D, Ross R: Cadaver validation of skeletal muscle measurements by magnetic resonance imaging and computerised tomography. J Apply Physiol 1998;85:115–122.

75   Sartorio A, Malavolti M, Agosti F, Marinone PG, Caiti O, Battistini N, Bedogni G: Body water distribution in severe obesity and its assessment from eight-polar bioelectrical impedance analysis. Eur J Clin Nutr 2005;59:155–160.

76   Planche T, Onanga M, Schwenk A, Dzeing A, Borrmann S, Faucher JF, Wright A, Bluck L, Ward L, Kombila M, Kremsner PG, Krishna S: Assessment of volume depletion in children with malaria. PLoS Med 2004;1:e18.

Jonathan C.K. Wells
Reader in Paediatric Nutrition, MRC Childhood Nutrition Research Centre
Institute of Child Health, 30 Guilford Street
London WC1N 1EH (UK)
Tel. + 44 207 905 2389, Fax + 44 207 831 9903, E-Mail J.Wells@ich.ucl.ac.uk

Ranke MB, Mullis P-E (eds): Diagnostics of Endocrine Function in Children and Adolescents, ed 4.
Basel, Karger, 2011, pp 483–498

Effect of Body Weight on Endocrine Parameters and Fat Hormones

Martin Wabitsch · Thomas Reinehr · Pamela Fischer-Posovszky

Division of Pediatric Endocrinology, Diabetes and Obesity Unit, University children's Hospital University of Ulm, Ulm, Germany

The first part of this chapter describes the typical alterations of endocrine parameters in individuals with increased body weight in response to increased fat mass. In the second part, information on biochemistry and the physiological role of clinically relevant hormones and other secretion products of adipose tissue is provided as well as reference values as far as such values currently exist.

Endocrine Parameters in Individuals with Increased Body Fat Mass

General Aspects

There are various endocrine diseases including defined genetic syndromes which are the underlying cause for obesity in children and adolescents. These cases are rare. However, there are very common alterations in endocrine functions in obese children and adolescents which are a characteristic of the increased body fat mass (fig. 1). These alterations include disturbances of insulin secretion and insulin sensitivity, alterations of the function of the adrenal gland, alterations of the growth hormone (GH)/IGF-1 axis and the thyroid gland as well as gastrointestinal hormones. In addition, obesity results in an altered profile of secretory products of the adipose tissue.

The observation of an increased glucocorticoid production and an impaired GH production in obese children suggests that these secondary endocrine changes may facilitate further weight gain. The altered secretory profile of adipose tissue and also the single fat cell in the obese state is responsible for various metabolic and endocrine disturbances resulting in clinical end points such as type 2 diabetes, steatosis hepatis, atherosclerosis and certain types of cancer. It should be stressed that almost all endocrine parameters which are affected by increased body fat mass can be normalized by caloric restriction, increased physical activity, and weight loss.

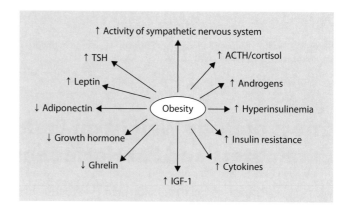

Fig. 1. Endocrine alterations in obesity.

Insulin Secretion and Action

Insulin resistance and hyperinsulinemia are hallmarks of obesity. In individuals whose β-cells are unable to compensate for insulin resistance, glucose tolerance is progressively impaired and type 2 diabetes develops. Interestingly, there is a large variability in insulin resistance in obese individuals which is associated with body fat distribution (increased visceral fat depots are associated with increased insulin resistance) and with the genetic background. Furthermore, insulin resistance aggravates during puberty.

Increased circulating concentrations of fatty acids contribute to peripheral insulin resistance. Fatty acids impair insulin-stimulated glucose uptake and oxidation in muscle and insulin-mediated suppression of hepatic glucose output. It has been suggested that fatty acids released from visceral adipose tissue play a key role in the impairment of liver and muscle insulin sensitivity. Muscular insulin resistance is characterized by fatty acid accumulation within the muscle.

In young children, extremely high insulin levels during oral glucose tolerance test may be measured together with still normal glucose tolerance. Some scientists suggest that the very high insulin levels observed in young children are contributing to the exaggerated weight gain [1]. In support of this idea, insulin levels are very high in patients with craniopharyngeoma and are associated with dramatic increases in weight gain [1].

GH/IGF Axis and Longitudinal Growth

The GH/IGF-1 axis shows typical changes in obese growing children (table 1).

Overweight and obese children and adolescents generally have an increased height and an accelerated bone age during childhood until the early pubertal period. Thus, reduced height and retarded bone age in obese pediatric patients should lead to further diagnostics.

Wabitsch · Reinehr · Fischer-Posovszky

Table 1. Typical changes of the GH/IGF-1 axis in overweight and obese children and adolescents

Impaired GH secretion in stimulation tests
Increased circulating levels of GH-binding protein
Increased circulation levels of IGF-1, IGFBP-1, IGFBP-2, IGFBP-3 in the pre- and intrapubertal period
Reduced levels of IGF-1, IGFBP-1, IGFBP-2, IGFBP-3 in the postpubertal stage
Reduced ghrelin secretion

The accelerated prepubertal longitudinal growth rate is followed by a slightly reduced pubertal growth spurt.

Several cohort studies have demonstrated that growing up in an obese state will lead towards an impaired final height. In obese children there was a negative correlation between the increase in BMI and peak height velocity [2]. The Swedish population-based longitudinal growth study [2] showed that an increase in BMI of one unit will lead to an increase in height of 0.23 and 0.29 cm in boys and girls in the age of 2–8 years. An increase in BMI of one unit leads to earlier puberty and to a reduced increase in height during puberty resulting in no beneficial effect in final height. There was a tendency to decreased final height in subjects that have been obese during childhood.

In a study of a large cohort of obese children, the analysis of growth and bone age showed in both genders that longitudinal growth was accelerated before puberty [3]. We found that a mean height SDS of +1 can lead to a gain in height of more than 6 cm in young children. The accelerated longitudinal growth in this cohort was also associated with an accelerated bone age [3]. In another study, a clear relationship between skeletal maturation and body fat mass determined by DEXA could be demonstrated in children aged 5–12 years. Further investigation of this phenomenon revealed that the only hormonal parameter significantly associated with the increase in bone age was IGF-1 [4].

IGF-1 is produced in large amounts in the liver as well as in adipose tissue. The increased circulating amounts of IGF-1 in obese children and adolescents results from an overproduction in both organs.

The accelerated linear growth in obese children and the alterations in the GH/IGF-1 axis have raised several hypotheses for mechanisms explaining this exaggerated growth without GH [5]. As mentioned before, GH secretion in obese children may be as low as in poorly growing GH-deficient children. Despite normal growth obesity is characterized by a reduced GH secretion in provocative tests, GHRH tests and 24-hour secretion profile. It has been shown that the half-life of endogenous GH is shorter in obese individuals and that there are fewer GH secretory bursts.

Factors that might be involved in GH-independent growth in obese children comprise leptin, adrenal androgens, GH-binding protein, IGF-1 and IGFBP-1, and insulin. Leptin may contribute to a stimulation of growth by its permissive role for puberty induction. The increased levels of adrenal androgens in obese children are able to stimulate longitudinal growth. Obese children have increased circulating levels of GH-binding protein possibly due to an increased density of GH receptors on peripheral cells. Increased circulating levels of IGF-1 have clearly been associated with increases in height-SDS and bone age in obese pre-pubertal children [4]. These children also have reduced levels of IGFBP-1 which would result in an increased amount of free IGF-1. The normal or accelerated growth rates in obese children might therefore be due to an increased disposal of free biologically active IGF-1 despite an impaired GH secretion. Following weight reduction, obese children and adolescents show a normalization (reduction) of the IGF-1:IGFBP-3 ratio [6]. This may result in a reduced amount of free IGF-1 explaining the reduction of longitudinal growth rate often seen during weight reduction. Furthermore, increased levels of insulin in obese children lead to an increased IGF-1 bioavailability due to low IGFBP-1 levels. Finally, leptin, insulin, and sex hormones locally activate the IGF system in the epiphyseal growth plate.

Despite low GH secretion in obesity and decreasing IGFBP-1 with increasing BMI, 24-hour mean bioactive IGF-1 levels were not reduced in obese women and did not correlate with BMI or IGFBP-1 levels [7]. This argues against elevated bioactive IGF-1 as the etiology of reduced GH secretion through a feedback mechanism in obesity.

It is suggested that the reduced levels of circulating GH in obese individuals result in a reduced lipolytic activity in adipose tissue and a reduced rate of protein synthesis in muscle tissue. The impaired central GH secretion rate is mainly due to a reduction in pulse amplitude and less to a reduction of pulse frequency. Higher levels of circulating free fatty acids in obesity are partially responsible for this, since they are able to reduce the GH response after application of GHRH. A reduction of body weight results in a normalization of these alterations.

A description of the alterations of the GH/IGF-1 axis in the obese state would be incomplete without mentioning ghrelin. Ghrelin is a strong GH secretagogue and stimulates GH secretion in a GHRH-independent way via the pituitary secretagogue receptors (GHS-R). Ghrelin consists of 28 amino acids and is secreted from neuroendocrine cells of the gut found mainly in the fundus of the stomach as well as in the nucleus arcuatus of the hypothalamus. Ghrelin secretion in the gut is increased in the fasted state and is significantly reduced in the postprandial state. Ghrelin has various biological effects. Within the gut, ghrelin stimulates motility and the production of acid. In the central nervous system, ghrelin stimulates appetite and is therefore an important link between the regulation of energy homeostasis and the activity of the GH/IGF-1 axis.

Thyroid Hormones

Children and adolescents with obesity often present with slightly increased TSH levels. Serum concentrations of T3 may be in the upper normal range or even increased. The latter finding may be seen in association with the increased basal metabolic rate in obese individuals. The elevation of TSH is not generally associated with iodine deficiency or autoimmune thyroiditis.

Table 2. Typical alterations of the hypothalamo-pituitary-adrenal axis in obesity

Increased stress-induced ACTH secretion
Increased cortisol secretion
Decreased cortisol-binding globulin levels
Increased cortisol clearance
Flattened cortisol profile
Lower cortisol morning peak
Disturbed dexamethasone suppression of the adrenal gland
Increased adrenal androgen production

The prevalence of positive thyroid autoantibodies was increased in the obese children, for the most part in those with elevated TSH [8]. Slightly increased TSH levels with normal or even increased T3 levels are not attributed to a latent hypothyroidism. It is suggested that the increased TSH levels are the result of increased circulating leptin levels, which are able to stimulate TRH-secreting neurons in the nucleus paraventricularis and thus stimulate TSH secretion.

The alterations of TSH and the peripheral thyroid hormones are reversible after weight reduction. In patients with slightly elevated TSH levels, treatment with levothyroxine does not show any effect on body weight. Thus, the substitution of L-thyroxin in obese children and adolescents with slightly increased TSH levels is not advisable.

Despite these clinical findings, it should be remembered that thyroid hormones are important regulators of energy homeostasis. During fasting, overnutrition and in the obese state, there are characteristic alterations of the hypothalamo-pituitary-thyroid axis. Experimental studies in men show that the nutritional status can affect the hypothalamo-pituitary-thyroid function. Overnutrition leads to an increase in serum concentrations of T3 and to a decrease of rT3 levels, whereas fasting results in reduced levels of free T3 and T4 in obese individuals. In addition, 5-deiodinase activity is regulated by energy consumption and itself regulates the conversion of T4 to T3. In summary, it can be concluded that the hypothalamo-pituitary-thyroid axis adapts to the nutritional status with the objective of keeping body weight and muscle mass in a normal range.

Adrenal Gland Function

Obesity is associated complex alterations of the hypothalamo-pituitary-adrenal axis such as increased steroid hormone production and clearance rates [4, 9] (table 2, fig. 2). In obese women, sex steroid production from both ovarian and adrenal origins is higher than their clearance, resulting in hyperandrogenemia and hyperestrogenemia [4]. Furthermore, there is an increased peripheral conversion of androgens to estrogens in the obese state, because adipose tissue is the major site of androgen aromatization.

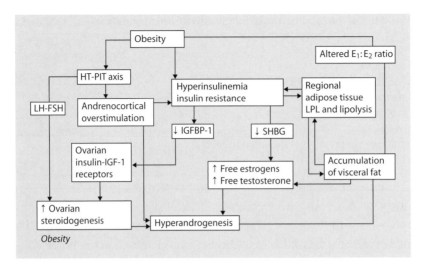

Fig. 2. Scheme of events seen in association with the development of obesity emphasizing a relationship between alterations in endocrine functions and visceral accumulation of body fat as well as the development of PCOS. Modified according to Kapelman [1998].

Studies have shown that an increased androgenic activity, often accompanied by hirsutism and menstrual abnormalities, is more frequent in adolescents with abdominal or upper body obesity than in adolescents with gluteal-femoral or lower body obesity [4]. The subgroup of abdominally obese patients is also more prone to metabolic disturbances such as hyperinsulinemia, disturbed glucose regulation, lipid abnormalities, and hypertension. It is now established that hyperandrogenic obese women frequently present this unfavorable metabolic syndrome and may be at particular risk of developing atherosclerotic complications.

In women with abdominal obesity, an increased activity of the hypothalamo-pituitary-adrenal axis has also been postulated, resulting in an exaggerated response of the adrenal cortex to ACTH [4]. In the latter studies, the cortisol clearance rates in patients with abdominal obesity were higher than those in patients with gluteal-femoral obesity, probably leading to a negative feedback on pituitary ACTH release.

Especially in individuals with preferential abdominal fat accumulation, an increased activity of this axis could be demonstrated in addition to an increased stress-induced cortisol response. The causal relationship between a high androgenic activity and hyperinsulinemia is still unexplained. Insulin may represent a regulatory factor for ovarian steroidogenesis by amplifying the stimulatory effect of LH [10]. The increased expression of β-hydroxysteroid dehydrogenase in visceral fat depot, an enzyme that facilitates the conversion of cortisone to cortisol, and the resulting increased local production of cortisol support the development of abdominal obesity.

Wabitsch · Reinehr · Fischer-Posovszky

Children with obesity may present with an accelerated growth rate and an increased bone age together with premature adrenarche [11]. Interestingly, already before puberty increased DHEAS levels correlate with leptin levels and BMI. We investigated growth and pubertal development in a large cohort study of 1,232 obese children and adolescents [3]. In this study, we found increased serum DHEAS levels from 8 years onwards until end of puberty in both genders. Interestingly, in boys from the ages of 8 to 18 years, we found reduced levels of serum testosterone, while testis volumes were normal compared to the reference values of Largo and Prader [12].

Pubertal and even prepubertal obese girls demonstrated increased testosterone levels. The production site of testosterone may be the ovaries as well as adrenal gland since DHEAS levels are also increased in prepubertal obese girls. Together with the decreased sex-hormone-binding globulin levels, obese adolescent girls may present with increased circulating free testosterone levels and signs of virilization. Also, these changes in the adrenal steroid hormone profile and the hyperandrogenemia in girls with obesity are reversible upon weight reduction [4].

Obese subjects have normal plasma and urinary cortisol levels but accelerated cortisol production and degradation rates. In addition, daytime variation is reduced with diminished morning peaks. A moderate elevation of plasma ACTH levels was demonstrated in obesity.

The obesity-related acceleration in adrenocortical function and cortisol clearance is associated with an increased adrenal androgen production and increased urinary 17-ketosteroid excretion.

Sex Hormone-Binding Globulin in Obesity
Sex hormone-binding globulin (SHBG) is produced by the liver and binds to sex steroids in high affinity but low capacity. It has been shown that body weight and waist-to-hip- ratio are inversely correlated with SHBG levels and directly correlated to free testosterone concentrations. The clearance of testosterone increases as SHBG decreases, which is the consequence of an increased fraction of unbound testosterone available for hepatic extraction and clearance.

Circulating SHBG is lower in obese children and increases with weight loss. The lower affinity of SHBG for estradiol compared to testosterone results in an estrogen amplification effect on sensitive tissues (particularly the liver) with decreasing SHBG levels. In obese children and adolescents, SHBG production is impaired by an inhibitory effect of insulin on SHBG synthesis. In addition, obesity-related hyperandrogenism may directly reduce SHBG levels.

Polycystic Ovary Syndrome
The polycystic ovary syndrome (PCOS) is a well-known finding in obese women. Endocrine alterations associated with PCOS are shown in table 3. Adolescents with obesity generally do not show the full picture of PCOS. Clinically, these adolescent

Table 3. Hormonal and metabolic alterations in obese patients with PCOS

Insulin resistance
Hyperinsulinemia
Disturbed glucose tolerance
Type 2 diabetes mellitus
Dyslipidemia
Increased adrenal androgen production
Increased ovarian testosterone production
Increased aromatisation of androstendione
Increased ratio of estrone/estradiol
Decreased levels of SHBG
Decreased levels of IGFBP-1
Increased free steroid hormone concentrations

girls may have acanthosis nigricans as a clinical sign of hyperinsulinemia, signs of hirsutism, and irregular menstrual bleeding.

In PCOS, the androgen-producing stroma cells of the ovaries are increased in number. There is a hyperplasia of the ovarian theca cells. The granulosa cells are not able to metabolize the increased androgen into estrogens. In patients with PCOS, the ovaries are the main production site of the increased circulating androgens. The production of these androgens is LH-dependent. PCOS is characterized by increased concentrations of androstendione and testosterone as well as reduced SHBG concentrations. In addition, there are increased levels of circulating estrone.

The etiology of PCOS is a subject of controversial discussions. There are recent data showing that insulin resistance and hyperinsulinemia play key roles in the development of PCOS.

Gastrointestinal Hormones
Ghrelin. Ghrelin is a peptide containing 28 amino acids and was identified in 1999 as a ligand for the secretion of the GH secretagogue receptor (GHSR) [13]. Ghrelin is produced principally by the stomach and, to a lesser extent, the duodenum, and is the only known circulating orexigen. Endogenous levels of ghrelin increase before meals and decrease after food intake, suggesting its role in both meal initiation and weight gain. It has been postulated that both the hyperphagia and potentially the GH deficiency in Prader-Willi syndrome may be related to ghrelin dysregulation, as high circulating levels of ghrelin have been observed in this disorder [13].

Obestatin. Is a recently identified peptide derived from the same gene (preproghrelin) as ghrelin and has the opposite effect on weight status, inhibiting food intake and gastrointestinal motility [13]. Obestatin is postulated to antagonize ghrelin's actions on homeostasis and gastrointestinal function. As obestatin and ghrelin are both derived from the same gene, one study hypothesized a possible cause of obesity to be an imbalance of circulating obestatin and ghrelin levels.

Peptide Tyrosine-Tyrosine (PYY). PYY is a 36-amino-acid peptide originally isolated and characterized in 1980 [13]. There are two endogenous forms, PYY_{1-36} and PYY_{3-36}, abundant in humans. PYY is a gut-derived hormone released postprandially by the L cells of the lower intestine that inhibits gastric acid secretion and motility through the neural pathways. PYY belongs to the family of peptides that include neuropeptide Y (NPY) and pancreatic polypeptide (PP) which mediate their effects via G-protein-coupled Y receptors (Y1, Y2, Y4, Y5 and Y6) and display different tissue distributions and functions. PYY_{1-36} binds to all known Y receptor subtypes, whereas PYY_{3-36} shows affinity for the Y1 and Y5 receptor subtypes and high affinity for the inhibitory Y2 receptor subtype. PYY_{3-36} binding to the Y2 receptor subtype inhibits orexigenic NPY in the hypothalamus causing short-term inhibition of food intake, especially high-fat meals. Studies in rodents identified the hypothalamus, vagus and brainstem regions as sites of action. In obese children, levels of the anorexigenic hormone PYY are low. After efficient weight loss, PYY levels significantly increase reaching levels comparable to normal-weight individuals [14]. Once effective weight loss has been achieved, the anorectic effect of PYY may help stabilize weight and thereby prevent later weight gain in patients whose PYY levels increased to normal levels.

Glucagon-Like Peptide-1 (GLP-1). GLP-1 is a gut hormone synthesized from enteroendocrine L cells of the small and large intestine and secreted in two major molecular forms [13], $GLP-1_{7-36}$amide and $GLP-1_{7-37}$, with equipotent biological activity. GLP-1 binds receptors in key appetite-related sites in the hypothalamus (e.g. arcuate and dorsomedial nuclei) and the brainstem (specifically the nucleus of the solitary tract). It is the most potent insulin-stimulating hormone known to date, it suppresses glucagon secretion, and inhibits gastric emptying and acid secretion. GLP-1 may also reduce energy intake and enhance satiety, likely through the aforementioned delay of gastric emptying and specific GLP-1 receptors in the CNS. Its role in childhood obesity is poorly understood with contradictory post-weight loss level changes reported in the literature.

Adipose Tissue as an Endocrine Organ

Many of the endocrine changes associated with overweight and obesity may be attributed to adipose tissue itself. For many years, adipose tissue was considered a passive organ playing a metabolic role in total energy homeostasis. Its only function was believed to be storage of excess energy as triglycerides and their release according to needs in the form of fatty acids.

Adipose tissue is the body's largest energy repository and it plays an important role in total energy homeostasis. Moreover, it is now well recognized as an endocrine organ. Nowadays, more than one hundred adipose tissue secretion products have

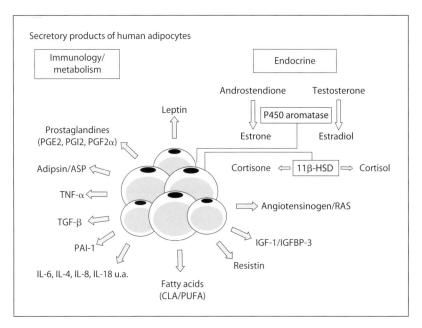

Fig. 3. Secretory products of adipose tissue.

been described [15] (fig. 3). These include complex proteins as well as fatty acids and prostaglandins. Steroids are either synthesized de novo or converted in adipose tissue and released into the bloodstream (fig. 3). Some of these factors primarily have local auto- or paracrine effects in adipose tissue, while others are released into the circulation and exert specific effects at target organs or systemic effects. These so-called adipokines contribute to the development of obesity-related disorders, particularly type 2 diabetes (T2D) and cardiovascular disease.

The endocrinology of adipose tissue remains an exciting research area in which epoch-making findings are still expected. The recently discovered new functions of adipose tissue have elucidated its important role in a complex cross-talk between organs regulating the body's energy homeostasis, insulin sensitivity, lipid metabolism, and the immune system. Thus, adipose tissue and its secretion products have also become a target for drug development. Improved knowledge on the endocrinology of adipose tissue will have implications for the treatment of obesity, diabetes, and cardiovascular diseases.

Leptin

The identification of the leptin (Greek, leptos, thin) gene and its cognate receptor started the endocrine era of the adipocyte. Leptin is the protein product of the *LEP* gene (also known as *OB*), which was first identified by positional cloning in 1994. Mice with mutations in the leptin (*ob/ob* mice) gene or the leptin receptor

Table 4. BMI (mean ± SD) and serum leptin levels in boys and girls according to pubertal stage [23]

Tanner stage	BMI	Leptin median	−1 SD to +1 SD
Boys			
1	16.79 ± 2.03	1.41	0.65–3.04
2	18.91 ± 2.32	2.19	0.91–5.28
3	18.53 ± 2.9	1.26	0.48–3.29
4	19.66 ± 1.73	0.79	0.38–1.64
5	21.25 ± 1.94	0.71	0.34–1.44
Girls			
1	16.3 ± 2.1	2.51	1.23–5.12
2	16.94 ± 1.59	2.86	1.51–5.44
3	18.11 ± 2.23	3.81	1.93–7.51
4	18.45 ± 1.63	4.39	2.67–7.23
5	21.2 ± 2.39	6.24	3.57–10.89

gene (*db/db* mice) are massively obese. Likewise, congenital leptin deficiency in humans causes severe obesity, which is reversed by leptin treatment. Leptin was first regarded as a promising anti-obesity drug, comparable to insulin for the treatment of diabetes mellitus. However, administration of recombinant leptin to overweight and obese subjects was not efficacious in terms of weight loss due to central leptin resistance.

Leptin is almost exclusively expressed in adipocytes and its secretion depends on the fat cell volume. Subcutaneous adipocytes secrete higher amounts of leptin than visceral adipocytes. There is a close relationship between body fat mass and leptin serum concentrations. Likewise, obese subjects have higher leptin levels than lean subjects. The main hormonal regulators of leptin secretion are insulin and cortisol [16]. In the circulation, leptin is bound to carrier proteins such as the soluble leptin receptor. Its main site of action is located in the arcuate nucleus within the hypothalamus, where hunger and satiety are regulated.

Reference values for leptin serum concentrations at different stages of puberty are given in table 4. There is a clear gender difference of circulating leptin levels becoming obvious during puberty. Gender dependency is explained by a lower body fat content of male subjects and a direct negative regulation of leptin secretion by androgens at the level of the adipocyte [17].

Besides its role in regulation of body weight, leptin regulates puberty and reproduction, placental and fetal function, immune response, and insulin sensitivity of muscle and liver. In hypoleptinemic patients with lipodystrophy, leptin replacement therapy resulted in a dramatic improvement in glucose metabolism, dyslipidemia and hepatic steatosis.

In *ob/ob* mice, treatment with leptin initiates fertility. In wild-type mice, leptin triggers the time of puberty. Administration of leptin to food-deprived animals blunts the drop of LH and FSH levels normally observed during starvation. Leptin has been shown to act both at the hypothalamic and at the pituitary level to stimulate LH-RH as well as LH and FSH secretion.

Female patients with mutations leading to either biologically inactive leptin or the leptin receptor are characterized by primary amenorrhea. It has been suggested that there is a leptin threshold level for menarche. In postmenarcheal women, a critical leptin level is seemingly a prerequisite for menstruation. Furthermore, studies in female adolescents with eating disorders or underweight showed that low leptin levels predicted amenorrhea. In a recent study, female adolescents with secondary amenorrhea due to acute anorexia nervosa were followed up during weight gain. It was found that the observed increments of LH levels generally tracked the increments of leptin levels. There was a critical serum leptin level of 1.85 µg/l, below which LH levels were insufficient to trigger menstruation [18].

Adiponectin

Adiponectin was first identified in 1995 by four independent groups. It is specifically expressed in mature adipocytes with higher levels detected in subcutaneous rather than visceral fat. It is released into the bloodstream and accounts for ~0.01% of all serum proteins. Adiponectin is a 30-kDa protein with an N-terminal collagen-like domain and a C-terminal globular domain. As such, it structurally belongs to the collagen superfamily, which is known to form characteristic multimers. Indeed, via its collagen domain it creates 3 major oligomeric forms: a low-molecular-weight (LMW) trimer, a middle-molecular-weight (MMW) hexamer, and a high-molecular-weight (HMW) 12–18-mer. In addition, a smaller, globular fragment of adiponectin has been detected, which accounts for ~1% of total circulating adiponectin.

Two receptors for adiponectin, AdipoR1 and AdipoR2 are known. Both contain seven-transmembrane domains, but are functionally and structurally different from G-protein-coupled receptors. AdipoR1 is expressed in muscle and binds with high affinity to globular adiponectin and with low affinity to full-length adiponectin. AdipoR2 is expressed primarily in liver and binds full-length adiponectin and, with relatively low affinity, the globular form. Thus, the biological effects of adiponectin not only depend on relative circulating concentrations, but also on tissue-specific expression of its receptor subtypes.

In contrast to other adipokines, serum adiponectin is reduced with obesity in conditions of insulin resistance and T2D, and in cardiovascular disease in correlation with increasing severity. This reduction seems to precede these disorders. Low levels of adiponectin, especially the HMW form, apparently predict the development of T2D and cardiovascular disease. In addition, a close correlation of adiponectin levels has been shown with risk factors and components of the metabolic syndrome. Weight loss results in an increase in adiponectin levels that is accompanied by an improvement in insulin sensitivity. These findings demonstrate the important role of adiponectin in the pathogenesis of the metabolic syndrome. This is further supported by adiponectin gene polymorphisms, which may result in hypoadiponectinemia, insulin resistance, T2D and cardiovascular disease.

In healthy lean boys, adiponectin levels significantly decline in parallel with pubertal development subsequently leading to significantly reduced adiponectin levels compared with girls (5.6 ± 0.5 vs. 7.1 ± 0.5 mg/l). This decline is inversely related to testosterone levels. In obese children and adolescents adiponectin levels are decreased as compared with lean peers of corresponding age and pubertal stage (5.2 vs. 7.1 mg/l) [19].

Retinol-Binding Protein 4 (RBP4)

In 2001, Abel et al. [20] postulated the existence of an adipocyte-secreted factor that causes insulin resistance when they found that mice with an adipose-specific GLUT4 knockout developed insulin resistance in muscle and liver. On the other hand, mice specifically over-expressing GLUT4 in adipose tissue exhibited an increased efficiency of glucose clearance. DNA arrays of these two mice identified RBP4. RBP4 is a specific circulating transport protein for retinol (vitamin A). RBP4 was upregulated in adipose tissue of adipose-*Glut4*$^{-/-}$ mice, and its serum levels were elevated in five independent mouse models of obesity and insulin resistance. Treatment with the insulin-sensitizing PPARγ agonist rosiglitazone lowered RBP4 levels and normalized insulin sensitivity in mice lacking GLUT4, and injection of recombinant RBP4 to normal mice, or overexpression of RBP4, induced insulin resistance. On the other hand, mice with a heterozygous or homozygous RBP4 knockout showed increased insulin sensitivity. The expression of GLUT4 is greatly reduced in adipocytes but not in muscle cells of obese and insulin-resistant mice and humans. Yang et al. [21] suggest that adipose tissue might act as a glucose sensor: adipocytes detect the absence of glucose by GLUT4 and respond by secreting RBP4. The latter inhibits insulin signaling by decreasing PI-3 kinase activity and insulin receptor substrate-1 (IRS-1) phosphorylation in muscle, while expression of the gluconeogenic enzyme phosphoenolpyruvate carboxykinase (PEPCK) is upregulated in the liver. Consequently, this might cause an increase in circulating blood glucose [21]. Intensive research on the regulation of RBP4 secretion is necessary to support this model.

A plethora of human studies have performed examining RBP4 levels in the circulation or within adipose tissue in subjects with obesity, insulin resistance, and type 2 diabetes mellitus. While some studies showed a positive association between RBP4 and obesity and insulin resistance, other have not found such a relationship.

Genetic study identified SNPs in the RBP4 gene that are associated with RBP4 levels, T2D and BMI.

Despite all controversy, RBP4 represents a curious new adipokine in mice and humans. Further studies will help understand its role in the pathogenesis of obesity-related disorders and show whether RBP4 might serve as a potential therapeutic target for the treatment of T2D.

Resistin

Resistin, a cysteine-rich protein, was first described as an adipokine in 2001. Murine studies suggested that resistin links obesity to insulin resistance since it was increased with obesity and downregulated upon TZD treatment. Resistin is differentially expressed between mice and humans. In mice, it is predominantly expressed in mature adipocytes, while the stromal vascular fraction is the primary source of resistin in humans. Although the clinical relevance of resistin has not been elucidated, it is an interesting cytokine.

During a hyperinsulinemic-euglycemic clamp, resistin administration in mice resulted in hepatic but not peripheral insulin resistance, suggesting that resistin blunts hepatic insulin action. In accordance, transgenic overexpression of resistin leads to insulin resistance, i.e. increased fasting glucose and decreased glucose tolerance, while knockout of resistin produced reciprocal results, i.e. decreased fasting glucose levels, hepatic glucose production, and gluconeogenic enzymes in the liver. Taken together, these studies suggest that the insulin-sensitizing effects of adiponectin in the liver might be counterbalanced by resistin.

Angiotensinogen/Angiotensin II

Adipose tissue is an important site of angiotensinogen (ANG) or angiotensin II (ANG II) production. Higher levels of ANG mRNA levels are detectable in adipose tissue of obese subjects in comparison to lean subjects. In addition, a positive association of BMI and circulating concentrations of ANG has been found in a clinical study. ANG II is a very potent vasoconstrictor and the risk for hypertension increases with BMI. Thus, it has been assumed that an increased synthesis of ANG II by adipose tissue might contribute to obesity-associated hypertension. In fact, overexpression of ANG in adipose tissue in mice resulted in elevated plasma ANG and hypertension. In addition, ANG II seems to exert different pro-inflammatory effects locally in adipose tissue. ANG II stimulates the production and secretion of PAI-1, leptin, IL-6 and IL8 in cultivated human adipocytes which can be abolished by the blocking of angiotensin-receptor subtype 1 (AT(1) receptor). In addition, ANG II increases oxidative stress and activates NFκB as well as NAD(P)H oxidase.

The clinical relevance of all these findings is still not completely understood. However, all these effects in summary might help understand why lowering ANG II production by angiotensin-converting enzyme inhibitors and AT(1) receptor blockade leads to improvement of chronic inflammation in practice.

Pro-Inflammatory Cytokines

Adipose tissue produces a plethora of other factors which have their origin from either mature adipocytes or other cell types. Pro-inflammatory cytokines are coming to the fore since obesity has been recognized as a state of low-grade inflammation, and adipose tissue has been accepted as a pathogenic site of obesity-related disorders.

Wabitsch · Reinehr · Fischer-Posovszky

In 1993, Hotamisligil et al. [22] showed an increased expression of TNF-α in adipose tissue of genetically obese rats. The idea that a factor produced from white adipose tissue is involved in the development of insulin resistance was revolutionary at that time. Since then, many other factors were described to be secreted from adipose tissue, including transforming growth factor-β), interferon-γ, interleukins, such as IL-1, IL-6, IL-10, and IL-8, monocyte chemotactic protein-1, and factors of the complement cascade (complement factor 3, metallothionein, angiopoietin-related proteins, plaminogen activator inihibitor-1, fibrinogen).

The circulating levels of these pro-inflammatory factors increase with the enlargement of fat mass. Many of these pro-inflammatory factors are produced by adipocytes and by activated macrophages. The relative amount of each remains unknown so far.

The increase of cytokines together with the finding that obesity is associated with macrophage infiltration in adipose tissue suggests that obesity should be considered as a state of low-grade inflammation.

Indeed, it has been shown that increasing adiposity activates two typical pro-inflammatory pathways, c-jun NH2-terminal kinase (JNK) and IκB-β. Concordantly, chemical or genetic inhibition of JNK or IκB-β/NFkB improves insulin resistance. Several mechanisms have been hypothesized to explain how obesity activates these receptor pathways (TNF receptor, IL-1 receptor, TLR, receptor for advanced glycation end products) and receptor-independent pathways (for example reactive oxygen species, endoplasmatic reticulum stress).

Obesity induced IκB-β activation results in NFκB translocation to the nucleus and to increased expression of potential mediators that could cause insulin resistance. On the other hand, obesity-induced JNK activation promotes phosphorylation of IRS-2, which in turn prevents normal insulin signal transduction.

The initial events of how obesity might activate inflammation in adipose tissue are not completely understood. One potential mechanism involves the initiation of a state of cellular stress by dietary excess and excess lipid accumulation in adipose tissue.

References

1   Lustig RH: Childhood obesity: behavioral aberration or biochemical drive? Reinterpreting the first law of thermodynamics. Nat Clin Pract Endocrinol Metab 2006;2:447–458.
2   He Q, Karlberg J: BMI in childhood and its association with height gain, timing of puberty, and final height. Pediatr Res 2001;49:244–251.
3   Denzer C, Weibel A, Muche R, Karges B, Sorgo W, Wabitsch M: Pubertal development in obese children and adolescents. Int J Obes (Lond) 2007;31:1509–1519.
4   Wabitsch M, Hauner H, Heinze E, Bockmann A, Benz R, Mayer H, Teller W: Body fat distribution and steroid hormone concentrations in obese adolescent girls before and after weight reduction. J Clin Endocrinol Metab 1995;80:3469–3475.
5   Phillip M, Moran O, Lazar L: Growth without growth hormone. J Pediatr Endocrinol Metab 2002; 15(suppl 5):1267–1272.
6   Wabitsch M, Blum WF, Muche R, Heinze E, Haug C, Mayer H, Teller W: Insulin-like growth factors and their binding proteins before and after weight loss and their associations with hormonal and metabolic parameters in obese adolescent girls. Int J Obes Relat Metab Disord 1996;20:1073–1080.

7 Frystyk J, Brick DJ, Gerweck AV, Utz AL, Miller KK: Bioactive insulin-like growth factor-i in obesity. J Clin Endocrinol Metab 2009;94:3093–3097.

8 Stichel H, l'Allemand D, Gruters A: Thyroid function and obesity in children and adolescents. Horm Res 2000;54:14–19.

9 Migeon CJ, Green OC, Eckert JP: Study of adrenocortical function in obesity. Metabolism 1963;12:718–739.

10 Poretsky L: On the paradox of insulin-induced hyperandrogenism in insulin-resistant states. Endocr Rev 1991;12:3–13.

11 l'Allemand D, Schmidt S, Rousson V, Brabant G, Gasser T, Gruters A: Associations between body mass, leptin, IGF-I and circulating adrenal androgens in children with obesity and premature adrenarche. Eur J Endocrinol 2002;146:537–543.

12 Largo RH, Prader A: Pubertal development in Swiss boys. Helv Paediatr Acta 1983;38:211–228.

13 Roth CL, Reinehr T: Roles of gastrointestinal and adipose tissue peptides in childhood obesity and changes after weight loss due to lifestyle intervention. Arch Pediatr Adolesc Med;164:131–138.

14 Roth CL, Enriori PJ, Harz K, Woelfle J, Cowley MA, Reinehr T: Peptide YY is a regulator of energy homeostasis in obese children before and after weight loss. J Clin Endocrinol Metab 2005;90:6386–6391.

15 Fischer-Posovszky P, Wabitsch M, Hochberg Z: Endocrinology of adipose tissue – an update. Horm Metab Res 2007;39:314–321.

16 Wabitsch M, Jensen PB, Blum WF, Christoffersen CT, Englaro P, Heinze E, Rascher W, Teller W, Tornqvist H, Hauner H: Insulin and cortisol promote leptin production in cultured human fat cells. Diabetes 1996;45:1435–1438.

17 Wabitsch M, Blum WF, Muche R, Braun M, Hube F, Rascher W, Heinze E, Teller W, Hauner H: Contribution of androgens to the gender difference in leptin production in obese children and adolescents. J Clin Invest 1997;100:808–813.

18 Ballauff A, Ziegler A, Emons G, Sturm G, Blum WF, Remschmidt H, Hebebrand J: Serum leptin and gonadotropin levels in patients with anorexia nervosa during weight gain. Mol Psychiatry 1999;4:71–75.

19 Bottner A, Kratzsch J, Muller G, Kapellen TM, Bluher S, Keller E, Bluher M, Kiess W: Gender differences of adiponectin levels develop during the progression of puberty and are related to serum androgen levels. J Clin Endocrinol Metab 2004;89:4053–4061.

20 Abel ED, Peroni O, Kim JK, Kim YB, Boss O, Hadro E, Minnemann T, Shulman GI, Kahn BB: Adipose-selective targeting of the Glut4 gene impairs insulin action in muscle and liver. Nature 2001;409:729–733.

21 Yang Q, Graham TE, Mody N, Preitner F, Peroni OD, Zabolotny JM, Kotani K, Quadro L, Kahn BB: Serum retinol binding protein 4 contributes to insulin resistance in obesity and type 2 diabetes. Nature 2005;436:356–362.

22 Hotamisligil GS, Shargill NS, Spiegelman BM: Adipose expression of tumor necrosis factor-alpha: direct role in obesity-linked insulin resistance. Science 1993;259:87–91.

23 Blum WF, Englaro P, Hanitsch S, Juul A, Hertel NT, Muller J, Skakkebaek NE, Heiman ML, Birkett M, Attanasio AM, Kiess W, Rascher W: Plasma leptin levels in healthy children and adolescents: dependence on body mass index, body fat mass, gender, pubertal stage, and testosterone. J Clin Endocrinol Metab 1997;82:2904–2910.

Prof. Dr. Martin Wabitsch
Division of Pediatric Endocrinology, Diabetes and Obesity Unit
University children's Hospital University of Ulm
Eythstrasse 24, DE–89075 Ulm (Germany)
Tel. +49 731 500 57401, Fax +49 731 500 57412, E-Mail martin.wabitsch@uniklinik-ulm.de

Ranke MB, Mullis P-E (eds): Diagnostics of Endocrine Function in Children and Adolescents, ed 4.
Basel, Karger, 2011, pp 499–501

Diagnostics: Appendix A

Appendix A: Reference table for the conversion of current units to SI units

To convert from current units to SI units, multiply by the conversion factor. To convert from SI units to current units, divide by the conversion factor. Information about concentrations must be taken with caution, since methods may vary considerably.

Substance	Gravimetric unit	Conversion factor	International system of units (SI units)
Metabolites			
Alanine	mg/dl	112.2	μmol/l
Bilirubin	mg/dl	17.10	μmol/l
Calcium (Ca)	mg/dl	0.25	mmol/l
Creatine	mg/dl	88.40	μmol/l
Creatinine	mg/dl	88.40	μmol/l
Fructose	mg/dl	0.05551	mmol/l
Galactose	mg/dl	0.05551	mmol/l
Glucose	mg/dl	0.0571	mmol/l
Glycerol	mg/dl	0.1086	mmol/l
β-Hydroxybutyrate	mg/dl	96.05	μmol/l
Hydroxyproline	mg/dl	76.26	μmol/l
Iodine (inorganic)	mg/l	7.88	μmol/l
Lactic acid	mg/dl	0.1110	mmol/l
Leucine	mg/dl	76.24	μmol/l
Magnesium (Mg)	mg/dl	0.411	nmol/l
Osmolality	mosm/kg	1	mmol/kg
Phosphate	mg/dl	0.3229	mmol/l

Substance	Gravimetric unit	Conversion factor	International system of units (SI units)
Pyruvate	mg/dl	113.6	μmol/l
Steroid hormones			
Aldosterone	ng/dl	0.0277	nmol/l
Androstenedione	ng/dl	0.0349	nmol/l
Androsterone	ng/dl	0.0349	nmol/l
Corticosterone	ng/ml	2.89	nmol/l
Cortisol	μg/dl	27.6	nmol/l
18-OH-corticosterone	ng/dl	0.0276	nmol/l
Dehydroepiandrosterone (DHEA)	ng/dl	0.0347	nmol/l
Dehydroepiandrosterone sulfate (DHEAS)	μg/dl	0.0271	μmol/l
11-Deoxycorticosterone	ng/dl	0.0289	nmol/l
11-Deoxycortisol	μg/dl	29	nmol/l
Dihydrotestosterone (DHT)	ng/dl	0.0344	nmol/l
17β-Estradiol (E$_2$)	pg/ml	3.671	pmol/l
Estriol (E$_3$)	ng/ml	3.47	nmol/l
Estrone (E$_1$)	pg/ml	3.70	pmol/l
Etiocholanolone	mg/24h	3.443	μmol/24h
17-OH-pregnenolone	ng/dl	0.03	nmol/l
17-OH-progesterone	μg/l	3.03	nmol/l
Pregnanediol	mg/24h	3.120	μmol/24h
Pregnanetriol	mg/24h	2.972	μmol/24h
Pregnenolone	ng/ml	3.16	nmol/l
Progesterone	ng/dl	0.0318	nmol/l
Testosterone	ng/dl	0.03467	nmol/l
Peptide hormones			
Adrenocorticotropic hormone (ACTH)	pg/ml	0.2202	pmol/l
Angiotensin II	pg/ml	0.957	pmol/l
Angiotensinogen	ng/ml	0.000772	nmol/l
Arginine vasopressin	pg/ml	0.926	pmol/l
Calcitonin (human)	ng/l	0.2926	pmol/l

Substance	Gravimetric unit	Conversion factor	International system of units (SI units)
Cholecystokinin (33)	pg/ml	0.2551	pmol/l
C-peptide	mg/dl	33.3	nmol/l
Gastric inhibitin peptide	pg/ml	0.2006	pmol/l
Gastrin	pg/ml	0.455	pmol/l
Glucagon	pg/ml	0.2869	pmol/l
Growth hormone (GH)	ng/ml	0.0465	pmol/l
Insulin-like growth factor I (IGF-I)	ng/ml	0.131	nmol/l
IGF-II	ng/ml	0.134	nmol/l
Insulin	mIU/l	7.175	pmol/l
Pancreatic polypeptide	pg/ml	0.2390	pmol/l
Placental lactogen (human)	mg/l	46.30	nmol/l
Prolactin	ng/ml	44.4	pmol/l
Secretin	pg/ml	0.3272	pmol/l
Vasopressin	pg/ml	0.99	pmol/l
Other substances			
1,25-Dihydroxyvitamin D [$1,25(OH)_2D$]	μg/dl	2.4	pmol/l
Dopamine	ng/l	6.53	pmol/l
Epinephrine	ng/l	5.91	pmol/l
25-Hydroxyvitamin D (25OHD)	μg/l	2.496	nmol/l
Norepinephrine	ng/l	5.91	pmol/l
Plasma renin activity (PRA)	ng/h/ml	0.77	pmol/h/ml
Serotonin	μg/dl	0.05675	μmol/l
Thyroxine (tetraiodothyronine) (T_4)	μg/dl	12.87	nmol/l
Thyroxine, free (FT_4)	ng/dl	12.87	pmol/l
Tri-iodothyronine (T_3)	ng/dl	0.01538	nmol/l
Tri-iodothyronine, free (FT_3)	pg/ml	1.54	pmol/l
Tryptophan	mg/dl	48.97	μmol/l
Vanillylmandelic acid (VMA)	mg/l	5.05	μmol/l
Vitamin D_3 (cholecalciferol)	ng/ml	2.599	nmol/l

http://www.globalrph.com/conv_si.htm

Ranke MB, Mullis P-E (eds): Diagnostics of Endocrine Function in Children and Adolescents, ed 4.
Basel, Karger, 2011, pp 502–522

Appendix B

M.B. Ranke

Tübingen

Appendix B: Diagnostic Pathways to Major Hormonal and Metabolic Disorders in Pediatric Patients

Making diagnostic decisions based on a key symptom is often a tedious process. In order to simplify and abbreviate this process, we have designed algorithms displayed here as flow charts for the diagnosis of major endocrine disorders. In designing these algorithms, we were guided by suggestions made by the authors of the relevant chapters in this volume.

Since, in practice, establishing a diagnosis may be more complex than is suggested by a flow chart, the reader is therefore always referred to the appropriate chapters in this book for a detailed analysis of the rationale underlying the diagnostic approach.

It should be noted that algorithms have an inherent weakness, since too much emphasis is placed on entrance criteria and/or decision branches that are based on quantitative criteria (e.g., cut-off levels of a hormone). However, it is our experience that difficult or unnecessary procedures can be avoided, and approaching a diagnosis becomes progressively easier once the entrance criteria are firmly established.

The flow charts make use of the following conventions:
- Diagnostic tests to be performed are shown in shaded boxes
- Diagnoses are displayed in unshaded boxes
- Dotted lines indicate alternative diagnostic pathways
- The symbol $\uparrow$ stands for 'increased', while the symbol $\downarrow$ stands for 'decreased'

Chart 1: Causes of Congenital Hypothyroidism

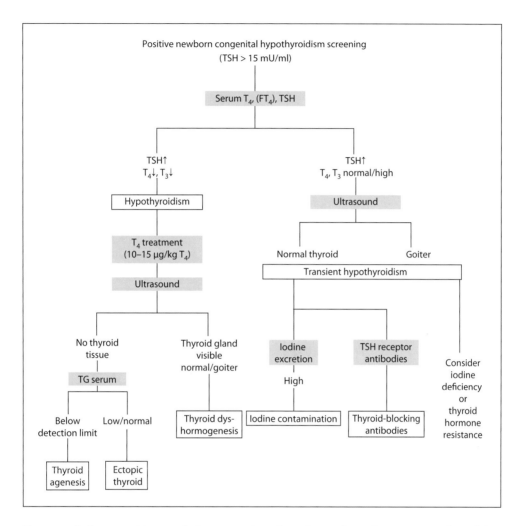

T_4, tetraiodothyronine; T_3, tri-iodothyronine; TSH, thyroid-stimulating hormone; TG, thyroglobulin.

Chart 2: Work-Up of Congenital Hypothyroidism

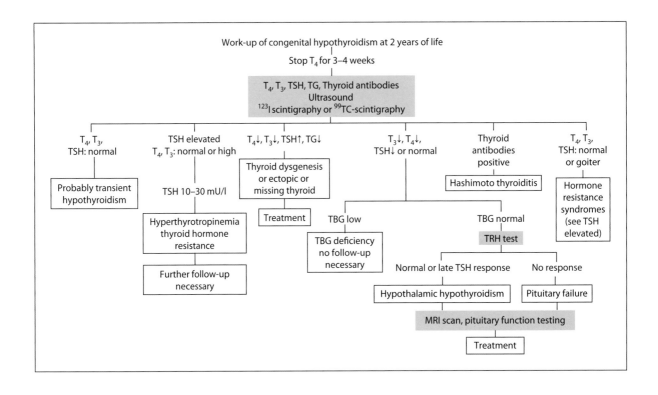

Chart 3: Hyperthyroidism

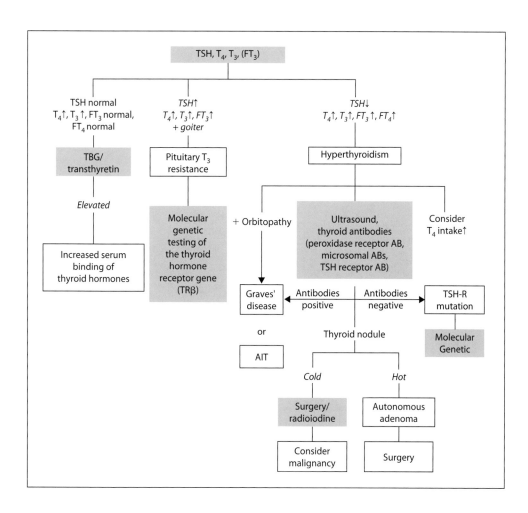

The clinical signs of hyperthyroidism include goiter, increased appetite, weight loss, heat intolerance, sweating, diarrhea, emotional lability, tachycardia, and restlessness.

Chart 4: Short Stature and/or Slow Growth Suggesting Growth Hormone Deficiency

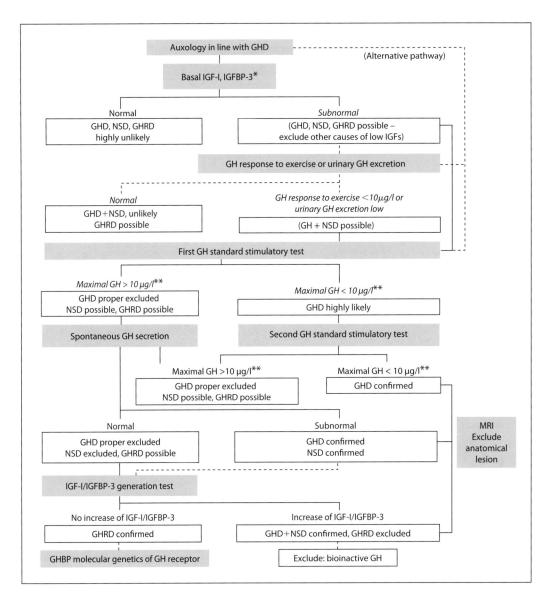

GHD, growth hormone deficiency; IGF-I, insulin-like growth factor I; IGFBP-3, insulin-like growth factor-binding protein 3; NSD, neurosecretory dysfunction; GHRD, growth hormone receptor defect; GH, growth hormone; MRI, magnetic resonance imaging; GHBP, growth hormone-binding protein.

* Normality of IGF-I =>−1.0 SDS for age; normality of IGFBP-3 => 0.0 SDS for age
** With modern assays cut-off levels may be lower (e.g. 8 µg/l)

Chart 5: Tall Stature and Suspicion of GH Hypersecretion

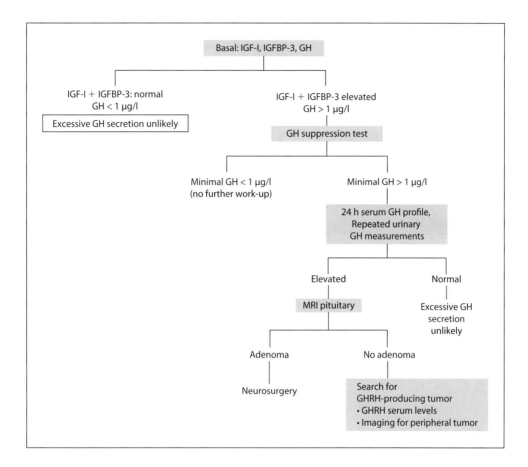

Note: Causes of tall stature other than GH hypersecretion should be ruled out. During puberty, acromegaloid features may be present. During normal and precocious puberty, levels of IGF-I and IGFBP-3 may be very high. Primary GH excess is very rare in childhood.

IGF-I, insulin-like growth factor I; IGFBP-3, insulin-like growth factor-binding protein 3; GH, growth hormone; MRI, magnetic resonance imaging; GHRH, growth hormone-releasing hormone.

Chart 6: Obesity

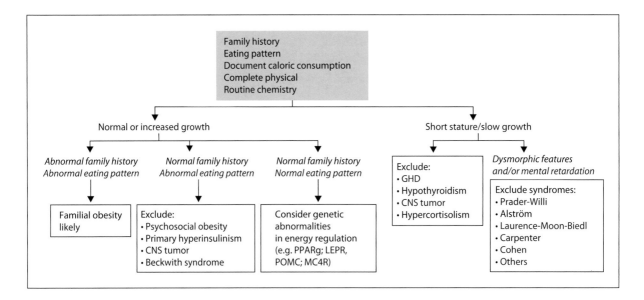

Obesity is defined as the condition where the body has accumulated an excessive amount of fat tissue. There are a multitude of methods to estimate the fat mass in children such as: hydrodensitometry (under water weighing), air-displacement plethysmography (ADP), anthropometry [e.g. skin fold thickness], measurement of total body water by means of isotope dilution [e.g. D^2O], bio-electric impedance (BIA), computed tomography (CT); dual energy absorptiometry (DEXA) and magnetic resonance tomography (MRT). Suitable references of all methods applied are required for children of various ages.

For clinical purposes the body mass index. BMI = weight [kg]/body surface [m²] is used in conjunction with appropriate references. Overweight is definded as: BMI >90th centile for age and sex ; obesity is defined as: BMI >97th centile for age and sex.

Chart 7: Polyuria

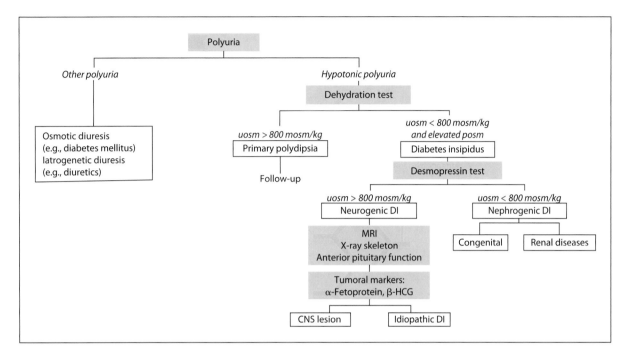

Polyuria is defined as an uninary volume exceeding 4 ml/kg BW and hour. This corresponds roughly to an urinary volume exceeding 2,500 ml/m² body surface in infants or exceeding 1,500 ml/m² in children.

A urinary osmolality (uosm) of <800 mosm/kg marks the lower limit. In the case of a plasma osmolality (posm) exceeding 300 mosm/kg there is usually ADH excretion leading to an increase of the urinary osmolality (uosm) >800 mosm/kg.

MRI, magnetic resonance imaging; ß-HCG, ß-human chorionic gonadotrophin; CNS, central nervous system.

Chart 8: Hyponatriemia

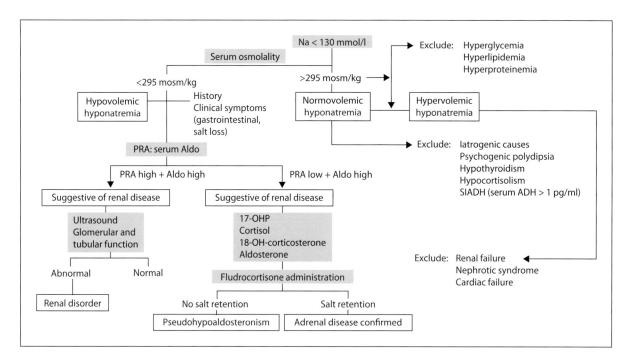

The definition of hyponatremia depends on the lower level of normality of serum/plasma sodium, which may range between 130 and 135 mmol/l. Osmolality (mosm/kg) is measured by means of osmometers which measure, e.g. the freezing-point depression. Osmolarity (mosm/l) is calculated on the basis of the molar concentartion of solutes like NaCl, glucose and BUN. The difference between the two is termed the 'osmolal gap'. If osmolality is measured a lower limit of 295 mosmol/kg is appropriate, while for osmolarity a level of about 275 mosmol/l is appropriate. In the case of normal sodium regulation and hyponatremia the urinary sodium concentration should be << 25 mEq/l.

PRA = plasma renin activity; Aldo = aldosterone; 17-OHP = 17-hydroxyprogesterone; SIADH = syndrome of inappropriate secretion of antidiuretic hormone; ADH = antidiuretic hormone.

Chart 9: Hypernatriemia

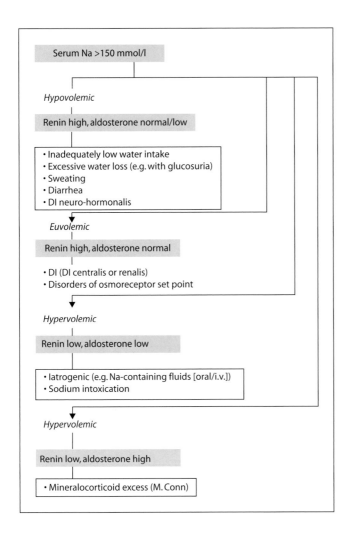

Serum Na >150 mmol/l

Hypovolemic

Renin high, aldosterone normal/low

- Inadequately low water intake
- Excessive water loss (e.g. with glucosuria)
- Sweating
- Diarrhea
- DI neuro-hormonalis

Euvolemic

Renin high, aldosterone normal

- DI (DI centralis or renalis)
- Disorders of osmoreceptor set point

Hypervolemic

Renin low, aldosterone low

- Iatrogenic (e.g. Na-containing fluids [oral/i.v.])
- Sodium intoxication

Hypervolemic

Renin low, aldosterone high

- Mineralocorticoid excess (M. Conn)

Chart 10: Rickets

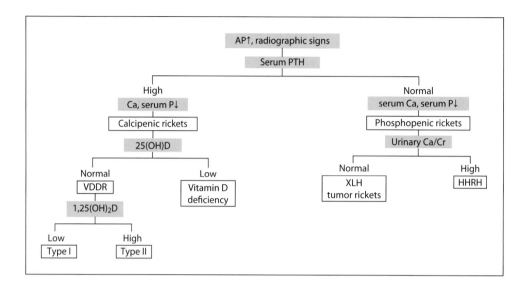

AP, alkaline phosphatase; PTH, parathyroid hormone; Ca, calcium; P, phosphate; 25(OH)D, 25-hydroxyvitamin D; VDDR, vitamin D-dependent rickets; 1,25(OH)$_2$D, 1,25-dihydroxyvitamin D; Cr, creatinine; XLH, X-linked hypophosphatemic rickets (phosphate diabetes); HHRH, hereditary hypophosphatemic rickets with hypercalciuria.

Chart 11: Hypocalcaemia with Normal Serum Albumin

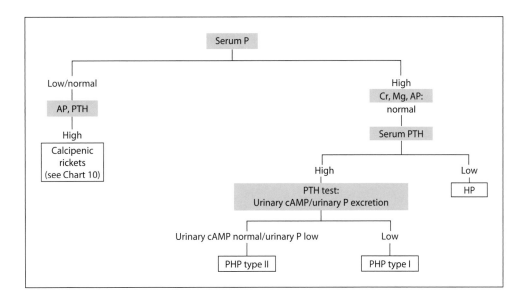

P, phosphate; AP, alkaline phosphatase; PTH, parathyroid hormone; Cr, creatinine; Mg, magnesium; cAMP, cyclic adenosine 3′,5′-monophosphate; HP, hypoparathyroidism; PHP, pseudohypoparathyroidism.

Chart 12: Hypocalcaemia in the Neonate

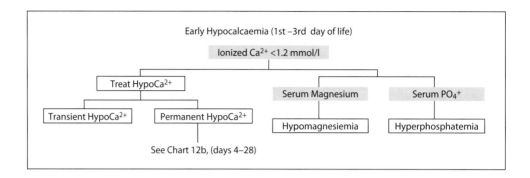

Hypocalcaemia is defined by a total serum calcium <2.2 mmol/l or an ionized serum calcium < 1.2 mmol/l.

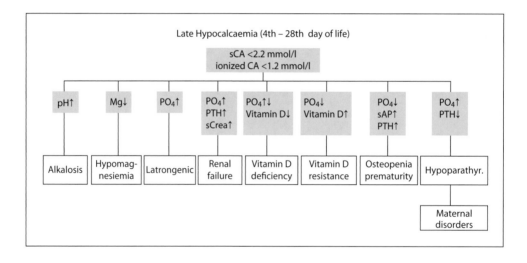

Chart 13: Hypoglycaemia in Infants and Children

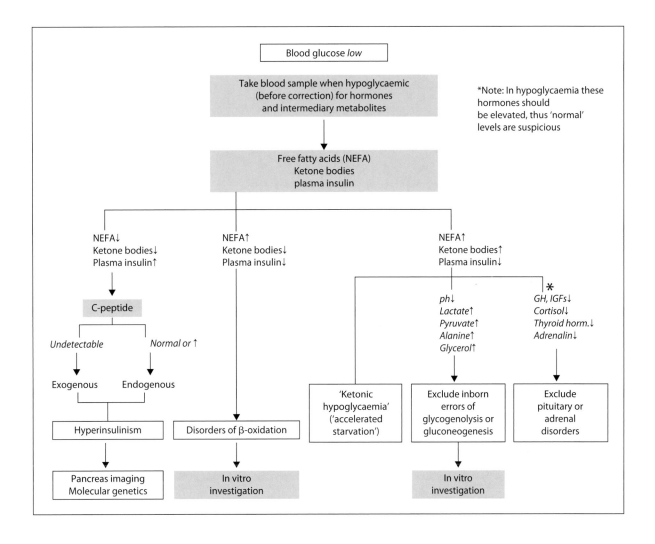

Chart 14: Hyperglycemia

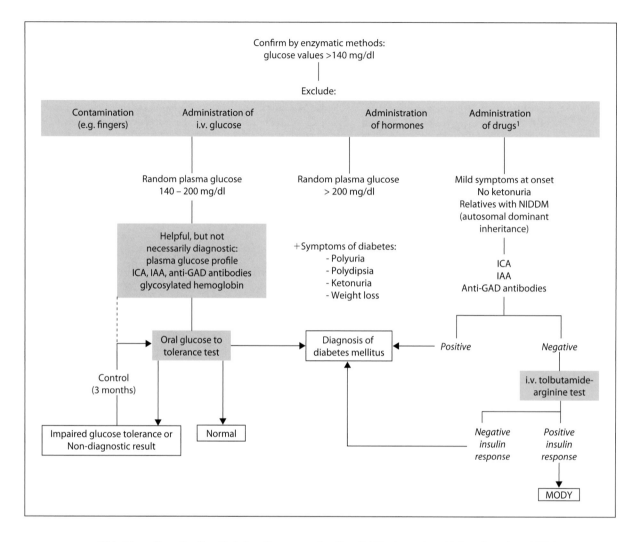

ICA, islet cell antibodies; IAA, insulin autoantibodies; GAD, glutamic acid decarboxylase; NIDDM, non-insulin-dependent diabetes mellitus; MODY, maturity-onset diabetes of the young.

[1]Including antihypertensive drugs, thiazide diuretics, estrogen preparations, psychoactive drugs, and sympathomimetic agents.

Chart 15: Delayed Puberty

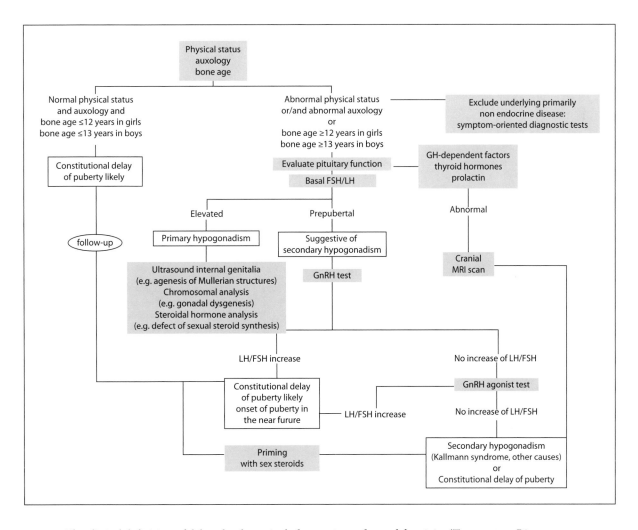

The clinical definition of delayed puberty includes no signs of gonadal activity (Tanner stage B2 or testicles >0.3 ml) after a chronological age of 12 years in girls or 14 years in boys.

Note: In more than 95% of patients, the diagnosis of constitutional delay of puberty can be made. In the remaining cases, an underlying systemic disease (e.g. Crohn's disease) is more likely than primary endocrine pathology.

FSH, follicle-stimulating hormone; LH, luteinizing hormone; GH, growth hormone; GnRH, gonadotropin-releasing hormone; MRI, magnetic resonance imaging.

Chart 16: Maldescended Testes

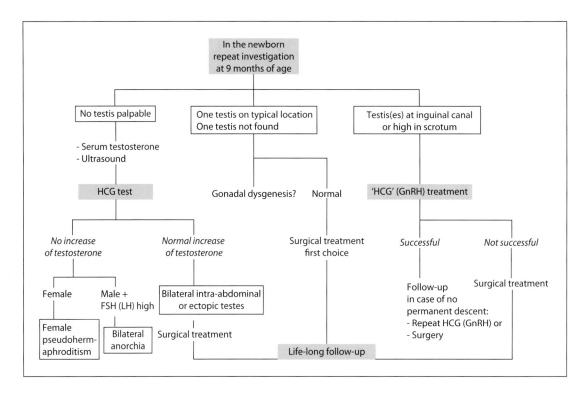

LH, luteinizing hormone; FSH, follicle-stimulating hormone; HCG, human chorionic gonadotropin; GnRH, gonadotropin-releasing hormone.

Chart 17: Newborn Child with Genital Ambiguity

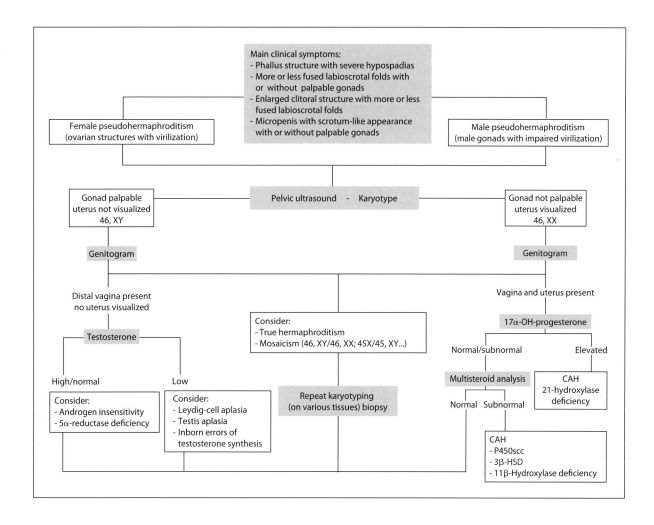

Genital ambiguity is an emergency. In this event, specialists including a pediatric endocrinologist, pediatric surgeon, radiologist, and geneticist should be consulted immediately. The aim of diagnosis is a speedy and correct gender assignment, with the potential for normal sexual functioning in adult life.

Note: Karyotype 46,XY is usually accompanied by a testicular anlage, if sex-determining genes are present. Karyotype 46,XX is usually accompanied by an ovarian anlage, but there may be occult testes-determining genes.

CAH, congenital adrenal hyperplasia; 3β-HSD, 3β-hydroxysteroid dehydrogenase.

Chart 18: Breast Development in Girls <8 Years of Age

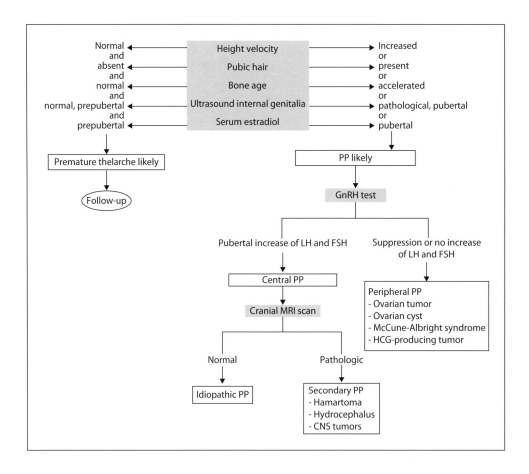

Note: There is not always a clear dividing line between premature thelarche and precocious puberty.

PP, precocious puberty; GnRH, gonadotropin-releasing hormone; LH, luteinizing hormone; FSH, follicle-stimulating hormone; MRI, magnetic resonance imaging; HCG, human chorionic gonadotropin; CNS, central nervous system.

Chart 19: Hypercortisolism

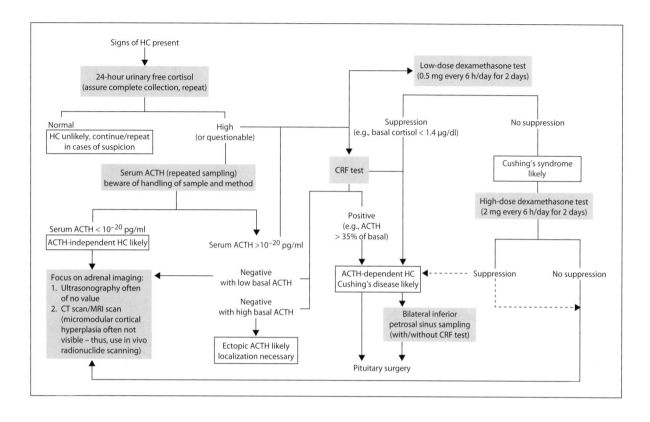

Obesity and suspicious basal serum cortisol levels are the most frequent reasons for submitting a child to a diagnostic work-up by a pediatric endocrinologist. Before embarking on tedious diagnostic procedures, the endocrinologist should verify that signs of hypercortisolism are indeed present.

The most typical signs of hypercortisolism in childhood include poor growth, development of truncal obesity with low muscle mass, and delayed bone age. In the presence of androgens (possibility of tumor!), there may be different, atypical signs.

HC, hypercortisolism; ACTH, adrenocorticotropic hormone; CRF, corticotropin-releasing factor; CT, computerized tomography; MRI, magnetic resonance imaging (cortisol: 1 μg/dl × 0.02759 = 1 nmol/l).

Chart 20: Hirsutism in Adolescent Girls

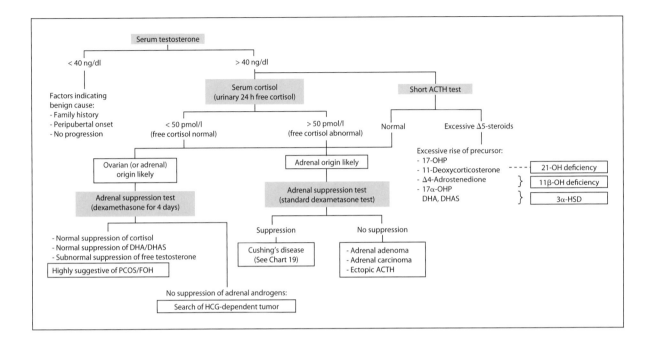

The clinical signs of hirsutism include coarse, stiff hair that is large in diameter and medullated, with a terminal pattern resembling that in males (upper lip, cheeks, sternum, and upper abdomen), as well as other signs of virilization (clitoromegaly, severe acne, deepened voice).

Note: Hirsutism is frequently confused with hypertrichosis, which occurs most often on the arms, legs, and back. Hypertrichosis shows considerable variability with respect to ethnic background and family history.

ACTH, adrenocorticotropic hormone; DHA, dehydroepiandrosterone; DHAS, dehydroepiandrosterone sulfate; PCOS, polycystic ovary syndrome; FOH, functional ovarian hyperandrogenism; HCG, human chorionic gonadotropin; 17-OHP, 17-hydroxyprogesterone; 3β-HSD, 3β-hydroxysteroid dehydrogenase. See also Chart 19, 'Hypercortisolism'.

Author Index

Subject Index

Hypothyroidism, *see* Thyroid gland

Idiopathic juvenile osteoporosis, bone turnover
    markers 442
Immunoassay, *see also specific assays*
    antibody production 6, 7
    antigen production 7, 8
    competitive versus noncompetitive 8–10
    detection systems and sensitivity 10–12
    interpretation 27–29
    principles 8
    quality management and assurance 22–25
    technical trends 16–18
    validation
        clinical validation 25, 26
        preanalytical performance and
            validation 18
        technical validation 18–22
Immunofunctional assay, applications 6
Inflammatory bowel disease, bone turnover
    markers 444, 445
Inhibins
    genital ambiguity in neonates 416, 417
    ovarian function assessment 340–342
    testicular function assessment 232
Insulin
    hyperinsulinism, *see* Hypoglycemia
    IGF-1/IGFBP-3 response 171
    induced hypoglycemia test for adrenal
        cortex function assessment 363, 364
    obesity effects on secretion and action
        484
Insulin-like growth factors (IGFs)
    assays
        acromegaly evaluation 177, 178, 188
        factors affecting IGF-1 levels
            circadian rhythm 169
            growth hormone 170
            illness 171
            insulin 171
            kidney function 171, 172
            liver function 171
            nutrition 171
        IGF1 163
        insulin-like growth factor-binding
            protein interference 161, 162
        overview 161
    functional overview 158–160
    IGFBP-3 relationship 160
    normal ranges 164–168
    obesity effects 484–486

separation from insulin-like growth factor-
    binding proteins
    functional separation 162, 163
    physical separation 162
stability 164
types 157, 158
Insulin-like growth factor-binding proteins
    (IGFBPs)
    functional overview 158, 160
    IGFBP-3
        acromegaly evaluation 177, 178, 188
        assay 163, 164
        factors affecting levels
            circadian rhythm 169
            growth hormone 170
            illness 171
            insulin 171
            kidney function 171, 172
            liver function 171
            nutrition 171
        growth hormone deficiency
            evaluation 172–177
        growth hormone therapy response
            monitoring 178, 179
        normal ranges 164–167
        relationship with insulin-like growth
            factors 160, 161
        stability 164
    insulin-like growth factor assay
        interference 161, 162
    separation from insulin-like growth factor
        functional separation 162, 163
        physical separation 162
    types 157, 158
Insulin resistance (IR)
    consequences of childhood insulin
        resistance 296–298
    definition 294, 295
    measurements of sensitivity
        fasting levels 298, 299
        hyperglycemic clamp 301, 302
        hyperinsulinemic-euglycemic
            clamp 299, 300
        Modified Minimal Model analysis 302,
            303
        overview 298
        surrogate measures
            Homeostasis Model Assessment 303,
                304
            Quantitative Insulin Sensitivity
                Check Index 304, 305

hypercalcemia 423–426
hypocalcemia 421–423
investigations 420, 421, 423, 426
dysmorphic syndrome association with
endocrine disease 404–407
endocrine disease signs 402, 403
genital ambiguity
anti-Müllerian hormone levels 416
assessment 411, 412
associated disorders 415
diagnostic algorithm 519
inhibin levels 416, 417
internal anatomy investigation 414
levels 417
testosterone response to human
chorionic 416
undervirilized males
evaluation 418–420
overview 414
virilized females 412–414
thyroid function
hypothyroxinemia of prematurity 408,
409
overview 403, 408
NKX2.1, mutation in hypothyroidism 93, 97
Nonalcoholic fatty liver disease (NAFLD),
childhood insulin resistance as risk
factor 297

Obesity, *see also* Body mass index
adipose tissue endocrine activity
adiponectin 494, 495
angiotensin II 496
inflammatory cytokines 496, 497
leptin 492–494
overview 491, 492
resistin 496
retinol-binding protein-4 495
endocrine effects
adrenal gland function 487–489
ghrelin 490
glucagon-like peptide-1 491
growth hormone/insulin-like growth
factor axis 484–486
insulin secretion and action 484
obestatin 490, 491
overview 483
peptide YY 491
polycystic ovary syndrome 489, 490
sex hormone-binding globulin 489
thyroid function 486, 487

insulin resistance risks 295, 296
investigative algorithm 508
Obestatin, obesity effects 490, 491
Online Mendelian Inheritance in Man
(OMIM) 50
Oral glucose tolerance test (OGTT), growth
hormone suppression 187
Ornithine tolerance test, growth hormone
function 117, 118
Osteocalcin, bone turnover marker
overview 432
reference range 437, 438
Osteodensitometric analysis, *see* Bone
densitometry
Osteogenesis imperfecta, bone turnover
markers 441
Osteopenia of prematurity, bone turnover
markers 442
Osteoprotegerin (OPG), bone turnover
marker 433, 434
Ovarian function
development and follicular depletion
331–333
hormone levels
anti-Müllerian hormone 342, 343
estradiol 340
follicle-stimulating hormone 343, 344
gonadotrophin-releasing hormone 343,
344
infants 339, 340
inhibins 340–342
luteinizing hormone 343–345
hypothalamic-pituitary-gonadal axis 333,
334
menstrual history in evaluation 339
premature ovarian failure, *see* Premature
ovarian failure
ultrasonography
diagnostic value 63
normal changes in aging 345, 346
normal findings 63
premature ovarian failure 345
technical requirements 61, 62

Pallister-Hall syndrome, endocrine disease in
neonates 406
Parathyroid gland
neoplasia 242, 243
scintigraphy
indications 78
radiopharmaceuticals 78